Handbook of Immunology and Aging

Handbook of Immunology and Aging

Editor: Isla Pierce

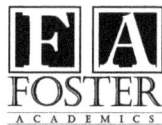

FA FOSTER
ACADEMICS

www.fosteracademics.com

www.fosteracademics.com

FA
FOSTER
ACADEMICS

Cataloging-in-Publication Data

Handbook of immunology and aging / edited by Isla Pierce.
    p. cm.
Includes bibliographical references and index.
ISBN 978-1-63242-685-7
1. Aging--Immunological aspects. 2. Older people--Diseases--Immunological aspects.
3. Geriatrics. 4. Gerontology. I. Pierce, Isla.
RC952.5 .H36 2019
618.97--dc23

Foster Academics,
118-35 Queens Blvd., Suite 400,
Forest Hills, NY 11375, USA

ISBN 978-1-63242-685-7 (Hardback)

Contents

Preface...IX

Chapter 1 **Cytomegalovirus viral load within blood increases markedly in healthy
people over the age of 70 years** 1
Helen M. Parry, Jianmin Zuo, Guido Frumento, Nikhil Mirajkar,
Charlotte Inman, Emma Edwards, Mike Griffiths, Guy Pratt and Paul Moss

Chapter 2 **CXCL-16, IL-17, and bone morphogenetic protein 2 (BMP-2) are associated
with overweight and obesity conditions in middle-aged and
elderly women Silvana Mara Turbino Luz** 11
Ribeiro, Laís Roquete Lopes, Guilherme de Paula Costa, Vivian Paulino Figueiredo,
Deena Shrestha, Aline Priscila Batista, Roney Luiz de Carvalho Nicolato,
Fernando Luiz Pereira de Oliveira, Juliana Assis Silva Gomes and Andre Talvani

Chapter 3 **Nutrition, aging and cancer: lessons from dietary intervention studies** 18
Giuseppe Carruba, Letizia Cocciadiferro, Antonietta Di Cristina,
Orazia M. Granata, Cecilia Dolcemascolo, Ildegarda Campisi,
Maurizio Zarcone, Maria Cinquegrani and Adele Traina

Chapter 4 **The inflammatory protein Pentraxin 3 in cardiovascular disease** 27
Francesco Fornai, Albino Carrizzo, Maurizio Forte, Mariateresa Ambrosio,
Antonio Damato, Michela Ferrucci, Francesca Biagioni, Carla Busceti,
Annibale A. Puca and Carmine Vecchione

Chapter 5 **Lifewide profile of cytokine production by innate and adaptive immune
cells from Brazilian individuals** 36
Gabriela Silveira-Nunes, Elaine Speziali, Andréa Teixeira-Carvalho,
Danielle M. Vitelli-Avelar, Renato Sathler-Avelar, Taciana Figueiredo-Soares,
Maria Luiza Silva, Vanessa Peruhype-Magalhães, Daniel Gonçalves Chaves,
Gustavo Eustáquio Brito-Melo, Glenda Meira Cardoso, Eric Bassetti Soares,
Silvana Maria Elói-Santos, Rosângela Teixeira, Dulciene Magalhães Queiroz,
Rodrigo Corrêa-Oliveira, Ana Maria Caetano Faria and
Olindo Assis Martins-Filho

Chapter 6 **Higher plasma levels of complement C3a, C4a and C5a increase the risk of
subretinal fibrosis in neovascular age-related macular degeneration** 49
Judith Lechner, Mei Chen, Ruth E. Hogg, Levente Toth, Giuliana Silvestri,
Usha Chakravarthy and Heping Xu

Chapter 7 **Evaluation of circulating sRAGE in osteoporosis according to BMI,
adipokines and fracture risk: a pilot observational study**...58
Emanuela Galliera, Monica Gioia Marazzi, Carmine Gazzaruso,
Pietro Gallotti, Adriana Coppola, Tiziana Montalcini, Arturo Pujia and
Massimiliano M. Corsi Romanelli

Chapter 8   **A pilot observational study on magnesium and calcium imbalance in elderly patients with acute aortic dissection**...70
E. Vianello, E. Dozio, A. Barassi, G. Sammarco, L. Tacchini,
M. M. Marrocco-Trischitta, S. Trimarchi and M. M. Corsi Romanelli

Chapter 9   **Altered activation state of circulating neutrophils in patients with neovascular age-related macular degeneration** 75
Marie Krogh Nielsen, Sven Magnus Hector, Kelly Allen,
Yousif Subhi and Torben Lykke Sørensen

Chapter 10   **Dietary phytochemicals and neuro-inflammaging: from mechanistic insights to translational challenges** 84
Sergio Davinelli, Michael Maes, Graziamaria Corbi, Armando Zarrelli,
Donald Craig Willcox and Giovanni Scapagnini

Chapter 11   **Efforts of the human immune system to maintain the peripheral CD8+ T cell compartment after childhood thymectomy**...101
Manuela Zlamy, Giovanni Almanzar, Walther Parson,
Christian Schmidt, Johannes Leierer, Birgit Weinberger,
Verena Jeller, Karin Unsinn, Matthias Eyrich,
Reinhard Würzner and Martina Prelog

Chapter 12   **Immunosenescence in persons with spinal cord injury in relation to urinary tract infections -a cross-sectional study**...114
David Pavlicek, Jörg Krebs, Simona Capossela, Alessandro Bertolo,
Britta Engelhardt, Jürgen Pannek and Jivko Stoyanov

Chapter 13   **Elastic band resistance training influences transforming growth factor-ß receptor I mRNA expression in peripheral mononuclear cells of institutionalised older adults: the Vienna Active Ageing Study (VAAS)**..128
Barbara Schober-Halper, Marlene Hofmann, Stefan Oesen,
Bernhard Franzke, Thomas Wolf, Eva-Maria Strasser, Norbert Bachl,
Michael Quittan, Karl-Heinz Wagner and Barbara Wessner

Chapter 14   **TLR-6 SNP P249S is associated with healthy aging in nonsmoking Eastern European Caucasians - A cohort study** 139
Lutz Hamann, Jasmin Bustami, Leonid Iakoubov, Malgorzata Szwed,
Malgorzata Mossakowska, Ralf R. Schumann and
Monika Puzianowska-Kuznicka

Chapter 15   **Expression of cellular protective proteins SIRT1, HSP70 and SOD2 correlates with age and is significantly higher in NK cells of the oldest seniors** 145
Lucyna Kaszubowska, Jerzy Foerster, Jan Jacek Kaczor, Daria Schetz,
Tomasz Jerzy Ślebioda and Zbigniew Kmieć

Chapter 16   **Nutraceutical effects of table green olives: a pilot study with *Nocellara del Belice* olives** 158
Giulia Accardi, Anna Aiello, Valeria Gargano, Caterina Maria Gambino,
Santo Caracappa, Sandra Marineo, Gesualdo Vesco, Ciriaco Carru,
Angelo Zinellu, Maurizio Zarcone, Calogero Caruso and
Giuseppina Candore

Chapter 17   **Immunological and non-immunological mechanisms of
allergic diseases in the elderly: biological and clinical characteristics**..164
Gabriele Di Lorenzo, Danilo Di Bona, Federica Belluzzo and
Luigi Macchia

Chapter 18   **Virtual memory cells make a major contribution to the response of aged
influenza-naïve mice to influenza virus infection** 172
Kathleen G. Lanzer, Tres Cookenham, William W. Reiley and
Marcia A. Blackman

Chapter 19   ***Porphyromonas gingivalis*, a periodontitis causing bacterium, induces
memory impairment and age-dependent neuroinflammation in mice**..185
Ye Ding, Jingyi Ren, Hongqiang Yu, Weixian Yu and Yanmin Zhou

Chapter 20   **Effects of a new nutraceutical combination on cognitive function in
hypertensive patients**..193
Giuseppe Giugliano, Alessia Salemme, Sara De Longis, Marialuisa Perrotta,
Valentina D'Angelosante, Alessandro Landolfi, Raffaele Izzo and
Valentina Trimarco

Chapter 21   **Anti-cytomegalovirus IgG antibody titer is positively associated with
advanced T cell differentiation and coronary artery disease in
end-stage renal disease**..202
Feng-Jung Yang, Kai-Hsiang Shu, Hung-Yuan Chen, I-Yu Chen,
Fang-Yun Lay, Yi-Fang Chuang, Chien-Sheng Wu, Wan-Chuan Tsai,
Yu-Sen Peng, Shih-Ping Hsu, Chih-Kang Chiang, George Wang and
Yen-Ling Chiu

Chapter 22   **Neuroinflammation and neurohormesis in the pathogenesis of
Alzheimer's disease and Alzheimer-linked pathologies: modulation by
nutritional mushrooms**..211
Angela Trovato Salinaro, Manuela Pennisi, Rosanna Di Paola, Maria Scuto,
Rosalia Crupi, Maria Teresa Cambria, Maria Laura Ontario,
Mario Tomasello, Maurizio Uva, Luigi Maiolino, Edward J. Calabrese,
Salvatore Cuzzocrea and Vittorio Calabrese

Chapter 23   **Immunosenescence and lymphomagenesis**..219
Salvatrice Mancuso, Melania Carlisi, Marco Santoro, Mariasanta Napolitano,
Simona Raso and Sergio Siragusa

Chapter 24   **NK cells of the oldest seniors represent constant and resistant to stimulation
high expression of cellular protective proteins SIRT1 and HSP70** 226
Lucyna Kaszubowska, Jerzy Foerster, Jan Jacek Kaczor, Daria Schetz,
Tomasz Jerzy Ślebioda and Zbigniew Kmieć

Chapter 25   **Crocetin attenuates inflammation and amyloid-β accumulation in
APPsw transgenic mice** 242
Jin Zhang, Yuchao Wang, Xueshuang Dong and Jianghua Liu

Chapter 26   **Ageing: from inflammation to cancer**..250
Giulia C. Leonardi, Giulia Accardi, Roberto Monastero,
Ferdinando Nicoletti and Massimo Libra

Chapter 27   **The association of high sensitivity C-reactive protein and incident Alzheimer disease in patients 60 years and older: The HUNT study, Norway** 257
Jessica Mira Gabin, Ingvild Saltvedt, Kristian Tambs and Jostein Holmen

Chapter 28   **Association of immunoglobulin GM allotypes with longevity in long-living individuals from Southern Italy** 265
Annibale A. Puca, Anna Ferrario, Anna Maciag, Giulia Accardi, Anna Aiello, Caterina Maria Gambino, Giuseppina Candore, Calogero Caruso, Aryan M. Namboodiri and Janardan P. Pandey

Permissions

List of Contributors

Index

Preface

Over the recent decade, advancements and applications have progressed exponentially. This has led to the increased interest in this field and projects are being conducted to enhance knowledge. The main objective of this book is to present some of the critical challenges and provide insights into possible solutions. This book will answer the varied questions that arise in the field and also provide an increased scope for furthering studies.

Immunology is a branch of biology concerned with the study of immune systems. Immunological studies have applications in the fields of oncology, organ transplantation, rheumatology, dermatology, etc. The disorders of the immune system can result in immunodeficiency diseases and autoimmune diseases. Immunodeficiency diseases are caused when the immune system fails to provide the adequate immune response. When the immune system attacks its own host's body, it leads to autoimmune diseases, some of which include rheumatoid arthritis, systemic lupus erythematosus, Hashimoto's disease, etc. The gradual accumulation of psychological, physical and social changes in a human being over time constitutes the process of aging. A less efficient immune function is a characteristic of old age. As the immune system weakens progressively with age, the organism becomes unable to fight infections and increasingly incapable of destroying old and neoplastic cells. This eventually leads to death. This book contains some path-breaking studies in immunology and aging. It unfolds the innovative aspects of the relationship between immunology and aging, which will be crucial for the understanding of these areas. The readers would gain knowledge that would broaden their perspective about these fields.

I hope that this book, with its visionary approach, will be a valuable addition and will promote interest among readers. Each of the authors has provided their extraordinary competence in their specific fields by providing different perspectives as they come from diverse nations and regions. I thank them for their contributions.

Editor

Cytomegalovirus viral load within blood increases markedly in healthy people over the age of 70 years

Helen M. Parry[1][*], Jianmin Zuo[1], Guido Frumento[1], Nikhil Mirajkar[2], Charlotte Inman[1], Emma Edwards[1,5], Mike Griffiths[3], Guy Pratt[1] and Paul Moss[1,4]

Abstract

Background: Cytomegalovirus (CMV) is a highly prevalent herpesvirus, which maintains lifelong latency and places a significant burden on host immunity. Infection is associated with increased rates of vascular disease and overall mortality in the elderly and there is an urgent need for improved understanding of the viral-host balance during ageing. CMV is extremely difficult to detect in healthy donors, however, using droplet digital PCR of DNA from peripheral blood monocytes, we obtained an absolute quantification of viral load in 44 healthy donors across a range of ages.

Results: Viral DNA was detected in 24 % (9/37) of donors below the age of 70 but was found in all individuals above this age. Furthermore, the mean CMV load was only 8.6 copies per 10,000 monocytes until approximately 70 years of age when it increased by almost 30 fold to 249 copies in older individuals ($p < 0.0001$). CMV was found within classical CD14+ monocytes and was not detectable within the CD14-CD16+ subset. The titre of CMV-specific IgG increased inexorably with age indicating that loss of humoral immunity is not a determinant of the increased viral load. In contrast, although cellular immunity to the structural late protein pp65 increased with age, the T cell response to the immediate early protein IE1 decreased in older donors.

Conclusion: These data reveal that effective control of CMV is impaired during healthy ageing, most probably due to loss of cellular control of early viral reactivation. This information will be of value in guiding efforts to reduce CMV-associated health complications in the elderly.

Keywords: Cytomegalovirus, Ageing, Monocyte, ddPCR, Lifespan

Background

Cytomegalovirus (CMV) is one of eight human herpesviruses and maintains a state of lifelong latency within the host following primary infection. CMV is highly prevalent in all parts of the world and infection rates increase with age, with seropositivity estimated between 50 and 95 % in those aged over 5 years [1, 2]. Viral replication is controlled by the development of a strong cellular and humoral CMV-specific immune response and this must be maintained throughout life in order to prevent episodes of clinically significant viral reactivation [3]. The magnitude of the CMV-specific immune response within the

blood is very large and higher than has been recorded against other pathogens [4, 5]. Moreover this immune response increases further with age in a phenomenon that has been termed 'memory inflation' [6]. This is associated with reduction in the CD4:8 ratio and accumulation of large numbers of late-differentiated memory cells [7]. However, there is now concern that CMV infection can serve to accelerate the development of immune senescence and several studies have shown that CMV seropositivity is associated with a range of clinical problems and increased risk of mortality in older people [8–12].

Although CMV rarely leads to overt clinical problems after primary infection, it is believed that subclinical episodes of CMV reactivation occur frequently during a lifetime but are rapidly controlled by the host immune response [13]. In order to understand more about the

* Correspondence: H.m.parry@bham.ac.uk
[1]Institute of Immunology and Immunotherapy, University of Birmingham, Vincent Drive, Birmingham B15 2TT, UK
Full list of author information is available at the end of the article

mechanisms by which CMV infection may impact on the health of elderly donors it is important to improve understanding of the level of CMV load within the blood and how this is related to specific features of the CMV-specific immune response. This information might then potentially be used to determine the optimal 'set point' of viral-host balance and as such serve as an aspiration to achieve within future interventional therapy, for instance with anti-viral or immune modulatory treatment.

The sites of CMV latency include haemopoietic stem cells, monocytes and epithelial cells. However the level of CMV within the blood is very low and conventional PCR assays are almost invariably negative in healthy donors [14–17]. Indeed this is a useful clinical finding, as a positive CMV PCR is generally interpreted as evidence of clinically significant reactivation in immune suppressed donors and can be used to guide anti-viral therapy. However, purification of discrete cell subsets that harbor viral infection, followed by PCR amplification, is one approach that can be taken to increase the sensitivity of viral detection [18]. Self-renewing CD34+ haemopoietic stem cells represent a reservoir for maintaining viral infection and it has been estimated that latent virus is present in 0.01–0.001 % of myeloid progenitor cells within bone marrow [15, 19, 20]. Monocytes are the major mature haemopoietic cellular host for CMV carriage and the frequency of infected cells is thought to be approximately 10 fold lower [21, 22]. Viral latency is maintained during monocytic carriage, whereas lytic viral replication can only arise following differentiation of monocytes into macrophages, due to changes in the pattern of chromatin binding to the immediate early promoter [23–25].

The use of highly sensitive PCR assays increases the frequency of CMV detection and nested PCR offers the advantage of substantial sensitivity but is poorly quantitative. Droplet digital PCR (ddPCR) is a new approach that provides a highly sensitive and direct method for detection of target DNA without the need for developing a 'standard curve'. ddPCR emulsifies an oil-based PCR reaction into thousands of droplets, each of which then acts as a PCR micro-reaction and increases the chances of a rare event being detected. Using Poisson's distribution, a direct measurement of the target DNA can then be determined. ddPCR does not therefore rely on any interpretation of rate-based data, as is the case with Q-PCR. The sensitivity and versatility of ddPCR for detection of low copy number events has been shown in several settings and is increasingly part of clinical practice for monitoring mutations levels in malignant disease [26, 27].

We have utilized purification of monocytes combined with droplet digital PCR to permit accurate quantification of the level of CMV within the blood of healthy donors. Our data showed that this provides a highly informative technique to quantify CMV viral load. Moreover they revealed that virus is found infrequently within the blood until the age of around 70 years when it becomes detectable in every donor. We showed that virus is present exclusively within the 'classical' CD14+ monocyte fraction and that the increase in viral load correlated with a decrease in the cellular immune response to immediate early protein. These findings have important implications for understanding the biology and clinical complications of CMV infection.

Results

Droplet digital PCR can be used for detection of CMV within the monocytes of healthy donors

Blood samples were obtained from 44 healthy donors between 25 and 86 years of age. CD14+ monocytes were purified by positive selection using magnetic beads and then DNA was extracted using miniprep kits. CMV-specific PCR primers and droplet digital PCR analysis (ddPCR) was then used to determine the number and proportion of CMV-positive droplets within each sample. Positive droplets were defined as those detectable above the set threshold (Fig. 1a) and Poisson's distribution was used to determine the absolute copy number of the reaction. Using this approach, CMV was detected in 16 of the 44 donors (36 %) and was confirmed in each case by 3 independent runs.

CMV viral load within monocytes increases markedly above the age of 70 years

When the results were assessed in relation to donor age it was clear that the proportion of donors in whom CMV was detectable increased markedly with age. Specifically, CMV was detected in 9 of 37 (24 %) of donors aged below 70 years whereas a positive test was seen in each of the 7 donors above this age (Fig. 1b). In those aged 20–30 years, only 1 out of 6 donors (16.7 %) had a detectable load, compared to 1 out of 4 (25 %) in 30–40 year olds, 1 out of 13 (7.7 %) in 40–50 year olds, 3 out of 8 (37.5 %) in 50–60 year olds and 3 out of 6 (50 %) in 60–70 year olds.

The absolute quantification of CMV viral load in relation to monocyte number was then determined by QuantaSoft® software in order to generate a value of 'viral load per 10,000 monocytes'. In those donors in whom CMV was detectable by ddPCR, the absolute viral load varied markedly from 3 copies per 10,000 monocytes to 353 copies per 10,000 monocytes, a range of 117 fold. This value was also found to increase with age, again with a marked increase observed in donors aged over 70 years (kruskal-wallis $p = 0.0005$). The mean viral load in donors aged below 70 years was 8.6 copies per 10,000 monocytes (SD 38), with a 29-fold increase in those over the age of 70, where the mean viral load was 249 copies per 10,000 monocytes (SD 59) (Fig. 1c).

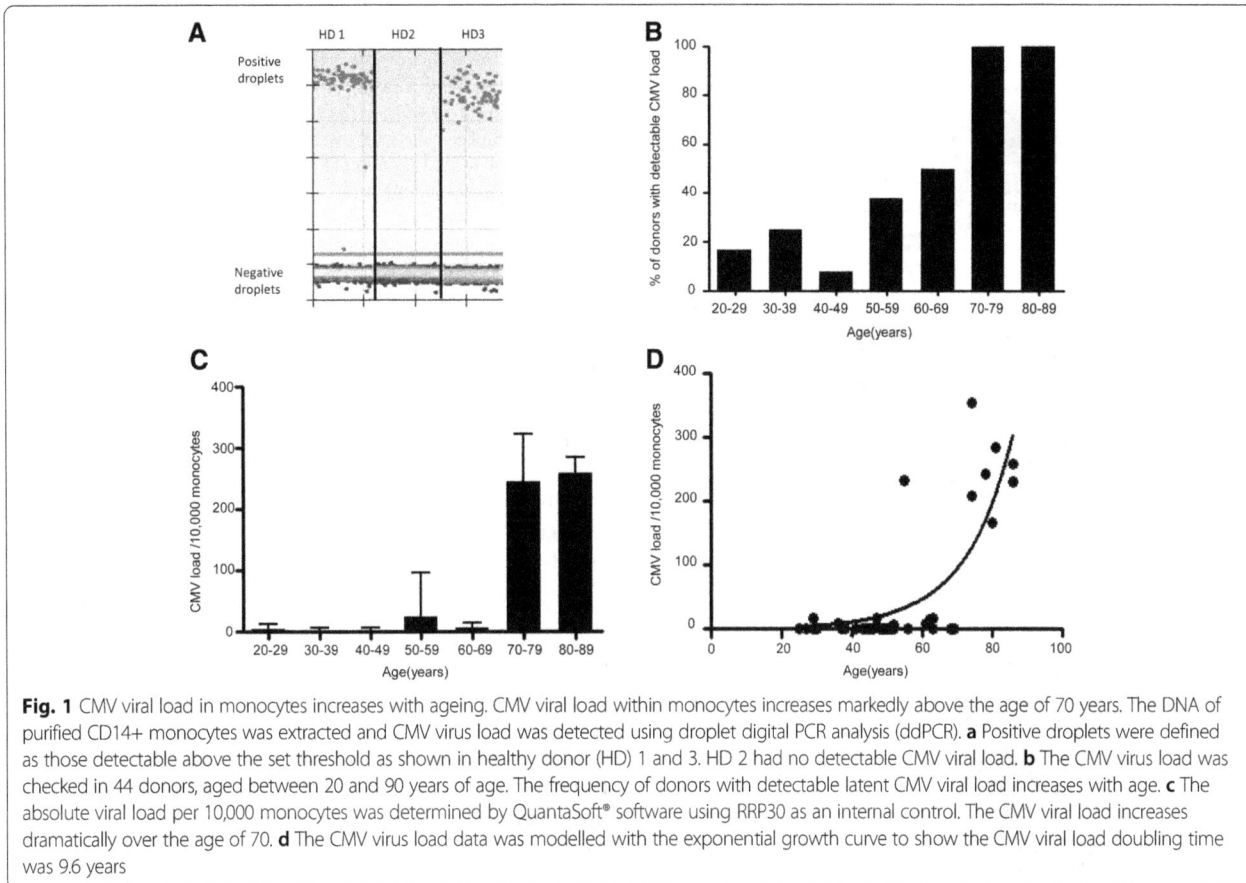

Fig. 1 CMV viral load in monocytes increases with ageing. CMV viral load within monocytes increases markedly above the age of 70 years. The DNA of purified CD14+ monocytes was extracted and CMV virus load was detected using droplet digital PCR analysis (ddPCR). **a** Positive droplets were defined as those detectable above the set threshold as shown in healthy donor (HD) 1 and 3. HD 2 had no detectable CMV viral load. **b** The CMV virus load was checked in 44 donors, aged between 20 and 90 years of age. The frequency of donors with detectable latent CMV viral load increases with age. **c** The absolute viral load per 10,000 monocytes was determined by QuantaSoft® software using RRP30 as an internal control. The CMV viral load increases dramatically over the age of 70. **d** The CMV virus load data was modelled with the exponential growth curve to show the CMV viral load doubling time was 9.6 years

Modelling of the data with an exponential growth curve showed that the CMV viral load doubling time was 9.6 years ($R^2 = 0.64$) (Fig. 1d).

The increase in CMV viral load with age is confirmed through the use of quantitative PCR

We next used a second method in order to confirm the observation of an increase in CMV load within monocytes in relation to age. Quantitative PCR (Q-PCR) was applied to the same sample cohort using an average plasmid series dilution, which produced an R^2 value of 0.983 ($p < 0.0001$) (Additional file 1: Figure S1A). Using triplicate runs, Q-PCR was sensitive down to a single copy of plasmid CMV per reaction. This same series of diluted plasmids was then verified using ddPCR and the absolute copy number of CMV was calculated through QuantaSoft® software. ddPCR was again capable of detecting 1 copy of CMV per reaction indicating that results generated from ddPCR and Q-PCR correlated very strongly ($R^2 = 0.995$; $p = <0.0001$) (Additional file 1: Figure S1B).

We then used Q-PCR to assess CMV load within the 44 samples of monocyte DNA from healthy donors. Thirteen of the 16 samples that were found to be positive by digital PCR were also detected as positive by Q-PCR (81 %). Twenty-seven out of the 28 samples that were negative by

ddPCR were also negative by Q-PCR and only one was reported positive by Q-PCR. The correlation between the two techniques using 13 results that were positive by both methods had a co-efficient of determination of $R^2 = 0.626$ ($p = 0.0013$). The Q-PCR technique also revealed a pronounced increase in viral load in association with age (Additional file 1: Figure S1C).

CMV viral load is detectable within CD34+ haemopoietic cells and is focused within 'classical' CD14+ monocytes

In order to determine the distribution of CMV load within different cells of the myeloid lineage we then went on to perform ddPCR on purified CD34+ haemopoietic stem cells and individual monocyte subsets. CD14 and CD16 expression can be used to subdivide the major subpopulations of monocytes into CD14 + CD16-, CD14 + CD16+ and CD14-CD16+ subsets (Fig. 2a). Fractions of G-CSF-mobilised peripheral blood were obtained from five haemopoietic stem cell donors and cells were sorted into CD34+ stem cells and monocytic subsets (Fig. 2b). CMV was detected in 3 of these 5 samples through the use of both ddPCR and Q-PCR. Interestingly, within the monocyte subsets, CMV was found only within classical monocytes with a CD14+ phenotype whereas the CD14-CD16+ subset was entirely negative by both assays (Fig. 2c).

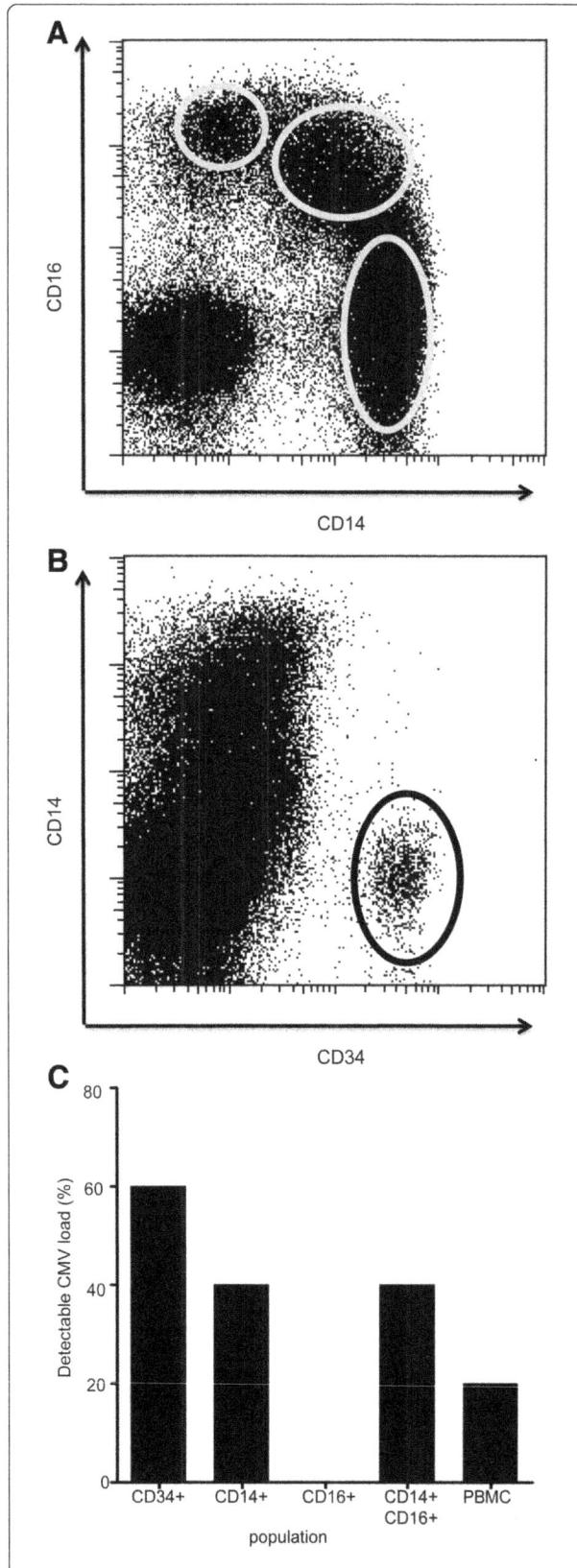

Fig. 2 CMV viral load is detectable in CD14 positive monocytes. CMV viral load is detectable within CD34+ haemopoietic cells and is focused within 'classical' CD14+ monocytes. DNA from CD34+, CD14+CD16-, CD14+CD16+ and CD14-CD16+ populations were used to detect CMV viral load using ddPCR. **a** Representation of flow plots used for selecting monocyte populations based on CD14+ and CD16+ antibody staining. **b** Representation of flow plots used for selecting CD34+ cells. **c** The frequency of detection of CMV viral load was compared between the different subpopulations

The titre of the CMV-specific IgG response increases with age

Our previous data showed an increase in CMV load within the peripheral blood during healthy ageing, so we next went on to determine the magnitude of the CMV-specific immune response in association with age. In particular, we assessed if the increase in viral load might result from a reduction in the magnitude of virus-specific immunity or if the immune response might actually increase as a response to the increased level of virus in the blood. We therefore determined the CMV-specific IgG titre using a quantitative ELISA assay against viral lysate. Interestingly, antibody titre increased substantially during ageing with a three fold increase in titre between the ages of 20 and 80 years (mean titre 65.1 in donors aged 20 years compared to 232 in those aged over 70); $r = 0.473$; $p = 0.001$). This increase in titre developed gradually during ageing and therefore had a different pattern to the quite dramatic elevation in viral load that was seen only after the age of 70 years (Fig. 3).

The CMV-specific T cell response to pp65 also increases with age whereas recognition of IE-1 is reduced in elderly donors

We next went on to assess the magnitude of the T cell immune response against CMV within the study cohort. Specifically, we focused on the cellular responses to pp65 and immediate early 1 (IE-1), which are two of the most immunodominant components of the CMV proteome. Several previous studies have reported the substantial magnitude of the CMV-specific T cell immune response within peripheral blood and have also identified that this can increase further with age [28, 29].

T cells were stimulated with peptide pools containing immunodominant epitopes from either pp65 or IE-1 and the IFN-γ release by peptide-specific CD4 and CD8 T cells was then determined by flow cytometry (Fig. 4a). The magnitude of the pp65-specific CD8+ T cell immune response ranged from 0 to 5.5 % of the CD8+ T cell pool, with a median value of 0.28 %. This value was over two-fold higher in those donors with detectable CMV viral load within monocytes compared to donors in whom the ddPCR was negative, but this did not reach statistical significance (0.5 vs 0.23 % respectively; $p = 0.087$). The pp65-specific T cell response also increased markedly with

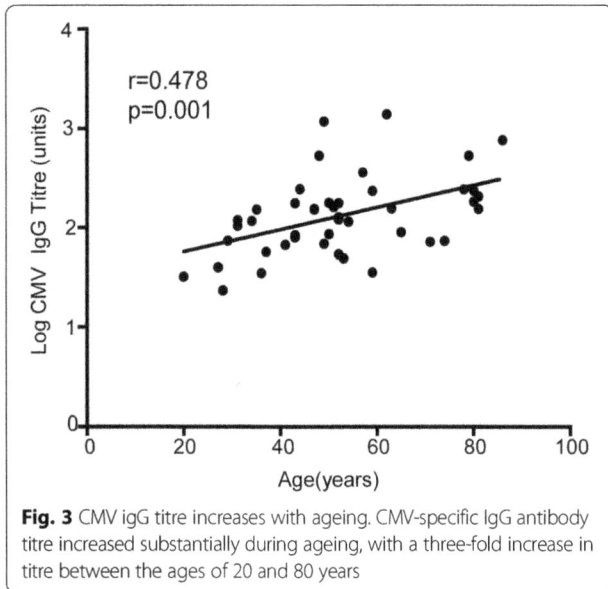

Fig. 3 CMV IgG titre increases with ageing. CMV-specific IgG antibody titre increased substantially during ageing, with a three-fold increase in titre between the ages of 20 and 80 years

age, from a median value of 0.17 % in 20–30 year olds to 1.17 % in those aged greater than 70 years ($r^2 = 0.146$, $p = 0.03$). A positive correlation with age was also noted following pp65 stimulation of CD4+ T cells, although this did not reach statistical significance.

In contrast to pp65, the frequency of CD8+ T cells recognizing IE-1 initially increased with age, but then peaked in people aged 50–60 years and actually decreased in older donors (median 0.01 % <50 years; 0.7 % 50–60 years and 0.1 % >70 years old; $R^2 = 0.05$; $p = 0.244$). The CD4+ T cell response to IE-1 peptide stimulation was of small magnitude but remained relatively constant across each age group, with a median frequency of 0.01 % (Fig. 4b).

In summary, the magnitude of the cellular immune response to the structural late protein pp65 increased with age, whilst the CD8+ T cell response to IE-1 peaked at the age of 50–60 years and reduced thereafter.

Discussion

Cytomegalovirus infection has been associated with a variety of health problems in elderly people and there is increasing interest in the mechanisms that underlie this association. A key determinant in this regard will be greater understanding of the balance of the viral load and the host immune response during healthy ageing. In this study we report, for the first time, that the level of cytomegalovirus viral load within the blood increased markedly in elderly people.

A novel feature of our work was the use of digital droplet PCR to provide an accurate quantitative measure of latent viral DNA. Previous methods for detection of CMV from monocytic DNA generally relied on nested PCR techniques, which made quantification challenging and also raised substantial problems with reproducibility

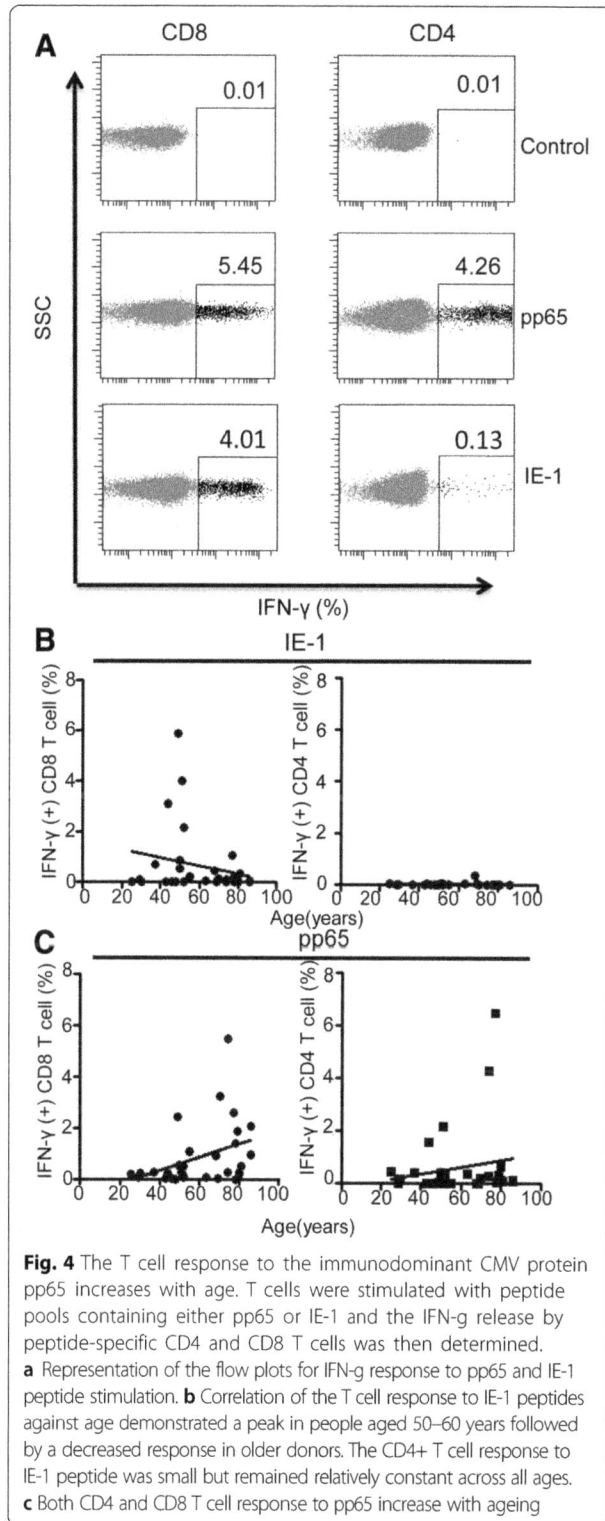

Fig. 4 The T cell response to the immunodominant CMV protein pp65 increases with age. T cells were stimulated with peptide pools containing either pp65 or IE-1 and the IFN-g release by peptide-specific CD4 and CD8 T cells was then determined. **a** Representation of the flow plots for IFN-g response to pp65 and IE-1 peptide stimulation. **b** Correlation of the T cell response to IE-1 peptides against age demonstrated a peak in people aged 50–60 years followed by a decreased response in older donors. The CD4+ T cell response to IE-1 peptide was small but remained relatively constant across all ages. **c** Both CD4 and CD8 T cell response to pp65 increase with ageing

[30]. Quantitative PCR is far more accurate but relies on interpretation of the cycle threshold of a sample against a known calibration standard. This is restricted by the lower limit of detection of the standards and the rate of amplification, which can vary between different PCR

runs. In contrast, digital PCR provides an absolute quantification and avoids these limitations. Our analysis included a direct comparison of ddPCR and Q-PCR and, as expected, we observed an extremely high concordance between the two technologies. However ddPCR was found to offer superior sensitivity and reliability of detection. Seventeen samples were found to be positive by either ddPCR or Q-PCR, 16 of these by ddPCR and 14 by Q-PCR.

Our work was performed using DNA isolated from monocytes, which are established as the most important haemopoietic site of viral latency [31, 32], and which in murine infection also serve to disseminate viral infection to distal sites such as salivary gland [33]. The first interesting finding was the observation that CMV was detectable in only a minority of donors, as 64 % of people remained negative by ddPCR despite the presence of chronic infection as confirmed by CMV-specific IgG positivity. Indeed, in younger people below the age of 50 years, the detection of CMV load in the blood was uncommon, being observed in only 13 % of donors tested. The lower limit of detection provided by ddPCR in our assay was for a single copy of virus within the total reaction volume (20 µl) and as such a negative result indicated absent or extremely low levels of virus. This low level carriage may reflect a lower intrinsic probability of viral reactivation in younger donors but is perhaps more likely to reflect the consequence of effective immune surveillance of viral replication in younger individuals.

The frequency of viral detection increased markedly with each decade above the age of 50 years to 37.5 and 50 % and finally became positive in every donor who was older than 70. Interestingly the amount of viral DNA detected within the blood also increased substantially with age with a 29 fold increase observed between donors aged less than 70 and those over this age. The use of nested PCR also detected viral DNA within the majority of healthy elderly donors [18]. These data indicate that a gradual impairment in the ability to control CMV load within blood starts around the age of 50 years and then deteriorates markedly beyond the age of 70. Importantly, our work did not address the number of CMV copies within individual monocytes, which has previously been shown to vary between 2 and 13 copies per cell [15]. Thus, it remains uncertain if ageing is associated with an increase in the number of viral copies within each infected monocyte or if there is an increase in the proportion of infected cells.

We were also interested to use the sensitivity of ddPCR to examine the presence of CMV within specific subsets of the myelo-monocytic lineage. CD14 and CD16 can be used to delineate three major subclasses of monocyte [34], classical monocytes (CD14 + CD16-) which account for >70 % of peripheral monocytes and are important for

innate immunity. These, together with intermediate monocytes (CD14 + CD16+) have more phagocytic properties than their non-classical CD14-CD16++ counterparts [35]. Our data suggested that CMV was not detectable within CD14-CD16+ monocyte cells, a finding which is in contrast to murine CMV, where CD16+ monocytes have been shown to exhibit higher levels of CMV latency than CD14+ cells [33].

We were also interested to compare levels of CMV load within haemopoietic precursors of the terminally differentiated monocytic lineage. As such we isolated CD34+ haemopoietic stem cells from G-CSF mobilized blood donations. CMV was detected in 3 of these 5 samples, which is comparable to a previous report of 8 positive samples out of 12 using an alternative PCR methodology [15]. This suggests that viral DNA may either pass selectively into cells that differentiate into the monocytic lineage or that some degree of viral replication occurs during myelopoiesis in order to sustain viral loads during the periods of cellular proliferation prior to monocyte formation.

Importantly, the ddPCR assay detects the level of viral DNA but does not assess the level of infectious virion. CMV was not detected by ddPCR within plasma samples taken from donors identified to have a positive monocyte viral load (n = 10). This indicated that viral DNA was retained within cells, with no evidence of production of extracellular virus (data not shown).

The direct measurement of viral DNA is a critical component in efforts to understand the balance of viral load and host immune response during natural CMV infection, an ambition that has been achieved so effectively for the study of HIV using RNA load. However, it is also important to correlate these values with assessment of the immune response to the virus.

Figure 5 gives a schematic overview of the parallel changes in immunity and viral load that arise following CMV infection over a lifetime. We observed that the humoral immune response to CMV increased steadily and markedly during ageing. Total immunoglobulin levels are known to fall with ageing and so our increase in CMV-specific antibody might appear somewhat surprising, but has in fact been reported previously [36, 37]. It is likely that episodes of subclinical viral reactivation serve to boost CMV-specific immunity and indeed this accumulation of CMV-specific immune memory may suppress the development of heterologous immune responses, which is a likely contributing factor towards immune senescence. Nevertheless these observations suggest that impairment in humoral immunity is not a major contributory factor towards the increase in viral load with ageing.

Studies have shown that the T cell immune response to CMV increases markedly with age such that the virus-specific CD8+ T cell response can come to dominate the

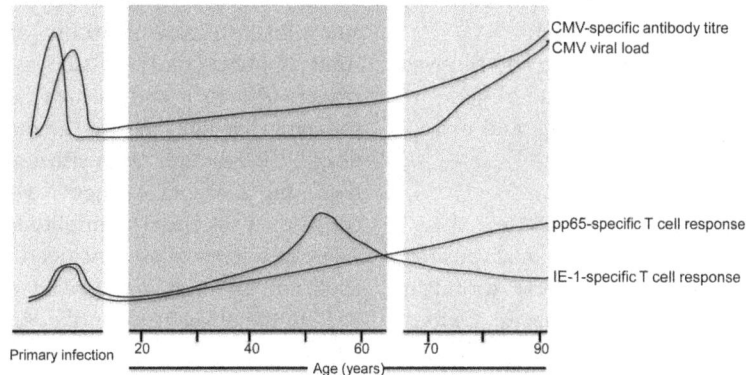

Fig. 5 An overview of the parallel changes in viral load and immunity during the lifetime of an individual infected with Cytomegalovirus. Schematic representation of the relative changes in the peripheral blood viral load as well as humoral and T cell immune response to CMV over the human life-course. Primary infection is shown as occurring during childhood, the most common age of infection. CMV viral load and CMV-specific IgG antibody titre increases during ageing. CD8 T cell responses to IE-1 peptides peaked in people aged 50–60 years and then decreased in older donors, while T cell response to pp65 peptides increase with ageing

CD8+ T cell repertoire in some donors [3, 38]. This profile of 'memory inflation' is also seen in murine CMV infection and is believed to be driven by recognition of viral peptides on non-haemopoietic cells. Relatively little is known about the specific profile of CMV proteins that drive CD8+ T cell expansion during ageing, although the importance of structural proteins such as pp65 are well documented [3, 29]. Indeed, the presence of CMV DNA within monocytic cells has been correlated with increased pp65-specific T cell immunity in elderly donors [18].

Our work also observed an expansion of pp65-specific T cells in relation to ageing, with an 8.4 fold increase between the youngest and most elderly donors and may reflect an incremental accumulation to recurrent subclinical episodes of viral reactivation. However, assessment of the T cell recognition of peptides derived from the immediate early protein IE-1 revealed an increase in middle aged individuals, with reduced recognition in those of an advanced age. This observation supports previous work, which has reported no significant increase in the IE-1 specific immune response with ageing [39].

It is currently unclear why IE-1 responses appear to wane with age. An important factor may relate to the frequency of T cell exposure to IE-derived epitopes, as these are presented to T cells repeatedly during the early period of viral replication and serve to elicit a cellular immune response that can prevent the late stages of viral infection before late viral proteins such as pp65 are produced. As such IE-1-specific T cells are exposed to very high levels of antigen stimulation and may be more susceptible to functional exhaustion than those directed against late-stage viral proteins such as pp65 [40]. However the explanation for the differing T cell responses to IE-1 and pp65 with ageing remains unclear and will require larger cross sectional and longitudinal study.

The concept that ageing leads to an alteration in the balance between viral load and the host immune response during chronic viral infection is supported by a variety of clinical and immunological observations. Herpes zoster, which represents reactivation of varicella zoster virus (VZV), is more common in the elderly and VZV titres increase with age, a pattern also reported for Epstein Barr Virus [41, 42]. Finally, levels of the persistent and highly prevalent Torque tenovirus are also known to increase markedly with ageing [43].

Conclusion

In conclusion, these data reveal the delicate balance that has evolved between chronic CMV infection and the host immune response and indicate that this symbiosis can break down during ageing, where an increase in CMV viral load occurs as the attritional effects of chronic surveillance and the impact of immune senescence become more apparent. It is likely that increased understanding of the clinical importance of chronic viral infection on human health will become an important health consideration in future years.

Methods
Healthy donors
Forty-four CMV positive healthy donors (confirmed by CMV ELISA) were recruited for study between the ages of 25 and 86 (mean 50.5). Healthy individuals below the age of 65 were recruited from The University of Birmingham, whilst those over 65 were recruited as part of the ongoing Birmingham 1000 elder's cohort which recruits elderly healthy donors from the local community. Following a 50 ml blood donation, plasma and PBMCs were extracted over a ficoll density gradient and stored at −160 °C. PBMCs were used for functional T cell studies

and monocyte extraction whilst plasma was used for CMV ELISA testing.

Five peripheral blood stem cell donors who had received G-CSF mobilization were also recruited and aliquots of PBMC stored at −160 °C prior to defrosting and extraction of myeloid cell subsets.

Extraction of cell subsets: CD14, CD34 and CD16

Enrichment of CD14, CD16, CD34 and dual positive CD14/16 cells from stem cell donations were sorted by flow cytometry (MoFLow sorter, BDBiosciences, Oxford, UK). Following defrosting, cells were washed in PBS and labeled for 15 min at 4° with LIVE/DEAD Fixable red dead cell stain kit (Life technologies, UK), PE anti-CD34 (BDBiosciences), anti-CD56 FITC (BDBiosciences), anti-CD14 FITC (BDBiosciences) and anti-CD16 Pe-Cy7 (Biolegend, San Diego, USA), prior to a further wash and sorting. For extraction of CD14 positive cells from healthy donor PBMC, positive selection using CD14 magnetically labeled beads was used and an average enrichment found to be 98.73 % (SD 0.39) by flow cytometry (Miltenyi Biotec, Surrey, UK). DNA extraction was then performed on the enriched cell populations according to the protocol for GenElute Mammalian Genomic DNA miniprep kit (Sigma-Aldrich, St. Louis, MO USA) and DNA concentration and purity checked using the Nanodrop 2000 (Thermo Scientific, Waltham, MA, USA).

CMV plasmid controls for standard curve generation

Human CMV HHV5 kit for Q-PCR amplification of glycoprotein B was purchased and used for all CMV PCR reactions within this work (PrimerDesign, Southampton, UK). Using the provided plasmid control, reconstituted aliquots were stored at −20 °C. Plasmid dilutions were then prepared fresh for Q-PCR to validate detection of the ddPCR assay and were diluted to produce the following copies per reaction: 50000, 10000, 2500, 500, 250, 100, 50, 10, 5 and 1.

Droplet digital PCR

Using the QX100 droplet digital PCR system (Bio-rad, Pleasanton, CA), a reaction mixture consisting of 5ul of either CD14 positive DNA (10 ng/ul) or plasmid standard made up to a volume of 8ul with PCR grade water, 10ul of 2 × ddPCR supermix for probes (Bio-rad), 1ul of reconstituted FAM labeled CMV primer and probe (Primer Design) and 1ul of HEX labeled RPP30 copy number assay for ddPCR (Bio-Rad) were loaded into a disposable plastic cartridge for droplet generation (Bio-Rad). Seventy microlitre of droplet generation oil (Bio-Rad) was also added before loading the cartridge into the droplet generator (Bio-Rad). After droplet generation, the sample was loaded into a 96 well PCR plate (Eppendorf, Hamburg, Germany) and PCR amplification carried out using the T100 thermocycler (Bio-Rad). PCR conditions consisted of 10 min at

95 °C, prior to 40 cycles at 94 °C for 30 s and 60 s at 60 °C and a finally 1 cycle at 10 min at 98 °C, ending at 12 °C. After amplification the plate was loaded onto the droplet reader (Bio-rad) and results analysed by QuantaSoft® software (Bio-Rad) to give the number of virus copies per ul of PCR reaction. A positive and negative control was used in each experiment, which also verified the consistency of droplet amplitude, and a well consisting solely of water was also included. Results were obtained in triplicate. As each mammalian cell contains 2 copies of RPP30, the absolute quantification of RPP30 was divided by two in order to determine the actual cell number. The CMV viral load was then divided by this figure to obtain the CMV load per cell.

Q-PCR

Using the 7500 Real Time PCR system (Applied Biosystems, California, USA), a PCR reaction mixture consisting of 5ul of standard plasmid or 5ul of CD14 positive DNA (10 ng/ul) made up to a volume of 9ul with PCR grade water, together with 10ul of 2 × Taqman Universal mastermix II with no UNG (Applied Biosystems) and 1ul of FAM labeled CMV primer and probe were loaded into a 96 well PCR plate (Eppendorf, Hamburg, Germany). PCR amplification consisted of 2 min at 95 °C, prior to 50 cycles at 95 °C for 10 s and 60 s at 60 °C. A positive and negative control plus water well were included in each experiment and the standard curve repeated in triplicate and averaged. Samples were only considered positive if present in triplicate.

Enzyme-linked immunosorbent assay (ELISA) testing for CMV IgG titre

As described by Kilgour et al, CMV ELISA testing (University of Birmingham, Birmingham UK) was used to ascertain participant's CMV status. Briefly, mock and viral lysate were used to coat 95 well plate overnight at 4 °C. Using plasma from 3 CMV positive donors, a standard was prepared and added to the plate in a 1 in 4 serial dilution, alongside 1ul of healthy donor samples. After 1 h incubation at room temperature, the plate was washed and anti-IgG horseradish peroxidase conjugated secondary antibody (Southern Biotech, Alabama, USA) added to each well and incubated for a further 1 h in the dark, RT. After repeat wash steps, 100 μL of TMB ELISA peroxidase substrate (Rockland Immunochemicals, Pennsylvania, USA) was added and incubated for 10 min in the dark, RT. To stop the reaction, 100 μL of 1 mM HCl was added, prior to reading on an ELISA plate reader at 450 nm [44].

CMV functionality testing

10^6 PBMC were resuspended in 500 ul RPMI plus 10 % FCS and incubated with either 10 ul Peptivator EI-1, 10 ul Peptivator pp65 (Miltenyi Biotech, Bergisch Gladbach,

Germany), 10 ul SEB (Sigma-Aldrich), or 10 ul RPMI. 0.5 ul of Brefeldin A was then added to all samples (Bio Legend) and incubated over night at 37 °C in 5 % CO_2. Afterwards, cells were washed and stained with viability dye-APC (Thermo Fisher Scientific) following manufacturer's instructions. After two washes, surface staining was performed, using anti-CD8 FITC, anti-CD4 PE-Cy7, anti-CD3 APC-Cy7 (BDBiosciences). Cells were then washed, fixed in 4 % paraformaldehyde (Sigma-Aldrich), washed again, and permeabilized with 0.5 % saponin (Sigma-Aldrich). After washing, cells were stained with anti-IFNγ PE (Miltenyi Biotech), washed and analysed using a FacsCanto II flow cytometer (BDBiosciences).

Statistical analysis

One way ANOVA (Kruskal-Wallis test) and post hoc Dunn's testing was used to compare CMV viral load with age. A growth exponential curve was used to assess the CMV load doubling time and linear regression used to assess the relationship between CMV copies (log_{10}) and the age of participants. For the standard dilution series ran in triplicate, the results were log transformed log_{10} and Pearson's correlation co-efficient was used to compare the quantitative agreement between ct value and plasmid copy number. Linear regression was used to examine the relationship between ddPCR copy number reading and that of the plasmid dilution and also to compare Q-PCR copy number with that of ddPCR in healthy donor samples. Pearson's correlation co-efficient was used to examine the relationship between CMV IgG titre and age. For comparison of age against functional T cell responses against Spearman's correlation co-efficient was used. Mann-Whitney testing was used to compare IFN-y responses in T cells following peptide stimulation in those with detectable viral load compared to those without. All analysis was performed using Prism version 6.0, Graphpad software, San Diego, USA.

Competing interests
The authors declare that they have no competing interests.

Authors' contributions
HP and JZ designed the study and carried out PCR experiments. NM optimized the ddPCR assay. GF performed the functional experiments and EE carried out the ELISA testing. Statistical analysis was performed by HP and CI. CI also provided donor information. Manuscript was written by HP and edited by PM and GP. All authors read and approved the final manuscript.

Acknowledgements
Many thanks to Jess Lander and Tasneem Khan at Birmingham Women's Hospital for their guidance and help using the ddPCR machine.
HP was funded for this work by a Wellcome Trust Clinical Fellowship Grant. JZ and GF were funded by Bloodwise.
All research was conducted in accordance with the declaration of Helsinki and ethical approval obtained by the Birmingham and South ethics committee.

Author details
[1]Institute of Immunology and Immunotherapy, University of Birmingham, Vincent Drive, Birmingham B15 2TT, UK. [2]University of Birmingham Medical and Dental School, Vincent Drive, Birmingham B15 2TT, UK. [3]West Midlands Regional Genetics Laboratories, Birmingham Women's NHS Foundation Trust, Mindelsohn Way, Edgbaston, Birmingham B15 2TG, UK. [4]University Hospitals NHS Foundation Trust, Birmingham, UK. [5]Charles Darwin Building, Henwick Grove, University of Worcester, Worcester WR2 6AJ, UK.

References
1. Lopo S, Vinagre E, Palminha P, Paixao MT, Nogueira P, Freitas MG. Seroprevalence to cytomegalovirus in the Portuguese population, 2002-2003. Euro Surveill. 2011; 16(25). http://www.eurosurveillance.org/ViewArticle.aspx?ArticleId = 19896
2. Staras SA, Dollard SC, Radford KW, Flanders WD, Pass RF, Cannon MJ. Seroprevalence of cytomegalovirus infection in the United States, 1988-1994. Clin Infect Dis. 2006;43(9):1143-51. doi:10.1086/508173.
3. Moss P, Khan N. CD8(+) T-cell immunity to cytomegalovirus. Hum Immunol. 2004;65(5):456-64. doi:10.1016/j.humimm.2004.02.014.
4. Elkington R, Shoukry NH, Walker S, Crough T, Fazou C, Kaur A, et al. Cross-reactive recognition of human and primate cytomegalovirus sequences by human CD4 cytotoxic T lymphocytes specific for glycoprotein B and H. Eur J Immunol. 2004;34(11):3216-26. doi:10.1002/eji.200425203.
5. Chidrawar S, Khan N, Wei W, McLarnon A, Smith N, Nayak L, et al. Cytomegalovirus-seropositivity has a profound influence on the magnitude of major lymphoid subsets within healthy individuals. Clin Exp Immunol. 2009;155(3):423-32. doi:10.1111/j.1365-2249.2008.03785.x.
6. Fulop T, Larbi A, Pawelec G. Human T cell aging and the impact of persistent viral infections. Front Immunol. 2013;4:271. doi:10.3389/fimmu.2013.00271.
7. Strindhall J, Skog M, Ernerudh J, Bengner M, Löfgren S, Matussek A et al. The inverted CD4/CD8 ratio and associated parameters in 66-year-old individuals: the Swedish HEXA immune study. Age (Dordrecht, Netherlands). 2012. doi: 10.1007/s11357-012-9400-3.
8. Schmaltz HN, Fried LP, Xue QL, Walston J, Leng SX, Semba RD. Chronic cytomegalovirus infection and inflammation are associated with prevalent frailty in community-dwelling older women. J Am Geriatr Soc. 2005;53(5): 747-54. doi:10.1111/j.1532-5415.2005.53250.x.
9. Strandberg TE, Pitkala KH, Tilvis RS. Cytomegalovirus antibody level and mortality among community-dwelling older adults with stable cardiovascular disease. Jama. 2009;301(4):380-2. doi:10.1001/jama.2009.4.
10. Aiello AE, Haan M, Blythe L, Moore K, Gonzalez JM, Jagust W. The influence of latent viral infection on rate of cognitive decline over 4 years. J Am Geriatr Soc. 2006;54(7):1046-54. doi:10.1111/j.1532-5415.2006.00796.x.
11. Roberts ET, Haan MN, Dowd JB, Aiello AE. Cytomegalovirus antibody levels, inflammation, and mortality among elderly Latinos over 9 years of follow-up. Am J Epidemiol. 2010;4:363-71.
12. Savva GM, Pachnio A, Kaul B, Morgan K, Huppert FA, Brayne C, et al. Cytomegalovirus infection is associated with increased mortality in the older population. Aging Cell. 2013;12(3):381-7. doi:10.1111/acel.12059.
13. Stowe RP, Kozlova EV, Yetman DL, Walling DM, Goodwin JS, Glaser R. Chronic herpesvirus reactivation occurs in aging. Exp Gerontol. 2007;42(6): 563-70. doi:10.1016/j.exger.2007.01.005.
14. Jordan MC. Latent infection and the elusive cytomegalovirus. Reviews of infectious diseases. 1983;5:205-15.
15. Slobedman B, Mocarski ES. Quantitative analysis of latent human cytomegalovirus. Journal of virology. 1999;73:4806-12.
16. Taylor-Wiedeman J, Sissons JG, Borysiewicz LK, Sinclair JH. Monocytes are a major site of persistence of human cytomegalovirus in peripheral blood mononuclear cells. The Journal of general virology. 1991;72(Pt 9):2059-64.
17. Stanier P, Kitchen AD, Taylor DL, Tyms AS. Detection of human cytomegalovirus in peripheral mononuclear cells and urine samples using PCR. Mol Cell Probes. 1992;6(1):51-8.
18. Leng SX, Qu T, Semba RD, Li H, Yao X, Nilles T, et al. Relationship between cytomegalovirus (CMV) IgG serology, detectable CMV DNA in peripheral monocytes, and CMV pp65(495-503)-specific CD8+ T cells in older adults. Age. 2011;33:607-14. doi:10.1007/s11357-011-9205-9.
19. Hahn G, Jores R, Mocarski ES. Cytomegalovirus remains latent in a common precursor of dendritic and myeloid cells. Proceedings of the National Academy of Sciences of the United States of America. 1998;95: 3937-42.

20. Kondo K, Kaneshima H, Mocarski ES. Human cytomegalovirus latent infection of granulocyte-macrophage progenitors. Proc Natl Acad Sci U S A. 1994;91(25):11879–83.

21. Goodrum FD, Jordan CT, High K, Shenk T. Human cytomegalovirus gene expression during infection of primary hematopoietic progenitor cells: a model for latency. Proc Natl Acad Sci U S A. 2002;99(25):16255–60. doi:10.1073/pnas.252630899.

22. Rossetto CC, Tarrant-Elorza M, Pari GS. Cis and trans acting factors involved in human cytomegalovirus experimental and natural latent infection of CD14 (+) monocytes and CD34 (+) cells. PLoS Pathog. 2013;9(5):e1003366. doi:10.1371/journal.ppat.1003366.

23. Reeves MB, MacAry PA, Lehner PJ, Sissons JG, Sinclair JH. Latency, chromatin remodeling, and reactivation of human cytomegalovirus in the dendritic cells of healthy carriers. Proc Natl Acad Sci U S A. 2005;102(11):4140–5. doi:10.1073/pnas.0408994102.

24. Bain M, Mendelson M, Sinclair J. Ets-2 Repressor Factor (ERF) mediates repression of the human cytomegalovirus major immediate-early promoter in undifferentiated non-permissive cells. J Gen Virol. 2003;84(Pt 1):41–9.

25. Stevenson EV, Collins-McMillen D, Kim JH, Cieply SJ, Bentz GL, Yurochko AD. HCMV reprogramming of infected monocyte survival and differentiation: a Goldilocks phenomenon. Viruses. 2014;6(2):782–807. doi:10.3390/v6020782.

26. Watanabe M, Kawaguchi T, Isa S, Ando M, Tamiya A, Kubo A, et al. Ultra-Sensitive Detection of the Pretreatment EGFR T790M Mutation in Non-Small Cell Lung Cancer Patients with an EGFR-Activating Mutation Using Droplet Digital PCR. Clin Cancer Res. 2015;21(15):3552–60. doi:10.1158/1078-0432.ccr-14-2151.

27. Kinz E, Leiherer A, Lang AH, Drexel H, Muendlein A. Accurate quantitation of JAK2 V617F allele burden by array-based digital PCR. Int J Lab Hematol. 2015;37(2):217–24. doi:10.1111/ijlh.12269.

28. Pourgheysari B, Khan N, Best D, Bruton R, Nayak L, Moss PA. The cytomegalovirus-specific CD4+ T-cell response expands with age and markedly alters the CD4+ T-cell repertoire. J Virol. 2007;81(14):7759–65. doi:10.1128/jvi.01262-06.

29. Khan N, Shariff N, Cobbold M, Bruton R, Ainsworth JA, Sinclair AJ, et al. Cytomegalovirus seropositivity drives the CD8 T cell repertoire toward greater clonality in healthy elderly individuals. J Immunol. 2002;169(4):1984–92.

30. Roback JD, Drew WL, Laycock ME, Todd D, Hillyer CD, Busch MP. CMV DNA is rarely detected in healthy blood donors using validated PCR assays. Transfusion. 2003;43(3):314–21.

31. Larsson S, Soderberg-Naucler C, Wang FZ, Moller E. Cytomegalovirus DNA can be detected in peripheral blood mononuclear cells from all seropositive and most seronegative healthy blood donors over time. Transfusion. 1998;38(3):271–8.

32. Soderberg C, Larsson S, Bergstedt-Lindqvist S, Moller E. Identification of blood mononuclear cells permissive of cytomegalovirus infection in vitro. Transplant Proc. 1993;25(1 Pt 2):1416–8.

33. Daley-Bauer LP, Roback LJ, Wynn GM, Mocarski ES. Cytomegalovirus hijacks CX3CR1(hi) patrolling monocytes as immune-privileged vehicles for dissemination in mice. Cell Host Microbe. 2014;15(3):351–62. doi:10.1016/j.chom.2014.02.002.

34. Ziegler-Heitbrock L, Ancuta P, Crowe S, Dalod M, Grau V, Hart DN, et al. Nomenclature of monocytes and dendritic cells in blood. Blood. 2010;116(16):e74–80. doi:10.1182/blood-2010-02-258558.

35. Stansfield BK, Ingram DA. Clinical significance of monocyte heterogeneity. Clin Transl Med. 2015;4:5. doi:10.1186/s40169-014-0040-3.

36. McVoy MA, Adler SP. Immunologic evidence for frequent age-related cytomegalovirus reactivation in seropositive immunocompetent individuals. J Infect Dis. 1989;160(1):1–10.

37. Alonso Arias R, Moro-Garcia MA, Echeverria A, Solano-Jaurrieta JJ, Suarez-Garcia FM, Lopez-Larrea C. Intensity of the humoral response to cytomegalovirus is associated with the phenotypic and functional status of the immune system. J Virol. 2013;87(8):4486–95. doi:10.1128/jvi.02425-12.

38. Wikby A, Johansson B, Olsson J, Löfgren S, Nilsson BO, Ferguson F. Expansions of peripheral blood CD8 T-lymphocyte subpopulations and an association with cytomegalovirus seropositivity in the elderly: the Swedish NONA immune study. Experimental gerontology. 2002;37:445–53.

39. Lachmann R, Bajwa M, Vita S, Smith H, Cheek E, Akbar A, et al. Polyfunctional T cells accumulate in large human cytomegalovirus-specific T cell responses. J Virol. 2012;86(2):1001–9. doi:10.1128/jvi.00873-11.

40. Tarrant-Elorza M, Rossetto CC, Pari GS. Maintenance and replication of the human cytomegalovirus genome during latency. Cell Host Microbe. 2014;16(1):43–54. doi:10.1016/j.chom.2014.06.006.

41. Ogunjimi B, Theeten H, Hens N, Beutels P. Serology indicates cytomegalovirus infection is associated with varicella-zoster virus reactivation. J Med Virol. 2014;86(5):812–9. doi:10.1002/jmv.23749.

42. Devlin ME, Gilden DH, Mahalingam R, Dueland AN, Cohrs R. Peripheral blood mononuclear cells of the elderly contain varicella-zoster virus DNA. J Infect Dis. 1992;165(4):619–22.

43. Haloschan M, Bettesch R, Gorzer I, Weseslindtner L, Kundi M, Puchhammer-Stockl E. TTV DNA plasma load and its association with age, gender, and HCMV IgG serostatus in healthy adults. Age (Dordr). 2014;36(5):9716. doi:10.1007/s11357-014-9716-2.

44. Kigour AH, Flrth C, Harrison R, Moss P, Bastin ME, Wardlaw JM et al. Seropositivity for CMV and IL-6 levels are associated with grip strength and muscle size in the elderly. Immun ageing. 2013;10(1):33. doi: 10.1186/1742-4933-10-33.

CXCL-16, IL-17, and bone morphogenetic protein 2 (BMP-2) are associated with overweight and obesity conditions in middle-aged and elderly women

Silvana Mara Turbino Luz Ribeiro[2,7†], Laís Roquete Lopes[2,7†], Guilherme de Paula Costa[2,7], Vivian Paulino Figueiredo[2,7], Deena Shrestha[2,7], Aline Priscila Batista[2], Roney Luiz de Carvalho Nicolato[5], Fernando Luiz Pereira de Oliveira[3,6], Juliana Assis Silva Gomes[8] and Andre Talvani[1,2,3,4,7*] (iD)

Abstract

Background: The current concept of overweight/obesity is most likely related to a combination of increased caloric intake and decreased energy expenditure. Widespread inflammation, associated with both conditions, appears to contribute to the development of some obesity-related comorbidities. Interventions that directly or indirectly target individuals at high risk of developing obesity have been largely proposed because of the increasing number of overweight/obese cases worldwide. The aim of the present study was to assess CXCL16, IL-17, and BMP-2 plasma factors in middle-aged and elderly women and relate them to an overweight or obese status. In total, 117 women were selected and grouped as eutrophic, overweight, and obese, according to anthropometric parameters. Analyses of anthropometric and circulating biochemical parameters were followed by plasma immunoassays for CXCL-16, IL-17, and BMP-2.

Results: Plasma mediators increased in all overweight and obese individuals, with the exception of BMP-2 in the elderly group, whereas CXCL16 levels were shown to differentiate overweight and obese individuals. Overweight and/or obese middle-aged and elderly individuals presented with high LDL, triglycerides, and glycemia levels. Anthropometric parameters indicating increased-cardiovascular risk were positively correlated with CXCL-16, BMP-2, and IL-17 levels in overweight and obese middle-aged and elderly individuals.

Conclusion: This study provides evidence that CXCL-16, IL-17, and BMP-2 are potential plasma indicators of inflammatory status in middle-aged and elderly women; therefore, further investigation of obesity-related comorbidities is recommended. CXCL16, in particular, could be a potential marker for middle-aged and elderly individuals transitioning from eutrophic to overweight body types, which represents an asymptomatic and dangerous condition.

Keywords: Inflammation, Elderly, Overweight, Obesity, CXCL-16, BMP-2, IL-17

* Correspondence: talvani@nupeb.ufop.br
†Equal contributors
[1]Department of Biological Sciences, Federal University of Ouro Preto, Ouro Preto, Minas Gerais, Brazil
[2]Post-graduation Program in Biological Sciences/NUPEB, Federal University of Ouro Preto, Ouro Preto, Minas Gerais, Brazil
Full list of author information is available at the end of the article

Background

Obesity is a worldwide epidemic and pathological condition resulting from contemporary lifestyles; it is characterized by lack of physical activity in addition to an energy-dense diet [1]. Adipose tissue was previously defined as a simple energy source used to manage energy flow in the body; however, it has taken on the integrative role of linking bioactive mediator release, homeostasis, and pathological conditions [2]. At least 24 typical inflammatory mediators such as leptin, resistin, IL-6, TNF, and chemokines, among others (e.g., C-reactive protein, haptoglobin, and amyloid A) are upregulated during obesity [3–5].

Natural ageing is currently associated with senescent immune remodeling, which occurs when innate barriers lose their abilities to restrict pathogen entry; in this condition, the internal organs become more vulnerable to metabolic disturbances resulting in a natural reduction in life expectancy [6, 7]. It is currently accepted that increased visceral omental, not abdominal subcutaneous adipose tissue, correlates the most with cardiovascular diseases, insulin resistance, and other obesity-related diseases [8, 9]. Overweight and obesity statuses often start early in child- or adulthood. These conditions become detrimental during senescence, when the human body requires balance to deal with age-associated changes. Accordingly, lifestyle and nutritional changes in infants and adults might prevent or postpone some adverse effects on the immune system and improve quality of life in elderly individuals. Both the inflammatory context and biological aging are crucial interrelated components of the understanding the association of clinical disturbances with overweight and obesity.

Based on the many potential biomarkers that have the capacity to predict obesity- and overweight-related diseases, we investigated the clinical role of three soluble mediators in human cardiac and metabolic diseases: (i) IL-17, a pro-inflammatory cytokine previously associated with obesity due to its role in the development of atherosclerosis, coronary syndromes, and glucose tolerance [10, 11], (ii) CXCL16, an interferon-gamma-regulated chemokine and scavenger receptor for oxidized low-density lipoprotein that is expressed in atherosclerotic lesions and described as a marker of acute coronary syndromes [12, 13], and finally, (iii) bone morphogenetic protein-2/BMP-2, a cytokine that promotes bone formation, but also is associated with potential adverse clinical effects including cyst-like bone formation, soft tissue swelling, and other anabolic activities in normal and osteoarthritic chondrocytes [14, 15]. Thus, the aim of the present study was to investigate the association between CXCL-16, BMP-2, and IL-17 plasma levels and overweight and obese conditions in middle-aged (35 to 55 years of age) and elderly (>60 years old) women to find possible targets to monitor early progression to obesity.

Methods

Study population

We performed this study using 46 healthy individuals (23 middle-aged and 23 elderly), 33 overweight individuals (20 middle-aged and 13 elderly), and 38 obese individuals (23 middle-aged and 15 elderly). All study participants were of the female sex and recruited at the UNIMED Inconfidentes, Ouro Preto, MG, Brazil. These women were undergoing a complete clinical examination and the following laboratory workup was performed: full blood count, free T4, TSH, glucose, cholesterol, VLDL, LDL, HDL, and triglycerides. Individuals with hypertension, diabetes, thyroid or renal disturbances, or any other cardiac or systemic diseases as well as those using steroidal drugs were excluded from this study. These conditions could prevent adequate interpretation of the association between obesity-related diseases and immune parameters. After blood collection and full clinical evaluation, all individuals were monitored weekly by health professionals (medical doctors, nutritionists, physiotherapist, and others) from UNIMED-Inconfidentes.

Definition of anthropometric measures

All study participants had body mass, triceps skinfold, and arm, waist, and hip circumference measurements collected by a trained staff member, in accordance with standardized protocols [16, 17]. Body mass index was calculated as weight divided by squared height (kg/m^2). The triceps skinfold was verified on the mid-line of the posterior surface of the arm (over the triceps muscle) at the level of the mid-point between the acromiale and the radiale. The subscapular skinfold was measured just below the angle of the scapula. Waist circumference was also measured at the midpoint between the lowest rib and the iliac crest.

Arm muscle circumference was the chosen indicator for elderly individuals, as the Third National Health and Nutrition Examination Survey (NHANES III) has presented reference data for this indicator [18]. All measurements were taken in a private room and conducted by an experienced nutritionist.

Biochemical analysis

Blood samples (7 ml) were drawn using S-Monovette tubes (Sarstedt Ltda, Nümbrecht Germany) between 7:00 and 9:00 AM, from all study participants after 12–14 h of overnight fasting. All blood tests (cholesterol, VLDL, LDL, HDL, triglycerides, and glycemia) were performed using conventional enzymatic methods at the certified Clinical Analysis Laboratory from the Pharmacy

School at Universidade Federal de Ouro Preto, MG, Brazil, on the day of blood collection.

Immunoassays for inflammatory mediators

Circulating levels of the inflammatory mediators, IL-17, CXCL16, and BMP-2, were detected in plasma samples that were previously stored at −80°C. Briefly, flat-bottom 96-well microtiter plates (Nunc) were coated with 100 μl/well of appropriate monoclonal antibodies for 18 h at 4°C and then washed with PBS buffer (pH 7.4) containing 0.05% tween-20 (wash buffer). Non-specific binding sites were blocked with 200 μl/well of 1% bovine serum albumin in PBS. Plates were washed and 100 μl/well of sample was added, which was followed by incubation for 18 h at 4°C. In addition, 100 μl/well of the appropriate biotinylated detection antibody, diluted in blocking buffer containing 0.05% tween-20, was added and samples were incubated for 1 h at 24°C. Streptavidin-horseradish peroxidase was added and after subsequent incubation and washing, 100 μl/well of the chromogen substrate o-phenylenediamine (Sigma-Aldrich Brasil Ltda, SP, Brazil), diluted in 0.03 M citrate buffer containing 0.02% of H_2O_2 was added for 30 min, which was followed by incubation in the dark at room temperature. The reaction was stopped through the addition of 50 μl/well of 1 M H_2SO_4 solution and plates were read at 492 nm in a spectrophotometer (Emax_Molecular Devices, Sunnyvale, CA, USA). All samples were simultaneously measured using Peprotech ELISA kits (Ribeirão Preto, SP, Brazil) in triplicate.

Statistical analysis

Graph Pad InStat and Prism statistical programs were used for analysis (GraphPad, San Diego, CA, USA). In cases of normal distribution, the independent t test was used, whereas the non-parametric Mann-Whitney test was used for non-Gaussian sample distributions. Correlations were verified using a Spearman test and results were confirmed by performing a linear regression test. Data were considered statistically significant when $p < 0.05$.

Results

Anthropometric characterization of subjects

Our study population consisted of 63 middle-aged (mean age of 40.9 years) and 54 elderly (mean age of 68.9 years) women, categorized according anthropometric parameters as eutrophic, overweight, and obese (Table 1). All anthropometric parameters such as body mass, triceps skinfold, arm circumference, arm muscle circumference, and waist and hip measurements were elevated in overweight or obese middle-aged and elderly individuals when compared to eutrophic individuals. Body mass index similarly increased with weight gain in both age groups, but the waist-to-hip ratio only increased in obese middle-aged individuals, and not in overweight or obese elderly individuals (data not shown).

An apparent reduction in immune and physiological activity in the senescent body was observed under natural conditions and without the presence of disease. Overweight and obese middle-aged individuals presented with anthropometric parameters that were worse than those in elderly eutrophic individuals, based on all analyzed parameters, except for arm muscle circumference. In addition, overweight and obese conditions were associated with similar anthropometric parameters, in both groups of women, with a minimum age difference of 30 years.

Cholesterol and glucose parameters in overweight and obese women

Blood biochemical parameters are shown in Table 2. VLDL cholesterol and glycemia levels were higher in eutrophic elderly individuals than in eutrophic middle-aged individuals.

However, when anthropometric parameters were taken into consideration for this biochemical analysis, overweight and/or obese individuals had total cholesterol,

Table 1 Baseline anthropometric parameters of the eutrophic, overweight and obesity subjects

	Eutrophic	Overweight	Obesity
	Adult ($n = 23$) / Elderly ($n = 23$)	Adult ($n = 20$) / Elderly ($n = 13$)	Adult ($n = 23$) / Elderly ($n = 15$)
Age	40,0 ± 1,2 / 71,5 ± 1,4	40,1 ± 1,5 / 64,0 ± 2,0	42,6 ± 1,5 / 71,4 ± 2,1
Body mass (kg)	57,3 ± 1,6 / 59,1 ± 1,6	68,8 ± 1,0* / 70,7 ± 2,1*	86,8 ± 2,6*# / 80,3 ± 1,6*A#
BMI (Kg/m2)	21,8 ± 0,4 / 23,6 ± 0,4	27,2 ± 0,2* / 28,26 ± 0,3*	34,0 ± 0,6*# / 33,2 ± 0,5*#
TSF (mm)	17,0 ± 1,1 / 18,4 ± 1,4	25,8 ± 1,3* / 24,0 ± 1,4	32,2 ± 1,5*# / 28,3 ± 1,5*
AC (cm)	27,1 ± 0,5 / 29,2 ± 0,5	31,3 ± 0,4* / 33,2 ± 0,6*	36,4 ± 0,7*# / 35,5 ± 0,6*
AMC (cm)	21,7 ± 0,5 / 23,4 ± 0,3	23,2 ± 0,4 / 25,7 ± 0,5*A	26,0 ± 0,5*# / 26,8 ± 0,5*
Waist (cm)	82,1 ± 1,6 / 87,1 ± 1,9	91,5 ± 1,5* / 101,1 ± 2,2*A	107,7 ± 2,4*# / 102,9 ± 1,7*

Values are shown as the mean ± SEM. *BMI* body mass index, *TSF* Triceps skinfold, *AC* arm circumference, *AMC* arm muscle circumference. * $p < 0.01$ when eutrophic groups were compared with their respective chronological overweight (OW) or obesity (OB) groups; A $p < 0.05$ when adult and elderly were compared among in terms of eutrophic, OW or OB; # $P < 0.01$ when OW were compared with OB inside the same chronological groups

Table 2 Biochemical parameters in eutrophic, overweight and obesity women

Eutrophic	Overweight	Obesity
Adult ($n = 23$) / Elderly ($n = 23$)	Adult ($n = 20$) / Elderly ($n = 13$)	Adult ($n = 23$) / Elderly ($n = 15$)
Cholesterol (mg/dL) $157,8 \pm 6,5$ / $211,0 \pm 12,0^A$	$194,0 \pm 9,3^*$ / $193,8 \pm 13,0$	$217,0 \pm 8,4^*$ '/ $195,9 \pm 11,0$
VLDL (mg/dL) $13,4 \pm 1,0$ / $18,8 \pm 2,1^A$	$17,9 \pm 2,8$ / $27,05 \pm 1,8^A$ *	$22,0 \pm 2,3^*$ '/ $28,1 \pm 2,9^A$ *
LDL (mg/dL) $125,9 \pm 6,1$ / $133,0 \pm 11,0^A$	$119,9 \pm 8,5$ / $121,3 \pm 12,1$	$143,2 \pm 7,7''$ / $125,8 \pm 11,6$
HDL (mg/dL) $58,3 \pm 1,8$ / $55,7 \pm 2,3$	$53,6 \pm 2,7$ / $54,7 \pm 3.2$	$51,5 \pm 2,2''$/ $46,5 \pm 2,1''$
Triglycerides (mg/dL) $67,5 \pm 5,1$ / $86,9 \pm 10,6^A$	$89,5 \pm 14,0$ / $85,6 \pm 9,1$	$111,4 \pm 11,5''$/ $115,1 \pm 10,9''$
Glycemia (mg/dL) $91,0 \pm 1,9$ / $103,2 \pm 9,3^A$	$91,3 \pm 1,8$ / $119,6 \pm 8,8^A$ *	$104,4 \pm 4,7^*$ '/ $117,5 \pm 11,9^A$ *

Values are shown as the mean ± SEM. *VLDL* very low density lipoproteins, *LDL* low density lipoproteins, *HDL* High density lipoproteins. Statistical differences are represented being that (*) $p < 0.05$ when the OW or OB were compared with the eutrophic individuals in the same age group; (^{A}) $p < 0.05$ when adult and elderly were compared in the same anthropometric group, ('') when OB is different from OW in the same age group

VDLL cholesterol, and glycemia levels that were higher than those in the respective age-matched eutrophic control groups. When we compared overweight and obese statuses, obese middle-aged individuals had higher total cholesterol, VLDL, LDL, HDL, triglycerides, and glycemia levels, whereas only HDL and triglycerides were different in the obese elderly group.

Interestingly, soluble CXCL16, but not IL-17 and BMP-2, was positively correlated with glycemia in middle-aged ($r = 0.734$, $p < 0.01$) and elderly ($r = 0.604$, $p < 0.05$) individuals, as well as with VLDL cholesterol in middle-aged ($r = 0.623$, $p < 0.05$) and elderly ($r = 0.546$, $p < 0.05$) individuals.

Plasma indicators of overweight and obesity

Plasma levels of the inflammatory chemokine CXCL16 (Fig. 1a) were markedly elevated in overweight and obese middle-aged and elderly individuals when compared to that in eutrophic individuals In addition, CXCL16 was capable of distinguishing overweight and obese individuals in the two age-related groups. CXCL16 production in overweight or obese middle-aged individuals was higher than that observed in 60-year old eutrophic individuals.

IL-17 (Fig. 1b) production was high in all overweight and obese individuals. However, obese elderly individuals presented with higher cytokine levels than overweight individuals of the same age group. In terms of IL-17 production, there were no differences between overweight and obese middle-aged and eutrophic elderly individuals.

BMP-2 (Fig. 1c) was higher in all overweight and obese middle-aged individuals, similar to that observed with the Il-17 pattern, but there was no difference observed between eutrophic and overweight elderly individuals. Increased production of this factor was observed in eutrophic and obese elderly individuals, suggesting natural degeneration of the bones.

Correlations among CXCL16, IL-17, and BMP-2 and anthropometric parameters

We assumed that body mass index, triceps skinfold, arm muscle circumference, and hip and waist circumferences are variables used to predict obesity-related comorbidities. The correlations among these anthropometric

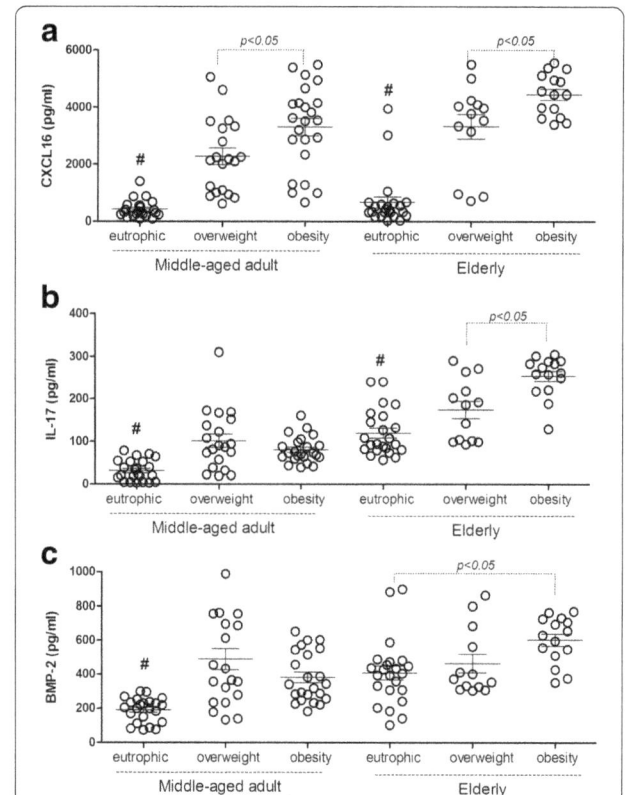

Fig. 1 Concentrations of the CXCL16, IL17 and BMP-2 plasma in middle-aged adult and elderly women. The concentrations (pg/ml) of chemokine CXCL16 plasma (**a**) The bone morphogenetic protein (BMP-2) (**b**) the inteleukin-17 (IL-17) (**c**) from middle-aged adult and elderly women presenting eutrophic, overweight and obesity conditions were measured through ELISA. The individual results were plotted in the graphic through mean ± SEM. # $P < 0.05$ when all groups were different from the eutrophic middle-aged adult or elderly subjects

parameters and plasma CXCL16, BMP-2, and IL-17 levels are shown in Table 3. Accordingly, CXCL16 showed the highest correlation with body mass index, triceps skinfold, and waist and hip circumference in middle-aged and elderly individuals, with Pearson's correlation coefficients (r) > 0.5.

Finally, IL-17 plasma levels were also positively correlated with body mass index, arm muscle circumference, and hip and waist circumferences in both age-related groups, whereas BMP-2 levels were only correlated with these anthropometric parameters in the elderly group.

Discussion

Results presented herein highlight the potential for CXCL16, IL-17, and BMP-2 plasma levels to be used as marker to discriminate overweight and obese individuals in both age groups. In particular, production of the chemokine CXCL16 was markedly high in the overweight and obese groups, and this correlated with anthropometric parameters that are considered comorbidity predictors.

The identification of biomarkers to predict obesity has become in important research area within the basic and clinical sciences, owing to the ability of these factors to predict cardiovascular and metabolic disturbances; this allows for proper treatment and lifestyle changes in individuals [19]. Unfortunately, the underlying complexity of biological pathway interactions demands further research before any of these potential biomarkers can be accurately used for diagnostic purposes. Many cellular inflammatory mediators come from white fat tissues, and they are often overproduced because of increased adiposity. In contrast, other regulatory factors or mediators of insulin sensitivity, such as adiponectin, are found in smaller amounts in similar conditions [20]. This imbalance between adipocyte products and other inflammatory mediators, caused by overweight and obese conditions might promote obesity-linked metabolic and cardiovascular disorders [1, 9]. Therefore, investigating biomarkers in overweight individuals should be a more common procedure in research and clinic. Ordinary individuals naturally gain a small amount of weight within a certain period-of-time; however, continuous chronic weight gain becomes problematic.

Interestingly, CXCL16 was shown to have a strong and exclusive association with overweight and obese conditions, regardless of subject age. Elderly women with higher VLDL and glycemia typically had higher levels of circulating CXCL16; these high circulating levels have previously been associated with the development of plaque deposits, artery walls, and/or diabetes [18, 20, 21]. Anthropometric parameters such as body mass index, triceps skinfold, and waist and hip circumference were positively correlated with CXCL16 levels in middle-aged and elderly women. CXCL16 is expressed in macrophages and aortic muscle cells. Expression increases in response to inflammatory stimuli and this enhances LDL uptake in favor of foam cell formation in human atherosclerotic plaques [11, 13]. Some chemokines have been described as effective adipokines and as biomarkers of obese conditions because of their inflammatory profile, which is associated with weight gain and adipose tissue accumulation, and the fact that their receptors are overexpressed in subcutaneous and visceral adipose tissues of obese individuals [22]. Previous studies have indicated an association between CXCL16 and obesity in C57BL6 mice [23] and coronary comorbidities in humans [24–26]. By assuming that obesity predisposes individuals to coronary and metabolic diseases, the present

Table 3 Correlation among CXCL16, IL-17 and BMP-2 and anthropometric parameters

ADULTS	BMI	TSF	AMC	WAIST	HIP	WHR
CXCL16	$R = 0.798*$	$R = 0,552*$	$R = 0.119$	$R = 0.860*$	$R = 0.555*$	$R = 0.2081$
	$p = 0.023$	$p = 0.5521$	$p = 0.1981$	$p = 0.016$	$p = 0.050$	$p = 0.1981$
IL-17	$R = 0.188*$	$R = 0.354$	$R = 0.371*$	$R = 0.341$	$R = 0.556*$	$R = 0.221*$
	$p = 0.047$	$p = 0.850$	$p = 0.010$	$p = 0.117$	$p = 0.050$	$p = 0.014$
BMP-2	$R = 0.1629$	$R = 0.0935$	$R = 0.1778$	$R = 0.2423$	$R = 0.1518$	$R = 0.1778$
	$p = 0.1034$	$p = 0,3523$	$p = 0.0752$	$p = 0.0146$	$p = 0.1295$	$p = 0.075$
ELDERLY	BMI	TSF	AMC	WAIST	HIP	WHR
CXCL16	$R = 0.798*$	$R = 0.552*$	$R = 0.198$	$R = 0.860*$	$R = 0.555*$	$R = 0.198$
	$p = 0.020$	$p = 0.050$	$p = 0.119$	$p = 0.016$	$p = 0.050$	$p = 0.110$
IL-17	$R = 0.184*$	$R = 0.332$	$R = 0.227*$	$R = 0.146$	$R = 0.542*$	$R = 0.371*$
	$p = 0.030$	$p = 0.090$	$p = 0.014$	$p = 0.110$	$p = 0.050$	$p = 0.020$
BMP-2	$R = 0.179*$	$R = 0.352$	$R = 0.187*$	$R = 0.242*$	$R = 0.251$	$R = 0.188*$
	$p = 0.050$	$p = 0,090$	$p = 0.050$	$p = 0.014$	$p = 0.129$	$p = 0.050$

BMI body mass index, *TSF* triceps skinfold, *AMC* arm muscle circumference, *WHR* waist-to-hip ratio
* positive correlation with $p < 0.05$

study included overweight and obese women. Regardless of this, high plasma levels of CXCL16 were observed in all middle-aged and elderly individuals presenting with an anthropometric status above overweight.

Overweight or obese individuals were expected to have increased adipocyte numbers, resulting from the recruitment of pluripotent stem cells to the vascular stroma of adipose tissue [27]. In our study, BMP-2 was investigated and was shown to be clearly elevated in overweight and obese middle-aged and elderly individuals. Regarding anthropometric parameters, this factor was positively correlated with body mass index, arm muscle circumference, and waist and waist-to-hip ratio in elderly women. These parameters are indicative of overweight or obese conditions, reinforcing the potential role BMP-2 to categorize individuals according to metabolic status. BMP-2 has been shown to promote osteogenic differentiation and adipogenesis in bone marrow stromal cells [28], and it could be partially responsible for increased obesity. A recent study suggested that increased demand to store excessive energy promotes BMP-2 expression and that adipocytes contribute to this phenomenon, due to energy storage in visceral and subcutaneous adipose tissues [29]. The present study reinforces such findings, since increased BMP-2 levels were observed in overweight and obese women and were associated with anthropometric parameters that indicate adipose tissue accumulation.

Unlike BMP-2, IL-17 has emerged as a negative regulator of adipogenesis and glucose metabolism in an experimental model. This cytokine acts in a complex network of inflammatory mediators that links adipose tissue to inflammatory cells such as neutrophils and adipocytes [10, 30, 31]. Indeed, excessive production of IL-17 during the initial stage of obesity could have a different effect on maintaining a prolonged inflammatory response and on associated long-term consequences. IL-17 was remarkably high in elderly individuals, and particularly in the obese and overweight middle-aged individuals; here, higher levels of VLDL and glycemia were observed. In addition, IL-17 was also positively correlated with classical anthropometric parameters (body mass index, arm muscle circumference, and hip and waist-to-hip ratio). These parameters have been described as anthropometric markers of poor prognosis in metabolic and cardiovascular diseases [19]. They have also been shown to contribute to the release of other inflammatory cytokines such as IL-6, IFN-gamma, and TNF [10], which reinforces the potential role of IL-17 in obesity-related diseases.

Our data reinforce the fact that obese individuals (middle-aged and elderly) present with higher cholesterol fractions, triglycerides, and glycemia, when compared to those parameters in eutrophic individuals, in accordance with the previous studies [1]. However, these overweight middle-aged individuals must receive follow-up care from health professionals when considering the relevance of visceral obesity, alongside soluble biomarkers. Nonetheless, integrated intervention programs based on weight reduction are demanding, since the immune conditions (systemic inflammation) in these patients are similar to those in elderly individuals. This might indicate the presence of accelerated damage due to the production of inflammatory mediators (e.g. CXCL-16, IL-17, and BMP-2), since high levels of these circulating factors clearly represent a risk for cardiovascular disease, cancer, and metabolic disturbances [12, 19, 25]. Preventing and reducing overweight and obese conditions depends on medical interventions, in addition to individual lifestyle changes; however, further research to motivate behavioral changes is required.

Conclusion

The present study provides complementary information regarding BMP-2, IL-17, and particularly CXCL-16, and their potential to be used as soluble markers capable of differentiating overweight and obese statuses in middle-aged and elderly women. These biomarkers were shown to be correlated with anthropometric (body mass index, triceps skinfold, arm muscle circumference, and hip and waist circumference) and biochemical (VLDL and glycemia) parameters. These factors might alter the inflammation axis observed in overweight and obese individuals, as well as in related disorders such as atherosclerosis, insulin resistance, and vascular damage. However, their clinical application needs to be investigated further in prospective population studies since its application in the clinical screening of overweight could help early in the preventive management of diseases associated with obesity.

Abbreviations
BMP-2: Bone morphogenetic protein-2; CXCL-16: CXC16 ligand; HDL: High density lipoprotein; IL-17: Interleukin-17; IL-6: Interleukin-6; LDL: Low density lipoprotein; T4: Thyroxine; TNF: Tumor necrosis factor; TSH: Thyroid-stimulating hormone; VLDL: Very low density lipoprotein

Acknowledgments
The authors thank Mr. Leonardo Mesquita for the donation of the S-Monovette tubes (Sarstedt LTDA) used in the present research.

Fundings
The present study was supported by granting from Conselho Nacional de Desenvolvimento Científico e Tecnológico (CNPq), Fundação de Amparo à Pesquisa do Estado de Minas Gerais (FAPEMIG) and Universidade Federal de Ouro Preto (UFOP). AT, FLPO and JASG are in credit with the CNPq for the fellowship applied to the development of the research.

Authors' contributions
SMTLR, LRL, GPC, DS, VPF and APB have helped conducting the experiments with patients and performing immunoassays and antropometric analysis; FLPO conducted the statistical analyses; RLCN was responsible for the biochemical analyses; AT has designed, supervised the project and the data analysis; JASG, FLPO and AT wrote the manuscript after the content was discussed and reviewed by all authors. All authors read and approved the final manuscript.

Competing interest

The authors declare that they have no competing interests regarding the publication.

Author details

[1]Department of Biological Sciences, Federal University of Ouro Preto, Ouro Preto, Minas Gerais, Brazil. [2]Post-graduation Program in Biological Sciences/NUPEB, Federal University of Ouro Preto, Ouro Preto, Minas Gerais, Brazil. [3]Post-graduation Program in Health and Nutrition, Federal University of Ouro Preto, Ouro Preto, Minas Gerais, Brazil. [4]Post-graduation in Ecology of Tropical Biomas, Federal University of Ouro Preto, Ouro Preto, Minas Gerais, Brazil. [5]Clinical Analyses Laboratory of the Pharmacy School, Federal University of Ouro Preto, Ouro Preto, Minas Gerais, Brazil. [6]Department of Statistics, Federal University of Ouro Preto, Ouro Preto, Minas Gerais, Brazil. [7]Laboratory of the Immunobiology of Inflammation, Federal University of Ouro Preto, Ouro Preto, Minas Gerais, Brazil. [8]Department of Morphology, Federal University of Minas Gerais, Belo Horizonte, Minas Gerais, Brazil.

References

1. Macpherson-Sánchez AE. Integrating fundamental concepts of obesity and eating disorders: implications for the obesity epidemic. Am J Public Health. 2015;105:271–85.
2. Lastra G, Sowers JR. Obesity and cardiovascular disease: role of adipose tissue, inflammation, and the renin-angiotensin-aldosterone system. Horm Mol Biol Clin Investig. 2013;15:49–57.
3. Luis DA, Sagrado MG, Conde R, Aller R, Izaola O, Romero E. Circulating adipocytokines in obese nondiabetic patients in relationship with cardiovascular risk factors, anthropometry and resting-energy expenditure. Ann Nutr Metab. 2007;51:416–20.
4. Fain JN. Release of inflammatory mediators by human adipose tissue is enhanced in obesity and primarily by the nonfat cells: a review. Mediators Inflamm. 2010;2010:1–20.
5. Jung UJ, Seo YR, Ryu R, Choi MS. Differences in metabolic biomarkers in the blood and gene expression profiles of peripheral blood mononuclear cells among normal weight, mildly obese and moderately obese subjects. Br J Nutr. 2016;9:1–11.
6. Frasca D, Landin AM, Lechner SC. Aging down regulates the transcription factor E2A, activation-induced cytidine deaminase, and Ig class switch in human B cells. J Immunol. 2008;180:5283–90.
7. Castelo-Branco C, Soveral I. The immune system and aging: a review. Gynecol Endocrinol. 2014;30:16–22.
8. Asrih M, Jornayvaz FR. Inflammation as a potential link between nonalcoholic fatty liver disease and insulin resistance. J Endocrinol. 2013;218:25–36.
9. Wali JA, Thomas HE, Sutherland AP. Linking obesity with type 2 diabetes: the role of T-bet. Diabetes Metab Syndr Obes. 2014;7:331–40.
10. Tarantino G, Costantini S, Finelli C. Is serum Interleukin-17 associated with early atherosclerosis in obese patients? J Transl Med. 2014;12:1–10.
11. Reinert-Hartwall L, Honkanen J, Salo HM. Th1/Th17 plasticity is a marker of advanced β cell autoimmunity and impaired glucose tolerance in humans. J Immunol. 2015;194:68–75.
12. Lehrke M, Millington SC, Lefterova M. CXCL16 is a marker of inflammation, atherosclerosis, and acute coronary syndromes in humans. J Am Coll Cardiol. 2007;49:442–9.
13. Kabir SM, Lee ES, Son DS. Chemokine network during adipogenesis in 3T3-L1 cells: Differential response between growth and proinflammatory factor in preadipocytes vs. adipocytes. Adipocyte. 2014;3:97–106.
14. Huang H, Song TJ, Li X. BMP signaling pathway is required for commitment of C3H10T1/2 pluripotent stem cells to the adipocyte lineage. Proc Natl Acad Sci USA. 2009;106:12670–5.
15. Hussein KA, Choksi K, Akeel S. Bone morphogenetic protein 2: a potential new player in the pathogenesis of diabetic retinopathy. Exp Eye Res. 2014;125:79–88.
16. WHO. Obesity: preventing and managing the global epidemic. Report of a WHO consultation, Geneva, 3-5 Jun 1997. Geneva: World Health Organization; 1998. WHO/NUT/98.1.
17. Felix HC, Bradway C, Chisholm L, Pradhan R, Weech-Maldonado R. Prevalence of moderate to severe obesity among U.S. Nursing Home Residents, 2000-2010. Res Gerontol Nurs. 2015;13:1–6.
18. Kuczmarski RJ, Ogden CL, Guo SS, Grummer-Strawn LM, Flegal KM, Mei Z, et al. CDC Growth charts for the United States: methods and development. Vital Health Stat. 2000;246:1–190.
19. Coffman E, Richmond-Bryant J. Multiple biomarker models for improved risk estimation of specific cardiovascular diseases related to metabolic syndrome: a cross-sectional study. Popul Health Metr. 2015;13:7–12.
20. Feng B, Zhang T, Xu H. Human adipose dynamics and metabolic health. Ann NY Acad Sci. 2013;1281:160–77.
21. Sorensen LP, Sondergaard E, Nellemann B, Christiansen JS, Gormsen LC, Nielsen S. Increased VLDL-tryglyceride secretion preceds impaired control of endogenous glucose production in obese, normoglycemic men. Diabetes. 2011;60:2257–64.
22. Huber J, Kiefer FW, Zeyda M. CC chemokine and CC chemokine receptor profiles in visceral and subcutaneous adipose tissue are altered in human obesity. J Clin Endocrinol Metab. 2008;93:3215–21.
23. Kurki E, Shi J, Martonen E, Finckenberg P, Mervaala E. Distinct effects of calorie restriction on adipose tissue cytokine and angiogenesis profiles in obese and lean mice. Nutr Metab. 2012;9:64–72.
24. Laugsand LE, Asvould BO, Vatten LJ, Janszky I, Platou C, Michelsen AE, et al. Soluble CXCL16 and risk of myocardial infarction: The HUNT study in Norway. Atherosclerosis. 2016;244:188–94.
25. Mitsuoka H, Toyohara M, Kume N, Haysashida K, Jinnai T, Tanaka M, et al. Circulating solube SR-PSOX/CXCL16 as a biomarker for acute coronary syndrome-comparison with high-sensitivity C-reactive protein. J Atheroscler Thromb. 2009;16:586–93.
26. Ma A, Yang S, Wang Y, Wang X, Pan X. Increased of serum CXCL16 levels correlates well to microembolic signals in acute stroke patients with carotid artery stenosis. Clinica Chimica Acta. 2016;460:67–71.
27. Zhang J, Li L. BMP signaling and stem cell regulation. Dev Biol. 2005;284:1–11.
28. Chen D, Ji X, Harris MA. Differential roles for bone morphogenetic protein (BMP) receptor type IB and IA in differentiation and specification of mesenchymal precursor cells to osteoblast and adipocyte lineages. J Cell Biol. 1998;142:295–305.
29. Guiu-Jurado E, Unthan M, Böhler N, Kern M, Landgraf K, Dietrich A, et al. Bone morphogenetic protein 2 (BMP2) may contribute to partition of energy storage into visceral and subcutaneous fat deposits. Obesity (Silver Spring). 2016. 12: doi: 10.1002/oby.21571
30. Zúñiga LA, Shen WJ, Joyce-Shaikh B. IL-17 regulates adipogenesis, glucose homeostasis, and obesity. J Immunol. 2010;185:6947–59.
31. Ahmed M, Gaffen SL. IL-17 in obesity and adipogenesis. Cytokine Growth Factor Rev. 2010;21:449–53.

Nutrition, aging and cancer: lessons from dietary intervention studies

Giuseppe Carruba[1*], Letizia Cocciadiferro[2], Antonietta Di Cristina[2], Orazia M. Granata[3], Cecilia Dolcemascolo[1], Ildegarda Campisi[1], Maurizio Zarcone[1], Maria Cinquegrani[2] and Adele Traina[4]

Abstract

There is convincing epidemiological and clinical evidence that, independent of aging, lifestyle and, notably, nutrition are associated with development or progression of major human cancers, including breast, prostate, colorectal tumors, and an increasingly large collection of diet-related cancers. Mechanisms underlying this association are mostly related to the distinct epigenetic effects of different dietary patterns. In this context, Mediterranean diet has been reported to significantly reduce mortality rates for various chronic illnesses, including cardiovascular diseases, neurodegenerative diseases and cancer. Although many observational studies have supported this evidence, dietary intervention studies using a Mediterranean dietary pattern or its selected food components are still limited and affected by a rather large variability in characteristics of study subjects, type and length of intervention, selected end-points and statistical analysis. Here we review data of two of our intervention studies, the MeDiet study and the DiMeSa project, aimed at assessing the effects of traditional Mediterranean diet and/or its component(s) on a large panel of both plasma and urine biomarkers. Both published and unpublished results are presented and discussed.

Background

Cancer represents today the second leading cause of death worldwide after cardiovascular diseases, despite the fact that cancer mortality rates have been declining since 90ies because of either early diagnosis/screening programs or an increasingly larger array of therapeutic options [1].

In this context, the continuous rise in life expectancy has significantly contributed to the steady increase of cancer risk among general population [2]. However, mechanisms underlying both aging and cancer processes are still subjects of controversies more than consensuses, though cancer and aging seem to share common, rather than antagonistic, etiologies [3]. Notwithstanding, it ought to be emphasized that the onset of many chronic illnesses, including cancer, is occurring today at an average age earlier than ever, with a progressive leftward shift in the age of onset of various diseases including diabetes, cancer and obesity [4, 5]. This alarming figure would implies that, at least as far as cancer is concerned, the increasing incidence of human malignancies is not only related to the current increase in life expectancy, but other key risk factors, mostly related to lifestyle and environment, must be taken into account.

A number of both epidemiological and clinical studies strongly support the association between nutrition and development or progression of major human cancers, including breast, prostate, and colorectal tumors, but also many other tumor types have been recently included in a hypothetical list of diet-related cancers (reviewed in [6]).

There are many dietary components that have been implicated as either protective or promoting factors in cancer development. Several bioactive food components, including polyphenols, selenium, methyl-group donors, retinoids, mono- and poly-unsaturated fatty acids, isothiocyanates and allyl compounds, have all been claimed to have cancer prevention potential [7]. Although these compounds may impact upon a variety of different cellular processes, such as DNA repair, growth and differentiation, programmed cell death, oxidative stress, inflammation and so forth, in recent years the epigenome has been implicated as the primary target for nutrition-induced changes of gene expression and function [8].

* Correspondence: giuseppe.carruba@arnascivico.it
[1]Division of Research and Internationalization, ARNAS-Civico Di Cristina e Benfratelli, Palermo, Italy
Full list of author information is available at the end of the article

By definition, epigenetics comprises heritable changes in gene expression with no alteration of DNA sequence [9]. Major epigenetic mechanisms include DNA methylation, histone modification and RNA interference (RNAi) [10]. There is mounting evidence that all these epigenetic processes can be implicated and act in synergy with genetic alterations during carcinogenesis and tumor progression [11, 12]. However, contrary to genetic mutations, epigenetic abnormalities are potentially reversible and can be targeted by both cancer prevention and therapeutic strategies [13].

Convincing evidence is accumulating that many bioactive dietary components may extensively modulate epigenetic mechanisms, eventually leading to a rapid and effective regulation of gene expression and function in response to nutritional changes. In this respect, the term epigenetic diet has been introduced to indicate the consumption of foods, such as soy, grapes, cruciferous vegetables and green tea, that affect epigenetic mechanisms to protect against cancer and aging [14].

It is noteworthy that unbalanced maternal nutrient intake may severely impact on fetal epigenome early during in utero development. There is increasing evidence that nutritionally-induced epigenetic alteration of the offspring's epigenome may be responsible for higher susceptibility to cancer development later in life [15] and that several epigenetic marks can be inherited and reshape developmental and cellular features over generations, a phenomenon referred to as epigenetic inheritance [16].

Mediterranean diet & disease risk: observational and intervention studies

The term Mediterranean Diet was originally coined after Angel Keys and his colleagues ascribed the significantly lower rates of coronary heart disease observed in Mediterranean countries, including Italy and Greece, as compared to "northern" countries, such as Netherlands, Finland and USA, to various factors and, most notably, to the protective role of what they later called the "good Mediterranean diet" and its typical food components [17, 18].

Although there are various definitions of the Mediterranean Diet (MD) in literature, it is difficult to describe in details a Mediterranean dietary pattern and its components. According to Simopoulos [19], the term "Mediterranean Diet" is in fact a misnomer, simply because there are many different "Mediterranean diets", based on cultural, ethnical, religious and economical diversities among different populations and countries belonging to the Mediterranean basin. However, the distinct Mediterranean Diets generally share some major features, precisely: (a) a high consumption of whole grains (over 60 % of total caloric intake), (b) a high consumption of vegetables, fruits, and legumes; (c)

extravirgin olive oil for over 70 % of dietary fat; (d) a regular consumption of fresh fish (especially marine blue species); (e) a low intake of saturated animal fats, red and processed meat, poultry, dairy products; and (f) with the exception of muslim populations, a regular but moderate consume of red wine during main meals.

Adherence to a Mediterranean dietary pattern has generally been associated with a decreased risk of dying for most non-communicable diseases, including cardiovascular diseases, cancer, neurodegenerative diseases. Despite the difficulty to assess the extent of adherence to this dietary pattern and the limited number of studies exploring in depth the impact of Mediterranean Diet on chronic diseases and relevant pathogenetic mechanisms, both meta-analyses and systematic reviews of the existing literature have highlighted that Mediterranean Diet has a significant protective role on risk of cardiovascular and neurodegenerative disease, diabetes and cancer [20–22].

As far as dietary interventions are concerned, the protective role of Mediterranean Diet against chronic diseases has been challenged in a variety of studies.

The Lyon Diet Heart Study, a randomized secondary prevention trial aimed at testing whether a Mediterranean diet may reduce the rate of recurrence after a first myocardial infarction, indicated that the adherence to a Mediterranean dietary pattern has a significant protective role against secondary cardiac events, including death and nonfatal myocardial infarction, and that this effect is maintained up to 4 years after the first infarction, independent of major traditional risk factors, such as high blood cholesterol and blood pressure [23].

After such a pioneering observation, a number of dietary intervention studies have investigated the potential role of Mediterranean diet in the prevention of cancer, obesity, cardiovascular and neurodegenerative diseases. Serra-Majem and Estruch [24], in a systematic review of 35 experimental studies, indicated that Mediterranean diet has favorable effects on lipoprotein levels, endothelium vasodilatation, insulin resistance, metabolic syndrome, antioxidant capacity, myocardial and cardiovascular mortality, and cancer incidence in obese patients and in those with previous myocardial infarction.

In a recent systematic review of 11 randomized clinical trials for the Cochrane Collaboration, Rees and colleagues [25] concluded that, despite the limited evidence available, Mediterranean diet positively affects cardiovascular risk factors, including total cholesterol and low-density lipoprotein (LDL) cholesterol. More recently, Sleiman and associates [22] systematically reviewed 24 studies (including cross-sectional, prospective and controlled clinical trials) to show that Mediterranean diet shows favorable effects on both glycemic control and cardiovascular disease, while some degree of controversy remains on other issues, such as obesity.

In the Moli-sani study, a large prospective cohort stud, a Mediterranean-like diet was significantly associated with lower values of glucose, lipids, CRP, blood pressure and 10-year cardiovascular risk, while the consumption of healthy foods with high content in antioxidant vitamins and phytochemicals correlated with lower blood pressure and CRP plasma levels [26].

The PREDIMED study, a multicenter, randomized, primary prevention trial, showed that Mediterranean Diet, supplemented with either extravirgin olive oil or nuts, has favorable effect on blood pressure, insulin sensitivity, lipid profiles, lipoprotein particles, inflammation, oxidative stress, and carotid atherosclerosis [27].

As reviewed by Ostan and colleagues [28], there is consisting evidence that nutrition modulates multiple interconnected processes that play a major role in both carcinogenesis and inflammatory responses, including free radical production, NF-κB activation, expression of inflammatory cytokines, and the eicosanoids pathway [29]. In particular, Mediterranean Diet may positively impact on the so called "inflammaging" through either epigenetic mechanisms (that include chromatin remodeling, DNA methylation and miRNAs) or preservation of gut microbiota homeostasis.

Primary prevention of breast cancer: The MeDiet study

Breast cancer is the commonest malignancy in women and the second most common neoplasm worldwide, accounting for over 25 % of all female cancers [30]. It is worth noting that breast cancer incidence and mortality rates vary greatly across several countries, respectively ranging from 25.6 to 95.3/100.000 and from 5.2 to 19.4/100.000. This large variations may be ascribed to differences in both lifestyle and, notably, dietary habits among different geographical areas. Results from migrant studies have indicated that breast cancer incidence dramatically changes in Asians migrating to USA and in their offspring, with a steady increase from first to second and third generation [31], suggesting that international variations in breast cancer incidence represent a consequence of differences in lifestyle or environmental factors rather than genetic differences.

Estrogens are primarily implicated in both development and progression of human breast cancer, as either genotoxic or promoting agents [32–34]. However, there is little information on the impact that lifestyle, especially nutrition, produces on estrogen levels and metabolism and, hence on breast cancer risk.

Some years ago, we conducted the MeDiet study, a randomized, dietary intervention trial aiming to determine the effects of a traditional Mediterranean diet on endogenous estrogens in healthy postmenopausal women [35].

Out of 230 healthy female volunteers, 115 women were found to be eligible and were enrolled in the study based on serum testosterone levels equal or greater than 0.14 mg/ml (median value), an arbitrary cut-off value that has previously been reported to identify women at higher risk of developing breast cancer [36, 37]. After recruitment, study subjects were randomized into a dietary intervention ($n = 58$) and a control ($n = 57$) group. Women in the intervention group adopted a traditional, controlled Mediterranean diet for 6 months, while women in the control group continued to follow their regular diet. The intervention group women were instructed, through a weekly cooking course, to use and cook food components of the traditional Sicilian (Mediterranean) diet, including: whole cereals, legumes, seeds, blue fish, extravirgin olive oil, vegetables, and other Mediterranean seasonal food. Conversely, these subjects were advocated to reduce and/or avoid use of refined carbohydrates and additional animal fat, and to limit the use of salt.

Before (baseline) and after dietary intervention, women in both control and intervention groups undertook the following: (a) compiled a food frequency questionnaire originally developed for the EPIC study [38]; (b) collected both fasting blood samples and 12 h urine samples; (c) measured anthropometric indexes, including height, weight, waist-to-hip ratio.

Urine samples were of special interest since our early studies have indicated that metabolic profiles of urinary estrogens could be used to discriminate breast cancer patients in relation to their estrogen status, response to hormone treatment and prognosis [39]. Furthermore, urinary profiles of estrogens appear to be representative of intratissue estrogen content, as defined in our previous studies [40].

Profiles of endogenous estrogens in urine of both intervention and control women were assessed using a high performance liquid chromatography (HPLC) system, with both a photodiode array and an on line electrochemical detection.

At baseline, no significant difference was observed in urinary levels of individual estrogens comparing intervention and control women. It is important to note that the majority of urinary estrogens was represented by hydroxy and methoxy derivatives of both estradiol (E2) and estriol (E3), rather than by parent estrogens (E2, E3, and estrone – E1), in both control (75 %) and intervention (84 %) groups. This finding is in accordance with results of our early studies indicating that a high proportion of estrogens in urines of breast cancer patients is represented by hydroxylated metabolites of circulating (mainly E2 and E1) estrogens, referred to as "minor" or "unusual" metabolites [39]. In addition, this picture is cognate to what we have observed when measuring intratissue profiles of estrogens in both normal and malignant human mammary gland, where hydroxy and/or methoxy derivatives of either E2 or E1 represent the vast majority of tissue estrogens while parent hormones (E2, E1 and E3) account for a mere 5.2 % and 4.3 % in *nontumoral* and malignant breast, respectively [40]. More importantly, some of these compounds, notably hydroxylated metabolites and semiquinone or quinone derivatives of either E2 or E1 have been implicated as cancer-initiating or –promoting agents in breast carcinogenesis and tumor progression [32–34].

After 6 months, as expected, control women did not show any major change, whilst women in the intervention group showed a significant reduction (over 40 %, $P < 0.02$) of total estrogen levels (Fig. 1). Interestingly, this modification was in consequence of a remarkable reduction of estrogen metabolites, including hydroxy- and keto-derivatives of E2 or E3, notably 2hydroxy-E2 (2OHE2), 17EpiE3 and 16KetoE2, whose concentrations decreased by 80, 70 and 27 %, respectively (Fig. 2). At baseline, these three compounds represented the majority of urinary estrogens in both control (57 %) and intervention (68 %) women; after 6 months their levels dropped drastically in the intervention group (54 %), while remained unchanged in the control group (91 %). Conversely, E2, which represented a mere 0.2 % of total urinary estrogens, showed a limited though statistically significant increase in the intervention group (see Fig. 2), presumably because of its decreased biotransformation into 2OHE2 and 16KetoE2 that occurs in the intervention group.

Overall, this MeDiet study has provided convincing experimental evidence of two-fold value. In the first place, it has further highlighted the fact that both hydroxy and methoxy estrogen derivatives account for the vast majority of endogenous estrogens in human urine and that urinary estrogen profiles can be considered

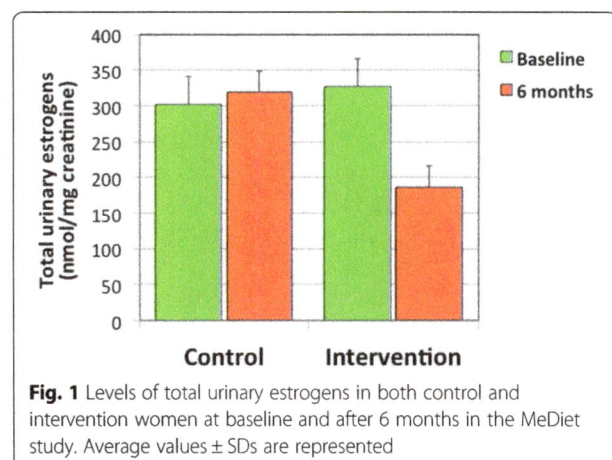

Fig. 2 Changes of estrogen concentrations in intervention women after 6 months in the MeDiet study. Data represent % of control, as compared with baseline values, ±SDs of estradiol (E2), 2hydroxy-estradiol (2OHE2), 17epi-estriol (17epiE3) and 16keto-estradiol (16ketoE2)

much closer to intratissue estrogen content than respective plasma values, where only parent estrogens (E2, E1, E3), that represent a limited fraction (5–8 %) of total endogenous estrogens, could be measured. Secondly, this study has clearly indicated that traditional Mediterranean diet may reduce the risk of developing breast cancer also through its effects on estrogen metabolism, whereby hydroxylation of E2 at C2, C16α and C16β position, a process eventually leading to the formation of genotoxic metabolites, is remarkably decreased in the intervention group but remains unchanged in the control group (Fig. 3).

Primary prevention of cancer and *noncommunicable* diseases: the DiMeSa project

Today the crisis of the agrifood sector across several geographical European areas, including our own, combined with the recent economic crisis running at regional, national and community level, is featured by extremely critical aspects, mainly residing in the limited innovation potential of companies and enterprises, the lack of integration with public-private research institutions, the insufficient systematization and organization of the existing resources in an extended territorial networking. This criticism results into increasing difficulties of small/medium enterprises (SMEs) to be present in both domestic and foreign markets with characteristics of quality and competitiveness.

On the other hand, several epidemiological studies clearly indicate that all Western regions, including our country, are facing a dramatic phenomenon consisting of real epidemics of chronic diseases (cardiovascular, cerebro-vascular, and respiratory diseases, diabetes, obesity, metabolic syndrome) and tumors, whose causes are largely attributable to (removable) lifestyle risk factors, notably diet [41]. In particular, the gradual abandonment

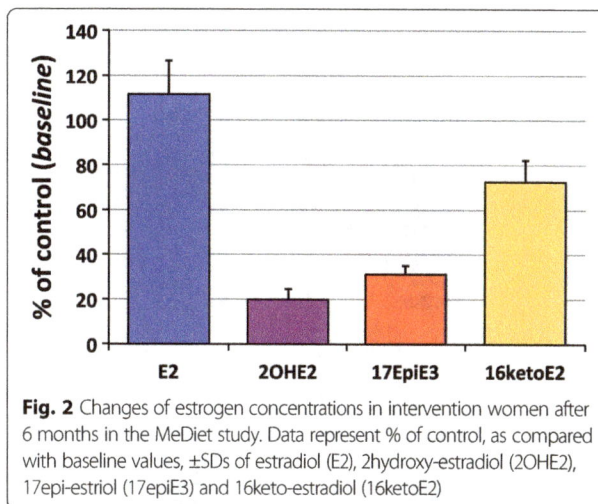

Fig. 1 Levels of total urinary estrogens in both control and intervention women at baseline and after 6 months in the MeDiet study. Average values ± SDs are represented

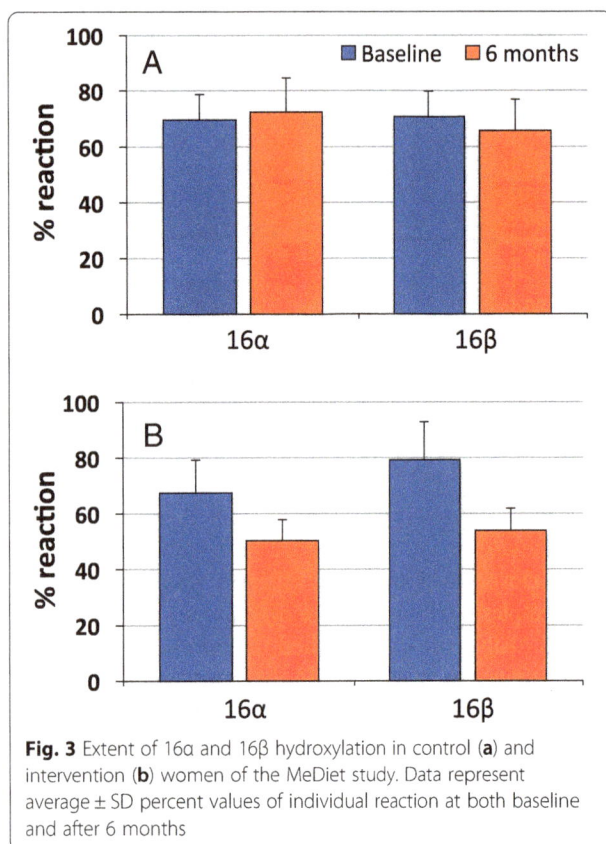

Fig. 3 Extent of 16α and 16β hydroxylation in control (**a**) and intervention (**b**) women of the MeDiet study. Data represent average ± SD percent values of individual reaction at both baseline and after 6 months

of the traditional principles and food of Mediterranean diet, that have protected for decades populations of Southern Europe, including Italy, Greece and Spain, is leading to a significant increase in incidence rates of these diseases in our region, where today, paradoxically, the highest European percentages of obese and/or overweight adolescents are being observed [42]. Since mortality from these diseases, that we might rightfully define lifestyle-based, is steadily declining since 90ies, thanks to more effective early diagnosis and to advancements in treatment options, we are witnessing an alarming "scissor" phenomenon, where a progressive increase in the number of new cases/year is accompanied by a significant reduction number of deaths, with a remarkable and continuous increase in the number of chronically ill individuals (prevalence) [41]. This phenomenon, has an economic, social and health impact of enormous importance worldwide, to the point that the World Health Organization (WHO), along with all major health institutions, have proposed primary prevention as the only effective approach to halt and eventually reverse it and launched a pluriannual (2013–2020) action plan for the prevention and control of non-communicable diseases based on a comprehensive intersectorial strategy targeting the removal of primary risk factors for these diseases,

notably western diet [43]. Based on this combined consideration, promoting both production and competitiveness of traditional food products in regional, domestic and foreign markets through a series of activities aimed at increasing their health and/or nutraceutical potential, to clinically validate their effects on both health and chronic disease(s), and to enable rapid technological transfer and industrial development of either processes or products would represent a systemic strategy of high impact in the short, medium and long term for the important expected outcome from an economic, technological and healthcare standpoint.

Armed with this conception, in October 2012 we embarked on a large regional project, funded by the Italian Ministry of University and Research (MIUR), leaded by the The AgroBioPesca Technology Cluster, called "DiMeSa - Valorization of typical products of Mediterranean Diet and their use for health and nutraceutical purposes", where DiMeSa stands for **Di**eta **ME**diterranea e **Sa**lute, simply Mediterranean Diet and Health.

This project was mainly aimed at multiplying the attractiveness and market capacities of the traditional products of Mediterranean diet in regional agriculture through the development and implementation of industrial research and experimental development activities that would eventually lead to improve their health potential and that, at the same time, would validate scientifically the relationship existing between selected Mediterranean food products and health, both in terms of maintaining a well-being state and, especially, of primary disease prevention.

The DiMeSa project is arranged into four major objectives, precisely:

1. the analysis and identification of traditional food processes and the development of innovative biotechnological protocols for the production of food with high nutritional and health potential, including extra virgin olive oil, cereals or vegetables and their derivatives;

2. the definition and implementation of procedures and methodological approaches for the production of functional foods (exra virgin olive oil, pasta, juices) through their enrichment (*functionalization*) with natural substances and/or plant/byproducts extracts having high health potential and their distribution through innovative vending machines;

3. the clinical validation of specific health claims through the conduction of randomized, controlled clinical trials to assess the health effects of selected *functional* food products on cohorts of either healthy, high-risk or diseased study-subjects through the evaluation of the impact of dietary intervention on some clinical and biomolecular end-points, such as: a) anthropometric measures; b) immunological

Table 1 The DiMeSa Project: partnerships

Public	SMEs
• University of Palermo	• CoRiSvl
- SAF	- Oleificio San Calogero
- DIFI	- Az. Agr. Angela Consiglio
- DIBIMEF	- Azienda "GeOlive" Belice
- DIMIS	- Pastificio Tomasello SpA
- STEMBIO	- Laboratorio di Ricerche
- CGA	Locorotondo
- DICGIM	• Innova Agro Sicilia
• University of Catania	- Molino di Sicilia SrL
- Dip. Scienze del Farmaco	- Agriplast SrL
- D3Di	- Medivis
• University of Messina	• Agroindustry Advanced
- Dip. Clinico-Sperimentale	Technologies (AAT)
di Medicina e Farm.	
• National Research Council (CNR)	
- IBF-Palermo	
- IBIM-Palermo	
- ISAFOM-UOS-Catania	
• Ballatore Consortium	
• CoRiSSIA	
• IZSS	

markers of inflammation; c) oxidative stress and endothelial function; d) hormonal profiles and gene expression;

4. the economic evaluation of the concept, traceability and industrial scale-up of either prototypal products or processes aiming to allow their immediate industrialization and successful marketing.

The project itself is a multicenter study, characterized by a rather large partnership, that included regional Universities and other public research institutions, on one end, and small/medium enterprises (SMEs), on the other (see Table 1). The project run for 39 months and ended just recently, by December 2015.

In this framework, we have conducted a randomized clinical trial for the assessment of the health impact of extravirgin olive oil (EVO) on 2 cohorts of study subjects represented by healthy postmenopausal women and patients with breast cancer. All study subjects were recruited at the Azienda di Rilievo Nazionale e di Alta Specializzazione (ARNAS) - Civico, Di Cristina, Benfratelli. Overall, 103 healthy postmenoausal women and 35 breast cancer patients were enrolled in the study. Two different mono-cultivar EVOs, one at lower (BL) and one at higher (CS) content of polyphenols and oleocantal, were used in the study; both EVOs were produced by the SAF (Scienze Agrarie e Forestali) Department of Palermo University, under the supervision of Prof. Tiziano Caruso. As regards healthy women, after an initial 1 week wash-out period ("no EVO" week), the subjects consumed a daily amount of 30 ml of the BL EVO for 4 weeks, followed by another 1 week wash-out period ("no EVO") and an additional 4 weeks intervention with the CS EVO, as illustrated in Fig. 4. Conversely, breast cancer patients were randomized into one BL EVO and one CS EVO intervention group that consumed daily amounts of 30 ml of either BL or CS EVO for 4 weeks (see Fig. 4). Both healthy and breast cancer study subjects, before and after any EVO intervention, undertook the following: (a) compiled a food frequency questionnaire originally developed for the EPIC study [38]; (b) measured anthropometric indexes, including height, weight, waist-to-hip ratio; (c) were administered psychometric tests (HADS, SF-36); (d)

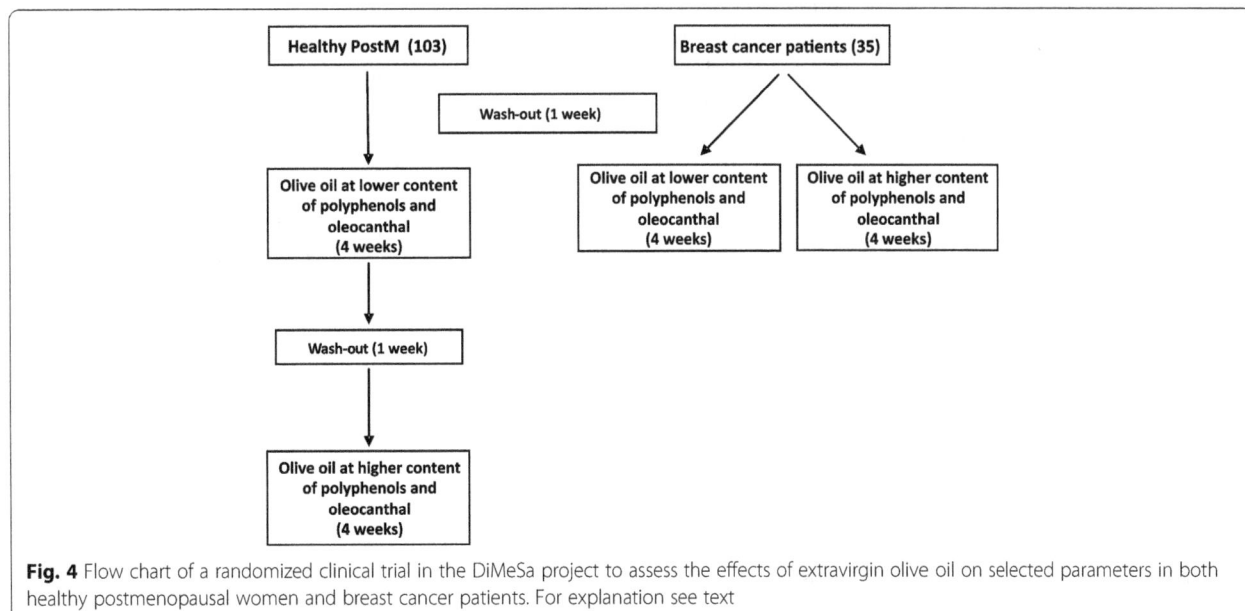

Fig. 4 Flow chart of a randomized clinical trial in the DiMeSa project to assess the effects of extravirgin olive oil on selected parameters in both healthy postmenopausal women and breast cancer patients. For explanation see text

Table 2 Effects of BL EVO on plasmatic biomarkers in both healthy postmenopausal women and breast cancer patients

Variable	Baseline	After	p-value[a]
Azotemia	30.85	28.48	0.002
Uricemia	4.17	4.29	0.001
Glycemia	85.35	83.59	0.021
Insulinemia	10.33	8.79	<0.001
Total cholesterol	207.48	197.12	<0.001
Gamma GT	21.90	24.50	0.001
Total Proteinemia	7.00	6.91	0.005
Sideremia	76.95	67.02	<0.001

[a]paired T test, ANOVA

collected both fasting blood samples and 12 h urine samples. These latter were collected to determine the potential effect of dietary intervention on an array of both plasmatic and serum biomarkers, the expression profiles of a set of previously selected genes, the whole miRNome and the urinary profile of sex steroid hormones.

Biological samples (plasma, serum, urine) were collected and stored in a biobank that, as far as the EVO clinical trial is concerned, included 5364 plasma/serum aliquots and 756 urine aliquots. A web-based study database was also created and data processed using advanced statistical analysis.

Currently, only preliminary results of the trial are available, concerning specifically a series of plasmatic biomarkers, before and after dietary intervention, in both healthy women and breast cancer patients. As reported in Table 2, consumption of BL EVO resulted in significant changes of various plasmatic biomarkers in both healthy subjects and breast cancer patients. In particular, the reduction of glycemia, insulinemia and total cholesterol levels appears of special interest. On the other hand, the consumption of CS EVO produced several modifications in selected biomarkers (see Table 3), including a significant increase of HDL cholesterol and reduction of LDL cholesterol. Interestingly, this EVO

Table 3 Effects of CS EVO on plasmatic biomarkers in both healthy postmenopausal women and breast cancer patients

Variable	Baseline	After	p-value[a]
Cretininemia	0.69	0.63	<0.001
Uricemia	4.23	4.43	0.002
Glycemia	89.16	88.48	0.023
Glycated hemoglobin	5.64	5.51	<0.001
HDL cholesterol	57.87	59.31	0.023
LDL cholesterol	119.62	102.12	0.047
Testosterone	0.39	0.36	0.033
Estradiol	31.40	23.95	0.002

[a]paired T test, ANOVA

also induced a marked decrease of plasmatic levels of estradiol. It appears noteworthy that, when comparing the two EVOs, BL EVO appeared to be more effective in reducing glycemia, while CS EVO proved to be more effective in decreasing plasmatic estradiol (see Table 4). This would imply that different EVOs may have a distinct impact on either glycemic control or hormonal (sex steroid) status, also depending on the cultivar and on the phenology of fruit ripening (the ealier the stage, the greater the content of polyphenols).

Results of gene expression, microRNA profiling and patterns of urinary sex steroids are currently under statistical analysis and are awaited with great expectation and interest.

Conclusions and perspectives

Doubtlessly, environment and lifestyle play a major role in human health and aging. An amazing array of environmental factors and nutrition may have in fact a major impact upon cellular and molecular processes, challenging severely cell adaptation capacities and the maintenance of tissue homeostasis. In this scenario, various aspects related to diet may be of crucial importance, including caloric intake, meal timing, balance of macro- and micro-nutrients, microbiome regulation [44]. Recently, WHO Europe launched a campaign for health promotion through a life-course approach, with the motto "Act Early, Act on Time, Act Together". This approach encompasses virtually all key health issues and relevant determinants throughout the entire life cycle, including pre- and perinatal life, adulthood and aging, as depicted in Fig. 5.

Data from our dietary intervention studies have underlined some interesting aspects related to both mechanisms underpinning biological and clinical effects of nutrition, on one hand, and specific activities of Mediterranean food components, on the other. In particular, the MeDiet study has provided evidence that Mediterranean diet may regulate estrogen metabolism in postmenopausal women in a way that the formation of potentially harmful genotoxic compounds is remarkably reduced, while levels of parent hormone estradiol are slightly increased; this would imply that traditional Mediterranean food reduces the risk of developing breast cancer while limiting the side-effects of estrogen withdrawal in menopause.

Table 4 Comparison of the effects of BL and CS EVO on glycemia and estradiol levels in both healthy postmenopausal women and breast cancer patients

Variable	BL EVO	CS EVO	p-value[a]
Glycemia	83.59	88.48	0.023
Estradiol	37.21	23.95	0.027

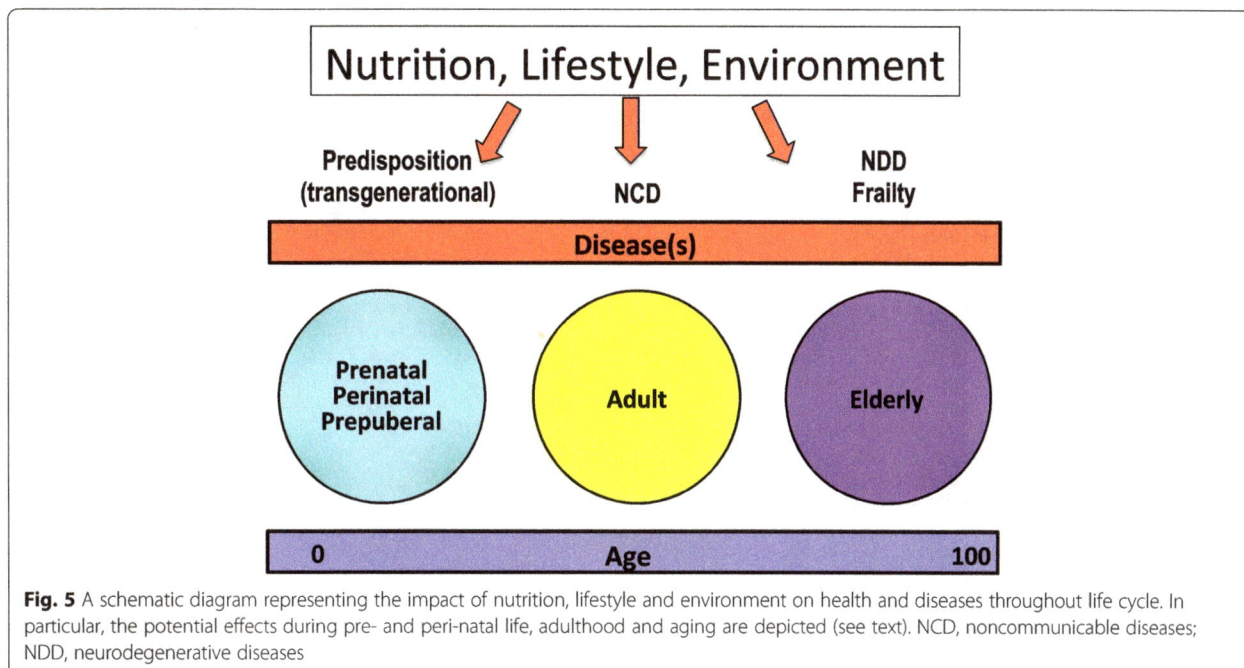

Fig. 5 A schematic diagram representing the impact of nutrition, lifestyle and environment on health and diseases throughout life cycle. In particular, the potential effects during pre- and peri-natal life, adulthood and aging are depicted (see text). NCD, noncommunicable diseases; NDD, neurodegenerative diseases

On the other hand, the DiMeSa project has indicated that technological innovation and prototypical industrialization of either processes or products could be used to obtain traditional Mediterranean food having high health potential and market capacities. Precisely, the production of mono-cultivar extravirgin olive oils (EVOs) has revealed that selected EVO(s) may have a differential activity on different cellular and metabolic processes, eventually leading to produce highly characterized EVOs with a preferential use for the prevention and care of distinct chronic diseases.

Nevertheless, further large, multicentric and long-term, prospective intervention studies are yet necessary to dissect the real effects of a strictly defined Mediterranean dietary pattern on both individual risk of noncommunicable diseases and the underpinning action mechanisms.

Competing interests
The authors declare that they have no competing interests.

Authors' contributions
GC designed both studies, supervised all clinical and experimental activities and drafted the manuscript; LC, ADC, OMG and MC did most of laboratory work; IC and AT presided over subjects' recruitment and dietary intervention; CD was responsible for psychometric testing; MZ was responsible for databasing and performed. All authors read and approved the final manuscript.

Acknowledgements
The MeDiet study was supported by a generous grant from both City and Province of Palermo. The DiMeSa project has been financed by a grant (PON02 00667 – PON02 00451 3361785) of the Italian Ministry of University and Research (MIUR) to the The AgroBioPesca Technology Cluster.
The authors are grateful to Ing. Antonio Giallanza, Project Manager, for his valued professional work. We also wish to thank Prof. Tiziano Caruso, for his precious collaborative efforts in preparation of monocultivar EVOs. Last not least, we are grateful to Dr. Nicola Locorotondo for his continuous enthusiastic support.

Author details
[1]Division of Research and Internationalization, ARNAS-Civico Di Cristina e Benfratelli, Palermo, Italy. [2]Research Laboratories Dr. Nicola Locorotondo, Palermo, Italy. [3]Clinical Pathology, "G. DI Cristina" Pediatric Hospital ARNAS-Civico Di Cristina e Benfratelli, Palermo, Italy. [4]The Diana Project, National Cancer Institute, Milan, Italy.

References
1. Stewart BW, Wild CP, editors. World cancer report 2014. Lyon: International Agency for Research on Cancer; 2014.
2. Niccoli T, Partridge L. Ageing as a risk factor for disease. Curr Biol. 2012;22: R741–752.
3. Finkel T, Serrano M, Blasco MA. The common biology of cancer and ageing. Nature. 2007;448:767–74.
4. Kurtz Z, Peckham CS, Ades AE. Changing prevalence of juvenile-onset diabetes mellitus. Lancet. 1988;2:88–90.
5. Gale EAM. The rise of childhood type 1 diabetes in the 20th century. Diabetes. 2002;51:3353–61.
6. World Cancer Research Fund/American Institute for Cancer Research. Food, nutrition, physical activity, and the prevention of cancer: a global perspective. Washington: American Institute for Cancer Research; 2007.
7. Milner JA. Molecular targets for bioactive food components. J Nutr. 2004; 134:2492S–8S.
8. Daniel M, Tollefsbol TO. Epigenetic linkage of aging, cancer and nutrition. J Exp Biol. 2015;218:59–70.
9. Waddington CH. The epigenotype. Int J Epidemiol. 2012;41:10–3.
10. Herceg Z. Epigenetics and cancer: towards an evaluation of the impact of environmental and dietary factors. Mutagenesis. 2007;22:91–103.
11. Ballestar E, Esteller M. Epigenetic gene regulation in cancer. Adv Genet. 2008;61:247–67.
12. Kanwal R, Gupta S. Epigenetic modifications in cancer. Clin Genet. 2012;81:303–11.
13. Ong TP, Moreno FS, Ross SA. Targeting the epigenome with bioactive food components for cancer prevention. J Nutrigenet Nutrigenomics. 2011;4:275–92.
14. Hardy TM, Tollefsbol TO. Epigenetic diet: impact on the epigenome and cancer. Epigenomics. 2011;3:503–18.
15. Thornburg KL, Shannon J, Thuillier P, Turker MS. In utero life and epigenetic predisposition for disease. Adv Genet. 2010;71:57–78.

16. Bohacek J, Mansuy IM. Epigenetic inheritance of disease and disease risk. Neuropsychopharm Rev. 2013;38:220–36.

17. Keys A, Menotti A, Karvonen MJ, Aravanis C, Blackburn H, Buzina R, Djordjevic BS, Dontas AS, Fidanza F, Keys MH, et al. The diet and 15-year death rate in the seven countries study. Am J Epidemiol. 1986;124:903–15.

18. Keys A. Mediterranean diet and public health: personal reflections. Am J Clin Nutr. 1995;61:1321S–3S.

19. Simopoulos AP. The Mediterranean diets: what is so special about the diet of Greece? The scientific evidence. J Nutr. 2001;131:3065S–73S.

20. Schwingshackl L, Hoffmann G. Adherence to Mediterranean diet and risk of cancer: a systematic review and meta-analysis of observational studies. Int J Cancer. 2014;135:1884–97.

21. Sofi F, Macchi C, Abbate R, Gensini GF, Casini A. Mediterranean diet and health status: an updated meta-analysis and a proposal for a literature-based adherence score. Public Health Nutr. 2014;17:2769–82.

22. Sleiman D, Al-Badri MR, Azar ST. Effect of Mediterranean diet in diabetes control and cardiovascular risk modification: a systematic review. Front Public Health. 2015;3:69. doi:10.3389/fpubh.2015.00069.

23. de Lorgeril M, Salen P, Martin J-L, Monjaud I, Delaye J, Mamelle N. Mediterranean diet, traditional risk factors, and the rate of cardiovascular complications after myocardial infarction. Final report of the Lyon diet heart study. Circulation. 1999;99:779–85.

24. Serra-Majem L, Roman B, Estruch R. Scientific evidence of interventions using the Mediterranean diet: a systematic review. Nutr Rev. 2006;64:S27–47.

25. Rees K, Hartley L, Hartley N, Clarke A, Hooper L, Thorogood M, Stranges S. 'Mediterranean' dietary pattern for the primary prevention of cardiovascular disease. Cochrane Database Syst Rev. 2013;8:CD009825. doi:10.1002/14651858.CD009825.pub2.

26. Bonaccio M, Cerletti C, Iacoviello L, de Gaetano G. Mediterranean diet and low-grade subclinical inflammation: the moli-sani study. Endocr Metab Immune Disord Drug Targets. 2015;15:18–24.

27. Martínez-González MA, Salas-Salvadó J, Estruch R, Corella D, Fitó M, Ros E, and PREDIMED INVESTIGATOR. Benefits of the Mediterranean diet: insights from the PREDIMED study. Prog Cardiovasc Dis. 2015;58:50–60.

28. Ostan R, Lanzarini C, Pini E, Scurti M, Vianello D, Bertarelli C, Fabbri C, Izzi M, Palmas G, Biondi F, Martucci M, Bellavista E, Salvioli S, Capri M, Franceschi C and Santoro A. Inflammaging and cancer: a challenge for the Mediterranean diet. Nutrients. 2015;7:2589–621.

29. Di Renzo L, Marsella LT, Carraro A, Valente R, Gualtieri P, Gratteri S, Tomasi D, Gaiotti F and De Lorenzo A. Changes in LDL oxidative status and oxidative and inflammatory gene expression after red wine intake in healthy people: a randomized trial. Mediators Inflamm. 2015;2015:317348. doi:10.1155/2015/317348.

30. International Agency for Research on Cancer. World cancer factsheet. World cancer burden 2012. Cancer Research UK 2014

31. Ziegler RG, Hoover RN, Pike MC, Hildesheim A, Nomura AM, et al. Migration patterns and breast cancer risk in Asian-American women. J Natl Cancer Inst. 1993;85:1819–27.

32. Liehr JG. Genotoxicity of the steroidal oestrogens oestrone and oestradiol: possible mechanism of uterine and mammary cancer development. Hum Reprod Update. 2001;7:273–81.

33. Cavalieri E, Rogan E. The molecular etiology and prevention of estrogen-initiated cancers. Mol Aspects Med. 2014;0:1–55. doi:10.1016/j.mam.2013.08.002.

34. Yager JD. Mechanisms of estrogen carcinogenesis: the role of E2/E1-quinone metabolites suggests new approaches to preventive intervention - a review. Steroids. 2015;99:56–60.

35. Carruba G, Granata OM, Pala V, Campisi I, Agostara B, Cusimano R, Ravazzolo B, Traina A. A traditional Mediterranean diet decreases endogenous estrogens in healthy postmenopausal women. Nutr Cancer. 2006;56:253–9.

36. Berrino F, Muti P, Micheli A, Bolelli G, Krogh V, et al. Serum sex hormone levels after menopause and subsequent breast cancer. J Natl Cancer Inst. 1996;88:291–6.

37. Dorgan JF, Stanczyk FZ, Kahle LL, Brinton LA. Prospective case–control study of premenopausal serum estradiol and testosterone levels and breast cancer risk. Breast Cancer Res. 2010;12:R98. http://breast-cancer-research.com/content/12/6/R98.

38. Pisani P, Faggiano F, Krogh V, Palli D, Vineis P, Berrino F. Relative validity and reproducibility of a food frequency dietary questionnaire for use in the Italian EPIC centres. Int J Epidemiol. 1997;26:S152–60.

39. Castagnetta L, D'Agostino C, Lo Casto M, Traina A, Leake RE. Breast cancer: a comparison of response to endocrine therapy and oestrogen excretion patterns including unusual metabolites. Br J Cancer. 1981;44:670–4.

40. Castagnetta LA, Granata OM, Traina A, Ravazzolo B, Amoroso M, et al. Tissue content of hydroxyestrogens in relation to survival of breast cancer patients. Clin Cancer Res. 2002;8:3146–55.

41. Hunter DJ, Reddy KS. Noncommunicable diseases. N Engl J Med. 2013;369:1336–43. doi:10.1056/NEJMra1109345.

42. Wijnhoven TMA, van Raaij JMA, Spinelli A, Starc G, Hassapidou M, Spiroski I, Rutter H, Martos E, Rito AI, Hovenger R, Pérez-Farinós N, Petrauskiene A, Eldin N, Braeckevelt L, Pudule I, Kunešová M and Breda J. WHO european childhood obesity surveillance initiative: body mass index and level of overweight among 6–9-year-old children from school year 2007/2008 to school year 2009/2010. BMC Public Health. 2014;14:806. http://www.biomedcentral.com/1471-2458/14/806.

43. World Health Organization. Global action plan for the prevention and control of noncommunicable diseases 2013–2020. WHO Press. Geneva: World Health Organization; 2013.

44. Fontana L, Partridge L. Promoting health and longevity through diet: from model organisms to humans. Cell. 2015;161:106–18. doi:10.1016/j.cell.2015.02.020.

The inflammatory protein Pentraxin 3 in cardiovascular disease

Francesco Fornai[1,2], Albino Carrizzo[2], Maurizio Forte[2], Mariateresa Ambrosio[2], Antonio Damato[2], Michela Ferrucci[1], Francesca Biagioni[2], Carla Busceti[2], Annibale A. Puca[3,4] and Carmine Vecchione[2,4*]

Abstract

The acute phase protein Pentraxin 3 (PTX3) plays a non-redundant role as a soluble pattern recognition receptor for selected pathogens and it represents a rapid biomarker for primary local activation of innate immunity and inflammation. Recent evidence indicates that PTX3 exerts an important role in modulating the cardiovascular system in humans and experimental models. In particular, there are conflicting points concerning the effects of PTX3 in cardiovascular diseases (CVD) since several observations indicate a cardiovascular protective effect of PTX3 while others speculate that the increased plasma levels of PTX3 in subjects with CVD correlate with disease severity and with poor prognosis in elderly patients.

In the present review, we discuss the multifaceted effects of PTX3 on the cardiovascular system focusing on its involvement in atherosclerosis, endothelial function, hypertension, myocardial infarction and angiogenesis. This may help to explain how the specific modulation of PTX3 such as the use of different dosing, time, and target organs could help to contain different vascular diseases. These opposite actions of PTX3 will be emphasized concerning the modulation of cardiovascular system where potential therapeutic implications of PTX3 in humans are discussed.

Keywords: Pentraxin 3, Acute phase protein of inflammation, Cardiovascular diseases, Myocardial infarction, Atherosclerosis, Angiogenesis

Abbreviations: AMI, Acute myocardial infarction; ApoE, Apolipoprotein E; CRP, C-reactive protein; CVD, Cardiovascular diseases; ECM, Extracellular matrix deposition; FGF2, Fibroblast growth factor 2; HF, Heart failure; IKK, IkB kinase; IL-6, Interleukin-6; LPS, Lipopolysaccharides; MI, Myocardial infarction; MMP, Matrix metalloprotease; NF-kB, Nuclear factor kappa-light-chain-enhancer of activated B cells; PTX3, Pentraxin 3; SAP, Serum amyloid protein; VEGFR2, Vascular endothelial growth factor receptor 2

Background

PTX3 belongs to a superfamily of phylogenically conserved multimeric proteins, which includes short and long pentraxins [1, 2]. All these proteins play a critical role in innate immunity and they are generally considered acute phase immunity proteins [2, 3]. However, their effects which are grounded on the modulation of the cardiovascular system influence a variety of phenomena such as inflammation, angiogenesis, tumorigenesis, cell adhesion [4, 5]. Short and long pentraxins possess a different protein size and they are synthesized by different genes under the influence of different gene promoters. In fact, short and long pentraxins are produced by different cell types in response to different stimuli and possess different molecular targets (Fig. 1). Among short pentraxins C-reactive protein (CRP) is well known. This protein is produced by hepatocytes and other cell types during inflammation. Release of CRP is induced by pro-inflammatory cytokines (mainly interleukin-6, IL-6). Similarly, a short pentraxin is the serum amyloid P-component (SAP), which is solely synthesized by hepatocytes [6].

In contrast, PTX3 belongs to long pentraxins and, as mentioned above, it possesses multifaceted properties extending beyond the fields of immunity and inflammation to CVD [7, 8].

---
* Correspondence: cvecchione@unisa.it
[2]I.R.C.C.S. Neuromed, Pozzilli, IS, Italy
[4]Department of Medicine and Surgery, University of Salerno, Via S. Allende, Baronissi, SA 84081, Italy
Full list of author information is available at the end of the article

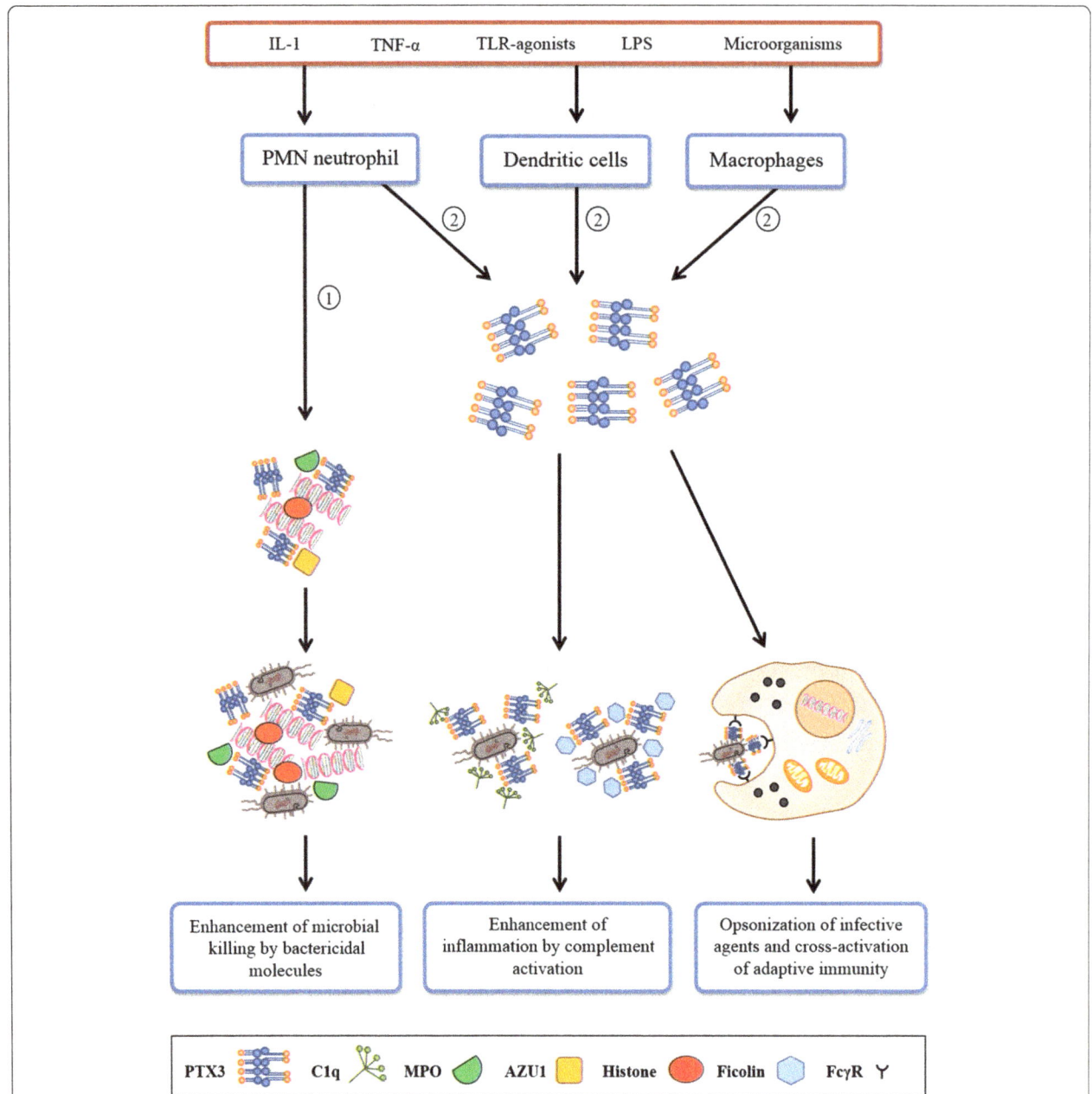

Fig. 1 Activity of PTX3 in innate immunity. PTX3 represents the humoral arm of the innate immunity. Inflammatory cytokines, Toll-like receptors (TLRs), microorganisms and microbial moieties stimulate secretion of PTX3 by polymorphonuclear (PMN) neutrophils, macrophages, and dendritic cells. (**1**) Release of PTX3 by PMN neutrophils occurs quickly and casts an immediate defensive response. In fact, these cells possesscytosolic granules containing a stored, ready- to-release, pool of PTX3. (**2**) Macrophages and dendritic cells are other effectors of the innate immunity, which neo-synthesize PTX3 upon stimulation. This newly synthesized pool of PTX3cells is responsible for a slower response to infective agents, which might persist even several days. Released PTX3 regulates inflammatory reactions by acting through several pathways/mechanisms: I) PTX3 released by PMN neutrophils localizesat level of neutrophil extracellular traps (NETs). NETs represent an extracellular fibrillary network, where some nuclear components, such as DNA and histones, are variously assembled with bactericidal proteins, such as azurocidin1(AZU1) andmyeloperoxidase(MPO). Within NETs, PTX3 and anti-microbial molecules converge and cooperate to enhance binding and killing of infective agents. II) PTX3 released in the extracellular space binds to specific microbial ligands and activates the complement cascade through interaction with C1q particles (classical pathway) or ficolins and mannose-binding lectins (lectin-mediated pathway). PTX3-induced complement activation enhances the inflammatory response. III) Finally, extracellular PTX3 opsonizes microorganisms binding to specific molecules on the cell surface (i.e. zymosan on *Aspergillusfumigatus*) and, in turn, it is recognized by Fcgamma receptors expressed by phagocytic cells, thus promoting microbial clearance. The interaction of PTX3with Fcgamma receptors indicates the antibody-like function of PTX3 and underlies its functional overlapping between innate and adaptive immunity during inflammation. (*FcγR* Fcgamma receptor, *IL-1* interleukin-1, *LPS* lipopolysaccaride, *PTX3* pentraxin 3, *TNF-alpha* tumor necrosis factor-alpha)

Interestingly, its multiple roles can be considered as site-specific since its production occurs in a variety of cell types, including endothelial cells, fibroblasts, hepatocytes, and monocytes. Moreover, during an acute phase response induced by LPS, PTX3 is expressed in a variety of organs, most prominently in the heart and skeletal muscle, unlike SAP, which is produced only in the liver [9]. Thus, this specific production pattern of PTX3, explains its involvement in multiple cardiovascular disorders.

The present review focuses on findings in humans and it discusses the molecular mechanisms encompassing experimental models and human beings.

PTX3 in cardiovascular diseases

Cardiovascular diseases (CVD) represent the major cause of death in the developed world [10]. In addition to well established risk factors such as diabetes, hypertension, dyslipidemia, recent evidence indicates that as it occurs for molecules belonging to the acute phase of inflammation, PTX3 may play a key role in the onset and progression of CVD [11–13].

Thus, PTX3 represents a specific and sensitive marker connecting inflammation with CVD since it is expressed and released by most cell compartments involved in the onset and progression of CVD.

PTX3 is involved in a variety of molecular mechanisms leading to vascular damage and its elevated plasma levels represent a significant predictor of frailty in elderly hypertensive patients [14]. In fact, blood vessels produce large amounts of PTX3 during inflammation, and the level of circulating PTX3 increases in several pathological conditions affecting the cardiovascular system [15, 16].

Here, we highlight the bad or good associations between PTX3 and CVD in humans. In addition, in experimental models we reported the mechanisms by which this inflammatory protein may exert itson the cardiovascular actions.

Atherosclerosis

Although cholesterol accumulation intimal layer is the major pathological feature of atherogenesis, growing evidence suggests that the inflammatory state represents the major detrimental factor for the progression of atherosclerosis both in young and in elderly subjects. In fact, the earliest stage of atherosclerotic damage is characterized by infiltration of macrophages and T-lymphocytes, which are progressively activated during the course of the damage [17, 18]. Based on the kind of cell phenotype being recruited (macrophages and vascular cells), which is known to produce PTX3, this protein was investigated as a potential modulator of atherosclerosis.

In fact, human sclerotic mammary arteries possess high levels of PTX3, which is mainly localized within endothelial cells and macrophages [19, 20]. In addition, smooth muscle cells, treated with inflammatory stimuli such as oxidized lipoproteins, increase their PTX3 mRNA level. This effect leads to a vascular acute-phase-response activating the classic pathway of complement [21], which represents one of the most important mechanisms leading to chemo tactic and pro-inflammatory effects. The link between PTX3 and complement system was confirmed by the occurrence of high PTX3 level within atherosclerosis-related coronary arterial thrombi that are mainly constituted by resident macrophages, neutrophils and foam cells [22].

Recently, epidemiological and clinical data candidate PTX3 as a valid biomarker for atherosclerosis [19, 22]. In particular, PTX3 plays a role in the regulation of innate resistance to inflammatory reactions, it is strongly expressed in atherosclerotic arteries [23] and its high plasma levels were found to be related with severity of coronary atherosclerosis [24]. Accordingly, PTX3 levels are significantly increased in patients with carotid stenosis [25], as well as in patients with acute coronary syndrome [26], in whom PTX3 is a candidate biomarker for plaque vulnerability [27]. Finally, PTX3 has been indicated also as a marker of neo-intimal thickening after vascular injury, since elevated levels of PTX3 have been found in patients with atherosclerosis, after 15 min from coronary stenting [28].

Although the presence of PTX3 in human atherosclerotic damage is well defined, its causal role in the onset and progression of atherosclerosis, remains unclear. Here, data obtained in experimental models are reviewed aimed at suggesting the mechanistic role of PTX3 in atherogenesis.

In particular, it has been reported that PTX3, by interacting with P-selectin, a cell-adhesion molecule involved in the tethering and rolling of leukocytes and platelets on activated endothelial cells, attenuates leukocytes recruitment at the site of inflammation [29]. These data clearly indicate a protective role of PTX3 in atherosclerosis. In keeping with this, in a double knockout mouse model for PTX3 and apolipoprotein E (ApoE), macrophages infiltration was enhanced, and a dramatic increase of atherosclerosis was reported. The molecular analysis indicates a dramatic rise in the pattern of inflammatory genes within vascular wall concomitant with up-regulation of pro-inflammatory mediators such as chemokines, cytokines, adhesion molecules, E-selectin and transcription factors, such as NF-kB [30].

In contrast, PTX3 was also reported to induce deleterious effects in the pathogenesis of atherothrombosis [31]. On this regard, it has been demonstrated that PTX3 increases the tissue factor (TF) expression in mononuclear and endothelial cells. The increased level of TF, the main orchestrator of the coagulation cascade, causes the thrombus formation, a feature of atherosclerosis [32]. PTX3 might also interfere with plaque stability by binding the fibroblast growth factor 2 (FGF2), that play a role in proliferation and migration of smooth muscle cells [33]. This evidence suggests a bad cop for PTX3, which promotes lesion progression through a stronger innate immune response. Recently, PTX3 has been proposed as a potential therapeutic target to limit the development of atherosclerosis. In fact, by using a cell model of atherosclerosis, it was shown that suppression of PTX3 reduces inflammation and apoptosis mediated by the IkB kinase (IKK)/IkB/nuclear factor-kB (NF-kB) pathway [34].

Actually, the role of PTX3 in the atherosclerosis is not well-understood. It will be interesting to examine the role of the protein in complement activation during atherogenesis to define the specific role of PTX3 in the atherosclerosis. Overall, PTX3 seems to exert detrimental effects on atherosclerotic process since it promotes plagues formation and leads to an amplification of vascular inflammation such as to be candidate it as a new possible biomarker for plaque vulnerability. However, only in those conditions in which it is able to reduce macrophages infiltration and the expression of adhesion molecules it exerts beneficial effects.

Endothelial dysfunction and hypertension

Endothelial dysfunction is a typical trait of several cardiovascular disorders including arterial hypertension. The impairment of the nitric oxide pathway and the enhanced smooth muscle vasoconstriction represent the main mechanisms leading to endothelial dysfunction in hypertension [35, 36].

A growing body of evidence attributes to local and systemic inflammation a key role in the development of endothelial dysfunction, thus suggesting a key role for acute phase proteins [37, 38].

On this regard, high plasma levels of the inflammatory molecule PTX3 were associated with endothelial dysfunction in different human diseases. Patients with chronic kidney diseases and with preeclampsia, a multi-systemic disorder associated with hypertension [39–41], show elevated PTX3 plasma levels which were correlated with the severity of endothelial dysfunction [39, 40, 42].

In addition, elevated plasma level of PTX3 have been found in patients with high systolic and diastolic blood pressure levels [16, 43] and in elderly hypertensive patients with high 24-h blood pressure levels [14]. In pulmonary arterial hypertension, PTX3 has been proposed as a more specific and sensitive biomarker compared with brain natriuretic peptide, which so far, was considered the gold standard marker for pulmonary hypertension [44, 45].

The evidence described so far in humans suggests a potential role of PTX3 in regulating vascular homeostasis. In experimental models, the absence of PTX3 is accompanied by massive suppression of tissue inflammation, cell injury and it determines decreased lethality after reperfusion of an ischemic superior mesenteric artery in mice, thus demonstrating that PTX3 is relevant in conditioning tissue damage [46]. In a recent study by Carrizzo et al. we investigated the molecular mechanisms recruited by PTX3 to induce damage of mesenteric artery. In particular, exogenous administration of PTX3 in mice impaired endothelial function in resistance vessels through a P-selectin/matrix metalloprotease1 pathway, thus producing morphological alterations of endothelial cells and disruption of nitric oxide signalling. These effects were associated with an increase in blood pressure in vivo. It is worth to be mentioned that PTX3, and its mediators of vascular damage are present at higher levels within plasma of hypertensive patients compared with normotensive subjects [47]. Based on these data, PTX3 could be considered as a novel biomarker for hypertension and a new target for future therapeutic strategy aimed to contain endothelial dysfunction and associated CVD.

Myocardial infarction

Myocardial infarction (MI) continues to be a significant cause of mortality and morbidity worldwide [48]. Over the past 50 years, it has become clear that the cascade of thrombotic events following atherosclerotic plaque rupture causes occlusion of the coronary artery, interrupting blood supply and oxygen supply to myocardium, thus producing infarction. The significance of occurrence of PTX3 expression in the heart from normal and hypertrophy human cardiac cells still needs to be clarified for its physiological pathological role [49, 50].

In older adults it was reported an association between PTX3 plasma levels, CVD and all causes of death, independently from CVD risk factors [25]. In particular, plasma level of PTX3 increases in patients with acute myocardial infarction (AMI) after about 7 h from the onset of symptoms, with a decrease at baseline levels after three days [50, 51]. Based on these data, PTX3 seems to be at the same time an early indicator of AMI, and also a prognostic marker for the outcomes of heart diseases. PTX3 level also predicts cardiac events in patients with heart failure (HF), suggesting a stratification of HF patients based on PTX3 plasma level [52]. This is fully supported by the identification of coronary circulation as the main source of PTX3 in HF patients with normal ejection fraction [53]. Moreover, in patients with MI, ST tract elevation and with chronic HF, PTX3, but not other cardiac biomarkers, modulating complement components, predicted 3 months mortality, after adjustment for major risk factors [12, 28, 54].

Recently, PTX3 was suggested to be a prognostic marker also in patients with coronary artery diseases after drug stent implantation, and in patients with angina pectoris [55–57], in whom adverse cardiac events were related with PTX3 plasma levels [58].

These studies in humans, do not allow to establish the specific action of PTX3 in the myocardium. Thus, to better characterize the cardiac action of PTX3, here we report data obtained in transgenic ptx3 deficient mice. After cardiac ischemia- reperfusion injury, ptx3 deficient mice develop increased myocardial damage, characterized by no-reflow area, increased neutrophil infiltration apoptotic cells and decreased number of capillaries. In addition, in the myocardium of these mice the C3 complement component increased focally being related with the area of damaged myocardium. The evidence that in PTX3-KO mice the administration of exogenous PTX3 reduces complement C3 deposition rescuing the phenotype, highlights the cardio-protective effect of PTX3, through the modulation of the complement cascade [59].

The discovery of PTX3 in the myocardial tissue and the characterization of its role lead to propose PTX3 as an early indicator of myocyte irreversible injury in ischemic cardiomyopathy. In addition, considering the local production and the rapid change in plasma concentration, PTX3 could be considered a novel potential biomarker of myocardial infarction.

Angiogenesis

Additional activities of PTX3 other than those related to innate immunity and inflammation have been described, such as extracellular matrix deposition (ECM), tissue remodeling, and angiogenesis. Several studies demonstrate that PTX3 is required for the secretion of extracellular matrix. This is critical for a number of functions such as maturation of the oophorus follicle, which explains why in PTX3-deficient mice sterility is observed. This condition seems to be related to a defective PTX3-dependent incorporation of the glycosaminoglycan hyaluronic acid into the matrix of the cumulus oophorus [60]. A similar molecular composition of the ECM, containing hyaluronan (HA), tumor necrosis factor-stimulated gene-6 (TSG-6), and inter-α-inhibitor (IαI), is observed in rheumatoid arthritis and other inflammatory infiltrates, suggesting a role of PTX3 also in these conditions [61].

Interestingly, PTX3 regulates angiogenesis via FGF2, thus interfering with a variety of conditions, including ontogenesis, growth, inflammation, tissue repair, atherosclerosis, and tumors [62]. The PTX3/FGF2 interaction prevents angiogenesis. Beyond the anti-angiogenetic

activity, the inhibitory effects of PTX3 on FGF2 possess a therapeutic rationale in the treatment of re-stenosis, the progressive occlusion of the coronary artery which occurs often following angioplastic surgery, due to anomalous FGF2-dependent proliferation and accumulation of smooth muscle cells on the vessel wall [63]. On the other hand, angiogenesis involves remodeling of ECM. In this respect, FGF2 modulates degradation of the ECM by inducing expression of urokinase-type plasminogen activator (uPA) and plasminogen activator inhibitor (PAI)-1 on endothelial cell surface, with opposite effects on matrix metalloprotease (MMP) activity. Moreover, FGF2 regulates expression and distribution of several integrins and cadherins on the plasma membrane of endothelial cells, thus promoting cell scattering or adhesion in different stages of angiogenesis [64]. Finally, in PTX3 deficient mice models a dramatic reduction of vascular endothelial growth factor receptor 2 (VEG-FR2)occurs. This contributes to worsening the outcome of cerebral ischemia associated with a reduction of vessels formation [65].

Retinal vasculature

Recently, some studies have investigated on the role of the PTX3 on the modulation of retinal vasculature [66]. In particular, Moon Woo and colleagues have demonstrated that human retinal pigment epithelial cells are the major source of PTX3 following pro-inflammatory cytokines stimulation and that its release exerts an important role in retinal injury against inflammation and infection. Diabetic Retinopathy (DR) represents the well-known microvascular complication of diabetes [67]. A recent study has demonstrated that PTX3 levels were significantly elevated in diabetic patients with DR compared to diabetic patients without DR and normal subjects. This association is correlated with an important retinal microvascular dysfunction, characterized by capillary leakage or closure, leading to ischemia [67, 68]. This study suggests that plasma PTX3 may be a better predictor for DR than CRP in diabetic patients. Moreover, Noma et al. have highlighted the relationship between PTX3 and retinal diseases such as age-related macular degeneration (AMD) and retinal vascular occlusion [69]. On this regards, it has been reported an interaction between PTX3 and the complement regulator factor H (CFH), a soluble molecule of the alternative pathway of the complement system involved in AMD pathogenesis. The authors hypothesize that aberrant expression of PTX3 could be associated with pathophysiology of AMD [69] because there is a loss of control of CFH activity. PTX3 has been evaluated also in the retinal vein occlusion (RVO), the second most common retinal vascular disease after diabetic retinopathy. This study demonstrate that PTX3 could be used as a useful diagnostic biomarker since patients with RVO have high plasma level of PTX3 [70]. Finally, during 2016 Zhou and Hu suggest that the use of PTX3 could be used as an anti-angiogenic molecule because PTX3 interacts specifically with FGF2 factor reducing the proliferative diabetic retinopathy thus ameliorating DR condition [68]. Although there are not specific evaluation of molecular signaling recruited by PTX3 in retinal vasculature, it could be represent another important field in which is possible to act modulating PTX3 to obtain favorable vascular results.

Genetics and epigenetics

Epigenetic modulation of PTX3 gene in cardiovascular diseases is increasingly emerging. A candidate modulator of PTX3 is TNFα. In fact, TNFα controls the expression of PTX3 by human adipose tissue, being potentially implicated in the development of atherosclerosis [71], and administration of antibodies against TNFα lowers the levels of PTX3 transcripts in Kawasaki disease (KD) patients with intravenous immunoglobulin resistance, thus reducing the risk to develop coronary artery aneurysms [72].

Another very recent study demonstrated that PTX3 gene is over expressed in the presence of Nogo-B, a member of the reticulon 4 protein family, which is critical in vessel regeneration [73, 74]. In rheumatoid

synoviocytes transcription of the PTX3 messenger RNA (mRNA) was found to be directly promoted by serum amyloid A [75]. Moreover, plasma analysis and gene expression profile revealed that PTX3 might be involved in the remote cardioprotective effects observed in mice after subcutaneous transplantation of heme oxygenase-1-overexpressing mouse mesenchymal stem cells [76]. Interestingly, in experimental brain stroke PTX3 is found locally increased in response to the pro-inflammatory cytokine interleukin-1 and it contributes to brain recovery by promoting glial scar formation and resolution of edema [77]. It is worth to be mentioned that the epigenetic regulation of long pentraxin 3 was demonstrated to recruit the PI3K/Akt pathway [78]. Remarkably, it was shown that HDL may increase the expression of PTX3 via activation of the PI3K/Akt pathway [79], which discloses a further beneficial effects of PTX3 under the regulation of HDL.

Conclusion

The multiple effects played by PTX3 are now of growing interest. Here we try to explain the mechanistic interactions of PTX3 in cardiovascular diseases discussing recent evidence coming from both cardiovascular and systemic studies showing the fine tuning of time, space, and organ context, which determine the final outcome

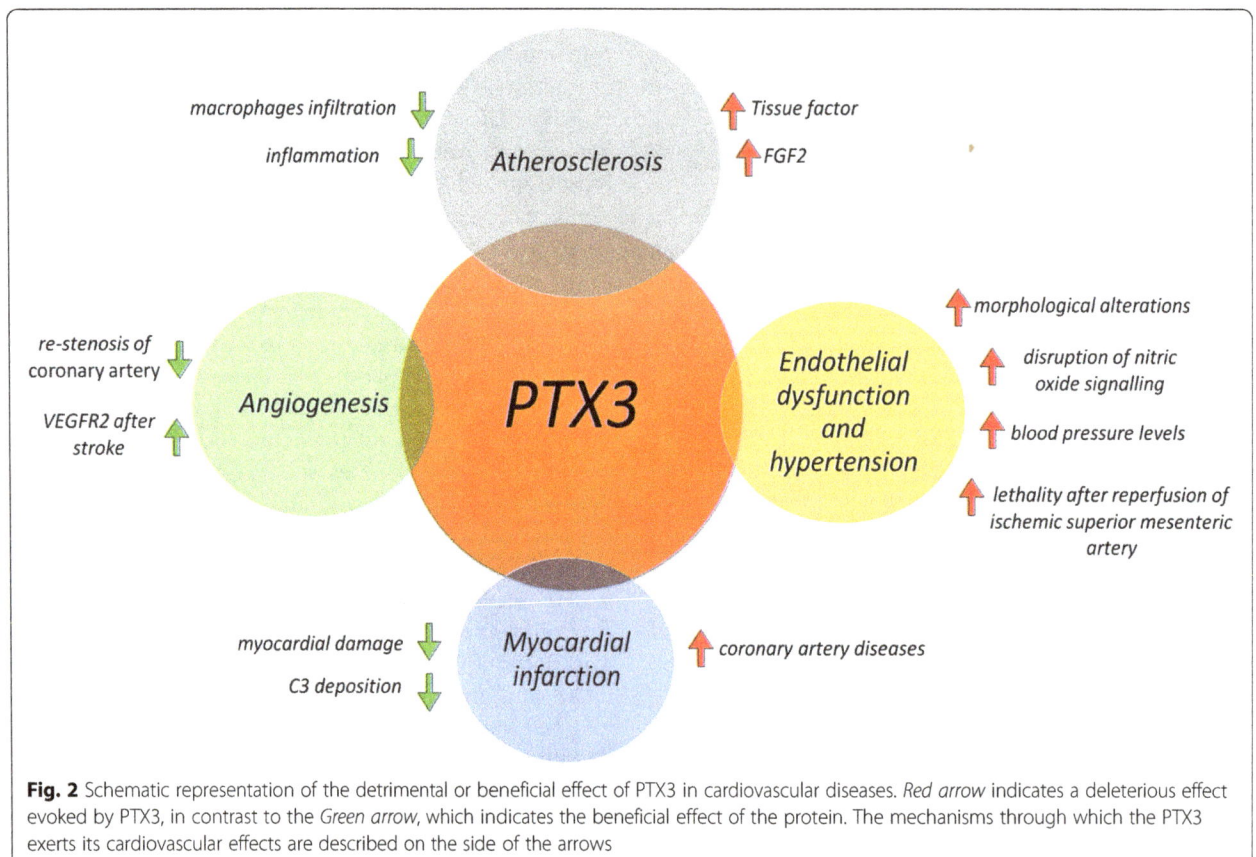

Fig. 2 Schematic representation of the detrimental or beneficial effect of PTX3 in cardiovascular diseases. *Red arrow* indicates a deleterious effect evoked by PTX3, in contrast to the *Green arrow*, which indicates the beneficial effect of the protein. The mechanisms through which the PTX3 exerts its cardiovascular effects are described on the side of the arrows

of PTX3 effects including either detrimental or beneficial effects (Fig. 2). Several studies have suggested PTX3 as a therapeutic tool for cardiovascular disorders although contradictory findings leave this point unresolved.

Nevertheless, considering that the ptx3-deficient mice have greater myocardial lesions following the coronary artery ligation/reperfusion damage due to activation of C1q [59], the PTX3 stimulation could be used as therapeutic tool to reduced AMI damage. Moreover, since HDL induces PTX3 through PI3K/Akt axis [80] exerting an atheroprotective effect, the positive modulation of PTX3 could counterbalancing the over activation of a proinflammatory atherogenic cascade thus protecting the vascular wall. Again, based on the interaction between PTX3 and complement factor H that contribute to maintain the retinal immunohomeostasis [81], the stimulation of PTX3 could reduce the pathophysiology of macular degeneration. Finally, in keeping with the detrimental vascular effects of PTX3 on endothelium, mediated by the activation of P-Selectin/MMP1, we wish to emphasize that PTX3 may represent a novel target to be blocked to protect blood vessels. Based on these data, we feel that the balance between the good and the bad cops of PTX3 must be kept in mind both kind of effects when planning further developments in human patients. In particular, the vascular-based therapeutic approach should be limited to block the vascular effects of PTX3 without affecting its beneficial effects in other organs. Alternatively one might theoretically plan to combine opposite actions in different systems. Opposite manipulations of PTX3 for future therapeutic strategies should be planned to block selectively PTX3-induced molecular cascade in blood vessel, while concomitantly increasing its effects in other selective district. These issues represent a challenge for future PTX3-based drug development.

Acknowledgements
Not applicable.

Funding
Not applicable.

Authors' contributions
FF, AC, MF, AAP, CV conceived and drafted the paper; MA, AD, MF, FB, CB, AAP, CV made critical revisions to the draft. All authors read and approved the final manuscript.

Competing interests
The authors declare that they have no competing interest.

Author details
[1]Department of Translational Research and New Technologies in Medicine and Surgery, University of Pisa, Pisa, Italy. [2]I.R.C.C.S. Neuromed, Pozzilli, IS, Italy. [3]Vascular Physiopathology Unit, I.R.C.C.S. Multimedica, Milan, Italy. [4]Department of Medicine and Surgery, University of Salerno, Via S. Allende, Baronissi, SA 84081, Italy.

References
1. Garlanda C, Bottazzi B, Bastone A, Mantovani A. Pentraxins at the crossroads between innate immunity, inflammation, matrix deposition, and female fertility. Annu Rev Immunol. 2005;23:337–66. doi:10.1146/annurev.immunol. 23.021704.115756.
2. Gewurz H, Zhang XH, Lint TF. Structure and function of the pentraxins. Curr Opin Immunol. 1995;7:54–64. doi:10.1016/0952-7915(95)80029-8.
3. Mantovani A, Garlanda C, Doni A, Bottazzi B. Pentraxins in innate immunity: from C-reactive protein to the long pentraxin PTX3. J Clin Immunol. 2008; 28:1–13. doi:10.1007/s10875-007-9126-7.
4. Bonacina F, Barbieri SS, Cutuli L, Amadio P, Doni A, Sironi M, et al. Vascular pentraxin 3 controls arterial thrombosis by targeting collagen and fibrinogen induced platelets aggregation. Biochim Biophys Acta. 2016. doi: 10.1016/j.bbadis.2016.03.007.
5. Bottazzi B, Inforzato A, Messa M, Barbagallo M, Magrini E, Garlanda C, et al. The pentraxins PTX3 and SAP in innate immunity, regulation of inflammation and tissue remodelling. J Hepatol. 2016. doi:10.1016/j.jhep.2016.02.029.
6. Agrawal A, Singh PP, Bottazzi B, Garlanda C, Mantovani A. Pattern recognition by pentraxins. Adv Exp Med Biol. 2009;653:98–116.
7. Fornai F, Carrizzo A, Ferrucci M, Damato A, Biagioni F, Gaglione A, et al. Brain diseases and tumorigenesis: the good and bad cops of pentraxin3. Int J Biochem Cell Biol. 2015;69:70–4. doi:10.1016/j.biocel.2015.10.017.
8. Dubin R, Li YM, Ix JH, Shlipak M, Whooley M, Peralta CA. Associations of Pentraxin-3 with cardiovascular events, incident heart failure and mortality among persons with coronary heart disease: data from the heart and soul study. Circulation. 2011;124.
9. Introna M, Alles VV, Castellano M, Picardi G, DeGioia L, Bottazzi B, et al. Cloning of mouse ptx3, a new member of the pentraxin gene family expressed at extrahepatic sites. Blood. 1996;87:1862–72.
10. Fuster V, Mearns BM. The CVD paradox: mortality vs prevalence. Nat Rev Cardiol. 2009;6:669. doi:10.1038/nrcardio.2009.187.
11. Willerson JT, Ridker PM. Inflammation as a cardiovascular risk factor. Circulation. 2004;109:II2–10. doi:10.1161/01.CIR.0000129535.04194.38.
12. Latini R, Maggioni AP, Peri G, Gonzini L, Lucci D, Mocarelli P, et al. Prognostic significance of the long pentraxin PTX3 in acute myocardial infarction. Circulation. 2004;110:2349–54. doi:10.1161/01.CIR.0000145167.30987.2E.
13. Inoue K, Kodama T, Daida H. Pentraxin 3: a novel biomarker for inflammatory cardiovascular disease. Int J Vasc Med. 2012;2012:657025. doi: 10.1155/2012/657025.
14. Yano Y, Matsuda S, Hatakeyama K, Sato Y, Imamura T, Shimada K, et al. Plasma Pentraxin 3, but not high-sensitivity C-reactive protein, is a useful inflammatory biomarker for predicting cognitive impairment in elderly hypertensive patients. J Gerontol A Biol Sci Med Sci. 2010;65:547–52. doi:10.1093/gerona/glq030.
15. Norata GD, Garlanda C, Catapano AL. The long pentraxin PTX3: a modulator of the immunoinflammatory response in atherosclerosis and cardiovascular diseases. Trends Cardiovasc Med. 2010;20:35–40. doi:10. 1016/j.tcm.2010.03.005.
16. Parlak A, Aydogan U, Iyisoy A, Dikililer MA, Kut A, Cakir E, et al. Elevated pentraxin-3 levels are related to blood pressure levels in hypertensive patients: an observational study. Anadolu Kardiyol Derg. 2012;12:298–304. doi:10.5152/akd.2012.092.
17. Libby P. Inflammation in atherosclerosis. Nature. 2002;420:868–74. doi:10. 1038/nature01323.
18. Libby P, Okamoto Y, Rocha VZ, Folco E. Inflammation in atherosclerosis: transition from theory to practice. Circ J. 2010;74:213–20.
19. Rolph MS, Zimmer S, Bottazzi B, Garlanda C, Mantovani A, Hansson GK. Production of the long pentraxin PTX3 in advanced atherosclerotic plaques. Arterioscler Thromb Vasc Biol. 2002;22:e10–14.

20. Zacho J, Tybjaerg-Hansen A, Nordestgaard BG. C-reactive protein and all-cause mortality–the Copenhagen City Heart Study. Eur Heart J. 2010;31: 1624–32. doi:10.1093/eurheartj/ehq103.

21. Klouche M, Peri G, Knabbe C, Eckstein HH, Schmid FX, Schmitz G, et al. Modified atherogenic lipoproteins induce expression of pentraxin-3 by human vascular smooth muscle cells. Atherosclerosis. 2004;175:221–8. doi: 10.1016/j.atherosclerosis.2004.03.020.

22. Savchenko A, Imamura M, Ohashi R, Jiang S, Kawasaki T, Hasegawa G, et al. Expression of pentraxin 3 (PTX3) in human atherosclerotic lesions. J Pathol. 2008;215:48–55. doi:10.1002/path.2314.

23. Mantovani A, Garlanda C, Bottazzi B. Pentraxin 3, a non-redundant soluble pattern recognition receptor involved in innate immunity. Vaccine. 2003;21 Suppl 2:S43–47.

24. Nerkiz P, Doganer YC, Aydogan U, Akbulut H, Parlak A, Aydogdu A, et al. Serum pentraxin-3 level in patients who underwent coronary angiography and relationship with coronary atherosclerosis. Med Princ Pract. 2015;24: 369–75. doi:10.1159/000381879.

25. Jenny NS, Arnold AM, Kuller LH, Tracy RP, Psaty BM. Associations of pentraxin 3 with cardiovascular disease and all-cause death: the Cardiovascular Health Study. Arterioscler Thromb Vasc Biol. 2009;29:594–9. doi:10.1161/ATVBAHA.108.178947.

26. Eggers KM, Armstrong PW, Califf RM, Johnston N, Simoons ML, Venge P, et al. Clinical and prognostic implications of circulating pentraxin 3 levels in non ST-elevation acute coronary syndrome. Clin Biochem. 2013;46:1655–9. doi:10.1016/j.clinbiochem.2013.08.014.

27. Soeki T, Niki T, Kusunose K, Bando S, Hirata Y, Tomita N, et al. Elevated concentrations of pentraxin 3 are associated with coronary plaque vulnerability. J Cardiol. 2011;58:151–7. doi:10.1016/j.jjcc.2011.04.005.

28. Kotooka N, Inoue T, Aoki S, Anan M, Komoda H, Node K. Prognostic value of pentraxin 3 in patients with chronic heart failure. Int J Cardiol. 2008; 130:19–22. doi:10.1016/j.ijcard.2007.07.168.

29. Deban L, Russo RC, Sironi M, Moalli F, Scanziani M, Zambelli V, et al. Regulation of leukocyte recruitment by the long pentraxin PTX3. Nat Immunol. 2010;11:328–34. doi:10.1038/ni.1854.

30. Norata GD, Marchesi P, Pulakazhi Venu VK, Pasqualini F, Anselmo A, Moalli F, et al. Deficiency of the long pentraxin PTX3 promotes vascular inflammation and atherosclerosis. Circulation. 2009;120:699–708. doi:10.1161/CIRCULATIONAHA.108.806547.

31. Shindo A, Tanemura H, Yata K, Hamada K, Shibata M, Umeda Y, et al. Inflammatory biomarkers in atherosclerosis: pentraxin 3 can become a novel marker of plaque vulnerability. PLoS One. 2014;9:e100045. doi:10.1371/journal.pone.0100045.

32. Napoleone E, di Santo A, Peri G, Mantovani A, de Gaetano G, Donati MB, et al. The long pentraxin PTX3 up-regulates tissue factor in activated monocytes: another link between inflammation and clotting activation. J Leukoc Biol. 2004; 76:203–9. doi:10.1189/jlb.1003528.

33. Bassi N, Zampieri S, Ghirardello A, Tonon M, Zen M, Cozzi F, et al. Pentraxins, anti-pentraxin antibodies, and atherosclerosis. Clin Rev Allergy Immunol. 2009;37:36–43. doi:10.1007/s12016-008-8098-6.

34. Qiu L, Xu R, Wang S, Li S, Sheng H, Wu J, et al. Honokiol ameliorates endothelial dysfunction through suppression of PTX3 expression, a key mediator of IKK/IkappaB/NF-kappaB, in atherosclerotic cell model. Exp Mol Med. 2015;47:e171. doi:10.1038/emm.2015.37.

35. Forstermann U, Munzel T. Endothelial nitric oxide synthase in vascular disease: from marvel to menace. Circulation. 2006;113:1708–14. doi:10.1161/CIRCULATIONAHA.105.602532.

36. Puca AA, Carrizzo A, Ferrario A, Villa F, Vecchione C. Endothelial nitric oxide synthase, vascular integrity and human exceptional longevity. Immun Ageing. 2012;9:26. doi:10.1186/1742-4933-9-26.

37. Carnevale D, Pallante F, Fardella V, Fardella S, Iacobucci R, Federici M, et al. The angiogenic factor PlGF mediates a neuroimmune interaction in the spleen to allow the onset of hypertension. Immunity. 2014;41: 737–52. doi:10.1016/j.immuni.2014.11.002.

38. Clapp BR, Hingorani AD, Kharbanda RK, Mohamed-Ali V, Stephens JW, Vallance P, et al. Inflammation-induced endothelial dysfunction involves reduced nitric oxide bioavailability and increased oxidant stress. Cardiovasc Res. 2004;64:172–8. doi:10.1016/j.cardiores.2004.06.020.

39. Witasp A, Ryden M, Carrero JJ, Qureshi AR, Nordfors L, Naslund E, et al. Elevated circulating levels and tissue expression of pentraxin 3 in uremia: a reflection of endothelial dysfunction. PLoS One. 2013;8:e63493. doi:10.1371/journal.pone.0063493.

40. Hamad RR, Eriksson MJ, Berg E, Larsson A, Bremme K. Impaired endothelial function and elevated levels of pentraxin 3 in early-onset preeclampsia. Acta Obstet Gynecol Scand. 2012;91:50–6. doi:10.1111/j.1600-0412.2011. 01238.x.

41. Cozzi V, Garlanda C, Nebuloni M, Maina V, Martinelli A, Calabrese S, et al. PTX3 as a potential endothelial dysfunction biomarker for severity of preeclampsia and IUGR. Placenta. 2012;33:1039–44. doi:10.1016/j.placenta. 2012.09.009.

42. Suliman ME, Qureshi AR, Carrero JJ, Barany P, Yilmaz MI, Snaedal-Jonsdottir S, et al. The long pentraxin PTX-3 in prevalent hemodialysis patients: associations with comorbidities and mortality. QJM. 2008;101:397–405. doi: 10.1093/qjmed/hcn019.

43. Jylhava J, Haarala A, Kahonen M, Lehtimaki T, Jula A, Moilanen L, et al. Pentraxin 3 (PTX3) is associated with cardiovascular risk factors: the Health 2000 Survey. Clin Exp Immunol. 2011;164:211–7. doi:10.1111/j.1365-2249. 2011.04354.x.

44. Tamura Y, Ono T, Kuwana M, Inoue K, Takei M, Yamamoto T, et al. Human pentraxin 3 (PTX3) as a novel biomarker for the diagnosis of pulmonary arterial hypertension. PLoS One. 2012;7:e45834. doi:10.1371/journal.pone.0045834.

45. Naito A, Tanabe N, Jujo T, Shigeta A, Sugiura T, Sakao S, et al. Pentraxin3 in chronic thromboembolic pulmonary hypertension: a new biomarker for screening from remitted pulmonary thromboembolism. PLoS One. 2014;9: e113086. doi:10.1371/journal.pone.0113086.

46. Souza DG, Amaral FA, Fagundes CT, Coelho FM, Arantes RM, Sousa LP, et al. The long pentraxin PTX3 is crucial for tissue inflammation after intestinal ischemia and reperfusion in mice. Am J Pathol. 2009;174:1309–18. doi:10. 2353/ajpath.2009.080240.

47. Carrizzo A, Lenzi P, Procaccini C, Damato A, Biagioni F, Ambrosio M, et al. Pentraxin 3 induces vascular endothelial dysfunction through a P-selectin/Matrix metalloproteinase-1 pathway. Circulation. 2015;131:1495–505. doi:10. 1161/CIRCULATIONAHA.114.014822. discussion 1505.

48. Okrainec K, Banerjee DK, Eisenberg MJ. Coronary artery disease in the developing world. Am Heart J. 2004;148:7–15. doi:10.1016/j.ahj.2003.11.027.

49. Haibo Liu, Xiaofang Guo, Kang Yao, Chunming Wang, Guozhong Chen, Wei Gao, Jie Yuan, Wangjun Yu, Junbo Ge. Pentraxin-3 Predicts Long-Term Cardiac Events in Patients with Chronic Heart Failure. BioMedResearch International. 2015;1-7.

50. Peri G, Introna M, Corradi D, Iacuitti G, Signorini S, Avanzini F, et al. PTX3, a prototypical long pentraxin, is an early indicator of acute myocardial infarction in humans. Circulation. 2000;102:636–41.

51. Duran S, Duran I, Kaptanagasi FA, Nartop F, Ciftci H, Korkmaz GG. The role of pentraxin 3 as diagnostic value in classification of patients with heart failure. Clin Biochem. 2013;46:983–7. doi:10.1016/j.clinbiochem.2013.04.026.

52. Suzuki S, Takeishi Y, Niizeki T, Koyama Y, Kitahara T, Sasaki T, et al. Pentraxin 3, a new marker for vascular inflammation, predicts adverse clinical outcomes in patients with heart failure. Am Heart J. 2008;155:75–81. doi:10. 1016/j.ahj.2007.08.013.

53. Matsubara J, Sugiyama S, Nozaki T, Sugamura K, Konishi M, Ohba K, et al. Pentraxin 3 is a new inflammatory marker correlated with left ventricular diastolic dysfunction and heart failure with normal ejection fraction. J Am Coll Cardiol. 2011;57:861–9. doi:10.1016/j.jacc.2010.10.018.

54. Latini R, Gullestad L, Masson S, Nymo SH, Ueland T, Cuccovillo I, et al. Pentraxin-3 in chronic heart failure: the CORONA and GISSI-HF trials. Eur J Heart Fail. 2012;14:992–9. doi:10.1093/eurjhf/hfs092.

55. Inoue K, Sugiyama A, Reid PC, Ito Y, Miyauchi K, Mukai S, et al. Establishment of a high sensitivity plasma assay for human pentraxin3 as a marker for unstable angina pectoris. Arterioscler Thromb Vasc Biol. 2007;27: 161–7. doi:10.1161/01.ATV.0000252126.48375.d5.

56. Helseth R, Solheim S, Opstad T, Hoffmann P, Arnesen H, Seljeflot I. The time profile of Pentraxin 3 in patients with acute ST-elevation myocardial infarction and stable angina pectoris undergoing percutaneous coronary intervention. Mediators Inflamm. 2014;2014:608414. doi:10.1155/2014/608414.

57. Matsui S, Ishii J, Kitagawa F, Kuno A, Hattori K, Ishikawa M, et al. Pentraxin 3 in unstable angina and non-ST-segment elevation myocardial infarction. Atherosclerosis. 2010;210:220–5. doi:10.1016/j.atherosclerosis.2009.10.033.

58. Haibo L, Xiaofang G, Chunming W, Jie Y, Guozhong C, Limei Z, et al. Prognostic value of plasma pentraxin-3 levels in patients with stable coronary artery disease after drug-eluting stent implantation. Mediators Inflamm. 2014;2014:963096. doi:10.1155/2014/963096.

59. Salio M, Chimenti S, De Angelis N, Molla F, Maina V, Nebuloni M, et al. Cardioprotective function of the long pentraxin PTX3 in acute myocardial

infarction. Circulation. 2008;117:1055–64. doi:10.1161/CIRCULATIONAHA.107.
749234.

60. Salustri A, Garlanda C, Hirsch E, De Acetis M, Maccagno A, Bottazzi B, et al.
PTX3 plays a key role in the organization of the cumulus oophorus
extracellular matrix and in in vivo fertilization. Development. 2004;131:1577–
86. doi:10.1242/dev.01056.

61. Day AJ, de la Motte CA. Hyaluronan cross-linking: a protective mechanism in
inflammation? Trends Immunol. 2005;26:637–43. doi:10.1016/j.it.2005.09.009.

62. Presta M, Oreste P, Zoppetti G, Belleri M, Tanghetti E, Leali D, et al.
Antiangiogenic activity of semisynthetic biotechnological heparins: low-
molecular-weight-sulfated Escherichia coli K5 polysaccharide derivatives as
fibroblast growth factor antagonists. Arterioscler Thromb Vasc Biol. 2005;25:
71–6. doi:10.1161/01.ATV.0000148863.24445.b4.

63. Camozzi M, Zacchigna S, Rusnati M, Coltrini D, Ramirez-Correa G, Bottazzi B, et al.
Pentraxin 3 inhibits fibroblast growth factor 2-dependent activation of smooth
muscle cells in vitro and neointima formation in vivo. Arterioscler Thromb Vasc
Biol. 2005;25:1837–42. doi:10.1161/01.ATV.0000177807.54959.7d.

64. Leali D, Inforzato A, Ronca R, Bianchi R, Belleri M, Coltrini D, et al. Long
pentraxin 3/tumor necrosis factor-stimulated gene-6 interaction: a biological
rheostat for fibroblast growth factor 2-mediated angiogenesis. Arterioscler
Thromb Vasc Biol. 2012;32:696–703. doi:10.1161/ATVBAHA.111.243998.

65. Rodriguez-Grande B, Varghese L, Molina-Holgado F, Rajkovic O, Garlanda C,
Denes A, et al. Pentraxin 3 mediates neurogenesis and angiogenesis after
cerebral ischaemia. J Neuroinflammation. 2015;12:15. doi:10.1186/s12974-
014-0227-y.

66. Woo JM, Kwon MY, Shin DY, Kang YH, Hwang N, Chung SW. Human retinal
pigment epithelial cells express the long pentraxin PTX3. Mol Vis. 2013;19:303–10.

67. Yang HS, Woo JE, Lee SJ, Park SH, Woo JM. Elevated plasma pentraxin 3
levels are associated with development and progression of diabetic
retinopathy in Korean patients with type 2 diabetes mellitus. Invest
Ophthalmol Vis Sci. 2014;55:5989–97. doi:10.1167/iovs.14-14864.

68. Zhou W, Hu W. Serum and vitreous pentraxin 3 concentrations in patients
with diabetic retinopathy. Genet Test Mol Biomarkers. 2016;20:149–53. doi:
10.1089/gtmb.2015.0238.

69. Min JK, Kim J, Woo JM. Elevated plasma pentraxin3 levels and its association
with neovascular age-related macular degeneration. Ocul Immunol Inflamm.
2015;23:205–11. doi:10.3109/09273948.2014.891755.

70. Park KS, Kim JW, An JH, Woo JM. Elevated plasma pentraxin 3 and its
association with retinal vein occlusion. Korean J Ophthalmol. 2014;28:460–5.
doi:10.3341/kjo.2014.28.6.460.

71. Alberti L, Gilardini L, Zulian A, Micheletto G, Peri G, Doni A, et al. Expression
of long pentraxin PTX3 in human adipose tissue and its relation with
cardiovascular risk factors. Atherosclerosis. 2009;202:455–60. doi:10.1016/j.
atherosclerosis.2008.05.015.

72. Ogihara Y, Ogata S, Nomoto K, Ebato T, Sato K, Kokubo K, et al. Transcriptional
regulation by infliximab therapy in Kawasaki disease patients with
immunoglobulin resistance. Pediatr Res. 2014;76:287–93. doi:10.1038/pr.2014.92.

73. Chick HE, Nowrouzi A, Fronza R, McDonald RA, Kane NM, Alba R, et al.
Integrase-deficient lentiviral vectors mediate efficient gene transfer to
human vascular smooth muscle cells with minimal genotoxic risk. Hum
Gene Ther. 2012;23:1247–57. doi:10.1089/hum.2012.042.

74. Acevedo L, Yu J, Erdjument-Bromage H, Miao RQ, Kim JE, Fulton D, et al. A
new role for Nogo as a regulator of vascular remodeling. Nat Med. 2004;10:
382–8. doi:10.1038/nm1020.

75. Satomura K, Torigoshi T, Koga T, Maeda Y, Izumi Y, Jiuchi Y, et al. Serum
amyloid A (SAA) induces pentraxin 3 (PTX3) production in rheumatoid
synoviocytes. Mod Rheumatol. 2013;23:28–35. doi:10.1007/s10165-012-0630-0.

76. Preda MB, Ronningen T, Burlacu A, Simionescu M, Moskaug JO, Valen G.
Remote transplantation of mesenchymal stem cells protects the heart
against ischemia-reperfusion injury. Stem Cells. 2014;32:2123–34. doi:10.
1002/stem.1687.

77. Rodriguez-Grande B, Swana M, Nguyen L, Englezou P, Maysami S, Allan SM,
et al. The acute-phase protein PTX3 is an essential mediator of glial scar
formation and resolution of brain edema after ischemic injury. J Cereb
Blood Flow Metab. 2014;34:480–8. doi:10.1038/jcbfm.2013.224.

78. Merchant S, Korbelik M. Upregulation of genes for C-reactive protein and
related pentraxin/complement proteins in photodynamic therapy-treated
human tumor cells: enrolment of PI3K/Akt and AP-1. Immunobiology. 2013;
218:869–74. doi:10.1016/j.imbio.2012.10.010.

79. Norata GD, Marchesi P, Pirillo A, Uboldi P, Chiesa G, Maina V, et al. Long
pentraxin 3, a key component of innate immunity, is modulated by high-
density lipoproteins in endothelial cells. Arterioscler Thromb Vasc Biol. 2008;
28:925–31. doi:10.1161/ATVBAHA.107.160606.

80. Moalli F, Doni A, Deban L, Zelante T, Zagarella S, Bottazzi B, et al. Role of
complement and Fc{gamma} receptors in the protective activity of the long
pentraxin PTX3 against Aspergillus fumigatus. Blood. 2010;116:5170–80. doi:
10.1182/blood-2009-12-258376.

81. Juel HB, Faber C, Munthe-Fog L, Bastrup-Birk S, Reese-Petersen AL, Falk MK, et al.
Systemic and ocular long pentraxin 3 in patients with age-related macular
degeneration. PLoS One. 2015;10:e0132800. doi:10.1371/journal.pone.0132800.

Lifewide profile of cytokine production by innate and adaptive immune cells from Brazilian individuals

Gabriela Silveira-Nunes[1], Elaine Speziali[2], Andréa Teixeira-Carvalho[2], Danielle M. Vitelli-Avelar[2], Renato Sathler-Avelar[2], Taciana Figueiredo-Soares[3,7], Maria Luiza Silva[2], Vanessa Peruhype-Magalhães[2,4,5], Daniel Gonçalves Chaves[2], Gustavo Eustáquio Brito-Melo[6], Glenda Meira Cardoso[2], Eric Bassetti Soares[2,3], Silvana Maria Elói-Santos[2,3], Rosângela Teixeira[2,3], Dulciene Magalhães Queiroz[2,3], Rodrigo Corrêa-Oliveira[4], Ana Maria Caetano Faria[1*] and Olindo Assis Martins-Filho[2]

Abstract

Background: Immunosenescence is associated with several changes in adaptive and innate immune cells. Altered cytokine production is among the most prominent of these changes. The impact of age-related alterations on cytokine global profiles produced by distinct populations of leukocytes from healthy Brazilian individuals was studied. We analysed frequencies of cytokine-producing lymphocytes and innate immune cells from individuals at several ages spanning a lifetime period (0–85 years).

Results: Healthy adult individuals presented a balanced profile suggestive of a mature immune system with equal contributions of both innate and adaptive immunity and of both categories of cytokines (inflammatory and regulatory). In healthy newborns and elderly, innate immune cells, especially neutrophils and NK-cells, contributed the most to a balanced profile of cytokines.

Conclusions: Our results support the hypothesis that ageing is not associated with a progressive pro-inflammatory cytokine production by all leukocytes but rather with distinct fluctuations in the frequency of cytokine-producing cells throughout life.

Keywords: Aging, Cytokine, Adaptive immune cells, Innate immune cells

Background

In the past decade, a new approach to the study of ageing emerged from the data collected from centenarians. The concept of successful or healthy ageing comes from these studies and it eliminated the confusion between ageing and age-related disorders. According to these studies, immunosenescence does not involve a simple unidirectional decline in all functions, but rather a remodeling of biological systems during the ageing process. In this sense, many immunological activities are

* Correspondence: anacaetanofaria@gmail.com
[1]Departamento de Bioquímica e Imunologia, Instituto de Ciências Biológicas, Universidade Federal de Minas Gerais, Avenida Antônio Carlos 6627, Belo Horizonte, Minas Gerais 31270-901, Brazil
Full list of author information is available at the end of the article

well preserved in the healthy elderly and they may compensate for other functions that are impaired [1–3].

Ageing is associated with several alterations in the phenotype, repertoire and activation status of leukocytes as well as in the cytokine profile produced by these cells. This complex age-related remodeling of the immune system is responsible for the profound changes within the cytokine network [3–8]. Cytokines are a key component in the communication among immune cells and they are responsible for differentiation, proliferation and survival of lymphoid cells, playing an important role in immune responses and inflammation. Age-related changes in the cytokine network is responsible for a chronic proinflammatory status, known as "inflammageing" [3, 5]. Inflammageing has been described as a combination of dysfunctional immunity with a state of low grade chronic inflammation and it has been considered as an universal phenomenon associated with frailty and morbidity in the elderly [3, 8–11]. This progressive increase in pro-inflammatory status is one of the major characteristics of immunosenescence [12–14].

Several ageing-associated immunological alterations have been already described in medical literature, mostly in the T-cell compartment. They include involution of the thymus, reduction in the number of naïve T-cells with a parallel increase of oligoclonaly expanded CD4+ T-cells with a memory phenotype, reduced potential to produce IL-2 and loss of CD28 expression [15–17]. Adaptive immunity undergoes severe deterioration with age and this represents the main problem in the elderly. However, evidence accumulated over the last decade supports the hypothesis that ageing has also a profound impact on innate immunity, which in turn markedly influences health and longevity of older people [3, 18–20].

In the complex scenario of immunosenescence, it has been generally accepted that some aspects of innate immunity, e.g., phagocytosis and natural killer (NK)-cell cytotoxicity, remain largely unaffected [19–21]. Innate immune responses are more resistant to change and NK-cells are well preserved in healthy elderly subjects. In fact, there is an age-related increase in CD16+ CD57-cells with high cytotoxicity capacity. This increase in NK cells has been correlated with successful ageing [21–24]. Our group reported a significant increase in frequency of CD16+ IFN-γ+ NK-cells in aged individuals in schistosomiasis endemic areas of Brazil who were protected from schistosome infection. Therefore, a high frequency of IFN-γ+ NK-cells correlated with "healthy ageing" in endemic areas [22].

Studies in aged mice showed functional decline of monocytes and macrophages, low expression level of Toll-like receptors from activated splenic and peritoneal macrophages and altered secretion of several chemokines and cytokines [25, 26]. Reduced class II major histocompatibility in aged macrophages also contribute to impaired proliferative response of activated peripheral T-lymphocytes [20, 27–29].

In humans, it has been described that although the elderly preserve the number and phagocytic capacity of neutrophils, other functional characteristics of these cells such as superoxide anion production, chemotaxis, and apoptosis are reduced during ageing [18, 30, 31].

In this sense, healthy immunosenescence is the net result of a continuous adaptation of the body to deteriorative changes occurring over time. According to this concept, body resources are continuously optimized, and successful immunosenescence must be considered a very dynamic process of immunological remodeling [32, 33].

Most of the studies investigating the influence of inflammageing in the elderly were obtained at particular age intervals and most of them come from Caucasian individuals from either Europe or the United States. Even among these reports, authors have observed variations and contrasting results as their samples vary demographically and geographically [34–36]. The study of various age groups should yield more meaningful data on immunosenescence that could be directly used by the geriatricians to restore or attenuate deregulated immune responses and assure a healthy longevity.

In this study, we described age-related changes in the frequency of cytokine-producing leukocyte populations in order to contribute to the establishment of new reference parameters for Brazilian individuals.

Methods
Aim of the study
The aim was to establish new reference parameters of cytokine production by leukocytes for Brazilian healthy individuals at different ages. Since there are controversies on the topic of cytokine production during ageing due to differences in experimental designs [37], this study is part of a broad effort to identify cell subsets involved in the production of distinct patterns of cytokines during healthy ageing.

Study population
The study population consisted of 181 healthy subjects: 35 children, 22 adolescents and 124 adults (age range 0–85 years). Blood samples were obtained from children visiting clinics for routine pediatric inspection. Adult samples were obtained from healthy individuals who accepted to participate in the study. Subjects were divided into 6 age categories: Newborn – 0 years ($n = 12$); Children – 6 – 10 years ($n = 23$); Adolescent – 11 – 20 years ($n = 22$); Adults – 21–50 ($n = 80$); Middle Aged – 51–60 ($n = 22$); Elderly – 61–85 ($n = 22$). These age ranges were set based on the main physiological changes occurring during lifetime (birth, childhood, adolescence, young and middle adulthood, senescence) as well as similar patterns of variation observed for cytokine-producing innate cells (Additional file 1: Figure S1) and lymphocytes (Additional file 2: Figure S2) throughout life. These volunteers were all residents in the state of Minas Gerais (Southeast Brazil).

All individuals were interviewed by a health practitioner using a health questionnaire, submitted to a physical exam and to hematological and biochemical tests to establish their health condition. The exclusion criteria for both populations were: infections, acute or chronic inflammation, autoimmune diseases, heart disease, undernourishment, anemia, leucopoenia, mood disorders, neurodegenerative disease, neoplasias and use of hormones (steroids) and drugs (alcohol, antidepressants, immunosuppressants, anticoagulants). Children were excluded of the study if they showed any evidence of congenital disease, infection, immunological disorder or were taking any concomitant medications. Written informed consent forms were obtained from each participant, their parents or guardians prior to their inclusion in our study. This work was approved by the Ethical Committees of FIOCRUZ (Ministry of Health, Belo Horizonte, Brazil) as well as the National Research Ethics Committees (CONEP) of Brazil.

Blood collection

Nine milliliters (9 mL) of blood were drawn from each individual always in the morning period to avoid circadian variations.

Short-term whole blood culture and intracytoplasmic cytokine staining

Aliquots of 500 µL peripheral blood were placed in 5 mL polypropylene tubes containing 500 µl RPMI-1640 added and incubated for six hours at 37 °C and 5% CO_2. Next, 10 µL Brefeldin A (BFA; Sigma Chemical Company, St. Louis, MO) (10 mg/mL final concentration) was added and incubated for four hours at 37 °C and 5% CO_2. Then, 110 µL ethylenediamine tetraacetic acid 20 mM (EDTA; Sigma Chemical Company), (final concentration of 2 mM) solution was added. Tubes were incubated for 15 min at room temperature. Next, 4 mL PBS-W (cell wash solution) was added and samples were centrifuged for 10 min at 400 x g and 18 °C. Supernatants were collected and aliquots stained with fluorescent-labeled anti-human cell surface monoclonal antibodies (to CD4, CD8, CD14, CD16 and CD19) for 30 min at room temperature and protected from light. After membrane staining, erythrocyte lysis, and leukocytes fixation, cell suspensions were permeabilized with PBS-P (PBS 0.05M pH 7.4 containing 0.5% BSA, 0.1% sodium azide and 0.5% saponin: SIGMA, St. Louis, MO, USA) and aliquots incubated for 30 min at room temperature, in the dark, with fluorescent-labeled anti-cytokine monoclonal antibodies to IL-4, IL-5, IL-10, TNF-α and IFN-γ (BD-Pharmingen, San Jose, CA). After intracytoplasmic cytokine staining, leucocytes were washed with PBS-W and fixed in fixative solution Macs Facs Fix (MFF). Samples were analyzed by flow cytometry for the production of TNF-α, IFN-γ, IL-4, IL-5 and IL-10 by CD4+ T-cells and CD8+ T-cells, and the production of TNF-α, IL-4 and IL-10 by CD19+ B cells. Additionally, production of TNF-α, IFN-γ, IL-4 and IL-10 by neutrophils, production of TNF-α and IL-10 by monocytes and production of TNF-α, IFN-γ and IL-4 by NK-cells were analyzed.

Flow cytometry acquisition and analysis

Flow cytometry acquisition and analysis were performed in a FACScalibur™ equipped with a four-color detection system (Becton Dickinson, San Jose, CA, USA), using the CELLQUEST software (Franklin Lakes, NJ, USA). After acquiring 30,000 events/tube, distinct gating strategies were used to analyze the different cytokine-expressing leukocytes subsets, including innate immune cells (neutrophils, monocytes and NK-cells) and adaptive immune cells (CD4+, CD8+ T-cell subsets and B-cells). Selective analysis of neutrophils was performed by establishing a specific scatter gate using the dot plot distribution of anti-CD16-FITC and laser side scatter (SSC) to discriminate the neutrophils as SSC high CD16high+. Analysis of monocytes was performed using the dot plot distribution of anti-CD14-TC and SSC to discriminate the monocytes as SSC int CD14high+ cells. Selection of NK-cells, T-cell subsets and B-cells was performed by gating lymphocytes on forward scatter (FSC) versus SSC dot plot distribution, followed by analysis based on anti-CD16-FITC, anti-CD19-FITC, anti-CD8-FITC or anti-CD4-TC labelling. Following the selection of leucocyte subsets, frequency of cytokine positive cells was determined using quadrant statistics over FL-1/anti-cell surface marker-FITC or FL-3/anti-cell surface marker-TC versus FL-2/anti-cytokine-PE dot plot distribution. Results were expressed as percentages of cytokine positive cells for different gated leucocyte subpopulations analyzed.

Cytokine signature analysis

Cytokine-mediated immune response elicited by leukocytes in each age group was assessed after short-term in vitro culture with no stimulation. Analysis of the intracytoplasmic cytokine profile of peripheral blood leukocytes initially yielded the percentage of cytokine positive cells. Cytokine profiles produced by leukocytes were assessed to identify low (≤ global median) and high (>global median) frequencies of cytokine-producing cells using the global median of each cytokine as a cut-off. For the calculation of the global median the whole universe of data obtained for the groups was considered. Leukocyte subpopulations assessed included neutrophils (NEU), monocytes (MON), NK-cells as well as lymphocyte subsets and the global median of each sub-population was described in Table 1. This strategy allows multiple comparative analyzes among groups, neither of which is excluded from the analysis. The high frequency of cells producing cytokines was used to evaluate the overall cytokine patterns from healthy individuals categorized by age ranges.

Comparative data analysis

The type of analysis that we have used in the present investigation is not a conventional statistical analysis. This novel concept of cytokine signature has been proposed by Luiza-Silva and colleagues [38]. It is a new strategy to evaluate the overall cytokine profile instead of analyzing single cytokine profiles. To reinforce our data we also used the Spearman correlation test in our

Table 1 Global median of the universe of data on cytokine-producing leukocytes

Immune Compartment	Cytokine-producing leukocytes	Median (%)
Innate	TNF-α+ Neutrophils	0.51
	IFN-γ+ Neutrophils	0.34
	IL-4+ Neutrophils	0.43
	IL-10+ Neutrophils	0.19
	TNF-α+ Monocytes	32.20
	IL-10+ Monocytes	3.00
	TNF-α+ NK-cells	0.18
	IFN-γ+ NK-cells	0.21
	IL-4+ NK-cells	0.19
Acquired	TNF-α+ CD4+ T-cells	0.28
	IFN-γ+ CD4+ T-cells	0.26
	IL-4+ CD4+ T-cells	0.32
	IL-5+ CD4+ T-cells	0.11
	IL-10+ CD4+ T-cells	0.75
	TNF-α+ CD8+ T-cells	0.34
	IFN-γ+ CD8+ T-cells	0.28
	IL-4+ CD8+ T-cells	0.27
	IL-5+ CD8+ T-cells	0.14
	IL-10+ CD8+ T-cells	0.40
	TNF-α+ B-cells	0.41
	IL-4+ B-cells	0.30
	IL-10+ B-cells	0.57

Silveira-Nunes et al.

relevant findings. The immune profile is represented as percentage of individuals with high frequency of cytokine-producing innate and acquired immune cells. Relevant differences were considered when the percentage of individuals with a high frequency of cells producing a given cytokine emerged above the 50th percentile (Figs. 1 and 2). This approach showed to be acurate to detect subtle changes in cytokine signatures not detectable by conventional statistical approaches. Then, considering the relevant production of cytokines, Spearman correlation was performed to evaluate increase or decrease in frequency of cytokine-producing cells among age groups.

Since lymphocytes are known to be at higher numbers in newborn and children than in adults, the absolute numbers of lymphocytes for each age group is provided in Table 2. In spite of the variation in the number of these cells, cell frequencies are reliable parameters to evaluate the relative contribution of each cytokine-producing cells within a population.

Radar charts
Radar charts were used to summarize the proinflammatory (■) versus regulatory (■) cytokine signatures in a range of leukocyte subsets of innate and adaptive immunity for each age group. This analysis highlights the contribution of different leukocytes subsets for the global balance of cytokines. On radar charts, each axis represents the percentage (%) of volunteers showing high frequency of cytokine-producing cells. The values of each axis can be connected to form a central polygonal area that represents the proinflammatory versus regulatory global balance. Increase or decrease of the central polygonal area reflects either a higher or a lower contribution of proinflammatory versus regulatory profile for each age group.

Ascendant cytokine profile
The high cytokine producing-cell strategy was also used to create, for each age group, an ascendant profile that allows to analyze the hierarchical behavior of cytokine-producing immune cells throughout life. For this analysis, a functional cytokine categorization was used: Inflammatory cytokines – red bars (TNF-α and IFN-γ) and regulatory cytokines – blue bars (IL-4, IL-5 and IL-10). Only those that had more than 50% frequency of cytokine-producing cells in the group were considered as relevant.

Results
To address the question of how ageing influences the global profile of cytokine production by acquired and innate immune cells, healthy individuals were categorized in carriers of either low or high frequency of cytokine-producing cells as previously described by Luiza-Silva and co-workers [38]. This allowed calculation of the percentage of individuals with high frequency of cytokine-producing cells for each age group. To assess a functional cytokine profile, we classified cytokines as proinflammatory (TNF-α and IFN-γ) and regulatory (IL-4, IL-5 and IL-10) according to its functional characteristics during the ageing process. We took into account for this classification that Th1 cytokines (TNF-α and IFN-γ) were mostly involved in chronic inflammatory disorders associated with ageing (such as cardiovascular, autoimmune and degenerative diseases) [39–41]. In addition, cytokines such as IL-4, IL-5 and IL-10 usually predominate in tolerogenic compartments such as gut mucosa and maternal-fetal interface [42–44].

There are distinct variations in frequency of cytokine-producing leukocyte subsets throughout life
To overview the production of proinflammatory and regulatory cytokines throughout life, we performed an evaluation of the cytokine profile produced by leukocyte subsets from the innate (neutrophils, monocytes and NK-cells) and adaptive (CD4+ T-cells, CD8+ T-cells and B-cells) immune compartments. In this analysis, individuals were categorized

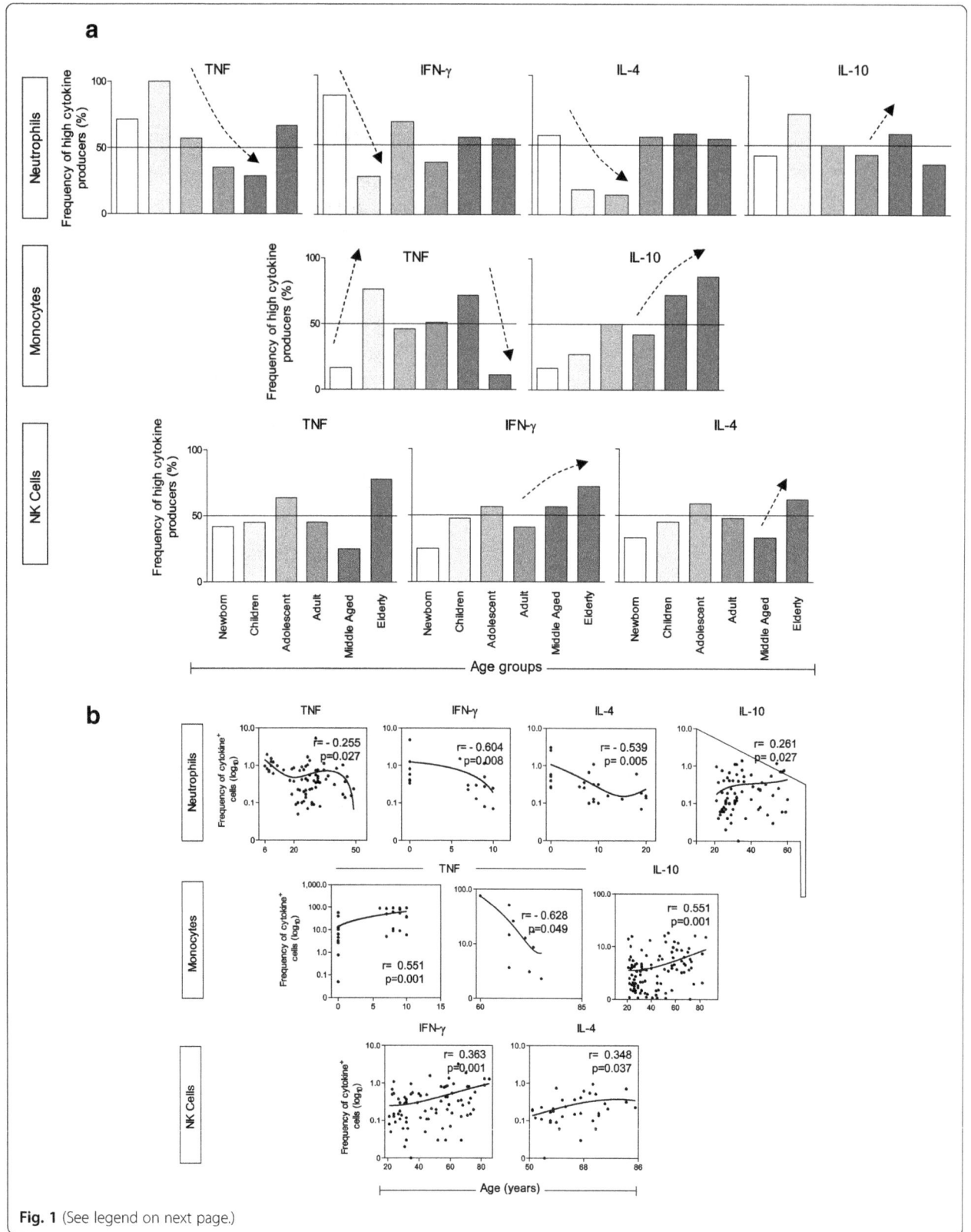

Fig. 1 (See legend on next page.)

(See figure on previous page.)
Fig. 1 Profile of subjects with high frequency of neutrophils, monocytes and NK-cells producing proinflammatory and regulatory cytokines. **a** The cytokine profile is presented as percentage of individuals with high frequency of cytokine-producing cells in each age group: Newborn – 0 years ($n = 12$); Children – 6–10 years ($n = 23$); Adolescent – 11–20 years ($n = 22$); Adults – 21–50 ($n = 80$); Middle Aged – 51–60 ($n = 22$); Elderly – 61–85 ($n = 22$). Bars represent the percentage of subjects with high frequency of neutrophils producing tumor necrosis factor (TNF)-α, interferon (IFN)-γ, interleukin (IL)-4 and IL-10, monocytes producing TNF-α and IL-10, and NK-cells producing TNF-α, IFN-γ and IL-4. Relevant differences were considered when the percentage of individuals with high frequency cells producing a given cytokine emerged above the 50th percentile (*continuous line*). Spearman correlation was performed to evaluate either increase or decrease in frequency of cytokine-producing cells among age groups. Significant positive or negative correlations were represented by *dotted arrows* (↑). **b** Spearman's rank correlation. Corresponding Pearson's correlation coefficient (r) and p value between cytokine-producing cell frequency and age in years is shown

as carriers of either low or high frequency of cytokine-producing cells, using the global median as a cut-off as previously described [38]. Therefore, it was possible to calculate the percentage of individuals with high frequency of cytokine-producing cells for each age group.

As mentioned in the methods section, establishment of age groups was performed according to the rhythmic variation of cytokine-producing cells from both innate and acquired immune compartments of peripheral blood of individuals throughout life (Additional file 1: Figure S1 and Additional file 2: Figure S2). Overall distribution of cytokine+ neutrophils, monocytes (CD14+) and NK-cells (CD16+) (Additional file 1: Figure S1) and of cytokine+ T-cells (CD4+ and CD8+) and B-cells (CD19+) (Additional file 2: Figure S2) were plotted as a function of age (ranging from 0 to 85). Age ranges were established based on the overall variation rhythm observed, considering the moving mean of all cytokine+ cell subsets (continuous lines). A similar strategy was used previously by our group in a study analyzing rhythmic variations in the frequency of different subsets of peripheral blood monocytes in individuals from 0 to 86 years of age. These age groups were shown to represent a homogenous profile suitable to identify immunologically meaningful periods in life [34].

Of note, in the innate cytokine profile, there was the significant decrease of TNF-α-producing neutrophils from childhood to adulthood when it reached a plateau. IFN-γ and IL-4 decreased early in life until childhood. On the other hand, IL-10-producing neutrophils increased during adulthood (adult and middle aged individuals). TNF-α-producing monocyte frequency increased from birth until childhood, then, maintained high during adolescence and adulthood decreasing in the elderly. Interestingly, monocytes maintained a low frequency of IL-10-producing cells during early life and shifted towards a progressive high production from adulthood to senescence. IFN-γ-producing NK-cells and IL-4-producing NK-cells increased in frequency from adult and middle-aged groups, respectively, until senescence (Fig. 1).

Frequency of TNF-α-producing CD4+ T-cells had an increase during the ageing process (significantly from adulthood to senescence), while TNF-α-producing CD8+ T-cells and B-cells decreased their frequencies.

Regarding IFN-γ production, only CD4+ T cells changed: they increased from adulthood to middle age. It could be observed a significant decrease of IL-4-producing CD8+ T cells throughout life (specially from adolescent to elderly groups). An interesting pattern could be found in the profile of IL-5-producing T-cells. At birth, there was a high frequency of both IL-5-producing CD4+ T-cells and CD8+ T-cells; then, these frequencies decreased during childhood to increase again in adolescence, being maintained at approximately 50% of frequency of high cytokine-producing cells during adulthood. From the fiftieth decade of life to senescence, the frequency of IL-5-producing CD4+ and CD8+ T-cells increased further. A remarkable finding is that all IL-10-producing lymphocytes (T and B-cells) had their frequency decreased from adolescence to senescence (Fig. 2).

Profiles of high frequencies of proinflammatory- and regulatory-cytokine-producing cells in innate and adaptive immune compartments vary throughout life

To further characterize the cytokine pattern of healthy individuals at distinct age groups, we have constructed radar charts for high frequency of cells producing proinflammatory and regulatory cytokines and an ascendant graph to characterize the hierarchical contribution of cytokine-producing cell types to the cytokine profile of each age group (Figs. 3 and 4).

Our data demonstrate that the cytokine pattern of newborns was characterized by a prominent participation of proinflammatory responses of the innate immune compartment (Fig. 3), especially driven by TNF-α and IFN-γ from neutrophils (Fig. 4). This profile seems to be counter-balanced by the presence of high frequencies of cells producing regulatory cytokines (mostly IL-5-producing T-cells) (Figs. 3 and 4).

According to our data, neutrophils had an important role in childhood. These innate cells, together with monocytes, produce large amounts of TNF-α, while neutrophils also produced high levels of IL-10, creating a compensatory circuit of cytokines (Figs. 3 and 4).

In the adolescent (11 to 20 years), we could observe a shift in the composition of the cytokine profile. In this age group, there was a predominance of adaptive

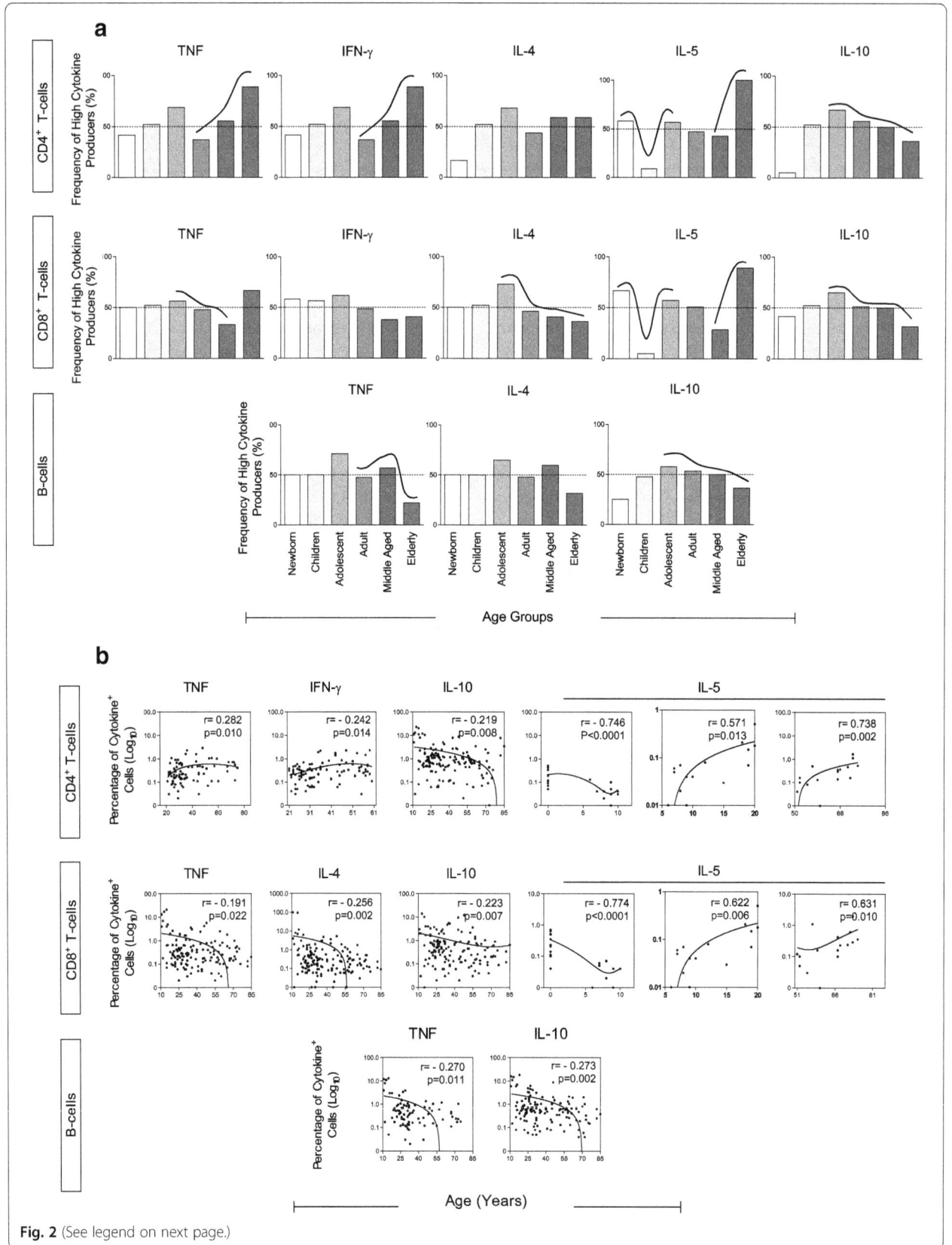

Fig. 2 (See legend on next page.)

(See figure on previous page.)
Fig. 2 Profile of subjects with high frequency of CD4+ T-cells, CD8+ T-cells and B-cells producing proinflammatory and regulatory cytokines. **a** Cytokine profile is presented as percentage of individuals with high frequency of cytokine-producing cells in each age group: Newborn – 0 years ($n = 12$); Children – 6–10 years ($n = 23$); Adolescent – 11–20 years ($n = 22$); Adults – 21–50 ($n = 80$); Middle Aged – 51–60 ($n = 22$); Elderly – 61–85 ($n = 22$). Bars represents the percentage of subjects with high frequency of CD4 T-cells producing tumor necrosis factor (TNF)-α, interferon (IFN)-γ, interleukin (IL)-4, IL-5 and IL-10. CD8 T-cells producing TNF-α, IFN-γ, IL-4, IL-5 and IL-10. B-cells producing TNF-α, IFN-γ, IL-4, IL-5 and IL-10. Relevant differences were considered when the percentage of individuals with high frequency of cells producing a given cytokine emerged above the 50th percentile (*continuous line*). Spearman correlation was performed to evaluate either increase or decrease in frequency of cytokine-producing cells among age groups. Significant positive or negative correlations were represented by *dotted arrows* (↑). **b** Spearman's rank correlation. Corresponding Pearson's correlation coefficient (r) and p value between cytokine-producing cell frequency and age in years is shown

immune responses, with participation of proinflammatory cytokines such as TNF-α from T and B-cells, and IFN-γ from CD4+ and CD8+ T-cells with a contribution of regulatory cytokines such as IL-4, IL-5 and IL-10 produced by T and B lymphocytes. Innate immune cells also influence the adolescent profile: TNF-α and IFN-γ produced by neutrophils and NK-cells, as well as IL-4 production by NK-cells (Figs. 3 and 4).

Interestingly, adults presented a profile well balanced between innate and adaptive immune responses with an equal contribution of proinflammatory and regulatory cytokine-producing cells (Figs. 3 and 4).

Another shift in the composition of the cytokine pattern could be observed from the fiftieth decade of life on. Middle aged group changed their profile from a balanced (seen in adulthood) to a higher contribution of the innate compartment of immune cells. Middle aged groups showed a high frequency of neutrophils producing TNF-α, IL-4 and IL-10, of monocytes producing TNF-α and IL-10, and of NK-cells producing IFN-γ. A prominent inflammatory profile of cytokines produced by lymphocytes was also observed in this age group (TNF produced by CD4+ T-cells and B-cells, IFN-γ produced by CD4+ T-cells and IL-4 produced by CD4 + T-cells and B-cells) (Figs. 3 and 4).

Changes in the cytokine pattern in the elderly group were characterized by a balanced profile with a prominent contribution of the innate immune response (driven by IL-10-producing monocytes, IL-4-producing neutrophils, TNF-α- and IFN-γ-producing neutrophils and NK-cells). Although innate immune cells are the most relevant element in the cytokine profile of this age group, the contribution of

adaptive immune cells could still be identified as IL-5- and TNF-α-producing T-cells and IL-4-producing CD4+ T-cells.

Discussion

Ageing influences the entire physiology of an organism, resulting in changes on functions at the molecular, cellular and systemic levels. Age-related physiological changes are well characterized in the immune system, which is continuously remodeled over the life course. One of these main remodeling changes during ageing occurs in the network of cytokine production [4, 8, 45].

In this study, we evaluated the profile of cytokine produced by major peripheral blood cells of individuals from various age groups. Interestingly, we observed that ageing was not associated with a progressive decline in cytokine production by all leukocyte subsets but it was rather characterized by distinct fluctuations of cytokines produced at various time points during a lifetime period. Furthermore, these variations were distinctive of each cell population examined.

Studies in this area are scarce and results are often contradictory. It is difficult to compare data among various studies owing to differences in experimental designs [37]. According to some reports, an increase of the plasma level of a variety of cytokines, in particular proinflammatory cytokines and their soluble receptors, occurs during ageing [2, 5, 7]. In this regard, it has to be considered that the production of most cytokines is not confined to one cell type and thus it is difficult to identify the cellular sources that contribute to their plasma levels [46–48]. The technique of intracellular cytokine staining [49] offers the possibility of evaluating the contribution of different cells to the production of cytokines in heterogeneous cell populations. Using this technique, it was possible to measure intracellular cytokines and cell surface markers simultaneously to identify specific subpopulations of human leukocytes and to characterize their cytokine production [50–55].

We evaluated the cytokine pattern of adaptive immune cells (CD4+ T-cells, CD8+ T-cells and B-cells), considering that this arm of the immune system is specially targeted during ageing. As expected, some cytokines, such as IL-10 produced by T-cells declined with ageing.

Table 2 Number of lymphocytes in peripheral blood of individuals from each age group

Age groups	Total lymphocytes (mean + SD)[a]
Newborn	2848 + 1725
Children	2984 + 1310
Adolescent	2180 + 678
Adult	2270 + 753
Middle aged	2553 + 658
Elderly	1324 + 515

[a]Numbers represent the total lymphocytes + standard deviation for each age group. Numbers of lymphocytes were obtained by blood count using an Abbott Cell-Dyn 1700 automatic analyzer

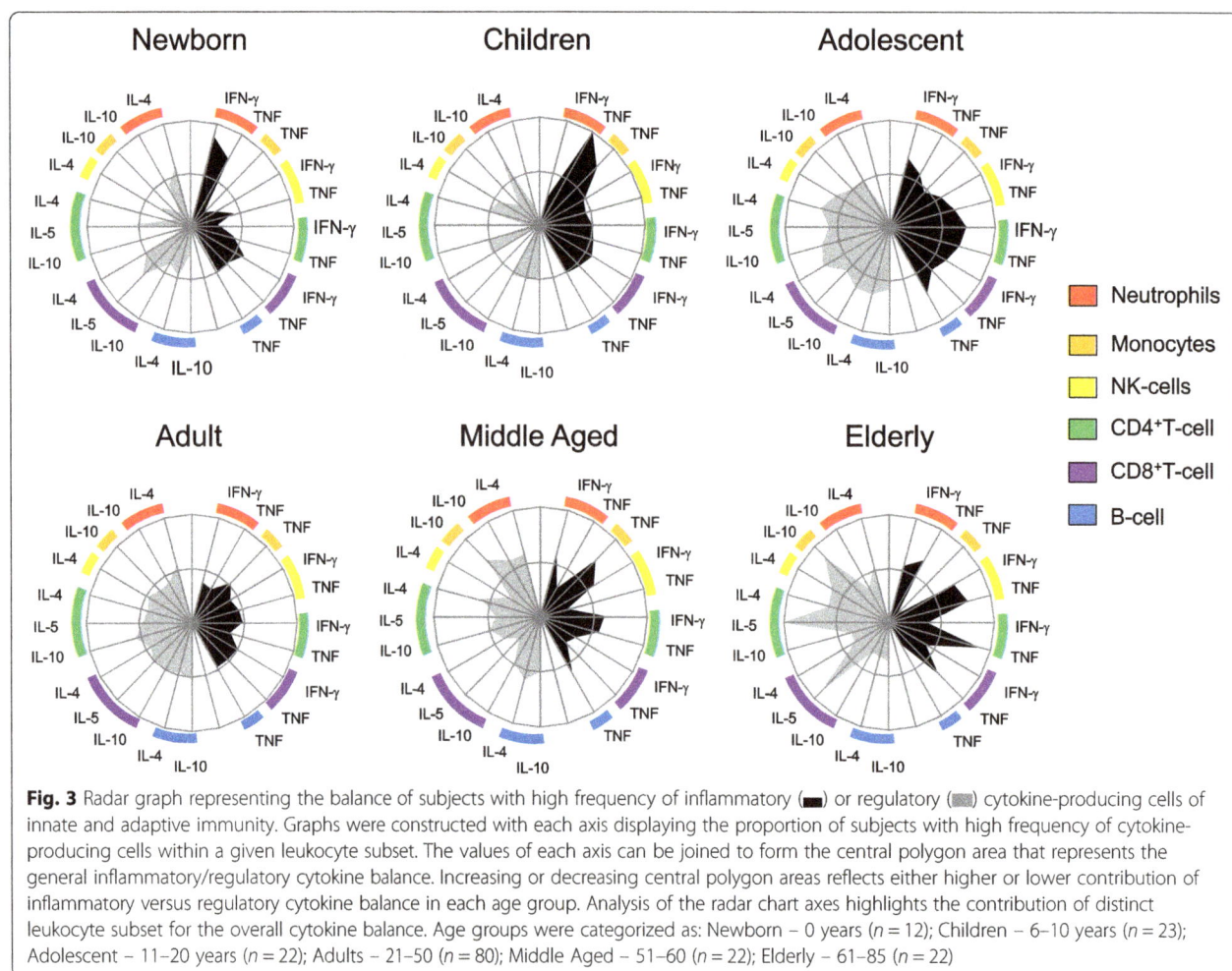

Fig. 3 Radar graph representing the balance of subjects with high frequency of inflammatory (■) or regulatory (▓) cytokine-producing cells of innate and adaptive immunity. Graphs were constructed with each axis displaying the proportion of subjects with high frequency of cytokine-producing cells within a given leukocyte subset. The values of each axis can be joined to form the central polygon area that represents the general inflammatory/regulatory cytokine balance. Increasing or decreasing central polygon areas reflects either higher or lower contribution of inflammatory versus regulatory cytokine balance in each age group. Analysis of the radar chart axes highlights the contribution of distinct leukocyte subset for the overall cytokine balance. Age groups were categorized as: Newborn – 0 years (n = 12); Children – 6–10 years (n = 23); Adolescent – 11–20 years (n = 22); Adults – 21–50 (n = 80); Middle Aged – 51–60 (n = 22); Elderly – 61–85 (n = 22)

However, production of TNF-α and IFN-γ by CD4+ T-cells and IL-5 produced by both CD4+ and CD8+ T-cells were unaffected. Our group demonstrated that the frequencies of T cells changes during ageing with maximum frequencies at the beginning of adulthood (19–40 years) and decreasing until elderly age. This is particularly observed for CD4+ T-cells. In contrast, the frequency of CD8+ T-cells is well preserved during ageing declining only in individuals at 41–65 and 61–75 age ranges [34]. Results obtained by Alberti and coworkers [8] from the analysis of 47 European subjects at different ages indicated that the percentage of IFN-γ+-positive CD4+ T-cells significantly decreased in old and nonagenarian individuals in comparison with young subjects while the percentage of TNF-α-positive activated/memory CD4+ T-cells significantly decreased in old subjects in comparison with young ones. Differences on the methodology, age ranges and genetic background of the population studied could explain these distinct findings.

Immunosenescence studies in humans have mainly focused on the impairment of the T-cell compartment.

However, changes are not limited to T-cells; B-cells have been studied as well. These cells showed a decreased production of TNF-α and IL-10 in adults and in the elderly group [12, 56, 57]. Our group has observed that frequencies of B-cells decline in Brazilian individuals of 19–40 age group and these data is compatible with the lower percentage of cytokine-positive B-cells in adulthood [34].

Although changes in T and B-cell functions were identified in healthy elderly, innate immune responses seem to be more resistant to age-associated changes [1]. NK-cells are one of the cellular mediators of innate defense and have been extensively studied in the elderly. The number and cytotoxicity activity of NK-cells are increased in healthy elderly and centenarians. Moreover, cumulative evidence in the last two decades supports the importance of NK-cell activity in maintaining good health during ageing. This is consistent with the well-preserved NK-cell cytotoxicity in centenarians fitting other criteria of healthy status such as physical fitness, independence to perform daily

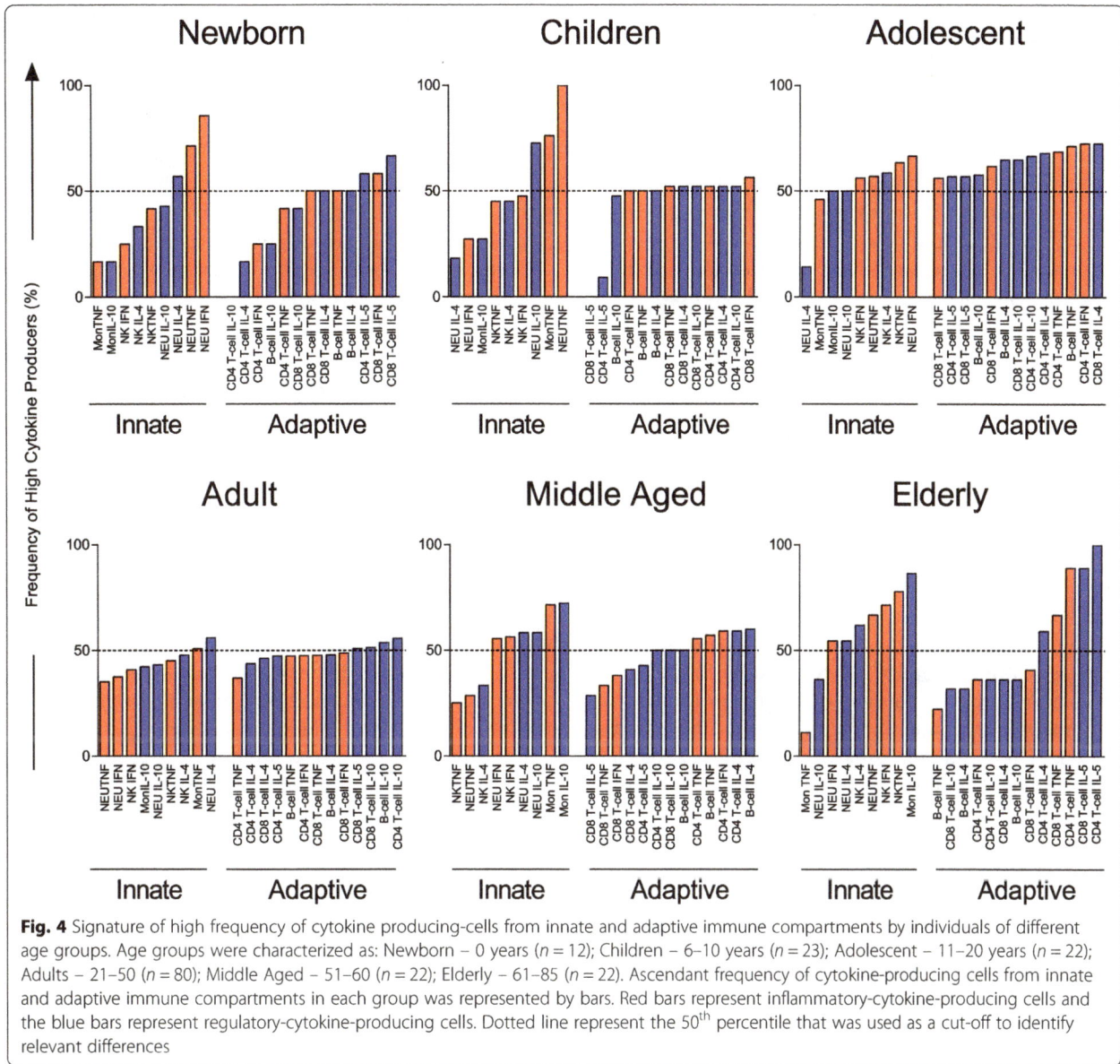

Fig. 4 Signature of high frequency of cytokine producing-cells from innate and adaptive immune compartments by individuals of different age groups. Age groups were characterized as: Newborn – 0 years (*n* = 12); Children – 6–10 years (*n* = 23); Adolescent – 11–20 years (*n* = 22); Adults – 21–50 (*n* = 80); Middle Aged – 51–60 (*n* = 22); Elderly – 61–85 (*n* = 22). Ascendant frequency of cytokine-producing cells from innate and adaptive immune compartments in each group was represented by bars. Red bars represent inflammatory-cytokine-producing cells and the blue bars represent regulatory-cytokine-producing cells. Dotted line represent the 50th percentile that was used as a cut-off to identify relevant differences

activities, or adequate cognitive function [18, 21, 23, 24]. Our group reported a significant increase in frequency of CD16+ IFN-γ+ NK-cells in non-infected individuals who inhabit schistosomiasis endemic areas of Brazil, and these cells are maintained at higher frequency in subjects over 70 years old. This suggests that the healthy individuals (who remain non-infected in endemic areas) are those who sustain a high frequency of IFN-γ+ NK-cells as they age [22]. In accordance with that, our results demonstrated that healthy ageing was related to a higher frequency of NK-cells that produce both a type 1 (IFN-γ) cytokine, and a counterbalancing type 2 (IL-4) cytokine.

Other innate immune cells seem to have a role in the immune-senescence process. Cellular components of the innate immune system, including neutrophils and macrophages, are the first to arrive at the site of injury. Their role is to initiate an inflammatory response, phagocyte the pathogen (in case of infection), recruit NK-cells, and facilitate the maturation and migration of dendritic cells (DCs) that regulate and determine the nature of the T-cell-mediated outcome [18]. Interestingly, frequencies of TNF-α-, IFN-gamma- and IL-4-producing neutrophils decreased from birth to adulthood and were maintained until senescence. On the other hand, frequency of TNF-α+ monocytes had a high plateau at childhood and decrease only at senescence. Of note, at this life stage, the reduced frequency of IL-10 production by adaptive immune cells was counter-balanced by an increase in the frequencies of IL-10+ cells from the innate compartment (neutrophils and monocytes).

Production of cytokines and their sources should not be evaluated alone during a complex process such as immunosenescence. The immune response is the result of several events that involves recruitment of cells, production of cytokines and chemotactic factors, establishment of immunoregulatory and proinflammatory factors. In this context, we performed a cytokine profile to assess a global picture of the immune response during the ageing process. This kind of analysis took into account the importance of the environment to an efficient immune response. This alternative strategy has been used by our group in a previous study [38], and it proved to be a useful tool to understand some of the complex immunological changes occurring during ageing.

Another important aspect of this study was the inclusion of a group of children. The childhood represents a critical period of immune development and there is a lack of data on the distributions of immunological parameters in healthy children [58]. We demonstrated that newborns had a high frequency of IL-5-producing T-cells, while neutrophils producing type 1 cytokines predominated in the innate immune compartment, a profile that remained in children. Exposure to an increasingly diverse range of antigens during the first years of life could be responsible for the environmentally driven type 1 response observed in the childhood period [59, 60]. These changes seem to promote a healthier immune profile, considering that failure in suppressing exacerbated type 2 immune responses and decreased capacity in producing type 1 cytokines during infancy are characteristic of individuals prone to develop allergic diseases [59–61].

Adolescents (11 to 20 years of age) presented an immunological profile characterized by balanced frequencies of adaptive cells able to produce both proinflammatory and regulatory cytokines. Adequate exposure to environmental antigens during infancy and the rise in sex hormones could explain the change into a robust and balanced immune profile with a predominant contribution of cytokine-producing adaptive immune cells in these individuals.

The immune system reached equilibrium in adulthood, when the cytokine profile was characterized by a balance contribution of innate and adaptive compartments to the production of both inflammatory and regulatory cytokines. Observing the overall cytokine production in individuals from the 25–51 age (Middle Aged) group, one could notice that it can be already observed a decline in cytokine production by adaptive immune cells and an expansion of the contribution of innate cells to cytokine secretion. It is widely accepted that T cells are specially targeted during immunosenescence. A number of factors have been linked to the decline in T-cell function with ageing. Age-related

thymic atrophy, decreased output of naïve T-cells and the resulting memory-type oligoclonal T-cell repertoire are of particular importance. All these changes are progressive and start at different time points of adulthood [15–17, 33].

As individuals age, major immunological events such as T-cell activation and cytokine production are progressively altered. Interestingly, in all analyses performed, the elderly group presented a balanced profile between regulatory and proinflammatory cytokines, with a prominent contribution of innate immune cells to this balance. Our results support the hypothesis that healthy immunosenescence involves remodeling and adaptation to the changes started in adulthood and aggravated by ageing [32, 33].

Conclusions

Taken together, our results showed a distinct pattern of changes in cytokine production by different leukocyte subsets during ageing. Furthermore, healthy ageing in this Brazilian population seems to involve alternative mechanisms to maintain an appropriate balance between regulatory and proinflammatory responses with well-preserved innate immunological activities compensating the impaired adaptive immune response at senescence.

The present study has limitations that should be acknowledged. First, we did not used Body Mass Index (BMI), body composition or nutritional behavior for this analysis, due to the unavailability of tools at the time of blood collection. Second, a small number of individuals was used preventing a definitive proposal of these profiles as representative of Brazilian individuals in general. One positive aspect about our cohort, however, is that the individuals are from the state of Minas Gerais, which is considered by demographic standards the most representative of the Brazilian population [62]. Therefore, despite the limitations, this study presents also important strengths. It is the first report describing changes in the profile of cytokine-producing leukocytes in Brazilian individuals within a large spectrum of age (0–85 years). These findings are an extension of another study from our group [34] that analyzed the frequency of sub-populations of leukocytes in Brazilian individuals at similar age range (0–85 years).

Data presented here may help to establish immunological reference values for future studies in Brazilian individuals at all ages. Longitudinal studies may reveal in more detail the role of innate immune cells in the elderly. Due to the progressive increase in the aged population in Brazil, these studies are critical for design and implementation of public policies aimed to optimize immune function and to improve the quality of life at advanced age.

Additional files

Additional file 1: Figure S1. Representative scatter distribution of cytokine-producing cell subsets from the innate immunity compartment of peripheral blood. Overall distribution of cytokine + neutrophils, monocytes (CD14+) and NK-cells (CD16+) was plotted as a function of age (ranging from 0 to 85). Age ranges were established based on the overall variation rhythm observed, considering the moving mean of all cytokine+ cell subsets (continuous lines). The selected age ranges were referred as: Newborn – 0 years; Children – 6–10 years; Adolescent – 11–20 years; Adults – 21–50 years; Middle Aged – 51–60 years and Elderly – 61–85 years. Dashed rectangles were used to

Additional file 2: Figure S2. Representative scatter distribution of cytokine-producing cell subsets from the adaptive immunity compartment of peripheral blood. The overall distribution of cytokine + T-cells (CD4+ and CD8+) and B-cells (CD19+) was plotted as a function of age (ranging from 0 to 85). Age ranges were established based on the overall variation rhythm observed, considering the moving mean of all cytokine + cell subsets (continuous lines). The selected age ranges were referred as: Newborn – 0 years; Children – 6–10 years; Adolescent – 11–20 years; Adults – 21–50 years; Middle Aged – 51–60 years and Elderly – 61–85 years. Dashed rectangles were used to

Abbreviations

IFN-γ: Interferon gamma; IL-10: Interleukin 10; IL-4: Interleukin 4; NK-cells: Natural killer cells; TNF-α: Tumor necrosis factor alpha

Acknowledgments

Not applicable.

Funding

This study was financially supported by a grant from Fundação de Amparo à Pesquisa do Estado de Minas Gerais, FAPEMIG (APQ-03593-13). Some of the authors are recipients of research fellowships (A.T.-C., R.C.-O., A.M.C.F., O.A.M.-F.) and a PhD scholarship (G.S.-N.) from Conselho de Desenvolvimento Científico e Tecnológico, CNPq, Brazil.

Authors' contributions

GS-N analysed, interpreted the data and was a major contributor in writing the manuscript; ES analysed and interpreted the data; AT-C coordinated the flow cytometry analysis of all data and was a major contributor to analyse and interpret the data; DMV-A and RS-A collected blood and performed flow cytometry analysis in samples from adult individuals; TF-S and MLS collected and analysed blood samples from children; VP-M, DGC, GEB-M, GMC and EBS collected blood samples, performed hematological, biochemical tests and flow cytometry analyses in samples from
individuals over 60; SME-S, RT, DMQ and RC-O coordinated study teams responsible for recruitment and sample collection as well as contribute with the analysis of the data; AMCF and OAM-F coordinated the study, analysed and interpreted the data and were major contributors in writing the manuscript. All authors read and approved the manuscript.

Competing interests

The authors declare that they have no competing interests.

Author details

[1]Departamento de Bioquímica e Imunologia, Instituto de Ciências Biológicas, Universidade Federal de Minas Gerais, Avenida Antônio Carlos 6627, Belo Horizonte, Minas Gerais 31270-901, Brazil. [2]Laboratório de Biomarcadores de Diagnóstico e Monitoração, Centro de Pesquisas René Rachou, FIOCRUZ, Belo Horizonte, Brazil. [3]Faculdade de Medicina, Universidade Federal de Minas Gerais, Belo Horizonte, Brazil. [4]Laboratório de Imunologia Celular e Molecular, Centro de Pesquisas René Rachou, FIOCRUZ, Belo Horizonte, Brazil. [5]Laboratório de Pesquisas Clínicas, Centro de Pesquisas René Rachou, FIOCRUZ, Belo Horizonte, Brazil. [6]Departamento de Farmácia, Universidade Federal dos Vales do Jequitinhonha e Mucuri, Diamantina, Minas Gerais, Brazil. [7]Maternidade Odete Valadares/Fundação Hospitalar do Estado de Minas Gerais (FHEMIG), Belo Horizonte, Brazil.

References

1. Cossarizza A, Ortolani C, Monti D, Franceschi C. Cytometric analysis of immunosenescence. Cytometry. 1997;27(4):297–313.
2. Franceschi C, Bonafe M, Valensin S, Olivieri F, De Luca M, Ottaviani E, De Benedictis G. An evolutionary perspective in immunosenescence. Ann NY Acad Sci. 2000;908:244–54.
3. Fülöp T, Dupuis G, Witkowski JM, Larbi A. The role of immunosenescence in the development of age-related diseases. Rev Invest Clin. 2016;68(2):84–91.
4. Franceschi C, Monti D, Barbieri D, Grassilli E, Troiano L, Salvioli S, Negro P, Capri M, Guido M, Azzi R, Sansoni P, Paganelli R, Fagiolo U, Baggio G, Donazzan S, Mariotti S, D'addato S, Gaddi A, Ortolani C, Cossarizza A. Immunosenescence in humans: deterioration or remodelling. Intern Rev Immunol. 1995;12:57–74.
5. Gerli R, Monti D, Bistoni O, Mazzone AM, Peri G, Cossarizza A, Di Gioacchino M, Cesarotti ME, Doni A, Mantovani A, Franceschi C, Paganelli R. Chemokines, sTNF-Rs and sCD30 serum levels in healthy aged people and centenarians. Mech Ageing Dev. 2000;121(1–3):37–46.
6. Franceschi C, Valensin S, Bonafe M, Paolisso G, Yashin AI, Monti D, De Benedictis G. The network and the remodeling theories of aging: historical background and new perspectives. Exp Gerontol. 2000;35:879–96.
7. Bruunsgaard H, Andersen-Ranberg K, Hjelmborg JB, Pedersen BK, Jeune B. Elevated levels of tumor necrosis factor alpha and mortality in centenarians. Am J Med. 2003;11:278–83.
8. Alberti S, Cevenini E, Ostan R, Capri M, Salvioli S, Bucci L, Ginaldi L, De Martinis M, Franceschi C, Monti D. Age-dependent modifications of type 1 and type 2 cytokines within virgin and memory CD4+ T cells in humans. Mech Ageing Dev. 2006;127(6):560–6.
9. Hobbs MV, Weigle WO, Noonan DJ, Torbett B, McEvilly E, Koch RJ, Cardenas GJ, Ernst DN. Patterns of cytokine gene expression by CD4+ T cells from young and old mice. J Immunol. 1993;150:3602–14.
10. Albright JW, Zuiga-Pflcker JC, Albright JF. Transcriptional control of IL-2 and IL-4 in T cells of young and old mice. Cell Immunol. 1995;164:170–5.
11. Shearer GM. Th1/Th2 changes in ageing. Mech Ageing Dev. 1997;94:1–5.
12. Franceschi C, Monti D, Barbieri D, Salvioli S, Grassilli E, Capri M, Troiano L, Guido M, Bonafè M, Tropea F, Salomoni P, Benatti F, Bellesia E, Macchioni S, Anderlini R, Sansoni P, Mariotti S, Wratten ML, Tetta C, Cossarizza A. Successful immunosenescence and the remodelling of immune responses with ageing. Nephrol Dial Transplant. 1996;11 Suppl 9:18–25.
13. Globerson A, Effros RB. Ageing of lymphocytes and lymphocytes in the aged. Immunol Today. 2000;21(10):515–21.
14. Pawelec G. Hallmarks of human "immunosenescence": adaptation or dysregulation? Immun Ageing. 2012;9(1):15.
15. Akbar AN, Fletcher JM. Memory T cell homeostasis and senescence during aging. Curr Opin Immunol. 2005;17(5):480–5.
16. Malaguarnera L, Ferlito L, Imbesi RM, Gulizia GS, Di Mauro S, Maugeri D, Malaguarnera M, Messina A. Immunosenescence: a review. Arch Gerontol Geriatr. 2001;32(1):1–14.
17. Pawelec G, Solana R. Immunoageing - the cause or effect of morbidity. Trends Immunol. 2001;22(7):348–9.
18. Solana R, Graham P, Raquel T. Aging and innate immunity. Immunity. 2006;24(5):491–4.
19. Solana R, Tarazona R, Gayoso I, Lesur O, Dupuis G, Fulop T. Innate immunosenescence: effect of aging on cells and receptors of the innate immune system in humans. Semin Immunol. 2012;24(5):331–41.
20. Pawelec G, Solana R, Remarque E, Mariani E. Impact of aging on innate immunity. J Leukoc Biol. 1998;64:703–12.
21. Sansoni P, Cossarizza A, Brianti V, Fagnoni F, Snelli G, Monti D, Marcato A, Passeri G, Ortolani C, Forti E, Fagiolo U, Passeri M, Franceschi C. Lymphocyte subsets and natural killer cell activity in healthy old people and centenarians. Blood. 1993;80:2767–73.
22. Speziali E, Bethony J, Martins-Filho O, Fraga LAO, Lemos DS, Souza LJ, Correa-Oliveira R, Faria AMC. Production of interferon-γ natural killer cells and aging in chronic human schistosomiasis. Mediat Inflamm. 2004;13(5/6):327–33.

23. Solana R, Alonso MC, Pena J. Natural killer cells in healthy aging. Exp Gerontol. 1999;34:435–43.

24. Solana R, Mariani E. NK and NK/T cells in human senescence. Vaccine. 2000;18:1613–20.

25. Lloberas J, Celada A. Effect of aging on macrophage function. Exp Geront. 2002;37:1325–31.

26. Renshaw M, Rockwell J, Engleman C, Gewirtz A, Katz J, Sambhara S. Cutting edge: impaired toll-like receptor expression and function in aging. J Immunol. 2002;169:4697–701.

27. Villanueva JL, Solana R, Alonso MC, Pena J. Changes in the expression of HLA-class II antigens on peripheral blood monocytes from aged humans. Dis Markers. 1990;8:85–91.

28. Herrero C, Marques L, Lloberas J, Celada A. IFN gamma-dependent transcription of MHC class II IA is impaired in macrophages from aged mice. J Clin Invest. 2001;107:485–93.

29. Plowden J, Renshaw-Hoelscher M, Engleman C, Katz J, Sambhara S. Innate immunity in aging: impact on macrophage function. Aging Cell. 2004;3:161–7.

30. Fulop T, Larbi A, Douziech N, Fortin C, Guerard KP, Lesur O, Khalil A, Dupuis G. Signal transduction and functional changes in neutrophils with aging. Aging Cell. 2004;3:217–26.

31. Larbi A, Franceschi C, Mazzatti D, Solana R, Wikby A, Pawelec G. Aging of the immune system as a prognostic factor for human longevity. Physiology (Bethesda). 2008;23:64–74.

32. De Martinis M, Franceschi C, Monti D, Ginaldi L. Inflamm-ageing and lifelong antigenic load as major determinants of ageing rate and longevity. FEBS Lett. 2005;579(10):2035–9.

33. Pawelec G, Barnett Y, Forsey R, Frasca D, Globerson A, McLeod J, Caruso C, Franceschi C, Fulop T, Gupta S, Mariani E, Mocchegiani E, Solana R. T cells and aging. Update. Front Biosci. 2002;7:d1056–183.

34. Faria AM, de Moraes SM, de Freitas LH, Speziali E, Soares TF, Figueiredo-Neves SP, Vitelli-Avelar DM, Martins MA, Barbosa KV, Soares EB, Sathler-Avelar R, Peruhype-Magalhães V, Cardoso GM, Comin F, Teixeira R, Elói-Santos SM, Queiroz DM, Corrêa-Oliveira R, Bauer ME, Teixeira-Carvalho A. Martins-Filho AO variation rhythms of lymphocyte subsets during healthy aging. Neuroimmunomodulation. 2008;15(4–6):365–79.

35. Rajilić-Stojanović M, Heilig HGHJ, Molenaar D, Kajander K, Surakka A, Smidt H, De Vos WM. Development and application of the human intestinal tract chip, a phylogenetic microarray: analysis of universally conserved phylotypes in the abundant microbiota of young and elderly adults. Environ Microbiol. 2009;11(7):1736–51.

36. Biagi E, Nylund L, Candela M, Ostan R, Bucci L, Pini E, Nikkila J, Monti D, Satokari R, Franceschi C, Brigidi P, De Vos W. Through ageing, and beyond: gut microbiota and inflammatory status in seniors and centenarians. PLoS One. 2010;5(5):e10667.

37. Gardner EM, Murasko DM. Age-related changes in type 1 and type 2 cytokine production in humans. Biogerontology. 2002;3(5):271–90.

38. Luiza-Silva M, Campi-Azevedo AC, Batista MA, Martins MA, Avelar RS, Da Silveira LD, Bastos Camacho LA, De Menezes MR, De Lourdes De Sousa MM, Guedes Farias RH, Da Silva FM, Galler R, Homma A, Leite Ribeiro JG, Campos Lemos JA, Auxiliadora-Martins M, Eloi-Santos SM, Teixeira-Carvalho A, Martins-Filho OA. Cytokine signatures of innate and adaptive immunity in 17DD yellow fever vaccinated children and its association with the level of neutralizing antibody. J Infect Dis. 2011; 204(6):873–83.

39. Hirsch EC, Breidert T, Rousselet E, Hunot S, Hartmann A, Michel PP. The role of glial reaction and inflammation in Parkinson's disease. Ann N Y Acad Sci. 2003;991:214–28.

40. Muñoz-Valle JF, Oregón-Romero E, Rangel-Villalobos H, Martínez-Bonilla GE, Castañeda-Saucedo E, Salgado-Goytia L, Leyva-Vázquez MA, Illades-Aguiar B, Alarcón-Romero LDC, Espinoza-Rojo M, Parra-Rojas I. High expression of TNF alpha is associated with −308 and −238 TNF alpha polymorphisms in knee osteoarthritis. Clin Exp Med. 2014;14(1):61–7.

41. Wojdasiewicz P, Poniatowski ŁA, Szukiewicz D. The role of inflammatory and anti-inflammatory cytokines in the pathogenesis of osteoarthritis. Mediators Inflamm. 2014;2014:561459.

42. Saito S. Cytokine network at the feto-maternal interface. J Reprod Immunol. 2000;47(2):87–103.

43. Gomes-Santos AC, Moreira TG, Castro-Junior AB, Horta BC, Lemos L, Cruz DN, Guimarães MA, Cara DC, McCafferty DM, Faria AM. New insights into the immunological changes in IL-10-deficient mice during the course of spontaneous inflammation in the gut mucosa. Clin Dev Immunol. 2012;2012:560817.

44. Lissauer D, Eldershaw SA, Inman CF, Coomarasamy A, Moss PA, Kilby MD. Progesterone promotes maternal-fetal tolerance by reducing human maternal T-cell polyfunctionality and inducing a specific cytokine profile. Eur J Immunol. 2015;45(10):2858–72.

45. Müller L, Pawelec G. Aging and immunity - impact of behavioral intervention. Brain Behav Immun. 2014;39:8–22.

46. Zanni F, Vescovini R, Biasini C, Fagnoni F, Zanlari L, Telera A, Di Pede P, Passeri G, Pedrazzoni M, Passeri M, Franceschi C, Sansoni P. Marked increase with age of type 1 cytokines within memory and effector/cytotoxic CD8+ T cells in humans: a contribution to understand the relationship between inflammation and immunosenescence. Exp Gerontol. 2003;38(9):981–7.

47. Franceschi C, Olivieri F, Marchegiani F, Cardelli M, Cavallone L, Capri M, Salvioli S, Valensin S, De Benedictis G, Di Iorio A, Caruso C, Prolisso G, Monti D. Genes involved in immune response/inflammation, IGF1/insulin pathway and response to oxidative stress play a major role in the genetics of human longevity: the lesson of centenarians. Mech Ageing Dev. 2005;126(2):351–61.

48. Testa R, Olivieri F, Bonfigli AR, Sirolla C, Boemi M, Marchegiani F, Marra M, Cenerelli S, Antonicelli R, Dolci A, Paolisso G, Franceschi C. Interleukin-6-174 G > C polymorphism affects the association between IL-6 plasma levels and insulin resistance in type 2 diabetic patients. Diabetes Res Clin Pract. 2006;71(3):299–305.

49. Collins DP, Luebering BJ, Shout DM. T-lymphocytes functionality assessed by analysis of cytokine receptor expression, intracellular cytokine expression and femtomolar detection of cytokine secretion by quantitative flow cytometry. Cytometry. 1998;33(2):249–55.

50. Jung T, Schauer U, Heusser C, Neumann C, Rieger C. Detection of intracellular cytokines by flow cytometry. J Immunol Meth. 1993;26:197–207.

51. Prussin C. Cytokine flow cytometry understanding cytokine biology at the single cell level. J Clin Immunol. 1997;17:195–203.

52. Prussin C, Metcalfe DD. Detection of intracytoplasmic cytokine using flow cytometry and directly conjugated anti-cytokine antibodies. J Immunol Methods. 1995;188(1):117–28.

53. Rostaing L, Tkaczuk J, Durand M, Peres C, Durand D, de Préval C, Ohayon E, Abbal M. Kinetics of intracytoplasmic Th1 and Th2 cytokine production assessed by flow cytometry following in vitro activation of peripheral blood mononuclear cells. Cytometry. 1999;35(4):318–28.

54. Moreira ML, Dorneles EM, Soares RP, Magalhães CP, Costa-Pereira C, Lage AP, Teixeira-Carvalho A, Martins-Filho OA, Araújo MS. Cross-reactivity of commercially available anti-human monoclonal antibodies with canine cytokines: establishment of a reliable panel to detect the functional profile of peripheral blood lymphocytes by intracytoplasmic staining. Acta Vet Scand. 2015;57:51.

55. Silveira AC, Santana MA, Ribeiro IG, Chaves DG, Martins-Filho OA. The IL-10 polarized cytokine pattern in innate and adaptive immunity cells contribute to the development of FVIII inhibitors. BMC Hematol. 2015;15(1):1.

56. Olsson J, Wikby A, Johansson B, Löfgren S, Nilsson BO, Ferguson FG. Age-related change in peripheral blood T-lymphocyte subpopulations and cytomegalovirus infection in the very old: the Swedish longitudinal OCTO immune study. Mech Ageing Dev. 2000;121(1–3):187–201.

57. Potestio M, Pawelec G, Di Lorenzo G, Candore G, D'Anna C, Gervasi F, Lio D, Tranchida G, Caruso C, Romano GC. Age-related changes in the expression of CD95 (APO1/FAS) on blood lymphocytes. Exp Gerontol. 1999;34(5):659–73.

58. Duramad P, Tager IB, Holland NT. Cytokines and other immunological biomarkers in children's environmental health studies. Toxicol Lett. 2007;172(1–2):48–59.

59. Prescott SL, Macaubas C, Smallacombe T, Holt BJ, Sly PD, Holt PG. Development of allergen-specific T-cell memory in atopic and normal children. Lancet. 1999;353(9148):196–200.

60. Tulic MK, Hodder M, Forsberg A, McCarthy S, Richman T, D'Vaz N, van den Biggelaar AH, Thornton CA, Prescott SL. Differences in innate immune function between allergic and nonallergic children: new insights into immune ontogeny. J Allergy Clin Immunol. 2011;127(2):470–8.

61. Yabuhara A, Macaubas C, Prescott SL, Venaille TJ, Holt BJ, Habre W, Sly PD, Holt PG. TH2-polarized immunological memory to inhalant allergens in atopics is established during infancy and early childhood. Clin Exp Allergy. 1997;27(11):1261–9.

62. De Carvalho JA, Garcia RA. The aging process in the Brazilian population: a demographic approach. Cad Saude Publica. 2003;19(3):725–33.

Higher plasma levels of complement C3a, C4a and C5a increase the risk of subretinal fibrosis in neovascular age-related macular degeneration

Complement activation in AMD

Judith Lechner, Mei Chen, Ruth E. Hogg, Levente Toth, Giuliana Silvestri, Usha Chakravarthy and Heping Xu*ⓘ

Abstract

Background: The aim of this study was to investigate the plasma levels of complement C3a, C4a, and C5a in different types of neovascular age-related macular degeneration (nAMD) and whether the levels were related to patients' responsiveness to anti-VEGF therapy.

Results: Ninety-six nAMD patients (including 61 with choroidal neovascularisation (CNV), 17 with retinal angiomatous proliferation (RAP), 14 with polypoidal choroidal vasculopathy (PCV) and 4 unclassified patients) and 43 controls were recruited to this case–control study. Subretinal fibrosis was observed in 45 nAMD patients and was absent in 51 nAMD patients. In addition, the responsiveness to anti-VEGF (Lucentis) therapy was also evaluated in nAMD patients. Forty-four patients were complete responders, 48 were partially responders, and only 4 patients did not respond to the therapy. The plasma levels of C3a, C4a and C5a were significantly higher in nAMD patients compared to controls. Further analysis of nAMD subgroups showed that the levels of C3a, C4a and C5a were significantly increased in patients with CNV but not RAP and PCV. Significantly increased levels of C3a, C4a and C5a were also observed in nAMD patients with subretinal fibrosis but not in those without subretinal fibrosis. Higher levels of C3a were observed in nAMD patients who responded partially to anti-VEGF therapy.

Conclusions: Our results suggest increased systemic complement activation in nAMD patients with CNV but not RAP and PCV. Our results also suggest that higher levels of systemic complement activation may increase the risk of subretinal fibrosis in nAMD patients.

Keywords: Age-related macular degeneration, Choroidal neovascularisation, Complement, Subretinal fibrosis

Background

Neovascular age-related macular degeneration (nAMD), or wet AMD, is the leading cause of blindness in the elderly population and is characterised by the growth of abnormal blood vessels in the macular region of the retina. There are different subtypes of nAMD and the most commonly encountered is choroidal neovascularisation (CNV) which is characterised by the infiltration of abnormal neovascular complexes into the space between the retinal pigment epithelium and Bruch's membrane or the subretinal space [1]. Neovascular complexes may also arise de novo from retinal vasculature known as retinal angiomatous proliferation (RAP) and these are known to fuse with CNV [2]. Another subtype of neovascularisation, polypoidal choroidal vasculopathy (PCV), is characterised by a branching vascular network arising from the choroid with polypoidal lesions underneath the RPE [3]. VEGF is elevated in eyes of nAMD

* Correspondence: heping.xu@qub.ac.uk
The Wellcome-Wolfson Institute of Experimental Medicine, Queen's University Belfast, 97 Lisburn Road, Belfast BT9 7BL, UK

patients and plays an important role in the neovascularisation process and vascular permeability in nAMD and intravitreal injection of anti-VEGF antibody is the standard care for nAMD [1].

The pathogenesis of AMD is complex and incompletely understood with genetic as well as clinical and environmental factors (such as age, family history of AMD, cardiovascular disease, body mass index and cigarette smoking) known to influence the risk of developing this disease, however, the underlying mechanisms remain elusive [4–6]. Compelling evidence suggests that inflammation plays a critical role in the aetiology of AMD [7, 8] and a number of studies have specifically highlighted the role of the complement system in AMD. Many of the genetic variants that have been associated with AMD lie in genes involved in the complement cascade, including complement factor H (CFH) [9], complement component 3 (C3) [10], complement component 2 (C2) and complement factor B (CFB) [11]. A number of studies have shown increased levels of complement expression in the maculae of AMD patients [12, 13]. Complement fragments, including C3a and C5a [14], and the membrane attach complex (MAC or C5b-9) [15] were found in drusen of patients with AMD as well as complement activating proteins such as amyloid beta [16] and lipofuscin [17]. Besides the local complement activation in AMD, systemic complement activation has also been detected in patients with AMD. Increased serum levels of complement fragments (e.g. Ba, C3d) [18–20] and changes in the expression of complement regulatory proteins (e.g. CD46, CD59) [21] have been reported in AMD. Complement activation and accumulation of MAC has been found in choriocapillaris, which are part of the systemic circulation, during normal aging and especially in patients with AMD [22]. It is clear that uncontrolled or dysregulated complement activation may contribute to macular lesion development in AMD, which offers the opportunities for complement-targeted immune therapy. Indeed a number of complement inhibitors are in phase I, II and III clinical trials for AMD [23, 24]. In view of the diversity of AMD phenotype, it is likely that different immune mechanisms may be involved in different types of AMD, and this is exemplified by the diverse response to anti-VEGF therapy observed in various clinical studies [25]. Therefore, it is important to understand which type(s) of AMD is associated with uncontrolled complement activation.

The complement system can be activated through the classical pathway (CP), the mannose-binding lectin (MBL) pathway and the alternative pathway (AP) [26]. Complement fragments C3a and C5a can be generated by any of these activation pathways, whereas C4a is generated when the CP or MBL pathway is activated.

Elevated levels of these complement fragments are indicatives of increased complement activation. In this study, we measured the plasma levels of C3a, C4a and C5a in nAMD patients and correlated the expression levels with clinical presentations as well as the responsiveness to anti-VEGF therapy. Ninety-six nAMD patients (including 61 CNV, 17 RAP, 14 PCV and 4 unclassified patients) and 43 controls were recruited to this case–control study.

Results

Clinical evaluation

Of the 139 study participants, 43 were controls and 96 had diagnosed nAMD. Despite our efforts to recruit age matched controls, there was a significant difference in age between controls and nAMD patients ($P = 0.002$) as shown in Table 1. There were no significant differences regarding gender distribution, family history of AMD, history of cardiovascular disease, history of hypertension, history of diabetes, BMI and smoking habits between controls and nAMD patients. There were more patients taking vitamins and low-dose aspirin compared to controls ($P = 0.011$ and 0.001 respectively) (Table 1).

The average duration between the last anti-VEGF treatment and the day of blood collection was 140.1 ± 223.8 days (interquartile range: 42.0–127.0 days). No participant had received anti-VEGF treatment within 4 weeks prior to blood collection. The average number of anti-VEGF injections received per nAMD patient prior to blood collection was 16.1 ± 10.7 (interquartile range 8.3–21.8). There was no correlation between the number of anti-VEGF injections received and the concentration of C3a (Pearson's correlation coefficient (r) = 0.08; $P = 0.448$), C4a (r = −0.03; $P = 0.771$) and C5a (r = −0.16; $P = 0.131$) (see Additional file 1).

Complement fragments in nAMD patients and controls

All three complement fragments, C3a, C4a and C5a were significantly increased in nAMD patients compared to controls in the univariate analysis ($P < 0.001$, $P = 0.005$ and 0.049 respectively) and these associations remained significant in the multivariate analysis after correction for age and gender ($P = 0.001$, 0.012 and 0.045 respectively) (Table 2). In the nAMD group, C3a and C4a were significantly increased in those with a family history of AMD ($P = 0.058$ and 0.011 respectively) compared to those without a family history of AMD. The plasma level of C5a was not associated with a family history of AMD. Due to this association, we included the confounder "family history of AMD" in the multivariate analysis.

When comparing nAMD patients and controls, after including the confounder "family history of AMD" in

Table 1 Demographic and clinical characteristics of nAMD patients and controls

	All	Controls	nAMD	P value
	(n = 139)	(n = 43)	(n = 96)	nAMD vs Control
Age (median (range)), years	78.6 (53–93)	74.0 (58–92)	80.1 (53–93)	**0.002**[a]
Female (number (%))	63 (45)	19 (44)	44 (46)	1.000[b]
Family history of AMD (number (%))	32 (23)	6 (14)	26 (27)	0.127[b]
History of cardiovascular disease (number (%))	36 (26)	9 (21)	27 (28)	0.528[b]
History of hypertension (number (%))	81 (58)	23 (53)	58 (60)	0.576[b]
History of diabetes (number (%))	15 (11)	2 (5)	13 (14)	0.150[b]
Body Mass Index (mean ± SD)	26.1 ± 4.4	26.1 ± 5.1	26.0 ± 4.0	0.980[c]
Smoking status				0.381[b]
Non-smoker (number (%))	56 (40)	20 (47)	36 (38)	
Former smoker (number (%))	70 (50)	20 (47)	50 (52)	
Current smoker (number (%))	12 (9)	2 (5)	10 (10)	
Taking cardiovascular medication (number (%))	102 (73)	28 (65)	74 (77)	0.212[b]
Taking vitamins (number (%))	28 (20)	3 (7)	25 (26)	**0.011**[b]
Taking low-dose aspirin (number (%))	43 (31)	5 (12)	38 (40)	**0.001**[b]

[a]Mann Whitney U test
[b]Pearson's chi-square test
[c]Independent samples t-test
SD standard deviation
Bold P < 0.05

the multivariate analysis for C3a and C4a, the increase in C3a and C4a in the nAMD group remained significant ($P = 0.005$ and 0.031 respectively) as shown in Table 2. The concentrations of complement components were not associated with vitamin or low dose aspirin intake or any other confounders.

Complement fragments in patients with CNV, RAP and PCV

Out of the 96 nAMD participants, 61 had CNV, 17 with RAP, 14 with PCV and 4 were unknown. There were no significant differences in complement components when comparing between neovascular AMD subtypes, although there was a trend for higher C3a, C4a and C5a concentrations in those classified as CNV. On comparing subgroups of nAMD participants

with controls, there was a significant increase in C3a, C4a and C5a in those with CNV when compared to controls in the univariate analysis ($P < 0.001$, $P = 0.003$ and 0.044 respectively; Table 3) and these associations remained significant in the multivariate analysis after correction for age and gender as well as family history of AMD for C3a and C4a ($P = 0.001$, 0.009 and 0.008 respectively). There were no significant differences in the plasma levels of C3a, C4a, and C5a between RAP or PCV versus controls (Table 3).

Complement fragments and subretinal fibrosis

Subretinal fibrosis was present in 45 (47 %) of nAMD patients (Table 4). When comparing complement fragments in patients with and without fibrosis to controls, C3a was significantly increased in both groups compared to the

Table 2 C3a, C4a and C5a plasma levels in nAMD patients and controls

Variables (ng/ml)	Controls (mean ± SD) n = 43	nAMD (mean ± SD) n = 96	Univariate analysis P value nAMD vs Controls[a]	Multivariate analysis (age and gender) P value nAMD vs Controls[b]	Odds ratio	95 % confidence interval for odds ratio	Multivariate analysis (age, gender and family history of AMD) P value nAMD vs Controls[c]	Odds ratio	95 % confidence interval for odds ratio
C3a	11.95 ± 3.30	14.65 ± 4.48	**<0.001**	**0.001**	241.44	8.44–6910.14	**0.005**	140.67	4.53–4372.57
C4a	68.91 ± 33.23	108.48 ± 83.83	**0.005**	**0.012**	5.81	1.46–23.05	**0.031**	4.79	1.15–19.88
C5a	8.34 ± 2.05	9.43 ± 2.73	**0.049**	**0.045**	20.55	1.07–396.06			

[a]Independent samples t-test
[b]Multinomial logistic regression corrected for age and gender
[c]Multinomial logistic regression corrected for age, gender and family history of AMD
Bold P < 0.05
SD standard deviation

Table 3 Univariate analysis of C3a, C4a and C5a plasma levels in nAMD patients with CNV, RAP and PCV

Variables (ng/ml)	Controls (mean ± SD) n = 43	CNV (mean ± SD) n = 61	RAP (mean ± SD) n = 17	PCV (mean ± SD) n = 14	P value controls vs CNV vs RAP vs PCV[a]	P value Bonferroni post hoc test
C3a	11.95 ± 3.30	15.29 ± 4.29	14.15 ± 5.93	12.55 ± 2.86	**<0.001**	**<0.001**[b]
						0.609[c]
						1.000[d]
C4a	68.91 ± 33.23	118.16 ± 93.41	84.73 ± 55.07	96.51 ± 63.71	**0.004**	**0.003**[b]
						1.000[c]
						1.000[d]
C5a	8.34 ± 2.05	9.92 ± 2.81	8.10 ± 2.53	8.68 ± 1.95	**0.016**	**0.044**[b]
						1.000[c]
						1.000[d]

[a]One-way ANOVA
[b]Controls vs CNV
[c]Controls vs RAP
[d]Controls vs PCV
Bold P < 0.05
SD standard deviation

controls in the univariate analysis ($P = 0.046$ and <0.001 respectively; Table 4). After adjustment for age, gender and family history of AMD the difference in C3a between controls and patients with fibrosis remained highly significant ($P = 0.001$), whereas the difference between controls and patients without fibrosis was insignificant ($P = 0.055$). C4a was significantly increased in participants with fibrosis when compared to controls in the univariate ($P = 0.003$; Table 4) and multivariate analysis ($P = 0.010$). For C5a, the univariate analysis did not detect any significant differences between participants with or without fibrosis when compared to controls, however in the multivariate analysis there was a significant difference in C5a when comparing participants with fibrosis to controls ($P = 0.018$).

Complement fragments and responsiveness to anti-VEGF therapy

Of the 96 nAMD patients, 44 (46 %) responded completely to the anti-VEGF therapy, 48 (50 %) partially responded to the therapy and 4 patients (4 %) did not respond to the therapy. Due to the limited number of non-responders in this study, this group was not included in the statistical analysis. When comparing the concentration of plasma complement fragments between partial and complete responders, we found a significant increase in C3a in partial responders in the univariate analysis ($P = 0.041$; Table 5) and the difference remained significant in the multivariate analysis after correcting for age, gender and family history of AMD ($P = 0.033$). No significant differences in plasma levels of C4a and C5a were identified when

Table 4 Univariate analysis of C3a, C4a and C5a plasma levels in participants with nAMD with and without subretinal fibrosis

Variables (ng/ml)	Controls (mean ± SD) n = 43	Fibrosis absent (mean ± SD) n = 51	Fibrosis present (mean ± SD) n = 45	P value Fibrosis absent vs present[a]	P value Fibrosis absent vs present vs controls[b]	P value Bonferroni post hoc test
C3a	11.95 ± 3.30	13.68 ± 3.05	15.75 ± 5.51	0.051	**<0.001**	**0.046**[c]
						<0.001[d]
C4a	68.91 ± 33.23	93.95 ± 59.44	124.94 ± 103.14	0.102	**0.004**	0.258[c]
						0.003[d]
C5a	8.34 ± 2.05	9.14 ± 2.66	9.75 ± 2.80	0.343	0.088	

[a]Independent samples t-test
[b]One-way ANOVA
[c]Controls vs Fibrosis absent
[d]Controls vs fibrosis present
Bold P < 0.05
SD standard deviation

Table 5 Univariate analysis of C3a, C4a and C5a plasma levels in nAMD patients not responding, partially responding and completely responding to anti-VEGF Ab therapy

Variables (ng/ml)	Controls (mean ± SD)	Non responders (mean ± SD)	Partial responders (mean ± SD)	Complete responders (mean ± SD)	P value
	$n = 43$	$n = 4$	$n = 48$	$n = 44$	Partial vs complete responders[a]
C3a	11.95 ± 3.30	13.97 ± 3.94	15.61 ± 5.18	13.67 ± 3.45	**0.041**
C4a	68.91 ± 33.23	79.97 ± 75.52	120.85 ± 98.30	97.57 ± 64.80	0.147
C5a	8.34 ± 2.05	8.62 ± 2.47	9.31 ± 2.72	9.63 ± 2.80	0.654

[a]Independent samples t-test
Bold $P < 0.05$
SD standard deviation

comparing complete responders with partial responders as shown in Table 5. The response to anti-VEGF therapy was not associated with the presence of subretinal fibrosis ($P = 0.682$; Pearson's chi-square test).

Discussion

In the present study we report that complement fragments C3a, C4a and C5a are significantly elevated in the plasma of nAMD patients when compared to controls. Hence our results confirm previous findings of increased systemic complement activation in nAMD [18, 19]. The systemic levels of C3a, C4a and C5a in different types of nAMD (e.g. CNV, RAP, PCV and fibrosis) or in different anti-VEGF therapy responder groups have not been investigated before, and such studies are important as different immunomechanisms may be involved in different types of nAMD. In this study we found that higher plasma levels of C3a, C4a and C5a are associated with subretinal fibrosis and with CNV rather than RAP and PCV and that C3a was significantly increased in patients partially responding to anti-VEGF therapy.

How the complement system is activated in nAMD patients and how this may contribute to the development of nAMD is currently not well understood. Circulating complement fragments such as C3a and C5a may be recruited to the macula in AMD. Complement deposition (e.g., C3a, C5a, C5b-9) has been detected in RPE, Bruch's membrane and choroid of AMD eyes [27]. Studies conducted in patient samples as well as in animal models of laser-induced CNV have shown that complement activation may contribute to CNV development at multiple levels. The membrane attack complex (MAC), the final product of complement activation, may directly induce CNV. C3-deficient mice are unable to form MAC and do not develop CNV after laser photocoagulation. In the same study, CNV was suppressed by inhibition of MAC formation through blockage of C3 or C6 [28]. In addition, MAC can upregulate proangiogenic factors such as VEGF, TGF-β2, and β-FGF in retinal cells [28, 29]. Furthermore, the expression of MAC is increased in choriocapillaris of the aging

macula and the expression is further enhanced in patients with AMD [30].

Anaphylatoxins were also shown to be involved in experimental CNV. C3a and C5a were increased in the RPE/choroid after laser injury and blockage of C3a or C5a resulted in reduced CNV formation. CNV was reduced in mice deficient in C3a or C5a receptors or in mice treated with C3a or C5a receptor antagonist [14]. C3a and C5a were among the complement fragments detected in the RPE of nAMD patients and both can induce the expression of VEGF [14].

Systemic complement activation may also be involved in the activation of choroidal endothelial cells. C5a receptor was shown to be expressed in the endothelium of human choriocapillaris and treatment of human choroidal endothelial cells with C5a resulted in increased expression of ICAM-1, an intercellular adhesion molecule involved in leukocyte trafficking [31]. Furthermore, anaphylatoxins have been shown to be potent inflammatory mediators. Stimulation of human umbilical vein endothelial cells with C3a or C5a resulted in upregulation of pro-inflammatory cytokine production (e.g. IL-8 and IL-1β) [32]. C5a has been shown to promote IL-22 and IL-17 expression from human T-cells and both cytokines were shown to be increased in the serum of AMD patients [33]. In monocytes, C5a stimulation was shown to enhance LPS-induced production of IL-6 and TNFα [34]. Systemic complement activation may pre-condition leukocytes to a pro-inflammatory phenotype and may contribute to the local inflammatory responses in nAMD when recruited to the aging macula.

The role of C4a in nAMD development remains poorly elucidated [35] and deficiency of C4 did not affect CNV formation following laser photocoagulation in mice [36]. Nevertheless, in the present study we detected elevated plasma levels of C4a in nAMD patients, particularly in patients with CNV and in patients with subretinal fibrosis. Further studies are necessary to investigate the role of C4a in the pathogenesis of nAMD.

Subretinal fibrosis is a common finding in patients with late stage nAMD leading to considerable impairment of visual function although the underlying mechanisms remain poorly defined [1]. In this study we report significantly elevated plasma levels of C3a, C4a and C5a in patients with subretinal fibrosis. Systemic alterations in the complement system have previously been linked to subretinal fibrosis in nAMD. Singh et al. found reduced expression of complement regulatory protein CD46, which inhibits the production of C5a, on peripheral lymphocytes in nAMD patients with subretinal fibrosis [21]. C5a has been implicated in the development of fibrosis in a mouse model of chronic pancreatitis, where loss of C5 or injection of a C5a-receptor antagonist significantly reduced the level of pancreatic fibrosis [37]. Our results suggest uncontrolled complement activation and the formation of anaphylatoxins such as C3a, C4a and C5a may contribute to the development of subretinal fibrosis in nAMD and further studies are necessary to understand the detailed mechanisms.

We observed increased plasma C3a levels in patients partially responding to the anti-VEGF therapy when compared to patients completely responding to the therapy, suggesting C3a plasma level may be a biomarker in predicting outcomes to treatment. Biological plausibility for such an association exists in that C3a can induce the expression of other pro-angiogenic factors including IL-8 [38] which may explain why patients with increased levels of C3a respond less well to the anti-VEGF treatment. Furthermore, a SNP in the C3 gene has previously been linked to reduced central retinal thickness following anti-VEGF treatment [39], although subsequent studies have failed to replicate these findings [40]. Polymorphisms of complement factor H, C2 as well as interleukins IL-6 and IL-10 or VEGF genes are known to be linked to nAMD risk and may affect the pathogenesis of the disease [41]. These additional factors might also contribute to the responsiveness to anti-VEGF therapy [41].

Why C3a but not C4a and C5a is associated with responsiveness to anti-VEGF therapy is not known. The complement system can be activated through at least three pathways i.e., the CP, AP, and MBL pathway. C3a is generated when any of the pathways is activated, whereas the generation of C4a is restricted to the CP or MBL pathway and C5a to the terminal pathway. In addition, a recent study has shown that C3 can be cleaved into C3a and C3b intracellularly by cathepsin L (i.e., independently of C3 convertase) [42]. Therefore, changes in plasma levels of C3a, C4a and C5a may not follow the same pattern. The serum levels of C3a were similar in complete and non-responders, although only 4 patients were recruited to the non-responder group. Nevertheless we contend that confirming our results in a larger patient cohort and exploring the temporal

associations between plasma levels of C3a and morphological changes after anti-VEGF therapy are likely to help elucidate the mechanisms of treatment responsiveness to these agents.

In this study, we also found significantly increased plasma levels of C3a, C4a and C5a in patients with CNV, but not RAP or PCV when compared to controls, suggesting that systemic complement activation may play a bigger role in CNV than in RAP or PCV. However, the results must be interpreted with caution as there were small numbers of participants in the RAP and PCV group ($n = 17$ and 14 respectively). Further studies using larger patient samples are necessary to confirm the results.

The strengths of the present study include independent grading of CNV type, fibrosis and anti-VEGF responsiveness, and systematic and extensive exploration of complement changes in different types of nAMD as well as in patients partially or completely responding to anti-VEGF treatment.

There are a number of limitations in the current study. Firstly, the number of controls enrolled in this study is relatively small and some of the analyses involved small groups of patients (i.e. patients with RAP $n = 17$, patients with PCV $n = 14$) with the attendant consequences of drawing conclusions based on small samples. Secondly, all participates were recruited from one location and the data only represent results from Northern Ireland population. Replication of the study findings in other locations and with much improved bigger numbers is necessary to confirm our results. Thirdly, there was a significant difference in age between nAMD patients and controls. Furthermore, patients were recruited at different times following diagnosis of nAMD. Consequently, some patients enrolled at an early stage of nAMD and classified as having no fibrosis, might still develop fibrosis during the course of the disease. Patients enrolled in this study were receiving anti-VEGF treatment prior to enrolment which may have altered systemic complement levels although there was no correlation with the number of anti-VEGF injections received and the levels of C3a, C4a or C5a. Furthermore the drug in use in our study site was ranibizumab which is cleared more rapidly from the systemic circulation and has the least effect on serum VEGF levels when compared to other anti VEGF agents [43]. Finally, the change of C3a and C5a in the whole study, while statistically significant, was small and the clinical and biological relevance of such a small difference warrants further investigations.

Conclusions

In this study, we have demonstrated systemic complement activation in nAMD, particularly in patients with

CNV or with subretinal fibrosis, and we have shown that higher plasma C3a levels are related to reduced responsiveness to anti-VEGF treatment. Our observations may have important implications in future management of nAMD. Complement inhibitors are currently in clinical trials for AMD [23, 24], and the identification of suitable patients is important for the success of this type of immune therapy. Our results provide evidence that nAMD patients with CNV and with subretinal fibrosis may benefit more from the complement inhibitor therapy compared to other subgroups of nAMD patients. Complement inhibitors may also be a supplement therapy for patients who partially respond to VEGF inhibitors.

Methods

Study participants

The study protocol was approved by the Research Ethics Committee of Queen's University Belfast and procedures were performed in accordance with the tenets of the Declaration of Helsinki on research into human volunteers. Participants were recruited from the macular disease clinics in Belfast (Belfast Health and Social Care Trust, UK) with written informed consent obtained from every participant. Spouses, relatives or friends who accompanied patients and who were confirmed to be without retinal disease (fundus photography and optical coherence tomography (OCT)) were recruited as controls. All participants were older than 50 years of age and structured questionnaires were used to ascertain a history of medical conditions, current medication, family history of AMD, smoking habits (current, ex-smoker, never smoker) and body mass index (BMI). Participants with systemic inflammatory or autoimmune disorders (e.g. patients with active rheumatoid arthritis or active chronic bronchitis), participants undergoing steroid therapy or chemotherapy were excluded from the study.

The diagnosis of nAMD was by clinical examination and confirmed by multimodal imaging consisting of fundus photography, autofluorescence, optical coherence tomography, fluorescein angiography and Indocyanine green angiography. Participants were further subcategorised into CNV, RAP and PCV. Responsiveness to treatment was defined based on the participant achieving a fluid free macula at any stage during follow up. Participants were classified into the following 3 categories: Complete responder: Resolution of leakage at any point in time during follow up; Partial responder: Exhibiting dependence on VEGF inhibitors but a fluid free macula never achieved; Non responder: No morphological improvement or worsening.

Sample collection

In this study most of the participants were receiving anti-VEGF therapy prior to enrolment. The number of anti-VEGF (ranibizumab, trade name Lucentis, Genentech, San Francisco, CA) injections received by each patient prior to blood collection was ascertained from the medical records. Peripheral blood samples were drawn in tubes containing ethylenediaminetetraacetic acid (EDTA) as an anticoagulant between 9:00 and 12:00 am and processed within three hours. The plasma was separated from the whole blood by centrifugation for 10 min at $300\,g$. The plasma fraction was collected and centrifuged again for 10 min at $2000\,g$ to remove any residual cells and platelets before it was aliquoted and stored at $-80\,°C$ until analysis.

Cytometric bead array

Complement fragments C3a, C4a and C5a were measured in the plasma by Cytometric Bead Array using a Human Anaphylatoxin Kit (BD Biosciences, Oxford, UK) according to the manufacturer's instructions. In order to avoid spontaneous complement activation, plasma samples were thawed rapidly at 37 °C until just thawed and immediately transferred to ice. Plasma samples were diluted 1:20 with assay diluent prior to analysis.

Briefly, capture beads were mixed and incubated with diluted plasma samples and standards for 2 h at room temperature. After the incubation, samples were washed with wash buffer and incubated with anaphylatoxin PE detection reagent for 1 h at room temperature protected from light. After another washing step, samples were resuspended in wash buffer and fluorescence intensities were measured by flow cytometry (FACS CANTO II; BD Biosciences). Concentrations were calculated using the FCAP Array software version 3.0 (BD Biosciences, Oxford, UK).

Statistical analysis

Statistical analysis was performed using the Statistical Package for the Social Sciences, Windows version 21 (SPSS Inc, Armonk, NY). Categorical demographic and clinical data were compared using Pearson's chi-square test. The distribution of continuous variables was assessed for normality using the Kolmogorov-Smirnov test and logarithmic transformation was performed if necessary to achieve normal distribution. Normally distributed continuous samples were then compared using the Independent samples t-test or one-way ANOVA. Age was not normally distributed and the difference between controls and nAMD patients was analysed using the Mann–Whitney U test.

For the associations that were significant in the univariate analysis, multinomial logistic regression was performed to adjust for age and gender. All variables were also tested for association with family history of AMD, history of cardiovascular disease, history of hypertension, history of diabetes, smoking habits, BMI, taking of cardiovascular medication, vitamins and low-dose aspirin using the Independent samples *t*-test, one-way ANOVA or Pearson's correlation. If significant associations were identified, adjustments were made in the multinomial logistic regression analysis. Pearson's correlation was used to assess the correlation between the number of anti-VEGF injections a patient had received prior to blood collection and the concentration of complement components. Data were presented as mean ± standard deviation (SD) calculated from untransformed variables even if the statistical analysis was performed on transformed variables. *P* values <0.05 were considered statistically significant.

Abbreviations
AMD: Age-related macular degeneration; CNV: Choroidal neovascularisation; MAC: Membrane attack complex; nAMD: Neovascular age-related macular degeneration; PVC: Polypoidal choroidal vasculopathy; RAP: Retinal angiomatous proliferation.

Competing interests
The authors declare that they have no competing interests.

Authors' contributions
JL, MC and HX conceived and designed the experiments, JL and MC conducted the experiments, JL and REH analysed the results, LT, GS and UC conducted clinical analysis and recruited patients. JL and HX wrote the paper and all authors reviewed the manuscript. All authors read and approved the final manuscript.

Acknowledgement
We thank the patients who participated in this study. Special thanks to the research nurses Rebecca Denham and Georgina Sterrett for their help in patient recruitment. The study was funded by the Dunhill Medical Trust (R188/0211) and Guide Gods for the Blind Association UK (2008-5a).

References
1. Chakravarthy U, Evans J, Rosenfeld PJ. Age related macular degeneration. BMJ. 2010;340:c981. doi:10.1136/bmj.c981.
2. Hunter MA, Dunbar MT, Rosenfeld PJ. Retinal angiomatous proliferation: clinical characteristics and treatment options. Optometry. 2004;75(9):577–88.
3. Ciardella AP, Donsoff IM, Huang SJ, Costa DL, Yannuzzi LA. Polypoidal choroidal vasculopathy. Surv Ophthalmol. 2004;49(1):25–37. doi: 10.1016/j. survophthal.2003.10.007.
4. Hogg RE, Woodside JV, Gilchrist SE, Graydon R, Fletcher AE, Chan W, et al. Cardiovascular disease and hypertension are strong risk factors for choroidal neovascularization. Ophthalmology. 2008;115(6):1046–52. doi:10.1016/j. ophtha.2007.07.031. e2.
5. Chakravarthy U, Wong TY, Fletcher A, Piault E, Evans C, Zlateva G, et al. Clinical risk factors for age-related macular degeneration: a systematic review and meta-analysis. BMC Ophthalmol. 2010;10:31. doi:10.1186/ 1471-2415-10-31.
6. Ambati J, Ambati BK, Yoo SH, Ianchulev S, Adamis AP. Age-related macular degeneration: etiology, pathogenesis, and therapeutic strategies. Surv Ophthalmol. 2003;48(3):257–93.
7. Ambati J, Atkinson JP, Gelfand BD. Immunology of age-related macular degeneration. Nat Rev Immunol. 2013;13(6):438–51. 10.1038/Nri3459.
8. Chen M, Xu H. Parainflammation, chronic inflammation, and age-related macular degeneration. J Leukoc Biol. 2015;98(5):713-25. doi: 10.1189/jlb. 3RI0615-239R.
9. Klein RJ, Zeiss C, Chew EY, Tsai JY, Sackler RS, Haynes C, et al. Complement factor H polymorphism in age-related macular degeneration. Science. 2005;308(5720):385–9. doi:10.1126/science.1109557.
10. Maller JB, Fagerness JA, Reynolds RC, Neale BM, Daly MJ, Seddon JM. Variation in complement factor 3 is associated with risk of age-related macular degeneration. Nat Genet. 2007;39(10):1200–1. doi:10.1038/ng2131.
11. Gold B, Merriam JE, Zernant J, Hancox LS, Taiber AJ, Gehrs K, et al. Variation in factor B (BF) and complement component 2 (C2) genes is associated with age-related macular degeneration. Nat Genet. 2006;38(4):458–62. doi:10.1038/ng1750.
12. Anderson DH, Mullins RF, Hageman GS, Johnson LV. A role for local inflammation in the formation of drusen in the aging eye. Am J Ophthalmol. 2002;134(3):411–31.
13. Johnson LV, Leitner WP, Staples MK, Anderson DH. Complement activation and inflammatory processes in Drusen formation and age related macular degeneration. Exp Eye Res. 2001;73(6):887–96. doi:10.1006/exer.2001.1094.
14. Nozaki M, Raisler BJ, Sakurai E, Sarma JV, Barnum SR, Lambris JD, et al. Drusen complement components C3a and C5a promote choroidal neovascularization. Proc Natl Acad Sci U S A. 2006;103(7):2328–33. doi:10.1073/pnas.0408835103.
15. Johnson LV, Ozaki S, Staples MK, Erickson PA, Anderson DH. A potential role for immune complex pathogenesis in drusen formation. Exp Eye Res. 2000;70(4):441–9. doi:10.1006/exer.1999.0798.
16. Johnson LV, Leitner WP, Rivest AJ, Staples MK, Radeke MJ, Anderson DH. The Alzheimer's A beta -peptide is deposited at sites of complement activation in pathologic deposits associated with aging and age-related macular degeneration. Proc Natl Acad Sci U S A. 2002;99(18):11830–5. doi:10.1073/pnas.192203399.
17. Zhou J, Jang YP, Kim SR, Sparrow JR. Complement activation by photooxidation products of A2E, a lipofuscin constituent of the retinal pigment epithelium. Proc Natl Acad Sci U S A. 2006;103(44):16182–7. doi:10.1073/pnas.0604255103.
18. Scholl HP, Charbel Issa P, Walier M, Janzer S, Pollok-Kopp B, Borncke F, et al. Systemic complement activation in age-related macular degeneration. PLoS ONE. 2008;3(7):e2593. doi:10.1371/journal.pone.0002593.
19. Silva AS, Teixeira AG, Bavia L, Lin F, Velletri R, Belfort Jr R, et al. Plasma levels of complement proteins from the alternative pathway in patients with age-related macular degeneration are independent of Complement Factor H Tyr(4)(0)(2)His polymorphism. Mol Vis. 2012;18:2288–99.
20. Smailhodzic D, Klaver CC, Klevering BJ, Boon CJ, Groenewoud JM, Kirchhof B, et al. Risk alleles in CFH and ARMS2 are independently associated with systemic complement activation in age-related macular degeneration. Ophthalmology. 2012;119(2):339–46. doi:10.1016/j.ophtha.2011.07.056.
21. Singh A, Faber C, Falk M, Nissen MH, Hviid TV, Sorensen TL. Altered expression of CD46 and CD59 on leukocytes in neovascular age-related macular degeneration. Am J Ophthalmol. 2012;154(1):193–9. doi:10.1016/j. ajo.2012.01.036. e2.
22. Chirco KR, Tucker BA, Stone EM, Mullins RF. Selective accumulation of the complement membrane attack complex in aging choriocapillaris. Experimental Eye Res. 2015. doi:10.1016/j.exer.2015.09.003.
23. Williams MA, McKay GJ, Chakravarthy U. Complement inhibitors for age-related macular degeneration. The Cochrane Database of Systematic Reviews. 2014;1:CD009300. doi:10.1002/14651858.CD009300.pub2.
24. Rhoades W, Dickson D, Do DV. Potential role of lampalizumab for treatment of geographic atrophy. Clin Ophthalmol. 2015;9:1049–56. doi:10.2147/OPTH. S59725.
25. Otsuji T, Nagai Y, Sho K, Tsumura A, Koike N, Tsuda M, et al. Initial non-responders to ranibizumab in the treatment of age-related macular degeneration (AMD). Clin Ophthalmol. 2013;7:1487–90. doi:10.2147/OPTH.S46317.

26. Zipfel PF, Skerka C. Complement regulators and inhibitory proteins. Nat Rev Immunol. 2009;9(10):729–40. doi:10.1038/nri2620.

27. Sparrow JR, Ueda K, Zhou J. Complement dysregulation in AMD: RPE-Bruch's membrane-choroid. Mol Aspects Med. 2012;33(4):436–45. doi:10.1016/j.mam.2012.03.007.

28. Bora PS, Sohn JH, Cruz JM, Jha P, Nishihori H, Wang Y, et al. Role of complement and complement membrane attack complex in laser-induced choroidal neovascularization. J Immunol. 2005;174(1):491–7.

29. Liu J, Jha P, Lyzogubov VV, Tytarenko RG, Bora NS, Bora PS. Relationship between complement membrane attack complex, chemokine (C-C motif) ligand 2 (CCL2) and vascular endothelial growth factor in mouse model of laser-induced choroidal neovascularization. J Biol Chem. 2011;286(23):20991–1001. doi:10.1074/jbc.M111.226266.

30. Mullins RF, Schoo DP, Sohn EH, Flamme-Wiese MJ, Workamelahu G, Johnston RM, et al. The membrane attack complex in aging human choriocapillaris: relationship to macular degeneration and choroidal thinning. Am J Pathol. 2014;184(11):3142–53. doi:10.1016/j.ajpath.2014.07.017.

31. Skeie JM, Fingert JH, Russell SR, Stone EM, Mullins RF. Complement component C5a activates ICAM-1 expression on human choroidal endothelial cells. Invest Ophthalmol Vis Sci. 2010;51(10):5336–42. doi:10.1167/iovs.10-5322.

32. Klos A, Tenner AJ, Johswich KO, Ager RR, Reis ES, Kohl J. The role of the anaphylatoxins in health and disease. Mol Immunol. 2009;46(14):2753–66. doi:10.1016/j.molimm.2009.04.027.

33. Liu B, Wei L, Meyerle C, Tuo J, Sen HN, Li Z, et al. Complement component C5a promotes expression of IL-22 and IL-17 from human T cells and its implication in age-related macular degeneration. J Transl Med. 2011;9:1–12. doi:10.1186/1479-5876-9-111.

34. Seow V, Lim J, Iyer A, Suen JY, Ariffin JK, Hohenhaus DM, et al. Inflammatory responses induced by lipopolysaccharide are amplified in primary human monocytes but suppressed in macrophages by complement protein C5a. J Immunol. 2013;191(8):4308–16. doi:10.4049/jimmunol.1301355.

35. Barnum SR. C4a: An Anaphylatoxin in Name Only. J Innate Immunity. 2015. doi:10.1159/000371423.

36. Bora NS, Kaliappan S, Jha P, Xu Q, Sohn JH, Dhaulakhandi DB, et al. Complement activation via alternative pathway is critical in the development of laser-induced choroidal neovascularization: role of factor B and factor H. J Immunol. 2006;177(3):1872–8.

37. Sendler M, Beyer G, Mahajan UM, Kauschke V, Maertin S, Schurmann C et al. Complement Component 5 Mediates Development of Fibrosis, via Activation of Stellate Cells, in 2 Mouse Models of Chronic Pancreatitis. Gastroenterology. 2015. doi:10.1053/j.gastro.2015.05.012.

38. Monsinjon T, Gasque P, Chan P, Ischenko A, Brady JJ, Fontaine MC. Regulation by complement C3a and C5a anaphylatoxins of cytokine production in human umbilical vein endothelial cells. FASEB J. 2003;17(9):1003–14. doi:10.1096/fj.02-0737com.

39. Francis PJ. The influence of genetics on response to treatment with ranibizumab (Lucentis) for age-related macular degeneration: the Lucentis Genotype Study (an American Ophthalmological Society thesis). Trans Am Ophthalmol Soc. 2011;109:115–56.

40. Hagstrom SA, Ying GS, Pauer GJ, Sturgill-Short GM, Huang J, Callanan DG, et al. Pharmacogenetics for genes associated with age-related macular degeneration in the Comparison of AMD Treatments Trials (CATT). Ophthalmology. 2013;120(3):593–9. doi:10.1016/j.ophtha.2012.11.037.

41. Finger RP, Wickremasinghe SS, Baird PN, Guymer RH. Predictors of anti-VEGF treatment response in neovascular age-related macular degeneration. Surv Ophthalmol. 2014;59(1):1–18. doi:10.1016/j.survophthal.2013.03.009.

42. Liszewski MK, Kolev M, Le Friec G, Leung M, Bertram PG, Fara AF, et al. Intracellular complement activation sustains T cell homeostasis and mediates effector differentiation. Immunity. 2013;39(6):1143–57. doi:10.1016/j.immuni.2013.10.018.

43. Avery RL, Castellarin AA, Steinle NC, Dhoot DS, Pieramici DJ, See R, et al. Systemic pharmacokinetics following intravitreal injections of ranibizumab, bevacizumab or aflibercept in patients with neovascular AMD. Br J Ophthalmol. 2014;98(12):1636–41. doi:10.1136/bjophthalmol-2014-305252.

Evaluation of circulating sRAGE in osteoporosis according to BMI, adipokines and fracture risk: a pilot observational study

Emanuela Galliera[1,2]*, Monica Gioia Marazzi[3], Carmine Gazzaruso[4], Pietro Gallotti[4], Adriana Coppola[4], Tiziana Montalcini[5], Arturo Pujia[5] and Massimiliano M. Corsi Romanelli[3,6]

Abstract

Background: Osteoporosis is a systemic metabolic disease based on age-dependent imbalance between the rates of bone formation and bone resorption. Recent studies on the pathogenesis of this disease identified that bone remodelling impairment, at the base of osteoporotic bone fragility, could be related to protein glycation, in association to oxidative stress. The glycation reactions lead to the generation of glycation end products (AGEs) which, in turn, accumulates into bone, where they binds to the receptor for AGE (RAGE). The aim of this study is to investigate the potential role of circulating sRAGE in osteoporosis, in particular evaluating the correlation of sRAGE with the fracture risk, in association with bone mineral density, the fracture risk marker FGF23, and lipid metabolism.

Results: Circulating level of soluble RAGE correlate with osteopenia and osteoporosis level. Serum sRAGE resulted clearly associated on the one hand to bone fragility and, on the other hand, with BMI and leptin. sRAGE is particularly informative because serum sRAGE is able to provide, as a single marker, information about both the aspects of osteoporotic disease, represented by bone fragility and lipid metabolism.

Conclusions: The measure serum level of sRAGE could have a potential diagnostic role in the monitoring of osteoporosis progression, in particular in the evaluation of fracture risk, starting from the prevention and screening stage, to the osteopenic level to osteoporosis.

Keywords: Circulating RAGE, Glycation end products, Osteoporosis, Fracture risk

Background

Osteoporosis is defined, according to 2001 NHI consensus conference, as a systemic disease characterized by loss of bone volume and resulting in a reduced skeletal integrity leading to a higher risk of bone fracture [1, 2]. Osteoporosis develops because of an age-dependent imbalance between the rates of bone formation and bone resorption [3] and is an emerging disease due to the increase of the population average age and its socioeconomic and public health impact is estimated to significantly increase in the next future. Due to the

association with bone fragility and fracture risk, this disease interferes not only with the quality of life but also with life expectancy, in particular in elder people [4, 5] . The current recommendation for osteoporosis screening is the diagnosis by Bone Densitometry or DXA (Dual-energy X-ray absorptiometry) Scan, but even though this approach correlates with fracture risk and it can considered a good fracture predictor, many additional factors play a role in determining risk of fracture. While the first diagnosis of osteoporosis is based on bone mineral density (BMD), the evaluation of the individual fracture risk should consider all the clinical risk factors, ranging from age, sex, metabolic status and bone remodelling status [6, 7].

* Correspondence: emanuela.galliera@unimi.it
[1]Department of Biomedical, Surgical and Oral Science, Università degli Studi di Milano, Milan, Italy
[2]IRCCS Galeazzi Orthopaedic Institute, Milan, Italy
Full list of author information is available at the end of the article

On the one hand, DXA scan gives the static measurement of bone density in specific bone sites, on the other hand, additional diagnostic tool, such as bone turnover biomarkers, reflects the dynamic changes of bone turnover in the whole skeletal [8–10]. Therefore, the comprehension of the biochemical mechanisms involved in the pathogenesis of osteoporosis could provide new diagnostic tool for improving the sensibility and specificity the prediction of fracture risk [7].

Osteoporosis is a systemic metabolic disease and recent studies on the pathogenesis of this disease identified that bone remodelling impairment, at the base of osteoporotic bone fragility, could be related to protein glycation, in association to oxidative stress [5]. The glycation reactions lead to the generation of glycation end products (AGEs) which, in turn, accumulates into bone, where they binds to the receptor for AGE (RAGE) [11]. The RAGE receptor belongs to the immunoglobulin superfamily of cell- surface molecules expressed in different cell types, including osteoclasts and osteoblasts. Upon binding AGEs, RAGE increase osteoclasts activity and decrease osteoblasts activity [12, 13], thus contributing to increase bone resorption and, ultimately, bone fragility [5, 14].

The negative action of AGEs-RAGE axis is compensated by the soluble form of RAGE receptor (sRAGE), which is a decoy receptor of AGEs . Being a soluble receptor, sRAGE binds AGEs but doesn't lead to any signaling pathway, thus competing with the signaling, cell-bound RAGE receptor and, as a consequence, limiting the AGEs-RAGE axis action [15].

RAGE may be bound by many ligands which include advanced glycation endproducts (AGEs), certain members of the S100/calgranulin family, extracellular HMGB1-amphoterin, the integrin Mac-1, amyloid beta-peptide and amyloid fibrils. Acting as counter-receptor for leukocyte integrins RAGE may also have an important role in cell adhesion and clustering as well as recruitment of inflammatory cells [16, 17]. Other important ligands for RAGE may be glycosaminoglycans (including chondroitin sulfate, dermatan sulfate and heparan sulfate) which are frequently attached to proteoglycans on the surface of cancer cells and play an important role in the malignant transformation of the tumor and metastasis [17].

Being involved in the inflammatory response [18], RAGE ligand (s)/RAGE system, in particular the axes AGE-RAGE is involved in the pathogenesis of a variety of inflammatory disorders, ranging from diabetes to renal disease, sepsis and cardiovascular disease [11]. In particular, the circulating soluble form of the RAGE receptor (sRAGE) has been recently described as a marker of disease in different pathologies, ranging from cardiovascular disease to acute liver failure [19] and metabolic disorder in obesity and diabetes [5, 20], but the diagnostic role of sRAGE in osteoporosis has not been described so far.

The aim of this study is to investigate the potential role of circulating sRAGE in osteoporosis, in particular evaluating the correlation of sRAGE with the fracture risk, in association with bone mineral density e and the fracture risk marker FGF23 (Fibroblast Growth Factor 23), involved in bone mineral metabolism. Since osteoporosis pathogenesis is strictly related with the metabolic status [21, 22], the aim of this study is also to evaluate the role of sRAGE as marker of osteoporosis in correlation with BMI and the adipokines leptin, adiponectin and visfatin.

Methods

Patients

The study involves 84 postmenopausal female volunteers (mean age 53 ± 6 years old) enrolled in the region of Lombardia and Calabria, as described in our previous work (Montalcini et al. 2015 [23]). All participants were evaluated for familiarity of osteoporosis and past fractures, medication use, physical exercise and smoke habits. Post menopausal status was defined as FSH level higher than 40 IU/l or one year at least of absence of natural mense.

Exclusion criteria were: presence of diabetes or any metabolic condition affecting bone metabolism (kidney, thyroid, rheumatic and hematological disease, malignant tumors) taking drug, hormone therapy or vitamin D affecting bone metabolism. The patients in our study was not under bisphosphonates therapy or other anti-osteoporotic therapy.

Written informed consent was obtained from all participants included in the study. All procedures followed were in accordance with the Helsinki of Declaration of 1975, as revised in 2000 and 2008 and it was approved by both the Ethic Committee ASL Milan 2 and The University Hospital Mater Domini, Catanzaro (Italy).

Trial registration number: 2631, name of registry: Comitato Etico indipendente della ASL Milano due. URL: http://www.aslm2.it, date of registration: September 19, 2011. Date of enrolment of the first participant 1 October 2011.

DXA assessment

BMD evaluation of lumbar spine and left femoral was assessed by DXA (Horologic QDR Inc., MA. USA). BMD was expressed as T -score (number of standard deviation from healthy young mean) and Z- score (number of standard deviations from healthy women of the same age) calculated on the basis of physiological reference values. On the basis of T-score value the patients was classified as having normal bone (T-score > −1), osteopenia (Tscore: −1 to −2.49) or osteoporosis (T-score ≤ − 2.5).

In vivo precision, calculated as repeated measurements on 30 women, was <1%.

Anthropometric measurement

Body weight and BMI was measured as described in Montalcini et al. 2015 [23]. Briefly, body weight was measured with a calibrated scale before breakfast subtracting the weight of clothes. Height was measured by wall- mounted stadiometer and BMI was calculated as weight (kg)/(height (m)) ^{2}. According to BMI values, patients were classified as obese (BMI > 30), overweight (BMI 25–30) or normal weight (BMI < 25).

Glomerular filtration rate

Glomerular filtration rate was calculated for the whole population and for each RAGE quartile by CKD-EPI formula:

GFR = 141 * min(Scr/κ,1)^α * max(Scr/κ, 1)$^{-1.209}$ * 0.993^{Age} * 1.018 [if female] * 1.159 [if black]Scr is serum creatinine (mg/dL), κ is 0.7 for females and 0.9 for males, α is −0.329 for females and −0.411 for males, min indicates the minimum of Scr/κ or 1, and max indicates the maximum of Scr/κ or 1.

sRAGE, FGF23 and adipokines ELISA assay

Blood was sampled from all patients and sera were separated from whole blood after complete coagulation, by centrifugation at 3000 rpm for 10 min. Sera were stored at −70 °C until ELISA assay analyses.

Levels of soluble RAGE, C-Terminal FGF23, Leptin, Adiponectin and Visfatin in serum were determined by commercial assays, according to the manufacturers' instructions (sRAGE: R&D Systems, Minneapolis, Minnesota, USA; C-Terminal FGF23: Imuunotopiscs, San Clemente, CA, USA; Leptin: Enzo Life Sciences, Farmingdale, New York, USA; Adiponectin and Visfatin: AdipoGen AG, Liestal, Switzerland).

For the sRAGE assay, the sensitivity was 4.44 pg/mL, and intra- and inter-assay coefficients of variation were 2.4% and 4.7%, respectively. For the FGF23 assay, the sensitivity was 1.5 RU /mL, and intra- and inter-assay coefficients of variation were2.4% and 4.7%, respectively. According to manufacturer (, Imuunotopiscs, San Clemente, CA, USA) 1RU roughly equates to 2 pg/mL. For the Leptin assay, the sensitivity was 23.4. pg/mL, and intra- and inter-assay coefficients of variation were 4.4% and 3.7%, respectively. For the Adiponectin assay, the sensitivity was 1 ng/mL, and intra- and inter-assay coefficients of variation were 3.3% and 2.75%, respectively. For the Visfatin assay, the sensitivity was 30.0 pg/mL, and intra- and inter-assay coefficients of variation were 2.3% and 4.6%, respectively.

Statistical analysis

For all parameters, the normality of distribution of the three groups was verified by KS (Kolmogorov-Smirnov) normality and results are reported as mean ± standard deviation (SD). Statistical analysis was done using one-way ANOVA, $p < 0.05$ being considered significant and $p < 0.001$ highly significant. The correlation of sRAGE with LBMD (lumbar bone mineral density) and FBMD (femoral bone mineral density) (expressed as T-score and Z-score) and with FGF23 was calculated as Spearman correlation (r) calculating the 95% confidence interval. All statistical analysis was performed using PRISM 3.0 software.

Results
Glomerular filtration rate and sRAGE

Glomerular filtration rate was calculated by CKD-EPI formula for the whole population and for each RAGE quartile, in order to evaluate whether it could affect sRAGE levels in our patients . The mean eGFR calculated on the whole patient group was 88,71 ± 11,86 mL/min per 1.73 m^2, while it resulted 85,05 ± 10,74, 89,45 ± 12,71, 88,91 ± 9,56, 84,85 ± 9,13 mL/min per 1.73 m^2 in the first, second, third and fourth sRAGE quartiles, respectively. Therefore, no significative differences in eGFR were observed among sRAGe quartiles and compared to total mean eGFR.

sRAGE and bone mineral density

A total of 12 subject present osteoporosis, while 32 had osteopenia and 40 normal bone density values, as assessed by T-score and Z- score.

The serum level of circulating s RAGE was measured in the three groups of patients (osteopenic, osteoporotic and normal bone, according to T-score values). sRAGE displays a significative increase in osteopenic patients (940.36 ± 206.79 pg/mL) and an even more significative increase in osteoporotic patients (1028,54 ± 223.83 pg/mL) compared to patients with normal bone (743.02 ± 204.91 pg/mL), (Fig. 1, panel a). The population was divided according to sRAGE quartiles, calculating in each quartiles the mean lumbar and femoral T-score and Z-score values (Fig. 1, panel b) and the amount of patients having osteopenia, osteoporosis and normal bone according to LMBD and FBMD T-score and T-score values ranges (Fig. 1 panel c and d, respectively). The first quartiles of sRAGE present no pathological T-score or Z-score, the second and third quartile present osteopenia according to T-score but normal bone according to Z-score, while the fourth quartile present a more severe osteopenia according to both T-score and Z-score mean value.. The first quartile of sRAGE showed the highest percentage of patients with normal bone

a

sRAGE

b

	RAGE Quartiles							
	I		II		III		IV	
	Mean	SD	Mean	SD	Mean	SD	Mean	SD
lumbar T-score	-0,65	0.12	-1,05	0.14	-1,21	0.02	-1,22	0.02
femoral T-score	-0,061	0.23	-1,25	0.01	-1,26	0.09	-1,34	0.08
lumbar Z-score	0,53	0.06	0,15	0.21	0,12	0.11	-0,21	0.05
femoral Zs-core	0,18	0.02	-0,22	0.05	-0,42	0.08	-0,39	0.17

c

% of bone defects (lumbar T score)

d

% of bone defects (femoral T score)

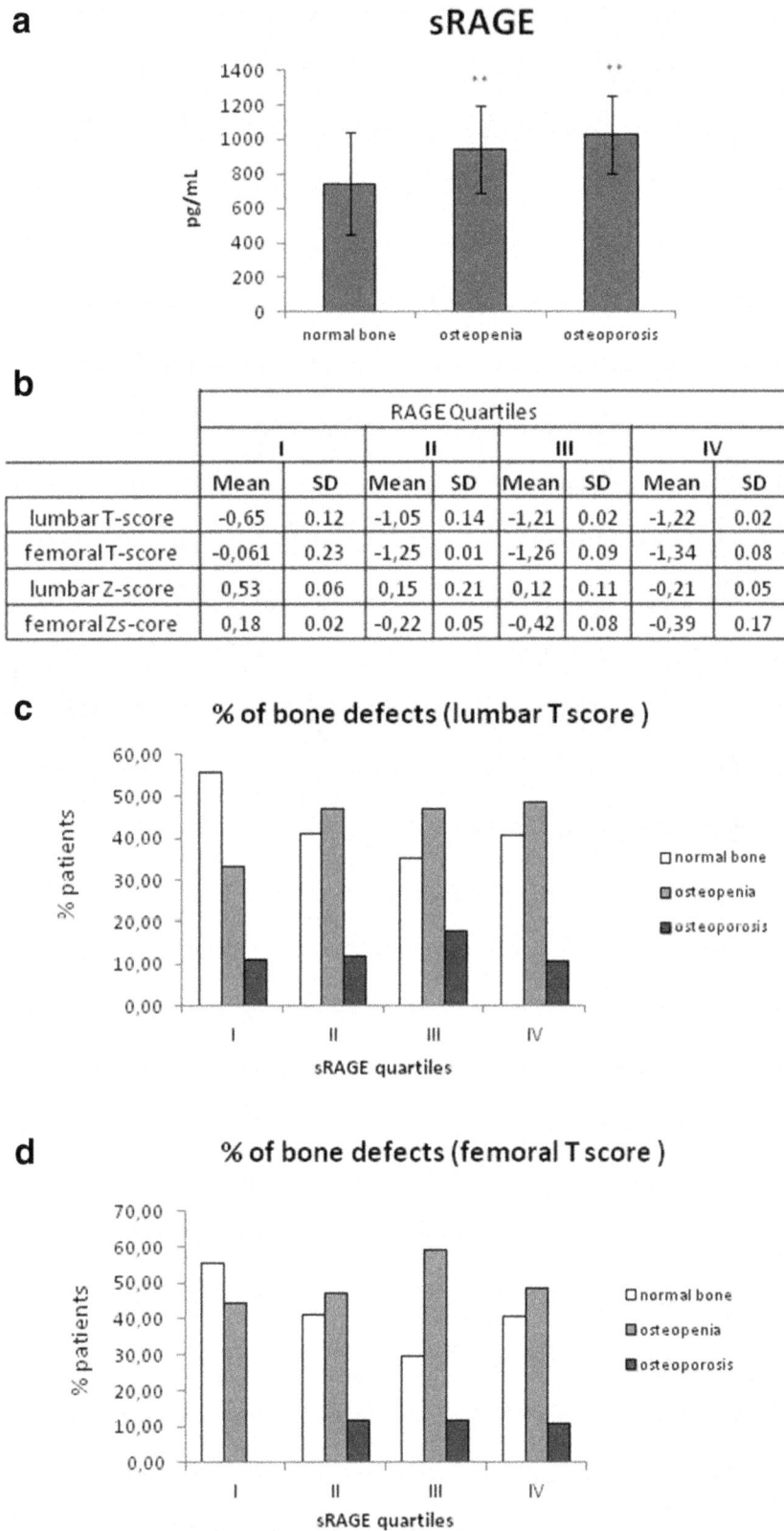

Fig. 1 (See legend on next page.)

(See figure on previous page.)
Fig. 1 Serum sRAGE and bone density. Panel **a**: serum sRAGE (pg/mL) in patients displaying normal bone, osteopenia and osteoporosis, according to Bone Mineral Density valuesPanel **b** bone mineral density, expressed as lumbar and femoral T- and Z-score, according to sRAGE quartiles Panel **c** and **d**: percentage of patients in each sRAGE quartiles displaying normal bone, osteopenia and osteoporosis, according to Bone Mineral Density values, expressed as lumbar T-score (panel **c**), and femoral T-score (panel **d**)

and the lower percentage of osteopenia and osteoporosis according to lumbar T-score (Fig. 1, panel c and d). More significantly, classification based on Femoral T-score (panel D) not only confirmed the percentage of normal and osteopenic patients, but resulted in no cases of osteoporosis in the lowest quartile of sRAGE. The second, third and fourth quartile of sRAGE display very similar classification, having higher percentage of osteopenic patient and a lower percentage of normal bone compared to the first quartile. More interestingly, while osteoporotic percentage is nearly constant in the three upper quartiles according to femoral T-score, lumbar T-score classification underlined a little increase of osteoporosis percentage in the fourth quartile of sRAGE. These results indicates increase of osteoporosis percentage according to sRAGE levels.

sRAGE and fracture risk

There is significative trend of increase of FGF23 according to bone defect classification (Fig. 2 panel a) and sRAGE quartiles (panel B), in particular the first quartile displaying the lowest FGF23 value, below the cutoff of fracture risk in the first quartile and reaching the highest and very significative value in the highest quartile of sRAGE.

The Spearman correlation analysis (Panel C) did not find a strong correlation between serum FGF23 and the whole sRAGE values, while after the classification into sRAGE quartile an increasing correlation with serum FGF23 emerged, reaching high value in the third and even more in the fourth sRAGE quartile. These results indicates a correlation between sRAGE and fracture risck marker FGF23.

sRAGE and BMI

The categorization into sRAGE quartiles was applied to analyze the metabolic status of the patients, evaluated by BMI calculation. There is a trend, even if not statistically significative, of decrease of BMI according to the increase of sRAGE (Fig. 3 panel a). In order to analyze this result in detail, we calculated the number of patients in each sRAGE quartile having normal (<25), overweight (25–30) or obese (>30) BMI (Fig. 3 panel b). According to sRAGE quartiles, there is a trend of decrease of obesity (BMI >30), reaching in the fourth sRAGE quartile the complete absence of obese subject and a very high prevalence of subjects with normal BMI. These results

indicates a trend of decrease of obesity according to sRAGE levels.

BMI and bone status

Figure 4 Panel a shows the mean FMBD and LBMD as Tscore and Z-score in three BMI group: normal (BMI < 25), overweight (BMI: 25–30) or obese (BMI > 30).Only in normal BMI group the mean lumbar T-score and femoral Z-score revealed a decrease of BMD but since the BMD values of the group are quite heterogeneous, Standard Deviation resulting in quite high. The percentage of normal bone, osteopenic and osteoporotic subject, according to lumbar (panel B) and femoral (panel C) T-score values, was evaluated into each BMI group. At the increase of BMI correspond a decrease of osteopenia and osteoporosis, and an increase of normal bone. In particular, according to femoral T-score, at BMI values over 30 there is a complete absence of osteoporotic subjects. These results indicates a decrease of osteopenia and osteoporosis according to BMI. Increase

sRAGE and Adipokines

Adiponectin and Visfatin (Fig. 5 panel a and b) displayed no significative differences among sRAGE quartiles, while Leptin and, as a consequence, Leptin/Adiponectin Ratio (Fig. 5 panel c and d) displayed a statistically significative decrease according to sRAGE quartiles.

Adiponectin and Visfatin display no significative correlation with total sRAGE or sRAGE quartiles, while Leptin and Leptin/Adiponectin Ratio displayed a good negative correlation ($p < 0.001$) with total sRAGE. This negative correlation increase according to sRAGE quartiles and it is particularly evident and significative ($p < 0.001$) n the forth quartile of sRAGE (panel E). These results indicates a negative correlation of sRAGE with leptin and Adiponectin.

Discussion

Several evidences indicated that AGEs are involved in the pathogenesis of osteoporosis [5] and AGEs-RAGE interaction modulates osteoclasts and osteoblasts activity [24, 25]. For this reason we aimed to investigate the potential diagnostic role of soluble RAGE in osteoporosis. Our result clearly indicates that circulating level of soluble RAGE correlate with osteopenia and osteoporosis level (Fig. 1). This correlation is particularly evident by scoring RAGE into four quartiles.. These results clearly

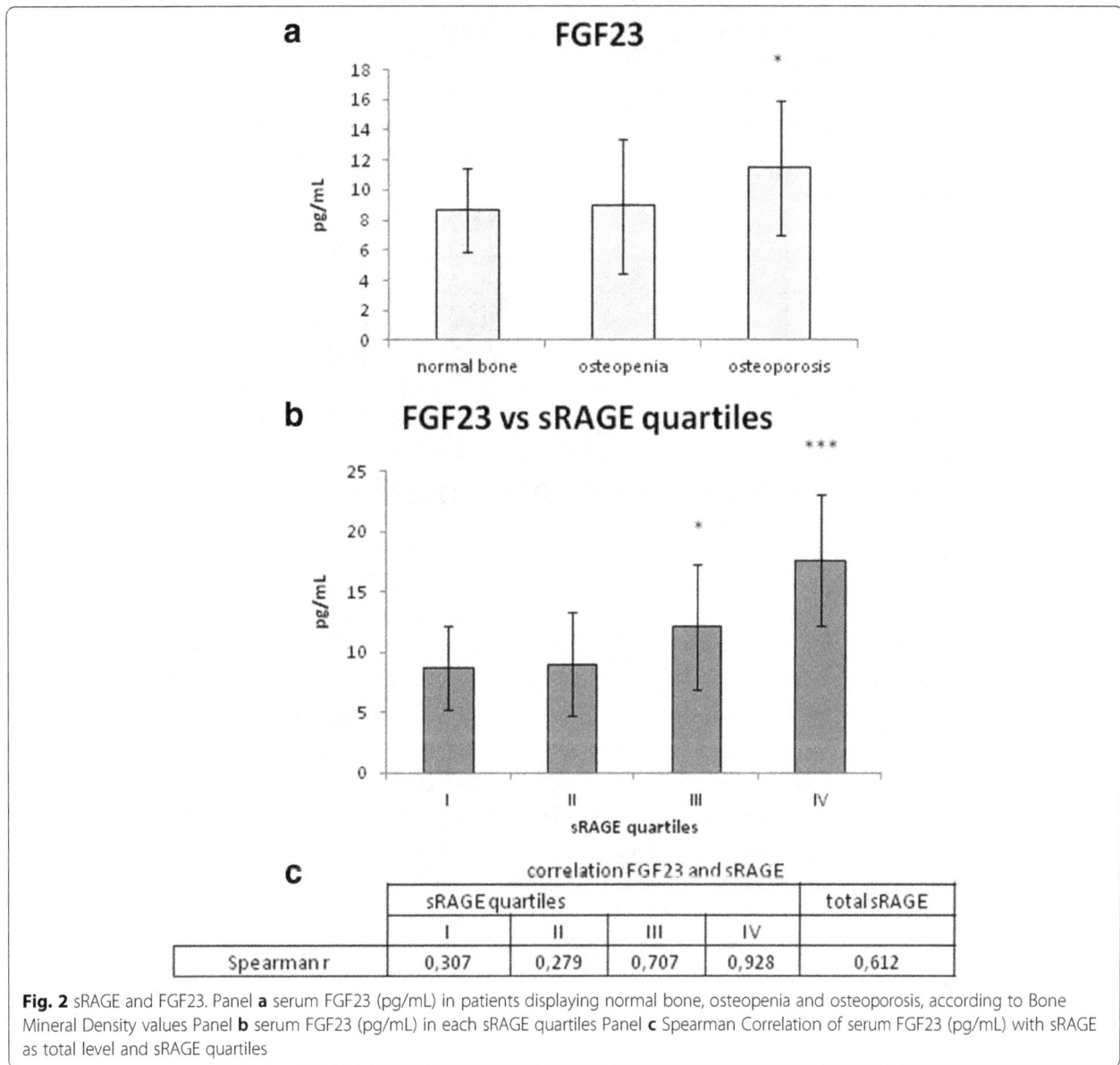

a FGF23

b FGF23 vs sRAGE quartiles

c correlation FGF23 and sRAGE

	sRAGE quartiles				total sRAGE
	I	II	III	IV	
Spearman r	0,307	0,279	0,707	0,928	0,612

Fig. 2 sRAGE and FGF23. Panel **a** serum FGF23 (pg/mL) in patients displaying normal bone, osteopenia and osteoporosis, according to Bone Mineral Density values Panel **b** serum FGF23 (pg/mL) in each sRAGE quartiles Panel **c** Spearman Correlation of serum FGF23 (pg/mL) with sRAGE as total level and sRAGE quartiles

indicate that sRAGE correlates with disease progression from osteopenic to osteoporosis level. Usually sRAGE is reported to be high in healthy patients and lower in pathological condition, but this is not the first case where sRAGE, on the contrary, correlates with disease progression, behaving as a marker of disease progression. Indeed very recent evidenced that sRAGE, as widely described by Kailash Prasad [26], is not always a marker of good prognosis, because it can be reduced in some disease [27–30] and elevated in others [30–33]. The biological function of sRAGE is to bind circulating AGE, which could have detrimental effect on tissues, thus playing a protective role. For this reason in most of the cases, such as cardiovascular disorders, sRAGE, as a protective factor, is elevated in healthy subject and low

in disease. On the contrary, in some cases such as diabetes renal disease, sRAGE is elevated compared to healthy controls as well as AGEs [5]. Similarly, recent evidences indicates a high level of sRAGE is present in acute respiratory distress and bronchiolitis [34], idiopathic pulmonary fibrosis [35] and it can correlate with disease severity in lung transplantation [35] and long term hemodyalisis patients [36].

It is known that AGEs accumulates in bone tissue at increasing ages, because bone tissue is susceptible to aGE accumulation due to its turnover. During bone remodelling bone cells are in close proximity to to AGE-modified proteins, such as collagen Type I and its degradation products. Bone cells express RAGE and can directly interact with Age, regulating differentiation maturation and function.

a   BMI vs sRAGE quartiles

b   BMI Range vs sRAGE quartiles

Fig. 3 sRAGE and BMI. Panel **a** BMI (mean ± SD) in patients in each sRAGE quartiles Panel **b** BMI classification (<25 normal weight, 25–30 overweight, >30 obese) in each sRAGE quartiles serum FGF23 (pg/mL) in each sRAGE quartiles

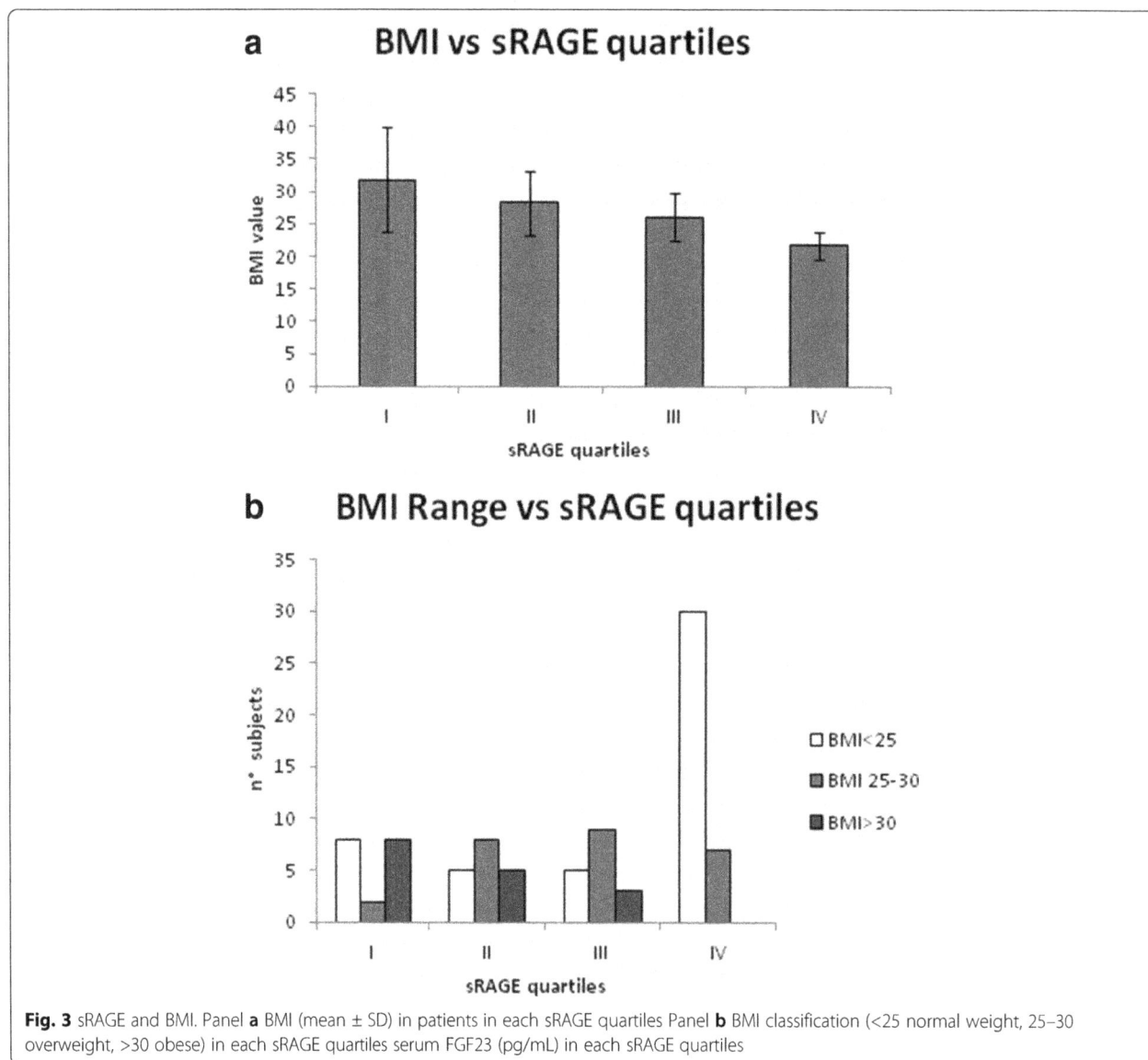

Therefore, protein glycation in clearly involved in age-regulating bone disorders [37]. Franke et al. reported that on the one hand AGE-RAGE binding activates inflammatory response by inducing NFkB and TNF-α, on the other hand NFkB upregulates RAGE expression, thereby activating a self-promoting cicle among RAGE, Age and inflammatory mediators [37]. AGEs induced a decrease of osteoblast proliferation and osteoblast apoptosis [38]. In addition circulating AGE are reported to decrease bone strength [39]. The circulating sRAGE is the direct effect of the proteolitic cleavage of RAGE by metalloproteinases, and recent evidences suggested that diseases characterized by high level of MMPs, such as diabetes and renal disease [40, 41] display high level of serum sRAGE compared to healthy controls. Osteoporosis is characterized by a high expression of MMPs, acting on bone matrix resorption,

and this can be the reason of high level of serum sRAGE in osteoporosis level. Therefore, circulating levels of sRAGE can be considered a direct indicator of circulating AGEs and, therefore, bone resorption status.

Consistently with this, our data indicates that serum sRAGE correlates with bone density decrease, ranging from the level of osteopenia to marked osteoporosis, confirming a correlation of serum sRAGE with the stage of bone fragility. This is also confirmed by the correlation of sRAGE quartiles with a strong marker of bone fracture risk, FGF23, as shown in Fig. 2. Being an important regulator of vitamin D and phosphorus, a key process in bone matrix turnover, Fibroblast growth factor-23 (FGF23) is considered a strong marker of bone fracture [42, 43]. In our patients there if we consider the whole population there is not a strong correlation of

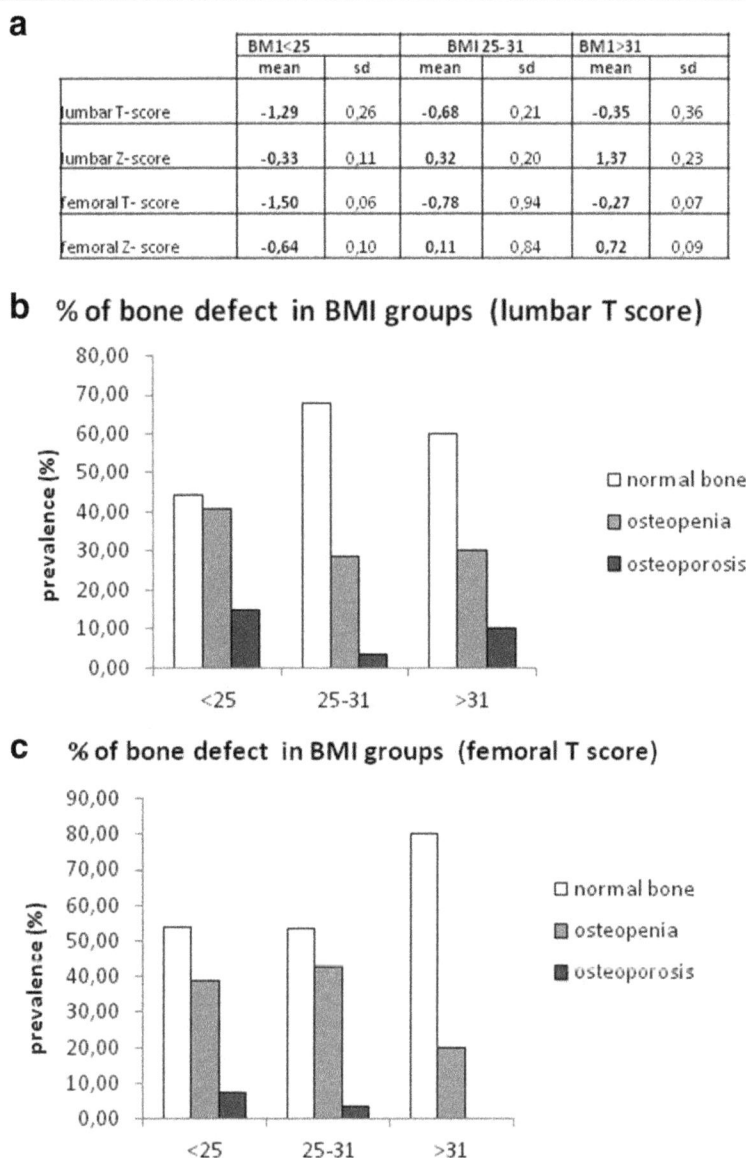

a

	BMI<25		BMI 25-31		BMI>31	
	mean	sd	mean	sd	mean	sd
lumbar T-score	-1,29	0,26	-0,68	0,21	-0,35	0,36
lumbar Z-score	-0,33	0,11	0,32	0,20	1,37	0,23
femoral T-score	-1,50	0,06	-0,78	0,94	-0,27	0,07
femoral Z-score	-0,64	0,10	0,11	0,84	0,72	0,09

b % of bone defect in BMI groups (lumbar T score)

c % of bone defect in BMI groups (femoral T score)

Fig. 4 BMI and bone status. Panel **a** Bone Mineral Density values, expressed as lumbar and femoral T-and Z. core, according to BMI classification (<25 normal weight, 25–30 overweight, >30 obese). Panel **b** and **c** percentage of patients displaying normal bone, osteopenia and osteoporosis, according to Bone Mineral Density values lumbar Tscore (panel **b**) and femoral T score (panel **c**), in BMI groups (<25 normal weight, 25–30 overweight, >30 obese)

FGF23 and total fracture risk, as reported by Montalcini et Al, 2015 [23]. If we consider the classification according to T-score into normal bone, osteopenic and osteoporotic patients, a slightly increasing concentration of FGF23 results in osteopenic and osteoporotic group. In particular the only significative difference is observed in osteoporotic patients, displaying higher bone fragility, while at the level of osteopenia the risk of fracture is still too low to induce a marked and significative increase of FGF23. In consistence with that, there is a strong significative increase of FGF23 according to sRAGE quartiles, with a significative increase in particular in the third and

even more in the highest quartile of sRAGE, suggesting a correlation of sRAGE with the increasing risk of bone fracture. This is also confirmed by the correlation analysis between serum FGF23 and sRAGE quartiles: even if the correlation with total sRAGE is not so strong, considering sRAGE quartiles classification a strong positive correlation emerges in the third and fourth quartiles. All these results clearly indicate that sRAGE can be considered a new biomarker of fracture risk in the osteoporosis.

It is well established that bone fracture risk is influenced not only by bone density but also by several metabolic factors, such as BMI and lipid metabolism [21, 22].

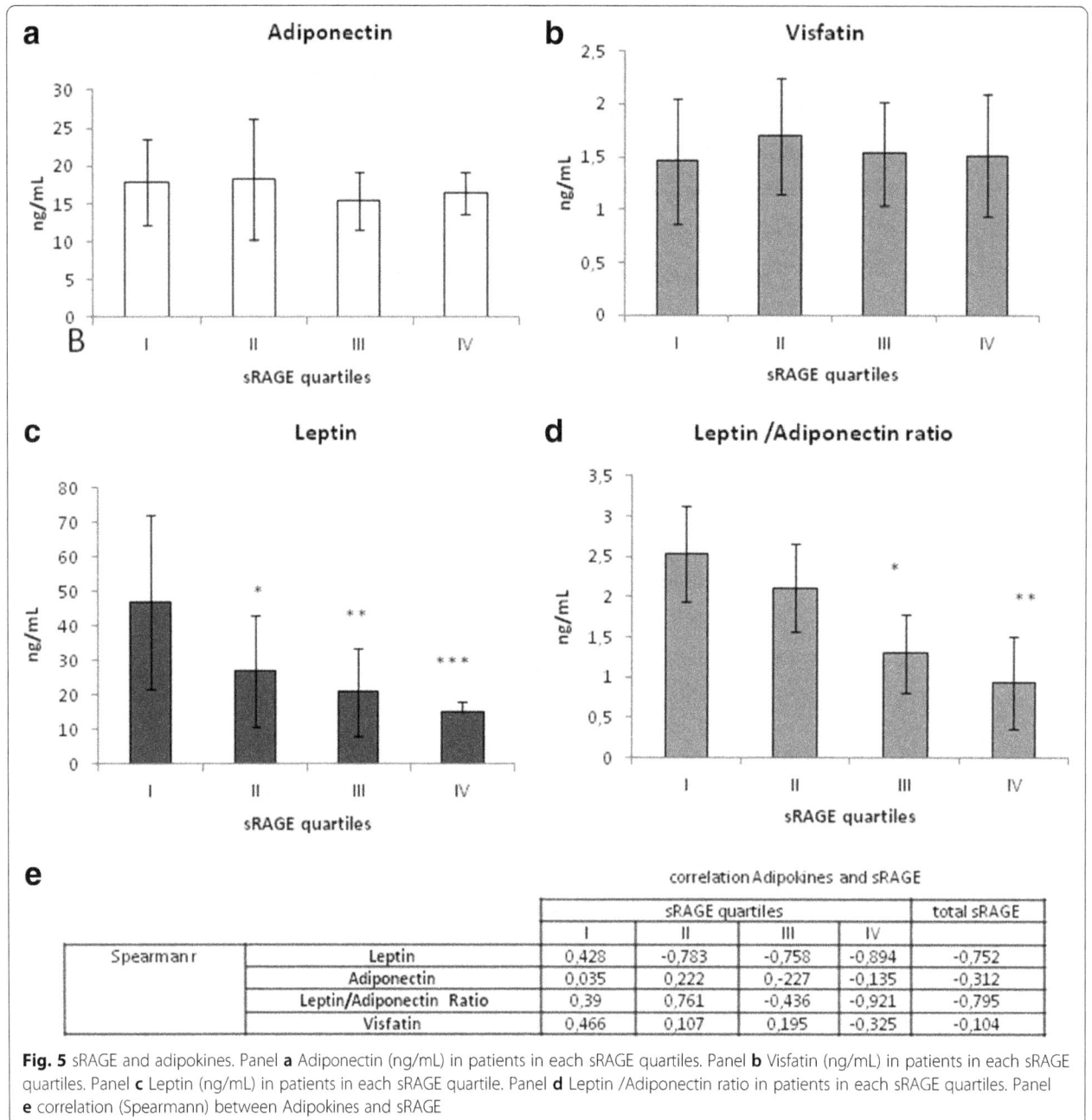

Fig. 5 sRAGE and adipokines. Panel **a** Adiponectin (ng/mL) in patients in each sRAGE quartiles. Panel **b** Visfatin (ng/mL) in patients in each sRAGE quartiles. Panel **c** Leptin (ng/mL) in patients in each sRAGE quartile. Panel **d** Leptin /Adiponectin ratio in patients in each sRAGE quartiles. Panel **e** correlation (Spearmann) between Adipokines and sRAGE

For this reason, we evaluated the association of BMI with the level of serum sRAGE. We observed a decrease of BMI according to sRAGE quartiles, and in particular if we categorize the patients into each sRAGE quartile according to the BMI standard classification (BMI < 25: normal weight, BMI 25–30 overweight, BMI > 30 obese) we observe a sticking prevalence of normal weight subject in the highest quartile of sRAGE. Accordingly, no obese subject is present in the highest quartile of sRAGE while the highest prevalence of obese subject results in the lowest quartile of sRAGE. This data indicate that there is a negative correlation with sRAGE and BMI.

In order to evaluate the relationship between BMI and bone status in our patients, we analyzed bone density score (lumbar and femora T-and Z-score) in the three BMI categories, as shown in Fig. 4. This result indicate that a lower bone density correspond to a lower BMI. This could appear contradictory, because, since BMI and lipid metabolism influences bone turnover, it could be supposed that elevated BMI and lipid metabolism correspond to a low bone density. However, it is well established that in obese patients there a counterbalancing mechanism: high body weight requires a stronger bone and, therefore, a higher bone density. Therefore, high

BMI level, as confirmed in our patients, correspond to a higher bone density. This result on the one hand confirmed the positive correlation between BMI and bone density already reported in literature [44–46], on the other hand, given the negative correlation between sRAGE and BMI, confirm the role of sRAGE as a marker of bone fragility and fracture risk. In order to deeply correlate the relationship between s RAGE and lipid metabolism me evaluated a panel of the main adipokine (adiponectin, visfatin and leptin) and correlated them to serum sRAGE. According to s RAGE quartile, no significative differences are observed for Adiponectin and Visfatin. These results confirm previous evidences indicating that adiponectin and visfatin are controversial in osteoporotic patient s and cannot be considered good markers of osteoporosis [47, 48]. On the contrary, leptin displayed a statistically significative decrease into sRAGE quartiles, in accordance with BMI data. In addition to the single adipokines, the leptin/adiponectin ratio (LAR) is usually used to analyzed the lipid metabolism [49] and in our patients LAR displays the same trend of decrease, with significative lower level in the highest sRAGE quartile. This result are confirmed by correlation analysis, indicating that leptin and leptin/adiponectin ratio display a strong correlation with sRAGE, both as total sRAGE and into quartiles, in particular in the highest sRAGE quartile.

Taken together these results indicates that s RAGE display a strong negative correlation with leptin and LAR ratio.

This is the first study to our knowledge evaluating serum sRAGE in normal, osteopenic and osteoporotic patients. The limit of the study is to evaluate only few of the great number of parameter in the global evaluation of bone and lipid metabolism in fracture risk. This is pilot study evaluating the association of sRAGE and bone fragility in osteoporosis, and further investigation could be performed on a wider panel of parameter. The study is performed on a selected population of a small number of patients, all belonging to female gender and recruited into a local area, but since osteoporosis affects also male, further investigation could be performed on both genders, in order to replicate and extend the analysis.

This marker resulted clearly associated on the one hand to bone fragility and, on the other hand, with BMI and leptin. Since the ultimate goal of osteoporosis diagnosis and monitoring is the evaluation of fracture risk, it is important to take into account all the aspect affecting bone fragility. In this context sRAGE is particularly informative because serum sRAGE is able to provide, as a single marker, information about both the aspects of osteoporotic disease, represented by bone fragility and lipid metabolism.

The exact mechanism connecting AGEs and bone fragility is still unclear, but the level of advanced glycation end products (AGEs) have been recently reported to be inversely correlated with bone toughness and rigidity, due to their role in the inhibition of the synthesis of type I collagen, [39, 50, 51]. In addition, it is known that obesity is connected with increased amounts of AGE in the body [52, 53], leading to decreased bone toughness. In this context, our results shows that sRAGE would play a role in regulating AGEs, also according to lipid metabolism.

Conclusion
The measure serum level of sRAGE could have a potential diagnostic role in the monitoring of osteoporosis progression, in particular in the evaluation of fracture risk, starting from the prevention and screening stage, to the osteopenic level to osteoporosis.

Acknowledgements
We acknowledge Fondazione di Piacenza eVigevano.for supporting this research.

Funding
The study was supported by Fondazione di Piacenza eVigevano.

Authors' contributions
EG and MMCR: study design, data analysis, article drafting; MG M ELISA Assay; CG, PG., AC,˙ TM, AP: patients recruitment DXA, antropometric measurements. All authors read and approved the final manuscript.

Competing interests
The authors declare they have no competing interests.

Author details
[1]Department of Biomedical, Surgical and Oral Science, Università degli Studi di Milano, Milan, Italy. [2]IRCCS Galeazzi Orthopaedic Institute, Milan, Italy. [3]Department of Biomedical Sciences for Health, Università degli Studi di Milano, Milan, Italy. [4]Internal Medicin, Diabetes, Vascular and Endocrine-Mtabolical Disease Unit and the Centre of Applied Clinical Research (Ce.R.C.A), Clinical Institute Betato Matteo, Vigevano, Italy. [5]Clinical Nutrition Unit, Department of Medical and Surgical Science, University Magna Grecia of Catanzaro, Catanzaro, Italy. [6]U.O.C SMEL-1 Patologia Clinica IRCCS Policlinico San Donato, San Donato, Milan, Italy.

References
1. Hein GE. Glycation endproducts in osteoporosis–is there a pathophysiologic importance? Clin Chim Acta. 2006;371:32–6.
2. Cockey CD. Coming to consensus on osteoporosis. AWHONN Lifelines. 2000;4:21.
3. Mohan S, Farley JR, Baylink DJ. Age-related changes in IGFBP-4 and IGFBP-5 levels in human serum and bone: implications for bone loss with aging. Prog Growth Factor Res. 1995;6:465–73.
4. Parsons LC. Osteoporosis: incidence, prevention, and treatment of the silent killer. Nurs Clin North Am. 2005;40:119–33.
5. Yamagishi S, Nakamura K, Inoue H. Possible participation of advanced glycation end products in the pathogenesis of osteoporosis in diabetic patients. Med Hypotheses. 2005;65:1013–5.

6. Camacho PM, Lopez NA. Use of biochemical markers of bone turnover in the management of postmenopausal osteoporosis. Clin Chem Lab Med. 2008;46:1345–57.

7. Vasikaran SD. Utility of biochemical markers of bone turnover and bone mineral density in management of osteoporosis. Crit Rev Clin Lab Sci. 2008; 45:221–58.

8. Tamaki J, Iki M, Kadowaki E, et al. Biochemical markers for bone turnover predict risk of vertebral fractures in postmenopausal women over 10 years: the Japanese population-based osteoporosis (JPOS) cohort study. Osteoporos Int. 2013;24(3):887–97. doi:10.1007/s00198-012-2106-7.

9. Biver E, Chopin F, Coiffier G, et al. Bone turnover markers for osteoporotic status assessment? A systematic review of their diagnosis value at baseline in osteoporosis. Joint Bone Spine. 2013;79:20–5.

10. Chopin F, Biver E, Funck-Brentano T, et al. Prognostic interest of bone turnover markers in the management of postmenopausal osteoporosis. Joint Bone Spine. 2012;79(1):20–5. doi:10.1016/j.jbspin.2011.05.003.1.

11. Schmidt AM, Yan SD, Yan SF, Stern DM. The biology of the receptor for advanced glycation end products and its ligands. Biochim Biophys Acta. 2000;1498:99–111.

12. Tanaka K, Yamaguchi T, Kaji H, Kanazawa I, Sugimoto T. Advanced glycation end products suppress osteoblastic differentiation of stromal cells by activating endoplasmic reticulum stress. Biochem Biophys Res Commun. 2013;438(3):463–7. doi:10.1016/j.bbrc.2013.07.126.

13. Okazaki K, Yamaguchi T, Tanaka K, et al. Advanced glycation end products (AGEs), but not high glucose, inhibit the osteoblastic differentiation of mouse stromal ST2 cells through the suppression of osterix expression, and inhibit cell growth and increasing cell apoptosis. Endocrinology. 2014;155(7): 2402–10. doi:10.1210/en.2013-1818.

14. Willett TL, Pasquale J, Grynpas MD. Collagen modifications in postmenopausal osteoporosis: advanced glycation endproducts may affect bone volume, structure and quality. Curr Osteoporos Rep. 2014;12(3):329–37. doi:10.1007/s11914-014-0214-3.

15. Sanguineti R, Puddu A, Mach F, Montecucco F, Viviani GL. Advanced glycation end products play adverse proinflammatory activities in osteoporosis. Mediators Inflamm. 2014;2014:975872. doi:10.1155/2014/975872.

16. Fritz G. RAGE: a single receptor fits multiple ligands. Trends Biochem Sci. 2011;36(12):625–32. doi:10.1016/j.tibs.2011.08.008.

17. Tesarova P, Kalousova M, Zima T, Tesar V. HMGB1, S100 proteins and other RAGE ligands in cancer - markers, mediators and putative therapeutic targets. Biomed Pap Med Fac Univ Palacky Olomouc Czech Repub. 2016; 160(1):1–10. doi:10.5507/bp.2016.003.

18. Balistreri CR, Candore G, Accardi G, Colonna-Romano G, Lio D. NF-kappaB pathway activators as potential ageing biomarkers: targets for new therapeutic strategies. Immun Ageing 2013 20;10(1):24. doi: 10.1186/1742-4933-10-24.

19. Santilli F, Blardi P, Scapellato C, et al. Decreased plasma endogenous soluble RAGE, and enhanced adipokine secretion, oxidative stress and platelet/coagulative activation identify non-alcoholic fatty liver disease among patients with familial combined hyperlipidemia and/or metabolic syndrome. Vasc Pharmacol. 2015;72:16–24. doi:10.1016/j.vph.2015.04.004.

20. Yang ZK, Shen Y, Shen WF, et al. Elevated glycated albumin and reduced endogenous secretory receptor for advanced glycation endproducts levels in serum predict major adverse cardio-cerebral events in patients with type 2 diabetes and stable coronary artery disease. Int J Cardiol. 2015;15(197): 241–7. doi:10.1016/j.ijcard.2015.06.003.

21. Cao JJ. Effects of obesity on bone metabolism. J Orthop Surg Res. 2011; 15(6):30. doi:10.1186/1749-799X-6-30.

22. Sharma S, Tandon VR, Mahajan S, Mahajan V, Mahajan A. Obesity: friend or foe for osteoporosis. J Midlife Health. 2014;5(1):6–9. doi:10.4103/0976-7800.127782.

23. Montalcini T, Gallotti P, Coppola A, et al. Association between low C-peptide and low lumbar bone mineral density in postmenopausal women without diabetes. Osteoporos Int. 2015;26(5):1639–46. doi:10.1007/s00198-015-3040-2.

24. Hein G, Wiegand R, Lehmann G, Stein G, Franke S. Advanced glycation end-products pentosidine and N epsilon-carboxymethyllysine are elevated in serum of patients with osteoporosis. Rheumatology (Oxford). 2003;42:1242–6.

25. Kume S, Kato S, Yamagishi S, et al. Advanced glycation end-products attenuate human mesenchymal stem cells and prevent cognate differentiation into adipose tissue, cartilage, and bone. J Bone Miner Res. 2005;20:1647–58.

26. Prasad K. Low levels of serum soluble receptors for advanced glycation end products, biomarkers for disease state: myth or reality. Int J Angiol. 2014; 23(1):11–6. doi:10.1055/s-0033-1363423.

27. Selvin E, Halushka MK, Rawlings AM, et al. sRAGE and risk of diabetes, cardiovascular disease, and death. Diabetes. 2013;62(6):2116–21. doi:10.2337/db12-1528.

28. Hudson BI, Moon YP, Kalea AZ, et al. Association of serum soluble receptor for advanced glycation end-products with subclinical cerebrovascular disease: the northern Manhattan study (NOMAS). Atherosclerosis. 2011; 216(1):192–8. doi:10.1016/j.atherosclerosis.2011.01.024.

29. Miniati M, Monti S, Basta G, Cocci F, Fornai E, Bottai M. Soluble receptor for advanced glycation end products in COPD: relationship with emphysema and chronic cor pulmonale: a case-control study. Respir Res. 2011;30(12):37. doi:10.1186/1465-9921-12-37.

30. Geroldi D, Falcone C, Emanuele E, et al. Decreased plasma levels of soluble receptor for advanced glycation end-products in patients with essential hypertension. J Hypertens. 2005;23:1725–9.

31. Challier M, Jacqueminet S, Benabdesselam O, Grimaldi A, Beaudeux JL. Increased serum concentrations of soluble receptor for advanced glycation endproducts in patients with type 1 diabetes. Clin Chem. 2005;51:1749–50.

32. Nin JW, Jorsal A, Ferreira I, et al. Higher plasma soluble receptor for advanced Glycation end products (sRAGE) levels are associated with incident cardiovascular disease and all-cause mortality in type 1 diabetes: a 12-year follow-up study. Diabetes. 2010;59(8):2027–32. doi:10.2337/db09-1509.

33. Fujisawa K, Katakami N, Kaneto H, et al. Circulating soluble RAGE as a predictive biomarker of cardiovascular event risk in patients with type 2 diabetes. Atherosclerosis. 2013;227(2):425–8. doi:10.1016/j.atherosclerosis.2013.01.016.

34. Rozycki HJ, Bradley J, Karam S. sRAGE is elevated in the lungs of premature infants receiving mechanical ventilation. Am J Perinatol. 2017;20 doi:10.1055/s-0037-1601311.

35. Manichaikul A, Sun L, Borczuk AC, et al. Plasma soluble receptor for advanced Glycation Endproducts in idiopathic pulmonary fibrosis. Ann Am Thorac Soc. 2017; doi:10.1513/AnnalsATS.201606-485OC.

36. Jung ES, Chung W, Kim AJ, et al. Associations between soluble receptor for advanced Glycation end products (sRAGE) and S100A12 (EN-RAGE) with mortality in long-term Hemodialysis patients. J Korean Med Sci. 2017;32(1): 54–9. doi:10.3346/jkms.2017.32.1.54.

37. Franke S, Ruster C, Pester J, Hofmann G, Oelzner P, Wolf G. Advanced glycation end products affect growth and function of osteoblasts. Clin Exp Rheumatol. 2011;29(4):650–60.

38. Alikhani M, Alikhani Z, Boyd C, et al. Advanced glycation end products stimulate osteoblast apoptosis via the MAP kinase and cytosolic apoptotic pathways. Bone. 2007;40:345–53.

39. Yang DH, Chiang TI, Chang IC, Lin FH, Wei CC, Cheng YW. Increased levels of circulating advanced glycation end-products in menopausal women with osteoporosis. Int J Med Sci. 2014;11(5):453–60. doi:10.7150/ijms.8172.

40. Yamagishi S, Takeuchi M, Inagaki Y, Nakamura K, Imaizumi T. Role of advanced glycation end products (AGEs) and their receptor (RAGE) in the pathogenesis of diabetic microangiopathy. Int J Clin Pharmacol Res. 2003;23:129–34.

41. Hagen I, Schulte DM, Muller N, et al. Soluble receptor for advanced glycation end products as a potential biomarker to predict weight loss and improvement of insulin sensitivity by a very low calorie diet of obese human subjects. Cytokine. 2015;73(2):265–9. doi:10.1016/j.cyto.2015.02.022.

42. Jovanovich A, Buzkova P, Chonchol M, et al. Fibroblast growth factor 23, bone mineral density, and risk of hip fracture among older adults: the cardiovascular health study. J Clin Endocrinol Metab. 2013;98(8):3323–31. doi:10.1210/jc.2013-1152.

43. Lane NE, Parimi N, Corr M, et al. Association of serum fibroblast growth factor 23 (FGF23) and incident fractures in older men: the osteoporotic fractures in men (MrOS) study. J Bone Miner Res. 2013;28(11):2325–32. doi: 10.1002/jbmr.1985.

44. Heidari B, Hosseini R, Javadian Y, Bijani A, Sateri MH, Nouroddini HG. Factors affecting bone mineral density in postmenopausal women. Arch Osteoporos. 2015;10:15. doi:10.1007/s11657-015-0217-4.

45. Jiang Y, Zhang Y, Jin M, Gu Z, Pei Y, Meng P. Aged-related changes in body composition and association between body composition with bone mass density by body mass index in Chinese Han men over 50-year-old. PLoS One. 2015;10(6):e0130400. doi:10.1371/journal.pone.0130400.

46. Zhang J, Jin Y, Xu S, et al. Associations of fat mass and fat distribution with bone mineral density in Chinese obese population. J Clin Densitom. 2015; 18(1):44–9. doi:10.1016/j.jocd.2014.03.001.

47. Tohidi M, Akbarzadeh S, Larijani B, et al. Omentin-1, visfatin and adiponectin levels in relation to bone mineral density in Iranian postmenopausal women. Bone. 2012;51(5):876–81. doi:10.1016/j.bone.2012.08.117.

48. Mohiti-Ardekani J, Soleymani-Salehabadi H, Owlia MB, Mohiti A. Relationships between serum adipocyte hormones (adiponectin, leptin, resistin), bone mineral density and bone metabolic markers in osteoporosis patients. J Bone Miner Metab. 2014;32(4):400–4. doi:10.1007/s00774-013-0511-4.

49. Lopez-Jaramillo P, Gomez-Arbelaez D, Lopez-Lopez J, et al. The role of leptin/adiponectin ratio in metabolic syndrome and diabetes. Horm Mol Biol Clin Investig. 2014;18(1):37–45. doi:10.1515/hmbci-2013-0053.

50. Roy B, Curtis ME, Fears LS, Nahashon SN, Fentress HM. Molecular mechanisms of obesity-induced osteoporosis and muscle atrophy. Front Physiol. 2016;29(7):439.

51. Roy B. Biomolecular basis of the role of diabetes mellitus in osteoporosis and bone fractures. World J Diabetes 2013 15;4(4):101-113. doi: 10.4239/wjd.v4.i4.101.

52. Unoki-Kubota H, Yamagishi S, Takeuchi M, Bujo H, Saito Y. Pyridoxamine, an inhibitor of advanced glycation end product (AGE) formation ameliorates insulin resistance in obese, type 2 diabetic mice. Protein Pept Lett. 2010; 17(9):1177–81.

53. de Andrade IS, Zemdegs JC, de Souza AP, et al. Diet-induced obesity impairs hypothalamic glucose sensing but not glucose hypothalamic extracellular levels, as measured by microdialysis. Nutr Diabetes. 2015;15(5): e162. doi:10.1038/nutd.2015.12.

A pilot observational study on magnesium and calcium imbalance in elderly patients with acute aortic dissection

E. Vianello[1*], E. Dozio[1], A. Barassi[2], G. Sammarco[3], L. Tacchini[1], M. M. Marrocco-Trischitta[4], S. Trimarchi[1,4] and M. M. Corsi Romanelli[1,3]

Abstract

Background: Magnesium (Mg) and calcium (Ca) are the principal essential elements involved in endothelial cell homeostasis. Extracellular changes in the levels of either alter endothelial contraction and dilatation. Consequently Mg and Ca imbalance is associated with a high risk of endothelial dysfunction, the main process observed during acute aortic dissection (AAD); in this clinical condition, which mainly affects elderly men, smooth muscle cell alterations lead to intimal tears, creating a false new *lumen* in the *media* of the aorta. AAD patients have a high risk of mortality as a result of late diagnosis because often it is not distinguished from other cardiovascular diseases. We investigated Mg and Ca total circulating levels and the associated pro-inflammatory mediators in elderly AAD patients, to gain further information on the pathophysiology of this disorder, with a view to suggesting newer and earlier potential biomarkers of AAD.

Results: Total circulating Mg and Ca levels were both lower in AAD patients than controls ($p < 0.0001$). Using Ca as cut-off, 90% of AAD patients with low Ca (<8.4 mg/dL) came into the type A classification of AAD. Stratifying AAD according to this cut-off, Mg was lower in patients with lower total Ca.
Compared to controls, both type A and B AAD patients had higher levels of all the pro-coagulant and pro-inflammatory mediators analyzed, including sP-sel, D-dimer, TNF-α, IL-6, and CRP ($p < 0.05$). Dividing types A and B using the Stanford classification, no significant differences were found ($p > 0.05$) The levels of both ICAM-1 and EN-1 were lower in AAD than in a control group ($p < 0.0001$ and $p < 0.05$ respectively).

Conclusions: These findings suggest that low Mg and Ca in AAD elderly patients may contribute to altering normal endothelial physiology and also concur in changing the normal concentrations of different mediators involved in vasodilatation and constriction, associated with AAD onset and severity.

Keywords: Magnesium (Mg), Calcium (Ca), Acute aortic dissection (AAD)

Background

Magnesium (Mg) and calcium (Ca) are involved in the most essential processes regulating cardiovascular function and their imbalance is a factor in the development of numerous disorders of the cardiovascular system, mostly linked to endothelial dysfunction and inflammation, mainly affecting vascular smooth muscle cells (VSMCs) [1]. In humans and animals extracellular Mg

has cardioprotective properties because it attenuates all the agonist-induced vasoconstriction molecules, including endothelin-1 (EN-1), helping preserve vascular tone and preventing coronary vasospasm [1–5]. These cardioprotective effects are reinforced by the fact that Mg assists the coagulation reactions, binding specific coagulation proteins in case of endothelial damage [6].

In the cardiovascular system, one of the main mechanisms that regulates VSMC activity during pressure load is the Ca channel block mediated by Mg [7–14]. This implies that Mg depletion is associated with a high risk of cardiovascular disease (CVD) [2] but little is known

* Correspondence: elena.vianello@unimi.it
[1]Department of Biomedical Sciences for Health, Chair of Clinical Pathology, Università degli Studi di Milano, via Luigi Mangiagalli 31, 20133 Milan, Italy
Full list of author information is available at the end of the article

about the Mg/Ca concentrations in acute aortic dissection (AAD), a dramatic cardiovascular disorder that is often fatal because of late diagnosis [15]. The etiology of AAD involves either genetic disorders affecting connective tissue, such as Marfan syndrome, or is a consequence of primary disorders, generally called non-Marfan AAD, both of which involve aortic stiffening, reduced coronary vessel flow, increased pulse pressure and left ventricular dysfunction [1, 15, 16].

Aging is one of the main risk factors leading to AAD: these include atherosclerosis, hypertension and calcification of the endothelial tunica [17–19]. In particular, patients younger than 65 years old with AAD, undergoing coronary bypass surgery, showed active formation of calcification in atherosclerotic plaques [16, 18, 19].

A discrete and temporary intracellular Ca increase, due to Na/K pump inhibition or blocking a natural Ca antagonist like Mg, may alter cell contraction and transcription and cause cell death [20]. This pathophysiological effect may evolve, at endothelial level, in pro-inflammatory mechanisms characteristic of AAD, including the release of pro-inflammatory mediators, pro-coagulant and endothelial factors from damaged vascular cells [1, 21, 22].

Our aim was to record total circulating Mg and Ca levels in AAD, looking for their possible implication in the severity of the disorder, which is also characterized by the release of mediators involved in endothelial dysfunction, including endothelial, pro-inflammatory and pro-coagulant factors.

Methods

Patients

At I.R.C.C.S. Policlinico San Donato in Milan we enrolled 33 males (age 40–86 years, mean 62.2 ± 18.6 years) with only non-Marfan AAD to exclude any genetic confounding factors, diagnosed within 24 h of symptom onset; 30 healthy age-matched individuals were enrolled as a control group. AAD patients were included in the International Registry of Aortic Dissection (IRAD) that was set up in 1996 by cardiovascular specialists committed to expanding current knowledge of aortic dissection with the goal of improving patient outcomes, with data from 1 January 1996 to 2015. The structure and methods of IRAD have been published [23, 24] and patients gave the hospital their written informed consent.

Patients were then classified according to the Stanford classification in two groups: type A, comprising 22 patients in whom the dissection involved the ascending aorta (proximal dissection) and type B, comprising 11 in whom the dissection was limited to the descending aorta (distal dissection). The type AAD in-patients had no prior aortic dissection and no prior mitral, bicuspid, cuspid or aortic valve diseases. All patients were non-smokers and had never used a drug of abuse (cocaine).

Assays

Serum and plasma were separated by 15 min centrifugation at 1000 g, and stored frozen at –20 °C until analysis. Total Mg was determined by a colorimetric method based on xylidyl blue reaction in alkaline medium to form a water-soluble purple-red chelate whose color intensity is proportional to the concentration of Mg ions in the sample. Calcium ion is excluded from the reaction by complexing with EGTA. For detection we used an RX Monza spectrophotometer (Randox Laboratories, Crumlin, County Antrim, United Kingdom) according to the manufacturer's protocol, with a clinical cut-off from 1.7 to 2.1 mg/dL. Intra- and inter-assay precision was respectively 0.70 and 2.71% (coefficient of variation - CV%). Total Ca was also determined using a colorimetric method with Vitros 5600 (VITROS Chemistry Products Ca Slides, Ortho Clinical Diagnostics, Rochester), and the clinical values ranged between 8.4 and 10.2 mg/dL. The CV% was 0.04 to 0.12%.

Human soluble P-selectin (s-Psel), interleukin-6 (IL-6), tumor necrosis factor-α (TNF-α), interleukin-1β (IL-1β), coagulation factor III (CFIII), endothelin-1 (EN-1), and intercellular adhesion molecule 1 (ICAM-1) were measured by enzyme-linked immunosorbent assays (ELISA) according to the manufacturer's directions (Quantakine Immunoassay, R&D System, Minneapolis, Minnesota, USA). Intra- and inter-assay precision (% CV) was as follows: s-Psel intra-assay mean precision 5.2% and inter-assay mean precision 8.86%; IL-6 intra-assay mean precision 2.6% and inter-assay mean precision 4.5%; TNF-α intra-assay mean precision 4.9% and inter-assay mean precision 7.6%; IL-1β intra-assay mean precision 5.4% and inter-assay mean precision 5.6%; CFIII intra-assay mean precision 2.83% and inter-assay mean precision 5.8%, EN-1 intra-assay mean precision 2.73% and inter-assay mean precision 6.26%, ICAM-1 intra-assay mean precision 4.63% and inter-assay mean precision 5.3%.

Human high-sensitive C-reactive protein (hCRP) was assayed by immunonephelometry (BN II, Dade Behring, Marburg, Germany) with intra- and inter-assay CV% less than 8 and 6% respectively. D-dimer was quantified by immunoreactions using Cobas® 6000 platform analyzer series (Roche Diagnostics, Milan, Italy) with intra- and inter-assay CV% 1.7 and 3.1%.

Statistical analysis

Data were expressed as mean $\pm$ standard deviation (SD) and analyzed using the GraphPad Prism 6.0 biochemical statistical package (GraphPad Software, Inc., San Diego, CA). The normality of data distribution was assessed by the Kolmogorov-Smirnoff test. Groups were compared using Student's two-tailed unpaired T-test or the Mann–Whitney U-test, as appropriate. Correlations between parameters were evaluated using the Spearman test. A p value <0.05 was considered statistically significant.

Results

Circulating Mg and Ca levels were significantly lower in AAD patients than in the control group ($p < 0.0001$) (Fig. 1a–b) but no significant correlation was found between the two parameters (data not shown). Using a clinical cut-off for Ca of 8.4–10.2 mg/dL, 90% of AAD patients with low total Ca (<8.4 mg/dL) were classified as type A (Fig. 1c). Dividing the patients using the 8.4 mg/dL Ca cut-off, total circulating Mg was significantly lower in patients with low total calcium ($p < 0.01$) (Fig. 1d).

Compared to controls, types A and B AAD patients all had higher levels of all pro-coagulant mediators including CFIII, s-Psel, and D-dimer ($p < 0.0001$ for all) (Fig. 2). Human TNF-α, IL-6, and CRP, as pro-inflammatory mediators, were higher in the overall AAD group than controls ($p < 0.05$, $p < 0.05$ and $p < 0.0001$ respectively) (Fig. 2). Dividing type A and B using the Stanford classification, no significant differences were seen in either group.

The endothelial mediators analyzed, including ICAM-1 and EN-1, were lower in AAD patients than controls ($p < 0.0001$ and $p < 0.05$ respectively) (Fig. 2). No significant differences were found between type A and B patients ($p > 0.05$).

No significant correlations were found between Mg and Ca circulating levels and the levels of any of the pro-inflammatory, pro-coagulator and endothelial parameters (data not shown).

Discussion

This study focusing on AAD found low total magnesemia and calcemia. Mg total circulating levels were markedly lower in AAD patients than controls (Fig. 1a) and the pattern was similar for total Ca (Fig. 1b). Because Mg is the natural antagonist of Ca and both these elements have a primary role in VSM tone [14], we also compared the Mg concentration with total Ca. On stratifying AAD patients on the basis of the lower total Ca cut-off (clinically established as less than 8.4 mg/dL), 90% were type A, which is recognized as having a worse prognosis and higher risk of death than type B (Fig. 1c) [17]. These outcomes suggest that in AAD patients the extracellular Mg deficiency, known as an indicator of severe intracellular Mg depletion,

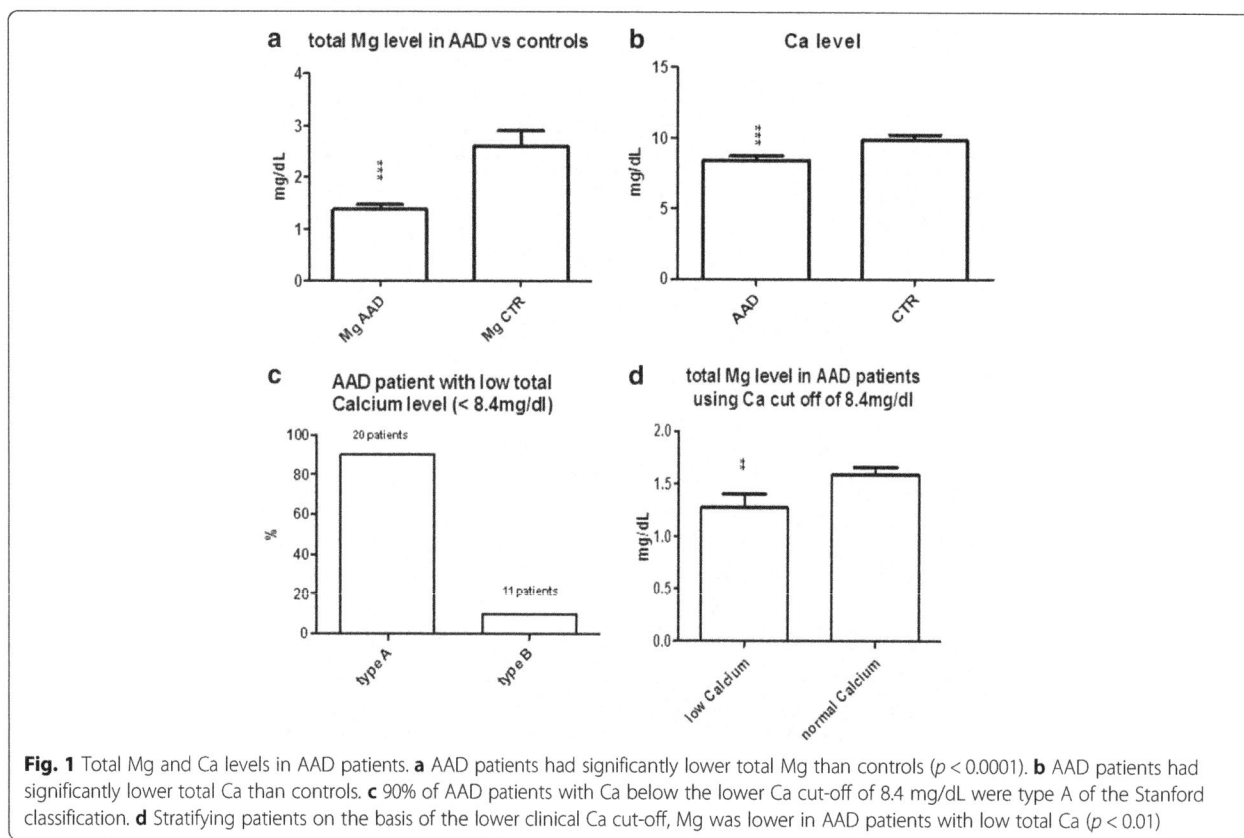

Fig. 1 Total Mg and Ca levels in AAD patients. **a** AAD patients had significantly lower total Mg than controls ($p < 0.0001$). **b** AAD patients had significantly lower total Ca than controls. **c** 90% of AAD patients with Ca below the lower Ca cut-off of 8.4 mg/dL were type A of the Stanford classification. **d** Stratifying patients on the basis of the lower clinical Ca cut-off, Mg was lower in AAD patients with low total Ca ($p < 0.01$)

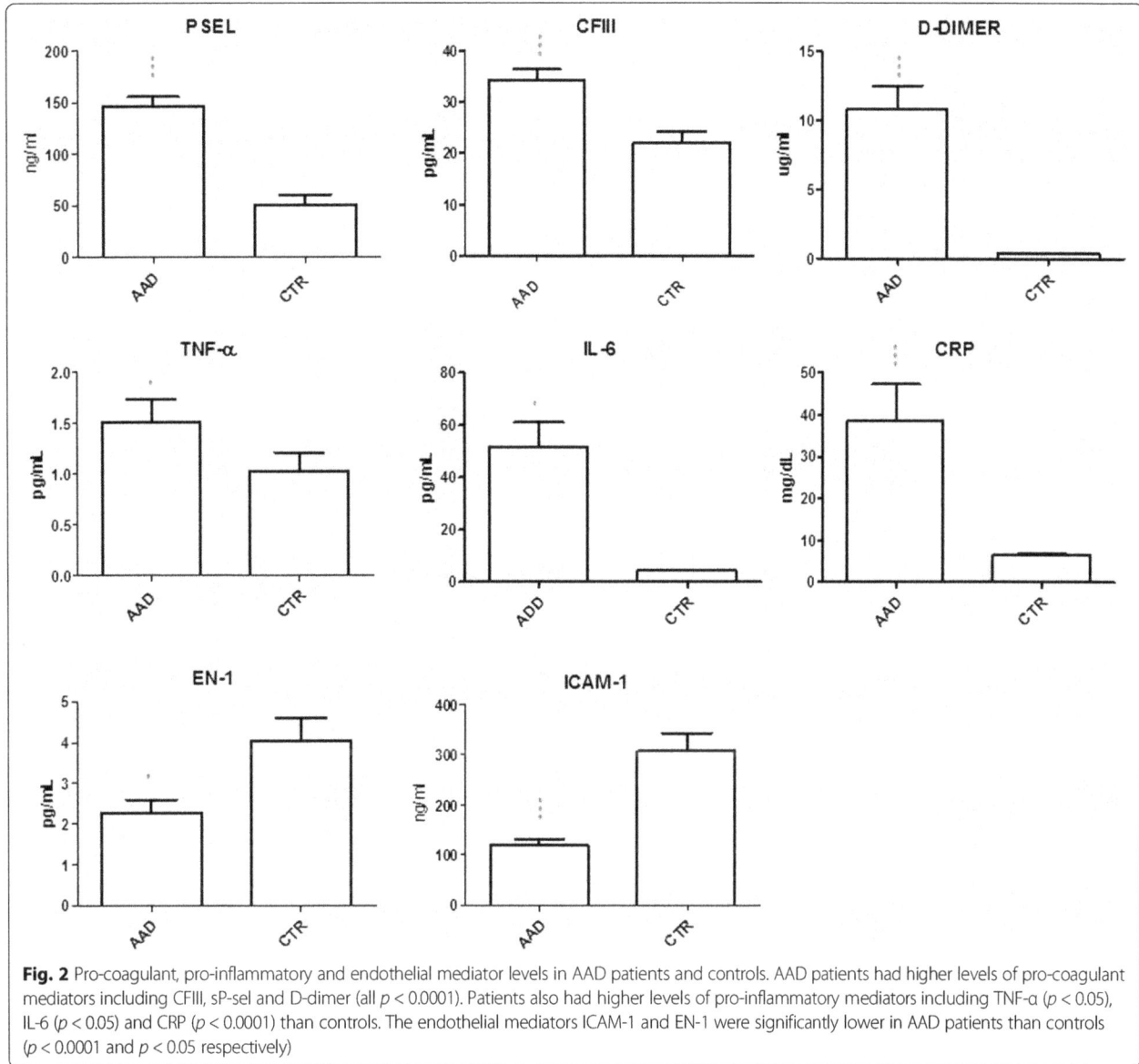

Fig. 2 Pro-coagulant, pro-inflammatory and endothelial mediator levels in AAD patients and controls. AAD patients had higher levels of pro-coagulant mediators including CFIII, sP-sel and D-dimer (all $p < 0.0001$). Patients also had higher levels of pro-inflammatory mediators including TNF-α ($p < 0.05$), IL-6 ($p < 0.05$) and CRP ($p < 0.0001$) than controls. The endothelial mediators ICAM-1 and EN-1 were significantly lower in AAD patients than controls ($p < 0.0001$ and $p < 0.05$ respectively)

directly influences total Ca. Therefore we assume that the lower extracellular Mg levels in AAD patients were too low to balance Ca entry into the cells, resulting in a total circulating Ca deficiency.

On the basis of this preliminary data we can only suggest that during the acute phase of AAD, within 24 h, the molecular mechanism may be driven by Mg/Ca deficiency promoting an imbalance among the concentrations of several mediators involved in inflammation and vasoconstriction of the endothelium. We therefore measured the circulating levels of the main pro-inflammatory mediators that can be directly affected by Mg/Ca and by endothelial dysfunction, including TNF-α, IL-6 and CRP [25–27]: they were all substantially higher in AAD patients than controls.

The systemic inflammation highlighted in AAD patients was also associated with an imbalance of pro-coagulant and vasoconstrictor factors including D-dimer, CFIII, s-Psel and EN-1, which are deregulated compared to controls, although we found no real differences between type A and B patients. Our findings with ICAM-1 agree with previous studies [28, 29], which reported that during the early phase of AAD deregulation of the production of soluble and intracellular forms of adhesion molecule could result in lower levels of the intracellular form, such as ICAM-1, to compensate the release of circulating mediators, as illustrated in Fig. 2.

The main limitation of this study is the small number of patients and further investigations are obviously needed to increase the power of our results.

Conclusion

Our findings suggest that hypomagnesemia may be one of the principal causes of AAD onset and development, which can result in different sub-events related to Mg depletion including first of all hypocalcemia and subsequently hypertension, then inflammation and vasoconstriction of the endothelium. Therefore it is plausible that besides the systemic Ca level intracellular calcium may increase too in AAD patients during Mg depletion, but this assumption needs to be verified by future analysis to better understand the pathophysiology of AAD and its direct relationship with Mg depletion.

Abbreviations

AAD: Acute aortic dissection; Ca: Calcium; CFIII: Coagulation factor III; CVD: Cardiovascular disease; ELISA: Enzyme-linked immunosorbent assays; EN-1: Endothelin-1; hCRP: Human high-sensitive C-reactive protein; ICAM-1: Intercellular adhesion molecule 1; IL-1β: Interleukin-1β; IL-6: Interleukin-6; Mg: Magnesium; SD: Standard deviation; s-Psel: Soluble P-selectin; TNF-α: Tumor necrosis factor-α; VSMC: Vascular smooth muscle cells

Acknowledgements

The authors are grateful to Dr. Elena Costa for clinical chemistry analysis and Dr. Judit Bagott for English edit.

Funding

The study was supported by the Italian Ministero dell'Istruzione, Università e Ricerca (MIUR) and Italian Ministero della Salute (R.C. no. 9.14.2).

Authors' contributions

CRMM, TL, DE and VE designed the study. VE did the research and analyzed the data. TS, MTMM and BA enrolled the patients and started the clinical study protocol. SG did part of the analysis. VE wrote the paper. All authors critically read, improved and approved the final manuscript.

Competing interests

The authors declare they have no competing interests.

Author details

[1]Department of Biomedical Sciences for Health, Chair of Clinical Pathology, Università degli Studi di Milano, via Luigi Mangiagalli 31, 20133 Milan, Italy. [2]Department of Health Sciences, Università degli Studi di Milano, Milan, Italy. [3]Laboratory Medicine Operative Unit-1, Clinical Pathology, I.R.C.C.S. Policlinico San Donato Milanese, Milan, Italy. [4]Thoracic Aortic Research Center, I.R.C.C.S. Policlinico San Donato, San Donato Milanese, Milan, Italy.

References

1. Wen D, Zhou XL, Li JJ, Hui RT. Biomarkers in aortic dissection. Clin Chim Acta. 2011;412:688–95.
2. Reffelmann T, Ittermann T, Dorr M, Volzke H, Reinthaler M, Petersmann A, Felix SB. Low serum magnesium concentrations predict cardiovascular and all-cause mortality. Atherosclerosis. 2011;219:280–4.
3. Shechter M. Magnesium and cardiovascular system. Magnes Res. 2010;23: 60–72.
4. Al-Ghamdi SM, Cameron EC, Sutton RA. Magnesium deficiency: pathophysiologic and clinical overview. Am J Kidney Dis. 1994;24:737–52.
5. Ko EA, Park WS, Earm YE. Extracellular Mg²⁺ blocks endothelin-1-induced contraction through the inhibition of non-selective cation channels in coronary smooth muscle. Eur J Physiol. 2004;449:195–204.
6. Tokutake T, Baba H, Shimada Y, Takeda W, Sato K, Hiroshima Y, Kirihara T, Shimizu I, Nakazawa H, Kobayashi H, Ishida F. Exogenous magnesium chloride reduces the activated partial thromboplastin times of lupus anticoagulant-positive patients. Plos One. 2016;11(6):e0157835.
7. Ma J, Zhao N, Zhu D. Biphasic responses of human vascular smooth muscle cells to magnesium ion. J Biomed Mater Res A. 2016;104:347–56.
8. Herencia C, Rodriguez-Ortiz ME, Munoz-Castaneda JR, Martinez-Moreno JM, Canalejo R, Montes De Oca A, Diaz-Tocados JM, Peralbo-Santaella E, Marin C, Canalejo A, Rodriguez M, Almaden Y. Angiotensin II prevents calcification in vascular smooth muscle cells by enhancing magnesium influx. Eur J Clin Invest. 2015;45:1129–44.
9. Bai Y, Zhang J, Xu J, Cui L, Zhang H, Zhang S, Feng X. Magnesium prevents beta-glycerophosphate-induced calcification in rat aortic vascular smooth muscle cells. Biomed Rep. 2015;3:593–7.
10. Veklich TO, Mazur I, Kosterin SO. [Mg2+, ATP-dependent plasma membrane calcium pump of smooth muscle cells. I. Structural organization and properties. Ukr Biochem J. 2015;87:5–20.
11. Song S, Yamamura A, Yamamura H, Ayon RJ, Smith KA, Tang H, Makino A, Yuan JX. Flow shear stress enhances intracellular Ca2+ signaling in pulmonary artery smooth muscle cells from patients with pulmonary arterial hypertension. Am J Physiol Cell Physiol. 2014;307:C373–383.
12. Denny JT, Pantin E, Chiricolo A, Tse J, Jan T, Chaudhry M, Barsoum S, Denny AM, Papp D, Morgan SL. Lower incidence of hypo-magnesemia in surgical intensive care unit patients in 2011 versus 2001. J Clin Med Res. 2015;7:253–6.
13. Edvinsson M, Ilback NG, Frisk P, Thelin S, Nystrom-Rosander C. Trace Element Changes in Thoracic Aortic Dissection. Biol Trace Elem Res. 2015; 169:159–63.
14. Kolte D, Vijayaraghavan K, Khera S, Sica DA, Frishman WH. Role of magnesium in cardiovascular diseases. Cardiol Rev. 2014;22:182–92.
15. Kharitonova M, Iezhitsa I, Zheltova A, Ozerov A, Spasov A, Skalny A. Comparative angioprotective effects of magnesium compounds. J Trace Elem Med Biol. 2015;29:227–34.
16. Cheuk BL, Chan YC, Cheng SW. Changes in inflammatory response after endovascular treatment for type B aortic dissection. PLoS One. 2012;7: e37389.
17. Kim WH, Bae J, Choi SW, Lee JH, Kim CS, Cho HS, Lee SM. Stanford type A aortic dissection in a patient with Marfan syndrome during pregnancy: a case report. Korean J Anesthesiol. 2016;69:76–9.
18. Yamada H, Sakata N, Wada H, Tashiro T, Tayama E. Age-related distensibility and histology of the ascending aorta in elderly patients with acute aortic dissection. J Biomech. 2015;48:3267–73.
19. Yeh YH, Su YJ, Liu CH. Acute aortic dissection (AAD) in the elderly. Arch Gerontol Geriatr. 2013;57:78–80.
20. de Jong PA, Helling WE, Takx RA, Išgum I, van Herwaarden JA, Mali WP. Computed tomography of aortic wall calcifications in aortic dissection. Plos One. 2014;9(7):e102036.
21. Vanhuyse F, Maureira P, Laurent N, Lekehal M, Grandmougain D, Villemot JP. Surgery for acute type A aortic dissection in octogenarians. J Card Surg. 2012;27:65–9.
22. Amico A, Caprili L, Fahim NA, Cristell D, Carbone C. Surgical strategy for acute type A aortic dissection in octogenarians. J Cardiovasc Med (Hagerstown). 2008;9:296–7.
23. Kwartler CS, Chen J, Thakur D, Li S, Baskin K, Wang S, Wang ZV, Walker L, Hill JA, Epstein HF, Taegtmeyer H, Milewicz DM. Overexpression of smooth muscle myosin heavy chain leads to activation of the unfolded protein response and autophagic turnover of thick filament-associated proteins in vascular smooth muscle cells. J Biol Chem. 2014;289:14075–88.
24. Giannitsis E, Mair J, Christersson C, Siegbahn A, Huber K, Jaffe AS, Peacock WF, Plebani M, Thygesen K, Mockel M, Mueller C, Lindahl B: How to use D-dimer in acute cardiovascular care. Eur Heart J Acute Cardiovasc Care. 2015. doi:10.1177/ 2048872615610870.
25. Hagan PG, Nienaber CA, Isselbacher EM, Bruckman D, Karavite DJ, Russman PL, Evangelista A, Fattori R, Suzuki T, Oh JK, Moore AG, Malouf JF, Pape LA, Gaca C, Sechtem U, Lenferink S, Deutsch HJ, Diedrichs H, Marcos y Robles J, Llovet A, Gilon D, Das SK, Armstrong WF, Deeb GM, Eagle KA. The International Registry of Acute Aortic Dissection (IRAD): new insights into an old disease. JAMA. 2000;283(7):897–903.
26. Mehta RH, Suzuki T, Hagan PG, Bossone E, Gilon D, Llovet A, Maroto LC, Cooper JV, Smith DE, Armstrong WF, Nienaber CA, Eagle KA. Predicting death in patients with acute type A aortic dissection. Circulation. 2002; 105(2):200–6.

Altered activation state of circulating neutrophils in patients with neovascular age-related macular degeneration

Marie Krogh Nielsen[1,2]*, Sven Magnus Hector[1], Kelly Allen[1], Yousif Subhi[1,2] and Torben Lykke Sørensen[1,2]

Abstract

Background: Neutrophil dysfunction plays a key role in the development of diseases characterized by inflammation and angiogenesis. Here, we studied the systemic expression of neutrophil markers reflecting activation, adhesion, and resolution of inflammation in patients with neovascular age-related macular degeneration (AMD).

Results: This was a prospective case-control study of patients with neovascular AMD and age-matched healthy control individuals. Patients were recruited from an outpatient program, and control individuals were recruited amongst patients' relatives. Current smokers and individuals with either active immune-disease or ongoing cancer were not included, as these factors are known to affect neutrophil function. Fresh-drawn venous blood was processed for flow cytometric analysis of neutrophil markers. We determined percentages of positive cells and compared expression levels using fluorescence intensity measures. We found conditional differences on marker expression between patients with neovascular AMD ($n = 29$) and controls ($n = 28$): no differences were found when looking broadly, but several differences emerged when focusing on non-smokers. Here, patients with neovascular AMD had increased expression of the activity marker cluster of differentiation (CD) 66b ($P = 0.003$; Mann-Whitney U test), decreased expression of adhesion marker CD162 ($P = 0.044$; Mann-Whitney U test), and lower expression of the resolution of inflammation marker C-X-C chemokine receptor 2 ($P = 0.044$; Mann-Whitney U test).

Conclusions: We present novel evidence suggesting that the activity of circulating neutrophils, sensitive to smoking, may differ in patients with neovascular AMD.

Keywords: Neutrophils, Age-related macular degeneration, Choroidal neovascularization, Flow cytometry, Inflammation

Background

Age-related macular degeneration (AMD) is a chronic progressive disease of the aged macula [1]. In the early stages, the disease is clinically characterized by drusen, which are yellow deposits between Bruch's membrane and the retinal pigment epithelium [1]. The late stages of AMD are characterized by localized atrophy of the retina or by choroidal neovascularizations (CNV) [1]. The latter instance is described as neovascular AMD due to its key feature where newly formed vessels of the choroid penetrate through Bruch's membrane into the subretinal space [1]. Consequently, fluid and blood leak into the retina, irreversibly impairing vision and visual function [2]. The treatment is only able to keep vision at a stable level for some years, and neovascular AMD still remains the most common reason for irreversible vision loss in the developed world [2–4].

The pathogenesis of neovascular AMD remains incompletely understood, but ageing and dysfunction of the immune system are believed to play a key role for the disease to develop in an aged macula [5–7]. A current developing area of interest is how neutrophils play a role in disease development. This is particularly interesting since aging is the highest risk factor of developing neovascular AMD and aged neutrophils are characterized by changed surface expression and activity [5–8]. Studies have found a higher neutrophil/lymphocyte ratio in patients with neovascular AMD [9–11], and studies of donor eyes have shown infiltrating lipocalin-2-positive neutrophils at

* Correspondence: mrrm@regionsjaelland.dk
[1]Department of Ophthalmology, Zealand University Hospital, Vestermarksvej 23, DK-4000 Roskilde, Denmark
[2]Faculty of Health and Medical Sciences, University of Copenhagen, Copenhagen, Denmark

significantly higher levels in retina and the choroid in both early and late stages of AMD [12]. Lipocalin-2 is a protein expressed in neutrophils, and levels of intravitreal lipocalin-2 are significantly elevated in eyes with neovascular AMD [13].

Neutrophils are the most prominent granulocytes and are part of the innate immune system practicing granulocyte release and phagocytosis [14]. Following stimuli, the activated neutrophils adhere to the endothelial cells in the area of inflammation and migrate their way to the site of injury and infection. Neutrophilic action is mediated through an effective combination of cytotoxic granules, antimicrobial peptides, and neutrophil extracellular traps [15]. Circulating neutrophils contains myeloperoxidase (MPO), which can form a hypochlourous acid that is an efficient killer of pathogens. In Parkinson's disease and Alzheimer's disease, MPO is redistributed into the extracellular space where it mediates tissue damage [16, 17], which is a mechanism suspected of contributing to the pathogenesis of AMD. Accumulated MPO is a two-edged sword: it may be beneficial by clearing toxic retinal lipofuscin deposits, but may be harmful by causing lysosomal stress that results in cell death [18].

Several chemokines are suggested to play a role in recruiting monocytes/macrophages and neutrophils resulting in the formation of CNVs [19]. Zhou et al. studied laser-induced CNV on mice and found that neutrophils infiltrate the retinal tissue from the first day after stimulation and that neutrophil-depleted mice had significantly smaller CNV-response. [20] Lavalette et al. found that neutrophils infiltrated the choroid 10 h after laser stimulation expressing the proangionetic interleukin 1β [21]. Taken together, these findings support the theory that neutrophils may play an important part in the early CNV-response. In humans, we previously described that systemic levels of neutrophils correlate with CNV-lesion size in patients with neovascular AMD [22], which further supports a role for neutrophils in CNV-development in AMD.

Based on these findings, we hypothesized that systemic neutrophil expression and properties could be altered in patients with wet AMD. To investigate this further, we selected markers of interest representing key steps of neutrophil activity: activation, adhesion, and inflammation [23]. Neutrophil migration is a process, which involves activation following interaction between adhesion molecules on the neutrophils and their ligands on the endothelial cells. Cluster of differentiation (CD) 63 and CD66b are activation-molecules expressed on the surface of neutrophils after appropriate stimulation [24, 25]. CD162 (P-selectin glycoprotein ligand-1) and CD62L (P-selectin) are mediators of the first step of rolling, after which integrin molecules CD11a (lymphocyte function-associated antigen-1) and CD11b (macrophage associated antigen-1) participate [23, 24, 26]. The process

of transmigration through the endothelial layer is mediated by CD54 and CD31 (platelet endothelial cell adhesion molecule-1) [27]. The degree of inflammatory activity of neutrophils can be studied by measuring the expression level of several markers. One such marker is the interleukin-1-receptor-2 (IL1-R2), which is the receptor of the highly proinflammatory cytokine interleukin-1 [28]. C-X-C chemokine receptor 2 (CXCR2) is also important in acute and chronic inflammation and is mainly regulated by interleukin-8 [29]. C-C chemokine receptor 5 (CCR5) is involved in resolution of inflammation [30]. The Duffy antigen receptor for chemokines (DARC) is suggested to play a role in inflammation since DARC seems to bind a large number of chemokines whereby it might have a protective role in preventing chemokine activation of neutrophils and inflammation [31].

In this study, we wished to study alterations of the innate immune system in neovascular AMD. We sampled blood from patients with neovascular AMD and compared them to that of aged-matched healthy control individuals. We did not include any participants who were actively smoking. Tobacco triggers acute inflammation mediated via Toll-like-receptors [32] and modulates the expression of pro-inflammatory cytokines and chemokines [33]. Also, tobacco smoking increases the risk of AMD significantly. The increase in risk is most pronounced in current smokers, but is also markedly higher in former smokers [34].

Methods
Study design
This was a prospective case-control study of patients with neovascular AMD and healthy controls. The study was approved by the Regional Committee of Ethics in Research in Region Zealand (SJ-142). Verbal and written informed consent was obtained from all participants prior to inclusion. The described project adhered to the tenets of the Declaration of Helsinki.

Participants
All participants were recruited from the Department of Ophthalmology, Zealand University Hospital, Roskilde, Denmark. Patients with neovascular AMD were recruited from our retinal clinic. Healthy age-matched control individuals were relatives of the participating patients. This was an intentional strategy to better match the control group (lifestyle, diet, exposure, etc.). Since this was a hypothesis-driven study, we were unable to perform power-calculations, but based on previous experience with flow cytometric studies of systemic leukocyte markers, we aimed at recruiting at least 20 participants and stopped recruitment after successfully analyzing 29 blood samples from each group.

All participants were interviewed regarding medical history and lifestyle. Smoking was considered active if the participants had smoked at any time within the last year regardless of whether or not they had decided to stop smoking [35]. Previous smokers and non-smokers were both defined as not having smoked within the last year, and previous and non-smokers were distinguished by the latter having smoked less than 100 cigarettes (5 packs) during their entire lifetime [35]. Self-reported alcohol consumption was noted as units (=12 g ethanol) per week. We calculated body mass index using weight and height. Physical activity was assessed using a single question for epidemiological studies which, has been validated previously on patients with neovascular AMD [36, 37].

We sampled fresh venous blood from the antecubital vein in two tubes: one 5 mL ethylenediamine-tetraacetic acid coagulant containing tube for flow cytometry and one 3 mL lithium-heparin coated tube for determining C-reactive protein (CRP) level.

Retinal diagnosis and eligibility

All participants had a comprehensive ocular examination including measurement of best-corrected visual acuity, slit-lamp examination, digital color fundus photography (Carl Zeiss, Jena, Germany), Spectral-Domain Optical Coherence Tomography, and fundus autofluorescence imaging (Spectralis HRA-OCT, SLO Heidelberg Engineering, Heidelberg, Germany). Retinal angiography using fluorescein and indocyanine green were performed where choroidal neovascularization was suspected. All retinal diagnosis was confirmed by an experienced ophthalmologist.

Healthy aged-matched controls individuals were only considered for inclusion if they had normal maculae with no more than 10 small drusen as defined in the Clinical Age-Related Maculopathy Grading System (CARMS) [38]. Any currently smoking participants were not included. Participants with any infectious diseases or immunological disorders were also not recruited, including those in immune-modulating therapy for any reason. We excluded any participant with a plasma CRP-level > 15 mg/L to avoid participants with possible ongoing infections [39]. To avoid interference with flow cytometric analyses, we did not recruit patients with neovascular AMD within 4 or 8 weeks respectively of Ranibizumab or Aflibercept therapy or immediately after retinal angiography [40].

Flow cytometry

All samples were analyzed within 4 h of phlebotomy. We used the white blood cell count (Sysmex KX-21N™, Sysmex Corporation, Kobe, Japan) to calculate a blood volume, that would contain 5×10^5 leukocytes, which we lysed in a 50 ml tube by adding red blood cell lysis buffer (Nordic Biosite AB, Täby, Sweden), and waiting

10 min in the dark at room temperature. The cells were washed three times; each time by centrifuging for 5 min at 500G, decanting the supernatant, and re-suspending in an isotonic buffer (IsoFlow Sheath Fluid, Beckman Coulter Inc., Brea, CA, USA). For each blood sample, we prepared four panels with monoclonal anti-human antibodies for cell population gating and for the markers of interest and two panels with fluorochrome-matched isotype controls: Phycoerythrin-Cyanine 7 (PC7) immunoglobulin G (IgG) 1 (Cat. No.: 400,126; BioLegend, San Diego, CA, USA), fluorescein isothiocyanate (FITC) IgG1 (Cat. No.: 400,108; BioLegend), phycoerythrin (PE) IgG1 (Cat. No.: 400,112; BioLegend), PC7 IgG2b (Cat. No.: 303,117; BioLegend), and PE IgG2b (Cat. No.: 400,212; BioLegend). We incubated samples in darkness and at room temperature, as recommended by the manufacturers. We then washed the cells, added 500 μL isotonic buffer, and re-suspended. Stained cells ($n = 100.000$) were analyzed using the flow cytometer BD FACS CANTO II (BD Biosciences, FranklinLakes, NJ, USA) and Kaluza Software (v. 1.5.20365.16139, Beckman Coulter Inc., Pasadena, CA,USA). All flow samples were analyzed using the same settings on the flow cytometer.

On a forward/side scatter plot, we isolated granulocytes, on which we used CD16 (Cat. No.: 360,712; BioLegend) and CD14 (Cat. No.: 325,616; BioLegend) for identifying neutrophils defined as $CD14^{dim}CD16^+$ (Fig. 1). On these neutrophils, we studied cell markers of three important functions of neutrophils: activation, adhesion, and resolution of inflammation:

- Activation: CD63 (Cat. No.: 353,009; BioLegend) and CD66b (Cat. No.: 305,103; BioLegend).
- Adhesion: CD11a (Cat. No.: 301,206; BioLegend), CD11b (Cat. No.: 301,306; BioLegend), CD31 (Cat. No.: 303,117; BioLegend), CD54 (Cat. No.: 533,107; BioLegend), CD62L (Cat. No.: 304,821; BioLegend), and CD162 (Cat. No.: 328,805; BioLegend).
- Resolution of inflammation: IL1-R2/CD121b (Cat. No: LS-C139986–100; LifeSpan BioSciences Inc., Seattle, WA, USA), CXCR2/CD182 (Cat. No.: 320,706; BioLegend), CCR5/CD195 (Cat. No.: 359,107; BioLegend), and Duffy antigen/chemokine receptor (DARC)/CD234 (Cat. No.: FAB4139P; R&D Systems Inc., Minneapolis, MN, USA).

We determined the percentage of neutrophils that were positive for the concerned marker. We gated the positive cells and defined the median fluorescence intensity (MFI).

Data analysis and statistics

First, we compared participant characteristics between patients with neovascular AMD and the healthy control

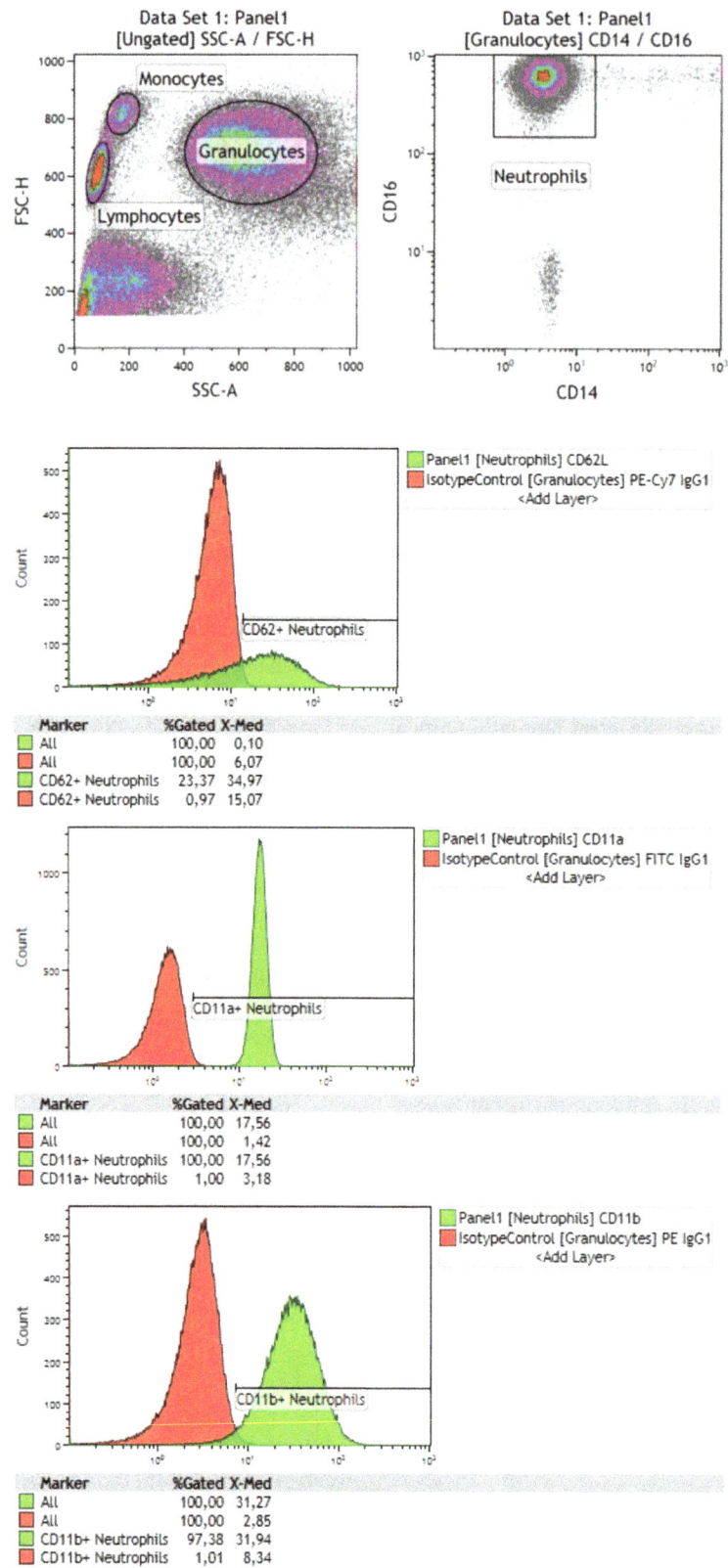

Fig. 1 Neutrophil gating and expression analysis. Here we analyze identify CD14^dim CD16^+ granulocytes (neutrophils) (Top) to study percentages of CD62, CD11a, and CD11b positives and their expression level in terms of median fluorescence intensity

individuals (demographics, co-morbidities, lifestyle factors, and basic blood values such as white blood cell count, neutrophil percentage and count, and plasma CRP). When dealing with continuous data, we checked for normal distribution using histograms and the Kolmogorov-Smirnov test. Where normal distribution was present, data was presented using mean and standard deviation (SD) and compared using the independent samples t-test. Otherwise, data was presented using median and interquartile range (IQR) and compared using the Mann-Whitney U test. For each category (activation, adhesion, and resolution of inflammation) of markers investigated, we compared the percentage of positive neutrophils and their expression

level in terms of MFI. Acknowledging the potential influence of smoking, we evaluated whether healthy controls differed in neutrophil markers between previous and non-smokers. Since this was the case, we decided to repeat all analyses on non-smokers only. All statistical analyses were made in SPSS version 23 for Mac (IBM, Armonk, NY, USA). P-values below 0.05 were interpret as sign of statistical significance.

Results

We recruited a total of 61 individuals, of which 58 provided blood sample for our neutrophil study. One of the healthy control individuals had a plasma CRP >15 mg/L

Table 1 Participant characteristics

	Healthy controls ($n = 28$)	Patients with neovascular AMD ($n = 29$)	P-value
Demographics			
Age, years, mean (SD)	77.2 (6.6)	79.4 (6.1)	0.192
Females, n (%)	12 (43)	20 (69)	0.047
Co-morbidities			
Hypertension, n (%)	13 (46)	14 (48)	0.889
Hypercholesterolemia, n (%)	9 (32)	10 (34)	0.851
Cardiovascular diseases, n (%)	12 (43)	10 (34)	0.516
Type 2 diabetes, n (%)	2 (7)	2 (7)	1.000
Lifestyle factors			
Body mass index, mean (SD)	25.8 (4.7)	26.7 (5.2)	0.506
Physically active, n (%)	6 (21)	9 (31)	0.410
Alcohol consumption, median (IQR)	7 (2 to 10)	3 (1 to 9)	0.126
Smoking status, n (%)			0.889
Previous smoker	15 (54)	15 (52)	
Non-smoker	13 (46)	14 (48)	
Blood measures			
C-reactive protein, mg/L			0.029
< 2.9 mg/L	23 (82)	16 (55)	
2.9–14.9 mg/L	5 (18)	13 (45)	
White blood cell count, 10^9 cells/L, mean (SD)	5.9 (1.2)	6.4 (1.6)	0.212
Lymphocytes, mean (SD)			
%	29 (8)	28 (9)	0.892
10^9 cells/L	1.7 (0.5)	1.8 (0.6)	0.654
Monocytes, mean (SD)			
%	7 (2)	6 (3)	0.457
10^9 cells/L	0.4 (0.1)	0.4 (0.2)	0.678
Neutrophils, mean (SD)			
%	64 (8)	65 (11)	0.618
10^9 cells/L	3.8 (1.0)	4.3 (1.5)	0.198
Neutrophils-to-lymphocytes, mean (SD)	2.52 (1.03)	2.80 (1.51)	0.422

Parametric continuous variables are presented using mean and standard deviation (SD) and tested using the independent samples t-test. Non-parametric continuous variables are presented using median and interquartile range (IQR) and tested using the Mann-Whitney U test. Categorical variables are presented using numbers (n) and percentages (%) and tested using the χ^2-test, but due to very small numbers is co-morbidity of type 2 diabetes tested using the Fisher's Exact test

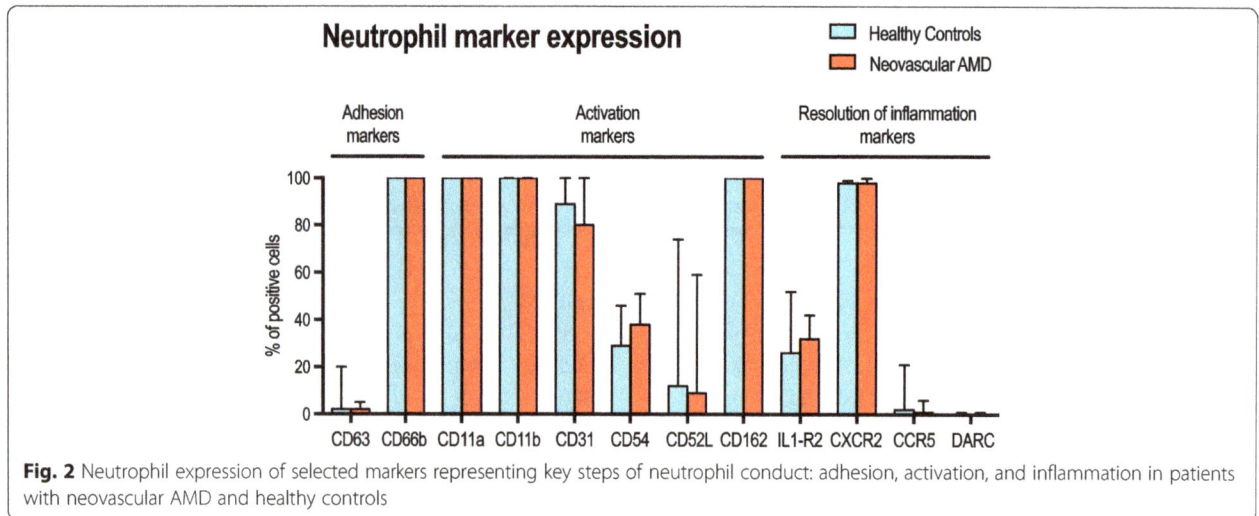

Fig. 2 Neutrophil expression of selected markers representing key steps of neutrophil conduct: adhesion, activation, and inflammation in patients with neovascular AMD and healthy controls

(22 mg/L) and was excluded from analyses. In total, 28 healthy control individuals and 29 patients with neovascular AMD were included for analyses. Mean age was 77.2 (SD: 6.6) years and 79.4 (SD: 6.1) years respectively for patients and controls ($P = 0.192$; independent samples t-test). Slightly more patients ($n = 20$, 69%) were female when compared to controls ($n = 12$, 43%) ($P = 0.047$, χ^2-test). The patients and the control groups were generally similar in their co-morbidities and lifestyle characteristics. White blood cell count, and leukocyte population percentages and counts also did not differ significantly between the groups. Increased plasma CRP was more likely in patients with neovascular AMD (odds ratio 3.7, $P = 0.033$) (Table 1).

Activation

Activation markers did not differ significantly in percentage of positive neutrophils (Fig. 2). Expression level of CD63 was also similar between groups. We observed a trend towards higher expression level of CD66b in patients with neovascular AMD, but this trend did not reach a level of statistical significance. However, we repeated the analyses on non-smokers only and found that among non-smokers, expression level of CD66b is significantly higher in patients with neovascular AMD when compared to healthy controls ($P = 0.003$; Mann-Whitney U test) (Fig. 3).

Adhesion

Adhesion markers did not differ significantly in percentage of positive neutrophils (Fig. 2). Expression level on the marker positive neutrophils were also similar between groups. Repeating the analyses on non-smokers only showed that CD162 expression was slightly lower in patients with neovascular AMD ($P = 0.044$; Mann-Whitney U test) (Fig. 4).

Resolution of inflammation

Resolution of inflammation markers did not differ significantly in percentage of positive neutrophils (Fig. 2). Expression level on the marker positive neutrophils were also similar for IL1-R2, CCR5, and DARC, but we observed a non-significant trend towards lower CXCR2 on neutrophils in patients with neovascular AMD. Repeating the analyses on non-smokers suggest that among non-smokers, patients with neovascular AMD have significantly lower expression of CXCR2 ($P = 0.044$; Mann-Whitney U test) (Fig. 5).

Discussion

We find that among non-smokers, patients with neovascular AMD had increased expression of the activity marker CD66b, decreased expression of the adhesion marker CD162, and lower expression of inflammation marker CXCR2. Our results suggest that neutrophils

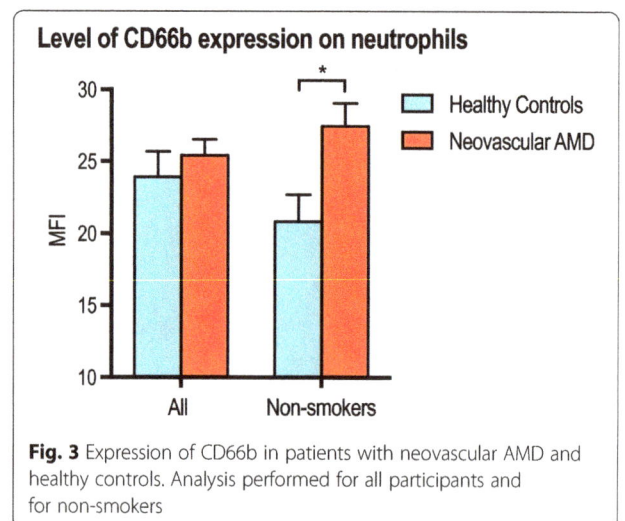

Fig. 3 Expression of CD66b in patients with neovascular AMD and healthy controls. Analysis performed for all participants and for non-smokers

Level of CD162 expression on neutrophils

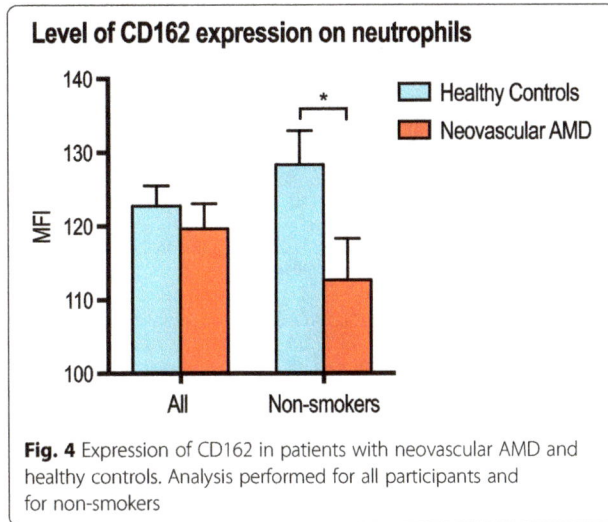

Fig. 4 Expression of CD162 in patients with neovascular AMD and healthy controls. Analysis performed for all participants and for non-smokers

may have specific components that play a role in neovascular AMD.

Complement activation plays a key role in the pathogenesis of AMD. Histopathological studies have found complement components in eyes with drusen [41], which are also reflected in altered levels of systemic complement markers in patients with AMD [42, 43]. Interestingly, complement activation induces CD66b overexpression and drastically reduces the neutrophils' phagocytic capacity [25]. In light of these findings, we hypothesize that CD66b overexpression on systemic neutrophils in patients with neovascular AMD may reflect an increased systemic level of complement components that in turn inhibit the phagocytic capacity of the neutrophils. Consequently, we speculate that the drusenoid macula may lack an appropriate neutrophil response to the increased inflammatory and angiogenic drive whereby CNV formation can proceed unhampered.

Level of CXCR2 expression on neutrophils

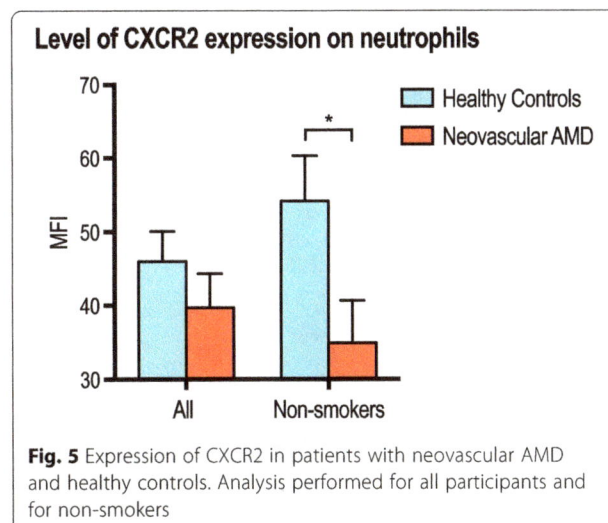

Fig. 5 Expression of CXCR2 in patients with neovascular AMD and healthy controls. Analysis performed for all participants and for non-smokers

Several studies suggest that AMD is associated with immunosenescence and systemic presence of low-grade inflammation [36, 44, 45]. We confirm this association in CRP, which were higher in patients with neovascular AMD. On neutrophils, such inflammatory environments influence the expression of CD162 [46, 47]. CD162 is a type 1 membrane protein that is constitutively expressed on human neutrophils and able to interact with all 3 types of selectins: P-selectin on activated platelets and endothelial cells, E-selectin on endothelial cells, and L-selectin on leukocytes [26]. This interaction between CD162 and its ligands is the first adhesion step and leads to neutrophils rolling on the endothelium prior to adhesion. Severe systemic inflammation in humans causes rapid downregulation of CD162 on neutrophils [46]. Inflammation of lesser degree have similar impact on CD162, exemplified by one study of surgical stress after cardiopulmonary bypass surgery [47]. Based on these considerations, we speculate that low-grade inflammation in patients with AMD may cause CD162 downregulation on neutrophils that in turn are less adherent.

CXCR2 is a chemokine receptor that regulates neutrophil recruitment in inflammatory contexts. Its function in inflammation and tumor-related inflammatory activities is vital and CXCR2 modulation has been suggested for treatment [48–50]. One study of CXCR2 deficient mice demonstrated that CXCR2 plays an important role for macrophage-dependent inflammatory response. In CXCR2 deficient mice, inflammatory responses were more excessive, more macrophages were recruited to sites of inflammation, and levels of anti- and pro-inflammatory cytokines were shifted towards relatively more pro-inflammatory levels [51]. Hence, CXCR2 controls the magnitude of macrophage response in inflammation. We and other groups have previously found that monocytes and macrophages may play a key role in AMD and particularly for CNV formation [22, 52–55]. Experimental laser-induced lesions on mice retinae show that macrophages are important for the CNV formation and systemic depletion of macrophages lead to significantly lower lesion size [55]. In patients with neovascular AMD, monocyte levels are increased in the first 30 days of new CNV diagnosis [22]. In light of these findings, we hypothesize that a lower expression of CXCR2 and the aged and drusenoid macula may be an ill-matched couple that orchestrates a more excessive macrophage activity and pro-inflammatory environment where CNV formation can occur. Interestingly, rheumatoid arthritis which is associated with CXCR2 deficiency is also associated with developing AMD later in life [56, 57].

Limitations of this study should be noted when interpreting its results. Importantly, this was an observational, case-control study, which can only associate but not infer on causality. Thus, we cannot exclude that these findings may also reflect a post-CNV state in the blood.

We can only speculate on causality. However, findings of previous studies suggesting that complement dysfunction, low-grade inflammation, and CXCR2 deficiency all comes prior to onset of AMD gives reasons to expect causality [45, 57, 58]. The exploratory approach in the study and the limited group sizes did not permit meaningful stratifications based on single nucleotide polymorphisms that could be interesting, e.g. in the complement system [58, 59] in light of our findings on CD66b. Our study design cannot determine whether the findings reflect immunological dysfunction that are seen in a broad range of retinal diseases or mechanisms that specifically lead to AMD. Future studies need to investigate other retinal and ophthalmological diseases to clarify such aspects.

Conclusions

In summary, we find that in non-smokers, patients with neovascular AMD present with neutrophils that have increased expression of the activity marker CD66b, decreased expression of the adhesion marker CD162, and lower expression of the resolution of inflammation marker CXCR2. Circulating neutrophils may play a role for neovascular AMD and experimental studies are warranted to fully clarify how and when these neutrophil dysfunctions contribute to disease development.

Abbrevations

AMD: Age-related macular degeneration; CNV: Choroidal neovascularization; CD: Cluster of differentiation; PC7: Phycoerythrin-Cyanine 7; IgG: Immunoglobulin G; FITC: Fluorescein isothiocyanate; PE: Phycoerythrin; CXCR2: C-X-C chemokine receptor 2; CCR5: C-C chemokine receptor 5; DARC: Duffy antigen receptor for chemokines; CARMS: Clinical Age-Related Maculopathy Grading System; CRP: C-reactive protein; MFI: Median fluorescence intensity; SD: Standard deviation; IQR: Interquartile range

Acknowledgements
None.

Funding
This project was supported by a grant from Synoptik-fonden, which had no influence on the design of the study, the analysis of data, the preparation of the manuscript, or the decision to publish.

Authors' contributions
TLS conceived the original idea. SH, KA and TLS designed the protocol. SH and KA acquired all data. MKN and YS analyzed and interpreted the data and drafted the manuscript. All authors revised the manuscript critically for important intellectual content and approved publication of the manuscript.

Competing interests
Author MKN has previously received travel grant for conference from Novartis. Author YS has previously received travel grants for conferences from Novartis and Bayer. The other authors declare that no competing interests exist.

References

1. Lim LS, Mitchell P, Seddon JM, Holz FG, Wong TY. Age-related macular degeneration. Lancet. 2012;379:1728–38.
2. Subhi Y, Henningsen GØ, Larsen CT, Sørensen MS, Sørensen TL. Foveal morphology affects self-perceived visual function and treatment response in neovascular age-related macular degeneration: a cohort study. PLoS One. 2014;9:e91227.
3. Krüger Falk M, Kemp H, Sørensen TL. Four-year treatment results of neovascular age-related macular degeneration with ranibizumab and causes for discontinuation of treatment. Am J Ophthalmol. 2013;155:89–95.
4. Bloch SB, Larsen M, Munch IC. Incidence of legal blindness from age-related macular degeneration in Denmark: year 2000 to 2010. Am J Ophthalmol. 2012;153:209–13.
5. Ambati J, Atkinson JP, Gelfand BD. Immunology of age-related macular degeneration. Nat Rev Immunol. 2013;13:438–51.
6. Ardeljan D, Chan CC. Aging is not a disease: distinguishing age-related macular degeneration from aging. Prog Retin Eye Res. 2013;37:68–89.
7. Subhi Y, Forshaw T, Sørensen TL. Macular thickness and volume in the elderly: a systematic review. Ageing Res Rev. 2016;29:42–9.
8. Zhang D, Chen G, Manwani D, Mortha A, Xu C, Faith JJ, et al. Neutrophil ageing is regulated by the microbiome. Nature. 2015;525:528–32.
9. Ilhan N, Daglioglu MC, Ilhan O, Coskun M, Tuzcu EA, Kahraman H, et al. Assessment of Neutrophil/lymphocyte ratio in patients with age-related macular degeneration. Ocul Immunol Inflamm. 2015;23:287–90.
10. Lechner J, Chen M, Hogg RE, Toth L, Silvestri G, Chakravarthy U, et al. Alterations in circulating immune cells in Neovascular age-related macular degeneration. Sci Rep. 2015;5:16754.
11. Sengul EA, Artunay O, Kockar A, Afacan C, Rasier R, Gun P, Yalcin NG, Yuzbasioglu E. Correlation of neutrophil/lymphocyte and platelet/lymphocyte ratio with visual acuity and macular thickness in age-related macular degeneration. Int J Ophthalmol. 2017;10:754–9.
12. Ghosh S, Shang P, Yazdankhah M, Bhutto I, Hose S, Montezuma SR, et al. Activating the AKT2-nuclear factor-κB-lipocalin-2 axis elicits an inflammatory response in age-related macular degeneration. J Pathol. 2017;241:583–8.
13. Rezar-Dreindl S, Sacu S, Eibenberger K, et al. The intraocular cytokine profile and therapeutic response in persistent Neovascular age-related macular degeneration. Invest Ophthalmol Vis Sci. 2016;57:4144–50.
14. Borregaard N. Neutrophils, from marrow to microbes. Immunity. 2010;33:657–70.
15. Urban CF, Lourido S, Zychlinsky A. How do microbes evade neutrophil killing? Cell Microbiol. 2006;8(11):1687–96.
16. Soubhye J, Aldib I, Delporte C, Prévost M, Dufrasne F, Antwerpen PV. Myeloperoxidase as a target for the treatment of inflammatory syndromes: mechanisms and structure activity relationships of inhibition. Curr Med Chem. 2016;23:3975–4008.
17. Ray RS, Katyal A. Myeloperoxidase:bridging the gap in neurodegeneration. Neurosci Biobehav Rev. 2016;68:611–20.
18. Yogalingam G, Lee AR, Mackenzie DS, Maures TJ, Rafalko A, Prill H, Berguig GY, Hague C, Christianson T, Bell SM, LeBowitz JH. Cellular uptake and delivery of Myeloperoxidase to Lysosomes promote Lipofuscin degradation and Lysosomal stress in retinal cells. J Biol Chem. 2017;292:4255–65.
19. Kauppinen A, Paterno JJ, Blasiak J, Salminen A, Kaarniranta K. Inflammation and its role in age-related macular degeneration. Cell Mol Life Sci. 2016;73:1765–86.
20. Zhou J, Pham L, Zhang N, He S, Gamulescu MA, Spee C, et al. Neutrophils promote experimental choroidal neovascularization. Mol Vis. 2005;11:414–24.
21. Lavalette S, Raoul W, Houssier M, Camelo S, Levy O, Calippe B, Jonet L, Behar-Cohen F, Chemtob S, Guillonneau X, Combadiére C, Sennlaub F. Interleukin-1β inhibition prevents Choroidal Neovascularization and does not exacerbate photoreceptor degeneration. Am J Pathol. 2011;178:2416–23.
22. Subhi Y, Lykke ST. New neovascular age-related macular degeneration is associated with systemic leucocyte activity. Acta Ophthalmol. 2016; doi:10.1111/aos.13330.
23. BD BioSciences. Human and Mouse CD Marker Handbook. https://www.bdbiosciences.com/documents/cd_marker_handbook.pdf. Accessed 26 July 2017.
24. Carlos TM, Harlan JM. Leukocyte-endothelial adhesion molecules. Blood. 1994;84:2068–101.
25. Schmidt T, Brodesser A, Schnitzler N, Grüger T, Brandenburg K, Zinserling J, et al. CD66b overexpression and loss of C5a receptors as surface markers for Staphylococcus Aureus-induced Neutrophil dysfunction. PLoS One. 2015;10:e0132703.

26. Hidari KI, Weyrich AS, Zimmerman GA, McEver RP. Engagement of P-selectin glycoprotein Ligand-1 enhances tyrosine Phosphorylation an activates Mitogen-activated protein Kinases in human Neutrophils. J Biol Chem. 1997;272:28750–6.

27. Woodfin A, Voisin MB, Nourshargh S. Recent developments and complexities in neutrophil transmigration. Curr Opin Hematol. 2010;17:9–17.

28. Shimizu K, Nakajima A, Sudo K, Liu Y, Mizoroki A, Ikarashi T, et al. IL-1 receptor type 2 suppresses collagen-induced arthritis by inhibiting IL-1 signal on macrophages. J Immunol. 2015;194:3156–68.

29. Murphy PM. Neutrophil receptors for interleukin-8 and related CXC chemokines. Semin Hematol. 1997;34:311–8.

30. Doodes PD, Cao Y, Hamel KM, Wang Y, Rodeghero RL, Kobezda T, et al. CCR5 is involved in resolution of inflammation in proteoglycan-induced arthritis. Arthritis Rheum. 2009;60:2945–53.

31. Pruenster M, Mudde L, Bombosi P, Dimitrova S, Zsak M, Middleton J, et al. The Duffy antigen receptor for chemokines transports chemokines and supports their promigratory activity. Nat Immunol. 2009;10:101–8.

32. Doz E, Noulin N, Boichbt E, Guenon I, Fick L, Le Bert M, et al. Cigarette smoke-induced pulmonary inflammation is TLR4/MyD88 and IL-1R1/MyD88 signaling dependent. J Immunol. 2008;180:1169–78.

33. Lerner L, Weiner D, Katz R, Reznick AZ, Pollack S. Increased pro-inflammatory activity and impairment of human monocyte differentiation induced by in vitro exposure to cigarette smoke. J Physiol Pharmacol. 2009;60:81–6.

34. Chakravarthy U, Augood C, Bentham CG, et al. Cigarette smoking and age-related macular degeneration in the EUREYE study. Ophthalmology. 2007;114(6):1157–63.

35. Freedman ND, Leitzmann MF, Hollenbeck AR, Schatzkin A, Abnet CC. Cigarette smoking and subsequent risk of lung cancer in men and women: analysis of a prospective cohort study. Lancet Oncol. 2008;9:649–56.

36. Subhi Y, Singh A, Falk MK, Sørensen TL. In patients with neovascular age-related macular degeneration, physical activity may influence C-reactive protein levels. Clin Ophthalmol. 2014;8:15–21.

37. Subhi Y, Sørensen TL. Physical activity patterns in patients with early and late age-related macular degeneration. Dan Med J. 2016;63:A5303.

38. Seddon JM, Sharma S, Adelman RA. Evaluation of the clinical age-related maculopathy staging system. Ophthalmology. 2006;113:260–6.

39. Rifai N, Ridker PM. Proposed cardiovascular risk assessment algorithm using high-sensitivity C-reactive protein and lipid screening. Clin Chem. 2001;47:28–30.

40. Burgisser P, Vaudaux J, Bart PA. Severe interference between retinal angiography and automated four-color flow cytometry analysis of blood mononuclear cells. Cytometry A. 2007;71:632–6.

41. Mullins RF, Russell SR, Anderson DH, Hageman GS. Drusen associated with aging and age-related macular degeneration contain proteins common to extracellular deposits associated with atherosclerosis, elastosis, amyloidosis, and dense deposit disease. FASEB J. 2000;14:835–46.

42. Reynolds R, Hartnett ME, Atkinson JP, Giclas PC, Rosner B, Seddon JM. Plasma complement components and activation fragments: associations with age-related macular degeneration genotypes and phenotypes. Invest Ophthalmol Vis Sci. 2009;50:5818–27.

43. Lechner J, Chen M, Hogg RE, Toth L, Silvestri G, Chakravarthy U, et al. Higher plasma levels of complement C3a, C4a and C5a increase the risk of subretinal fibrosis in neovascular age-related macular degeneration. Immun Ageing. 2016;13:4.

44. Faber C, Singh A, Krüger Falk M, Juel HB, Sørensen TL, Nissen MH. Age-related macular degeneration is associated with increased proportion of CD56(+) T cells in peripheral blood. Ophthalmology. 2013;120:2310–6.

45. Klein R, Myers CE, Cruickshanks KJ, Gangnon RE, Danforth LG, Sivakumaran TA, et al. Markers of inflammation, oxidative stress, and endothelial dysfunction and the 20-year cumulative incidence of early age-related macular degeneration: the beaver dam eye study. JAMA Ophthalmol. 2014;132:446–55.

46. Marsik C, Mayr F, Cardona F, Schaller G, Wagner OF, Jilma B. Endotoxin down-modulates P-selectin glycoprotein Ligand-1 (PSGL-1, CD162) on neutrophils in humans. Clin Immunol. 2004;24:62–5.

47. Holmannova D, Kolackova M, Mandak J, Kunes P, Holubcova Z, Holubec T, et al. Effects of conventional CPB and mini-CPB on neutrophils CD162, CD166 and CD195 expression. Perfusion. 2017;32:141–50.

48. Jamieson T, Clarke M, Steele CW, Samuel MS, Neumann J, Jung A, et al. Inhibition of CXCR2 profoundly suppresses inflammation-driven and spontaneous tumorigenesis. J Clin Invest. 2012;122:3127–44.

49. Schinke C, Giricz O, Li W, Shastri A, Gordon S, Barreyro L, et al. IL8-CXCR2 pathway inhibition as a therapeutic strategy against MDS and AML stem cells. Blood. 2015;125:3144–52.

50. Highfill SL, Cui Y, Giles AJ, Smith JP, Zhang H, Morse E, et al. Disruption of CXCR2-mediated MDSC tumor trafficking enhances anti-PD1 efficacy. Sci Transl Med. 2014;6:237ra67.

51. Dyer DP, Pallas K, Ruiz LM, Schuette F, Wilson GJ, Graham GJ. CXCR2 deficient mice display macrophage-dependent exaggerated acute inflammatory responses. Sci Rep. 2017;7:42681.

52. Singh A, Falk MK, Hviid TV, Sørensen TL. Increased expression of CD200 on circulating CD11b+ monocytes in patients with neovascular age-related macular degeneration. Ophthalmology. 2013;120:1029–37.

53. Calippe B, Augustin S, Beguier F, Charles-Messance H, Poupel L, Conart JB, et al. Complement factor H inhibits CD47-mediated resolution of inflammation. Immunity. 2017;46:261–72.

54. McLeod DS, Bhutto I, Edwards MM, Silver RE, Seddon JM, Lutty GA. Distribution and quantification of Choroidal macrophages in human eyes with age-related macular degeneration. Invest Ophthalmol Vis Sci. 2016;57:5843–55.

55. Sakurai E, Anand A, Ambati BK, van Rooijen N, Ambati J. Macrophage depletion inhibits experimental choroidal neovascularization. Invest Ophthalmol Vis Sci. 2003;44:3578–85.

56. Jacobs JP, Ortiz-Lopez A, Campbell JJ, Gerard CJ, Mathis D, Benoist C. Deficiency of CXCR2, but no other chemokine receptors, attenuates autoantibody-mediated arthritis in a murine model. Arthritis Rheum. 2010;62:1921–32.

57. Keenan TD, Goldacre R, Goldacre MJ. Associations between age-related macular degeneration, osteoarthritis and rheumatoid arthritis. Retina. 2015;35:2613–8.

58. Despriet DD, Klaver CC, Witteman JC, Bergen AA, Kardys I, de Maat MP, et al. Complement factor H polymorphism, complement activators, and risk of age-related macular degeneration. JAMA. 2006;296:301–9.

59. Haines JL, Hauser MA, Schmidt S, Scott WK, Olson LM, Gallins P, Spencer KL, Kwan SY, Noureddine M, Gilbert JR, et al. Complement factor H variant increases the risk of age-related macular degeneration. Science. 2005;308:385–9.

Dietary phytochemicals and neuro-inflammaging: from mechanistic insights to translational challenges

Sergio Davinelli[1][*], Michael Maes[2,3], Graziamaria Corbi[1], Armando Zarrelli[4], Donald Craig Willcox[5,6] and Giovanni Scapagnini[1]

Abstract

An extensive literature describes the positive impact of dietary phytochemicals on overall health and longevity. Dietary phytochemicals include a large group of non-nutrients compounds from a wide range of plant-derived foods and chemical classes. Over the last decade, remarkable progress has been made to realize that oxidative and nitrosative stress (O&NS) and chronic, low-grade inflammation are major risk factors underlying brain aging. Accumulated data strongly suggest that phytochemicals from fruits, vegetables, herbs, and spices may exert relevant negative immunoregulatory, and/or anti-O&NS activities in the context of brain aging. Despite the translational gap between basic and clinical research, the current understanding of the molecular interactions between phytochemicals and immune-inflammatory and O&NS (IO&NS) pathways could help in designing effective nutritional strategies to delay brain aging and improve cognitive function. This review attempts to summarise recent evidence indicating that specific phytochemicals may act as positive modulators of IO&NS pathways by attenuating pro-inflammatory pathways associated with the age-related redox imbalance that occurs in brain aging. We will also discuss the need to initiate long-term nutrition intervention studies in healthy subjects. Hence, we will highlight crucial aspects that require further study to determine effective physiological concentrations and explore the real impact of dietary phytochemicals in preserving brain health before the onset of symptoms leading to cognitive decline and inflammatory neurodegeneration.

Keywords: Brain, Aging, Diet, Phytochemicals, Inflammation, Oxidative stress

Background

Over the next few decades, given the rising life expectancy within the older population, the incidence of developing age-related neurodegenerative diseases is predicted to increase dramatically. A critical factor that plays a crucial role in brain aging is the exceptionally high energy demand of neurons to preserve neuronal processes and maintain cognitive ability. The high consumption of oxygen for the generation of energy may reflect more vulnerability of the brain to reactive species attack and subsequent inflammation [1]. In addition, normal brain metabolism is associated with more than one process contributing to functional impairment in brain aging. For instance, high content of polyunsaturated fatty acids (PUFAs) in neuronal membranes (easily peroxidizable), limited amount of endogenous antioxidant defences, low rate of cell turnover, and high production of reactive oxygen and nitrogen species (ROS/RNS) put the brain at risk to oxidative and nitrosative (O&NS) damage [2]. It should be also mentioned that the age-related redox imbalance underlying the pathophysiological basis of neurodegeneration is accompanied by many types of cellular damages, including oxidative DNA and lipid damage, oxidative and nitrosative protein damage, mitochondrial damage, telomere attrition and accumulation of macromolecular waste [2, 3]. Growing studies suggest that a bidirectional communication between brain and immune system is crucial to maintain central nervous system (CNS) homeostasis. To date, one of most recognized effects of brain aging is

* Correspondence: s.davinelli@gmail.com
[1]Department of Medicine and Health Sciences, School of Medicine, University of Molise, Campobasso, Italy
Full list of author information is available at the end of the article

the dysregulation of the immune system as a result of uncontrolled production of reactive species and pro-inflammatory cytokines [4, 5]. This chronic condition has been defined as "oxi-inflammaging" and may contribute to neuronal loss in different neurodegenerative diseases, culminating in accelerated neurodegeneration [6–9]. During brain aging, the generation of ROS and RNS increases the synthesis of numerous chemokines and pro-inflammatory cytokines, including interleukin (IL)-1, IL-6, and tumor necrosis factor- α (TNF-α). These inflammatory mediators activate microglia and astrocytes to generate large amounts of ROS/RNS. Recent studies showed that neuroinflammatory processes may be considered as a consequence of chronic oxidative stress [10, 11]. Moreover, the neuropathological alterations associated with oxidative stress and pro-inflammatory state include deposition of insoluble materials such as amyloid-β (Aβ) plaques and neurofibrillary tangles (NFTs), which are the main factors of cell death and age-related dementia [12].

However, it is now becoming clear that the consumption of diets rich in phytochemicals can influence neuroinflammation and mediate the activation of signaling pathways, leading to the expression of cytoprotective and restorative proteins [13, 14]. There is substantial evidence supporting the notion that bioactive dietary components may contribute to develop novel therapies capable of preventing the progressive dysfunction of neuronal populations that underlie neurodegeneration [15, 16]. A large variety of foods including fruit, vegetables, cereals, nuts and cocoa/chocolate as well as tea, coffee and wine contain a wide range of plant secondary metabolites, better known as phytochemicals, which have been shown to be effective in increasing antioxidant enzymes, neurotrophic factors and anti-apoptotic proteins. Several mechanisms have been proposed for the health benefits of phytochemicals, however, their ability to modulate signal transduction cascades and activate transcription factors that antagonize neuroinflammation and O&NS has attracted considerable interest [17]. Despite various beneficial biological activities, phytochemicals may have carcinogenic or genotoxic effects at high doses or concentrations [18]. Therefore, the challenge is to establish the exact dose range and perform human intervention studies to develop effective nutritional strategies capable of counteracting neuroinflammatory processes that accompany brain aging. Here, we discuss some of the new findings that provide insight into how phytochemicals positively affect neuroinflammation and brain aging. Specifically, we will discuss the main neuroprotective activities of phytochemicals that have been studied in cells, animals and humans emphasizing the importance of dosage, which is crucial to establish endpoints for clinical studies and develop dietary recommendations.

Oxidative stress, microglial redox activation and neuroinflammation

Aging is associated with an imbalance in redox status in a variety of cells and tissues, including the brain. Increasing O&NS stress is thought to be one of the main aging processes causing direct cell loss and cell damage within the brain architecture [19–21]. An age-associated increase in O&NS damage has been shown in neurons of human and rodent brains, and a selective susceptibility of different neuronal populations to oxidative stress has been demonstrated. For instance, oligodendrocytes are particularly vulnerable to oxidative activity due to their role in myelin maintenance and production and limited repair mechanisms [22]. Neuronal oxidation can lead to the destruction of subcellular structures and membranes. Indeed, during brain aging, in addition to the impaired function of many intracellular components such as mitochondrial electron transport chain, various important classes of macromolecules are particularly liable to the deleterious effects of oxidative modification. Several studies have indicated that oxidative damage to nucleic acids can actively contributes to the background, onset, and development of neurodegenerative disorders [23]. Age-associated accumulation of oxidative DNA damage such as the presence of the modified base 8-hydroxydeoxyguanosine (8-OHdG), was observed in many neuron types, including cerebellar granule cells, retinal ganglion, and amacrine, and horizontal cells [24]. Interestingly, it has been recently demonstrated in human neurons that oxidative RNA modification can occur not only in protein-coding RNAs but also in non-coding RNAs, leading to activate inappropriate cell fate pathways [23]. Oxidative damage of the brain is also characterized by increased lipid peroxidation and it has been shown that redox changes in membrane fatty acid composition contribute to the deterioration of neuronal functions. PUFAs, such as arachidonic acid (AA), are abundant in the brain and are highly susceptible to free radical attack during brain aging [25].

Hypernitrosylation may inhibit the functions of many different proteins involved in critical cell functions leading to apoptosis, dysfunctions in intracellular signalling, inhibition of cell growth, mitochondrial functions, cell death, etc. [20]. Another consequence of nitrosative stress is the formation of immunogenic neoepitopes, e.g. nitroso (NO)-tyrosine and NO-tryptophan which may mount autoimmune responses, e.g. IgM-mediated autoimmune responses to NO-cysteinyl [20]. The latter autoimmune responses may have neurotoxic effects and cause demyelination. Hypernitrosylation is tightly coupled to nuclear factor (NF)- κB activation which induces and supports inflammaging and induction of inducible NO-synthase (iNOS). An age-related NF-κB constitutive activation was observed in many tissues including brain [26]. Increased nitration of proteins, e.g. the formation of immunogenic nitro (NO2)-tyrosine, accompanies the aging process [27]. Besides oxidation of nucleic acids, lipids, and proteins, and nitrosylation, nitrosation and nitration of proteins, an excess of free radical generation is associated with chronic low-grade inflammation and the onset of age-related brain disorders [28]. The role of an excessive free radical production linked to persistent low-basal inflammation and brain aging is schematized in Fig. 1. In the CNS, reactive species, glial cells and inflammatory mediators form a co-ordinated network to maintain a proper equilibrium between physiological and pathological processes. In the brain, glial cells (mainly microglia) provide the first line of defense against noxious agents or injurious processes [29]. Microglial cells are the resident macrophages of the CNS and under physiological conditions they exhibit a deactivated phenotype. A tight control of microglial inflammatory response is essential for CNS homeostasis to promote the clearance of pathogens, toxic cellular debris and stimulate repair processes after brain damage. However, microglia are a potent cellular source of oxidation products and inflammatory molecules during brain aging. Microglia respond to oxidative damage, as a result of aging or neurodegeneration, by releasing a large spectrum of neuroactive mediators. The accumulation of oxidative damage in microglia during aging results in the increased production of ROS. Disproportional increase in intracellular ROS can activate the

redox-sensitive NF-κB and provoke excessive neuroinflammation [30]. A sustained activation of microglia may lead to neuronal degeneration and dysfunction, as observed in brain aging, cognitive and neuropsychiatric disorders [31]. An interruption in microglial homeostasis, a process referred to as microglial priming, makes the microglia more susceptible to inflammatory stimuli and neurodegeneration and may be an early events leading to oxidative damage and depletion of endogenous antioxidants [32]. The causal relationship between oxidative damage and neuroinflammatory response is exemplified by the cytokine TNF-α, which is released by activated microglia. Although TNF-α can ameliorate immune responses and promote neuroprotection, under uncontrolled conditions TNF-α is a powerful pro-inflammatory and neurotoxic molecule. In particular, TNF-α can contribute to neuroinflammation by activating the transcription factor NF-κB in glia cells, but also promoting the generation and release of ROS through the NADPH oxidase system and RNS [4, 33, 34]. In addition, recent findings suggest that the dysregulation of Toll-Tike receptors (TLRs) participate to generate a hyperactivated state of microglia. A persistent activation of TLRs, their signalling pathways and downstream effector molecules, may contribute to cytotoxic compounds accumulation such as ROS, RNS, cytokines, complements and proteases causing neuronal loss and damage [35, 36]. The formation of redox-derived damage-associated molecular patterns (DAMPs), may further activate the TLR4

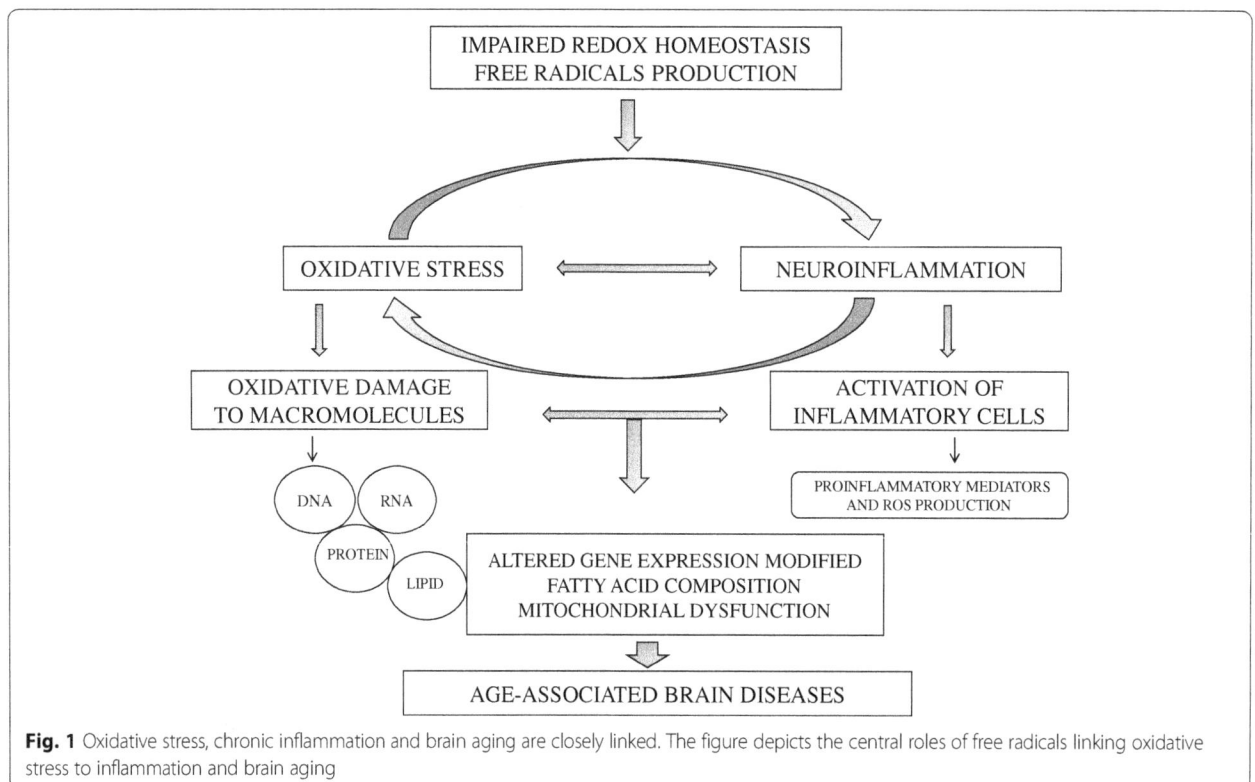

Fig. 1 Oxidative stress, chronic inflammation and brain aging are closely linked. The figure depicts the central roles of free radicals linking oxidative stress to inflammation and brain aging

complex leading to a chronic activation of the TLR-radical cycle, thereby causing chronic IO&NS [37]. Additional pro-inflammatory markers, including interleukin (IL)-6, C-reactive protein (CRP), matrix metalloproteinases (MMPs), cytosolic phospholipase A2 (cPLA2), cyclooxygenase-2 (COX-2) and TNF-α are consistently elevated in neuro-degenerative diseases, which are largely associated with chronically elevated levels of ROS [5, 38]. Moreover, it has been hypothesized that IL-6 is a central regulator of the neuroinflammatory responses in brain aging. Animal models and patients with neurodegenerative diseases had higher levels of IL-6 and CRP, providing evidence that peripheral inflammatory mediators can increase ROS production and also interfere with neurocognitive functions [39–41]. There is growing interest in the redox pathophysiology of neuroinflammation and emerging concepts open new ways to restore the inactive state of microglia and modulate the low-grade chronic neuroinflammation that characterizes brain aging.

Neuroprotective signaling pathways

Dietary phytochemicals exert their beneficial effects on the nervous system modulating cellular stress response signaling pathways [42]. At low doses, several phytochemicals are known to enhance neuronal stress resistance, whereas at high doses many different phytochemicals can be toxic. This is an example of biphasic dose–response relationship with stimulatory or beneficial effects at low doses and inhibitory or adverse effects at high doses (hormesis) [43]. Therefore, dietary phytochemicals act as mild stressors to induce adaptive expression of stress-protective genes in neuronal cells and enhance resistance to the mechanisms that determine brain aging. In the next sections, we highlight the major signaling pathways by which dietary phytochemicals offer neuroprotection in an exposure-related manner.

The Nrf2 antioxidant response pathway

The transcription factor nuclear factor E2-related factor 2 (Nrf2) has emerged as a key cytoprotective regulator against O&NS stress and neuroinflammation [44]. Nrf2 is a member of the cap'n'collar (CNC) family of stress-sensing transcription factors. Nrf2 is a basic leucine zipper protein that in the nucleus heterodimerizes with small Maf protein followed by binding to specific DNA sites termed antioxidant response elements (AREs) or electrophile response elements (EpRE) [45]. In basal conditions, Nrf2 is kept transcriptionally inactive and sequestered in the cytoplasm by its repressor protein, the Kelch-like ECH-associated protein 1 (Keap1). This binding provides the turnover of Nrf2 through proteasomal degradation. Keap1, a sulfhydryl-rich protein, is a specialized sensor to quantify stress in presence of oxidative stressors and electrophilic xenobiotics. In response to oxidative and/or electrophilic stress, Nrf2-Keap1 dissociation is triggered with consequent translocation of Nrf2 to the nucleus, where the formed heterodimer with Maf binds ARE sequence in the promoter regions of genes involved in phase II detoxification and antioxidant defense [46]. Nrf2 is ubiquitously present in all tissues but is widely expressed in the CNS where it promotes cell survival and coordinates the transcription of neuroprotective proteins. Some examples include various superoxide dismutase (SOD) isoforms, catalase (CAT), glutathione peroxidase, glutathione reductase, various glutathione-S-transferase (GST) isoforms, NAD(P)H:quinone oxidoreductase 1 (NQO1), and heme oxigenase-1 (HO-1). However, recent findings have linked the activation of the Nrf2 signaling not only to phase II detoxifying enzymes and antioxidants proteins but also to expression of other cytoprotective proteins such as the growth factor brain-derived neurotrophic factor (BDNF), the anti-inflammatory IL-10, the mitochondrial transcription (co)-factors Nrf-1 and peroxisome proliferator-activated receptor gamma coactivator 1-alpha (PGC-1α) [44]. Aging is associated with Nrf2 dysfunction and a dysregulation of this pathway has been linked to the pathogenesis of several chronic disorders, including neurodegenerative, cardiovascular, metabolic, infectious, and pulmonary diseases as well as chronic inflammatory conditions [47–49]. Accumulating evidence suggests that the decline in the Nrf2 signaling system plays a key role in the accumulation of pro-inflammatory mediators and oxidative damage during brain aging [50, 51]. Although the underlying mechanisms behind the impairment of Nrf2 pathway in neurodegeneration are not known, elevated levels of oxidative stress and inflammation in patients with neurodegenerative diseases have been reported. Studies have established that the nuclear translocation of Nrf2 is reduced in the hippocampus of Alzheimer's disease (AD) patients. Also mRNA and protein levels of Nrf2 are reduced in the motor cortex and spinal cord of amyotrophic lateral sclerosis (ALS) patients [52]. It appears also from studies with genetic deletion of Nrf2 that the absence of Nrf2 may be detrimental during brain aging and contribute to neurodegeneration. However, there are several promising compounds that at least in vitro are able to restore Nrf2 and induce neuronal protection, as discussed below. Indeed, recent findings suggest that Nrf2 may be a therapeutic target for the alleviation of neuroinflammation associated with neurodegeneration [53].

The NF-κB signaling pathway in brain inflammation

NF-κB is a ubiquitous stress response pathway and one of the well-described transcription signaling mechanisms. NF-κB transcriptional activity has been associated with neuronal plasticity and neurodegeneration [54]. Indeed, NF-κB is a crucial signal transducer for maintaining CNS homeostasis, particularly in neuronal and glial cells. In response to a wide range of biological stimuli, NF-κB coordinates the expression of numerous genes, encoding pro-inflammatory cytokines, chemokines, and inducible growth factors [55]. The number of target genes of NF-κB is continuously expanding and the deregulation of NF-κB signaling has been detected in multiple disease states, including neurodegenerative diseases and chronic inflammatory conditions. NF-κB orchestrates a broad range of physiological stimuli through canonical and non-canonical pathways. In CNS, NF-κB exists in a latent and a constitutively active form. Constitutively activated NF-κB is mostly detected within the nucleus of glutamatergic neurons and is regulated by synaptic activity. In glia, NF-κB has a lower basal activity and is heavily inducible [56]. Although NF-κB signalling is tightly regulated at multiple levels, in most unstressed cells is located in the cytoplasm in an inactive complex consisting of two subunits of 50 kDa (p50) and 65 kDa (p65) and an inhibitory subunit called IkB (IkBα or IkBβ). In response to activating stimuli, IkB is phosphorylated, ubiquitinated and degraded by the proteasome, which in turn allows the nuclear translocation of NF-κB to regulate gene expression. The most fundamental aspects of NF-κB regulation in the brain have been extensively discussed elsewhere [57–61]. Given that a fundamental goal for future studies is to determine whether activation of NF-κB is important for neuroprotection, in the present paragraph, we would like to highlight some data to demonstrate that NF-κB may be an activator of neuroprotective programs. Neuroprotective effects of NF-κB have been described in several experimental models, indicating the potential protective value of this essential transcription factors in the treatment of neuroinflammation and neurodegeneration [62]. Despite this, the role of NF-κB in mechanisms of brain tolerance is complex because it is involved in both protective and damaging pathways. NF-κB supports neuronal survival by increasing the expression of antioxidants, growth factors, and anti-apoptotic molecules. In contrast, glial NF-κB activation promotes neuronal death by inducing production of pro-inflammatory cytokines [63, 64]. However, it is noteworthy to mention that NF-κB signaling pathway has been identified as one of the major neuroprotective mechanism against AD [62]. The dual role of NF-κB in neuronal death and survival is intriguing but we still have limited knowledge on the molecular details underlying its actions as activator of neuroprotective programs or inducer of neurodegenerative processes. Understanding which determinants are implicated in switching NF-κB from a neuroprotective to a neurotoxic activity may help the development of new treatments for neuroinflammation. In this context, preconditioning/hormesis has been therapeutically linked to activation of NF-κB and inhibition of neuronal apoptosis [65, 66]. Therefore, a low dose of a toxic agent may trigger an adaptive stress-response program mediated by NF-κB and provide neuroprotection. Conversely, high doses of noxious compounds can exacerbate NF-κB activity and induce a neurotoxic response [60, 67]. Furthermore, experimental studies have also demonstrated that neuronal response to external stimuli is dependent on a differential activation of NF-κB dimers. Neurotoxic stimuli or the absence of NF-κB p50 depletes neuronal pro-survival gene products, including anti-apoptotic proteins [68, 69]. Finally, it is remarkable to mention that the identification of NF-κB binding sites in the promoter region of the Nrf2 gene suggests a potential relationship between these two transcription factors [70]. Moreover, it has been demonstrated that HO-1 induced by the Nrf2 inhibits the NF-κB transcriptional apparatus, and thereby HO-1 is one of the key mediator for the interplay between Nrf2 and NF-κB [71]. As already indicated above, increased NF-κB activity during brain aging is associated with enhanced production of pro-inflammatory cytokines such as IL-6, TNF-α, and COX-2. Reduced Nrf2 activity is characterized by decline in HO-1, SOD, and NQO1 leading to increased levels of oxidative stress and neuroinflammation. A schematic illustration of the crosstalk between Nrf2 and NF-κB in the brain is depicted in Fig. 2.

MAPK signal transduction and its role in brain aging

Mitogen-activated protein kinases (MAPKs) belong to the super-family of serine/threonine kinases that mediate a wide range of cellular responses. MAPKs have emerged as critical players that connect various extracellular signals into intracellular response. Based on the degree of sequence homology, MAPK transduction cascades are organised into at least three subfamilies: the extracellular signal regulated kinases (ERKs), the stress activated protein kinase/c-Jun N terminal kinase (JNK), and the p38 MAPK [72]. These kinases are involved in both survival and death pathways in response to different stresses to regulate cellular processes such as cell proliferation, survival, differentiation, and metabolism. The role of ERKs is usually associated with pro-survival signaling, however, depending on the type and function of a particular neuron, activation of ERKs can either be neuroprotective or can promote cell death [73]. For instance, in vivo studies of neurons derived from the hippocampal tissue revealed that BDNF regulates synapse formation and plasticity by a mechanism involving ERKs, Nrf2 and forkhead box O (FoxO) transcription factors [74]. Furthermore, ERK activation is required for consolidation and reconsolidation of hippocampal-dependent memory [75]. Dysregulation of ERK signaling has been implicated in both neuropsychiatric and neurodegenerative disorders including, schizophrenia, Huntington's disease (HD), Parkinson's disease (PD), and AD [76–78]. JNK and p38 are well-

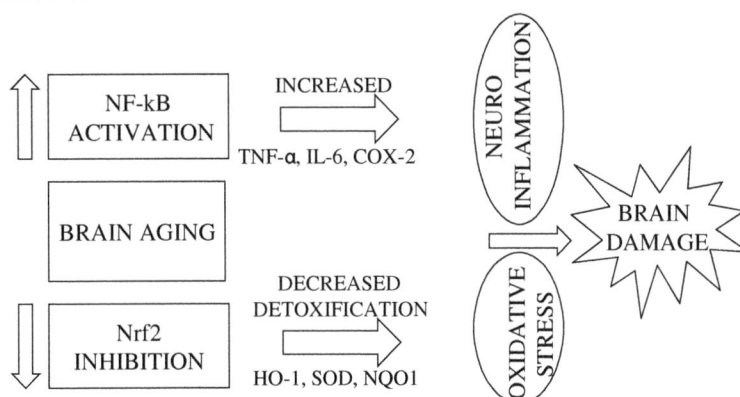

Fig. 2 Schematic illustration on the role of Nrf2–NF-κB axis in bran aging. An imbalance between Nrf2 and NF-κB can lead to increased levels of oxidative stress and neuroinflammation, resulting in structural and functional damage to nervous tissue

known stress-activated MAPKs, because are potently activated by stress signals such as UV light, inflammatory cytokines, and DNA damaging agents. In particular, a large body of evidence indicates that JNK is a key regulator of apoptotic and inflammatory pathways which are activated during neuro-inflammaging, PD, HD, and AD. Indeed, JNK is involved in inflammatory responses in astrocytes and in primary glial cells. JNK is activated by TNF, IL-1, UV light, and heat shock. Moreover, JNK activation in the brain is associated with intracellular Aβ accumulation and neuronal death in AD patients. It has been also reported that JNKs activity is involved in the regulation of neuronal survival via the maintenance of mitochondrial homeostasis [79–81]. Finally, evolving evidence suggests that p38 plays specific roles in inflammation, cell death, and senescence. Disruption of p38 signaling in neural cells contributes to the pathogenesis of many neurodegenerative diseases including AD, HD, and PD [82]. p38 has been shown to be essential for the maintenance of dopaminergic neurons and oxidative stress and p38 signalling cascade regulate pro and anti-apoptotic phenotypes of dopaminergic neurons [83]. Several studies have investigated the function of p38 in the context of neuroinflammation. Astrocytic p38 signalling is activated by inflammatory cytokines such as IL-1β and TNF-α. It has also been found that p38 in AD is one of the main kinases responsible for excessive tau phosphorylation.

Moreover, accumulation of Aβ plaques is partially mediated through misregulated activity of p38 cascade [84]. Inhibitors of p38 confirm that an elevated activation of this pathway is a critical contributor to neuronal damage and neuroinflammation [85].

Sirtuin-FoxO longevity pathway
Sirtuins (SIRTs) are members of the class III histone deacetylases, and so far seven sirtuin genes (sirtuins 1–7) have been characterized in mammals [86]. A large number of studies have shown that SIRT1 can alter the fate of a neuron promoting cell survival against stress. SIRT1 appears to be a crucial component for neuronal plasticity and cognitive functions because it is also involved in dendritic and axonal growth. In the brain, SIRT1 regulates numerous neuroprotective functions, including antioxidant and anti-inflammatory response, antiapoptosis, and mitochondrial biogenesis [87, 88]. An emerging target of the sirtuins is the family of FoxO transcription factors [89]. The mammalian FoxOs are composed of four members: FoxO1, FoxO3, FoxO4, and FoxO6. Temporal and tissue specific differences in expression can be observed with FoxO1 and FoxO3 almost ubiquitously expressed, FoxO4 highly expressed in kidney, colorectal and muscle tissue and FoxO6 mainly expressed in the liver and brain. FoxOs are involved in a myriad of cellular processes and programs including energy metabolism, cell cycle regulation, apoptosis, autophagy, immunity, inflammation, resistance to oxidative stress, stem cell maintenance and appear to play a conserved "prolongevity" role observed in worms through to human beings [90]. FoxOs also modulate key aspects of stress response and survival pathways in neurons [91]. Therefore, FoxOs have dual roles in survival and cell death and gene-specific contexts determine the effects of FoxOs on gene expression. Although the effects of SIRT1 on the FoxO target genes are complex, FoxOs can recognize and bind to different sites within the SIRT1 promoter region to induce transcription. SIRT1 activates several members of the FoxO family. Notably, SIRT1 positively controls FoxO transcription by shifting FoxO-dependent response away from cell death and toward stress resistance, particularly in the case of oxidative stress [92]. Three FoxO isoforms are commonly expressed in the brain. FoxO1 is strongly expressed in neuronal subsets of the hippocampus, whereas FoxO6 is highly enriched and expressed throughout the entire adult hippocampus, and

appears important for memory consolidation and neur-onal connectivity [93]. Of the isoforms, FoxO3 is the most diffusely expressed in the brain and has been shown to be strongly associated with human longevity including a re-duced risk for cognitive decline with age for those who possess the protective "G" allele. [94]. SIRT1 deacetylates FoxO3, reducing FoxO-mediated apoptosis but potenti-ates FoxO-induced cell cycle arrest [95]. SIRT1 and FoxO3 form a complex in response to oxidative stress, and the sites of FoxO3 that appear to be deacetylated by SIRT1 are K242, K245, and K262 [96, 97]. Therefore, the effect of acetylation on FoxO3 has a dual role on function because SIRT1 can increase the ability of FoxO3 to induce cell cycle arrest and resistance to oxidative stress but can also inhibit FoxO3 to induce cell death [89, 98]. Further-more, the SIRT1-FoxO3 network is associated with the induction of DNA repair proteins. In the context of be-havioural adaptations to cocaine, new findings have dem-onstrated that the induction of SIRT1 deacetylates and activates FoxO3, which then induces many gene targets involved in DNA repair in the brain [99]. Another SIRT widely expressed in neurons and astrocytes is SIRT3. It has been shown to have a major involvement in ROS regulation, deacetylating FoxO3 with consequent expres-sion of CAT and mnSOD [100, 101]. Recently, Rangarajan et al. reported for the first time that SIRT3 expression is induced in activated microglia in vivo and activates antioxidant genes through nuclear translocation of FoxO3 [102].

Neuroprotective activity of phytochemicals against neuro-inflammaging

Dietary phytochemicals may have a profound effect on many aspects of neuro-inflammaging. Several studies have revealed that the neuroprotective activities of phy-tochemicals typically occur in dose- and time-dependent manner [42, 103]. A variety of mechanisms appear to underlie the neuroprotective action of phytochemicals. Although research has focused predominantly on anti-oxidant properties of dietary phytochemicals, the ability of these compounds not only has the potency to scav-enge free radical effects in the brain but it has also demonstrated that specific phytochemicals target key stress-activated signaling pathways involved in neuro-protection (Fig. 3). Substantial in vitro and in vivo evi-dence have suggested that many phytochemicals can affect the expression of numerous genes encoding pro-survival proteins, including antioxidant enzymes, neuro-trophic or anti-apoptotic factors. In the next sections, we will present the main classes of food phytochemicals and their emerging role as hormetic inducers of neuro-protective pathways relevant for brain aging.

Curcumin

Curcuma species, particularly *C. longa* (turmeric) have been used in Southeast Asian countries for thousands of years as a food preservative and for medical conditions. Among curcuminoids, the main components in *Cur-cuma* species, curcumin is the most studied and shows a

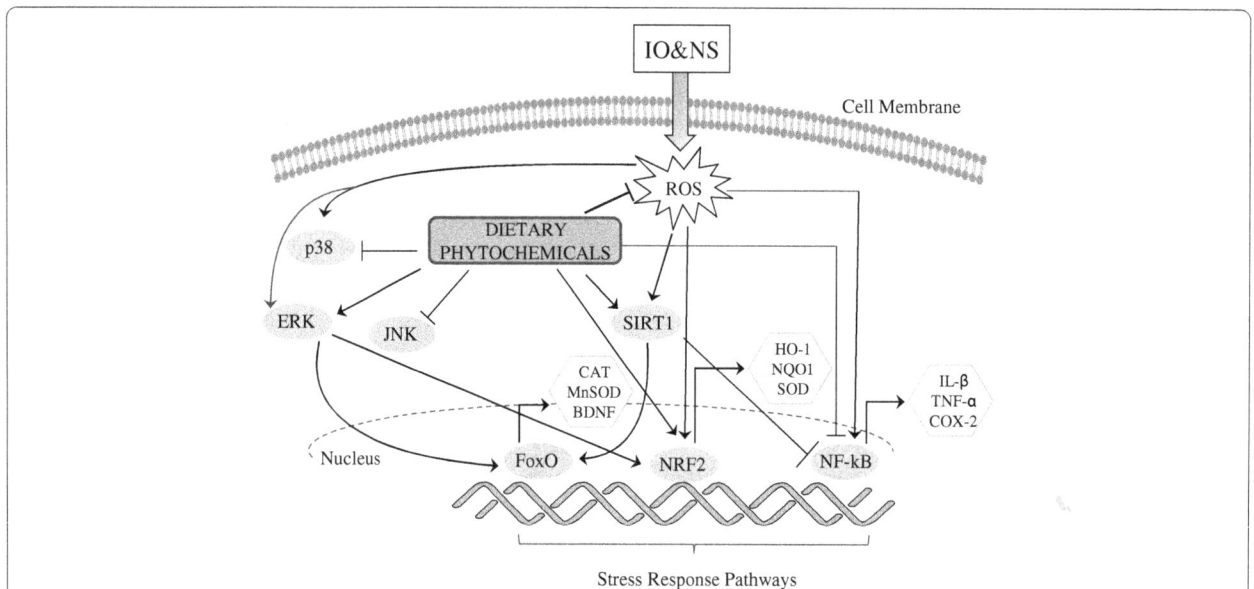

Fig. 3 The main intracellular targets involved in the neuroprotective effects of phytochemicals. Most of the phytochemicals with neuroprotective activity seem to converge in the modulation of stress response pathways. For example, phytochemicals can interact directly with Nrf2, allowing the expression of phase II detoxifier genes. The kinases p38, ERK and JNK are also modulated by phytochemicals, regulating both survival and death pathways in response to different stresses. Activation of SIRT1 can regulate FoxO, which modulate genes that encode antioxidant and other stress-response proteins. FoxO is also regulated by ERK in response to a variety of stimuli, including IO&NS and phytochemicals. ERK activation often leads to the activation of Nrf2. Phytochemicals and/or activated SIRT1can also inhibit NF-κB, reducing the expression of inflammatory mediators

broad range of pharmacological activities [104]. Its immuomodulatory activity is well-documented and in vivo (100 mg/kg) and in vitro (10 µM) studies have also demonstrated that curcumin can protect dopaminergic neurons against microglia-mediated neurotoxicity and reduce brain inflammation in a concentration-dependent manner [105–108]. Recent studies also indicate an epigenetic role of curcumin, which inhibits the expression of pro-inflammatory mediators by affecting histone acetylation of transcription factors and methylation pattern of gene promoters associated with inflammatory response [109]. Curcumin treatment (2–8 µM) inhibits in a dose-dependent manner the activation of microglial cells by diminishing the production of NO and reducing the secretion of IL-1β, IL-6 and TNF-α (5–20 µM) [110, 111]. Moreover, curcumin blocks the LPS-mediated induction of COX2 via inhibition of NF-κB, activator protein 1 (AP1) (2–16 µM), and signal transducers and activators of transcription (STATs) (5 or 10 µM) [112, 113]. DNA-microarray analyses revealed that 20 µM of curcumin has a strong impact on the microglial transcriptome, leading to an anti-inflammatory and neuroprotective phenotype in LPS-triggered microglia [114]. These concentrations may be indicative of clinical efficacy, since curcumin preparations with enhanced bioavailability (delivered orally) can cross the blood–brain barrier and reach therapeutic concentrations up to 3 µM [115, 116]. Moreover, it should be mentioned that peak plasma concentrations (approximately 1.6 µM) in mice were achieved 15 min after the intraperitoneal administration of 100 mg/kg curcumin, followed by brain accumulation within one hour [117]. In an experimental animal model of chronic epilepsy, 60–100 mg of daily curcumin are effective in attenuating glial immuno-reactivity with ameliorative effects on cognitive deficits [118]. Curcumin administration (100 mg/kg) to rats under hypoxic conditions attenuated the upregulation of NF-κB, thereby leading to concomitant downregulation of pro-inflammatory cytokine levels (IL-1, IL-2, IL-18 and TNF-α) and cell adhesion molecules (P-selectin and E-selectin) [119]. Also, repeated intrathecal injection of curcumin (50, 100, 200 mg/kg) dose-dependently attenuates glial activation and spinal neuroinflammation in a rat model of monoarthritis [120]. The TLR4 complex is an important mediator of neuroinflammatory events and treatment with curcumin (50, 100, 200 mg/kg) attenuated TLR4-mediated acute activation of microglia/macrophages, pro-inflammatory mediator release and neuronal apoptosis in the injured brain tissue of rats via inhibition of the MyD88/NF-κB signaling cascade [121]. As reviewed elsewhere, curcumin is also a Nrf2 inducer that upregulates antioxidant defence mechanisms [15]. Recent cell and animal studies have shown that the neuroprotective effects of curcumin (approximately at concentrations of 5 to 25 µM) involves the Akt/Nrf2 pathway, which is consistent with the fact that Nrf2 participates in the neuroprotective effects of curcumin against oxidative damage [122, 123]. Pretreatment with curcumin (5–30 µM) induces neuroprotective antioxidant effects against hemin-induced neuronal death, regulating the expression of Nrf2, HO-1 and glutathione synthesis [124]. Axon degeneration is mediated by microglial MyD88/p38 MAPK signalling and JNK phosphorylation. A new quantitative approach for monitoring axon degeneration found that curcumin (10 µM) protects axons from degeneration during neuroinflammation, inhibiting axonal JNK phosphorylation [125]. The neuroprotective action of curcumin also involves the modulation of SIRT1. Recent observations indicate that SIRT1 signaling activation is associated with the neuroprotective effect of curcumin and preatreatment of curcumin (50 mg/kg) attenuated inflammation, apoptosis, and mitochondrial dysfunction in a rat model of ischemic brain [126]. Curcumin (5–10 µM) was also effective in inducing FoxO3a activity in monocytes/macrophages, suggesting a potential protective mechanism against oxidative damage in the inflammatory cells of the vascular system [127].

Anthocyanins

Anthocyanins are a class of flavonoids consisting of water-soluble colored pigments. Berry fruits with red, blue or purple colors constitute one of the most important sources of dietary anthocyanins [128]. These compounds are consumed as part of a normal diet and in the United States the human intake of anthocyanins has been approximately estimated to be 180–255 mg/day. Anthocyanins after ingestion reach the circulatory system within 0.25–2 h [129]. Several studies have indicated that anthocyanins from berries may enhance cognitive and motor function during aging due primarily to their antioxidant and neuroprotective properties [130, 131]. Although only a few studies have explored the specific actions of anthocyanins in the context of neuroinflammation, it was recently reported in an experimental model of multiple sclerosis (MS) that anthocyanins (100 mg/kg) suppress the secretion of pro-inflammatory mediators and protect cellular components against oxidative damages induced by demyelination [132]. Moreover, in high-fat-fed animals chronic intake of an anthocyanin extract from blackberry (25 mg/kg) may be capable of preventing the detrimental effects of neuroinflammation with positive effects on synaptogenesis and synaptic plasticity [133]. Anthocyanins protect neuronal cells from pro-oxidant and pro-inflammatory damage via diverse mechanisms, including modulation of Nrf2 and inhibition of NF-κB pathways [134]. For instance, an anthocyanin-rich açaí extract (1 µg/mL) attenuated oxidative stress in rat primary astrocyte cultures through modulation of Nrf2 pathway, thereby restoring the GSH/GSSG ratio and protecting the astrocytic membranes from lipid peroxidation [135].

Furthermore, Aboonabi et al. propose that anthocyanins are efficient inducers of Nrf2 activation and can be considered a good treatment option for inflammation-mediated disorders such as atherosclerosis [136]. Anthocyanins from blueberry, blackberry, and blackcurrant exhibited a similar degree of anti-inflammatory effects and these compounds suppressed the expression and secretion of pro-inflammatory mediators in macrophages by inhibiting nuclear translocation of NF-κB [137]. In another study, the neuroprotective effects of anthocyanins have also been reported in the hippocampus of postnatal rat brain. Anthocyanins (100 mg/kg) inhibited the ethanol-activated expression of JNK, NF-κB, COX-2, as well as attenuated neuronal apoptosis [138]. A blueberry anthocyanin fraction significantly inhibited the LPS-induced production of pro-inflammatory mediators NO, iNOS and COX2 in BV2 microglial cell and this effect was due to the attenuation of NF-κB nuclear translocation [139]. Berries also contain high levels of proanthocyanidins that have neuroprotective effects similar to those of anthocyanins. Findings in primary hippocampal neuronal cells treated with various blueberry fractions (anthocyanins 15 μg/mL; proanthocyanidins 14 μg/ml) and exposed to $A\beta_{42}$ and LPS showed that the major neuroprotective effects of blubbery involve reduction of NF-κB, p38, and JNK [140]. Also bilberry and lingonberry contain high amounts of anthocyanins and proanthocyanidins. At final concentrations of 1–10 μM these molecules exert protective effects against blue light-emitting diode (LED) light-induced retinal photoreceptor cell damage by regulating the activation of NF-κB, p38 MAPK, autophagy and pro-apoptotic proteins [141]. In senescence-accelerated mice prone 8 (SAMP8) mice, blueberry extracts (200 mg/kg) and cyanidin-3-O-galactoside (Cy-3-GAL) (50 mg/kg) may reverse the declines of cognitive and behavioural function, increasing SOD activity, reducing MDA levels in brain tissues and promoting hippocampal ERK expression [142]. Red wine contains a broad spectrum of anthocyanins (Delphinidin-3-glucoside 1.6 mg/L; Petunidin-3-glucoside 2.8 mg/L; Peonidin-3-glucoside 3.8 mg/L; Malvidin-3-glucoside 28.9 mg/L) and a recent study supports the notion that the enhanced myelination after wine treatment in an in vitro mouse model of peripheral nerve system may be induced by SIRTs activation, particularly SIRT1 [143]. Although there are no studies demonstrating that anthocyanins affect the activity of members of the FoxO class of transcription factors, exposure of *Caenorhabditis elegans* to anthocyanin-rich purple wheat (100 μg/mL) leads to a translocation of DAF-16/FoxO to the nucleus, where it stimulates the expression of stress resistance and longevity-related genes [144].

Flavanols: catechin and epicatechin

Flavanols (also referred to as flavan-3-ols) are one of the largest subclass of flavonoids consisting of monomers, oligomers, and polymers. Catechin and epicatechin are examples of monomeric flavanols and these compounds were found in higher concentrations in cocoa than in other plant-based foods. Flavanol concentrations found in cocoa products are dependent on the cocoa cultivar type, post-harvest handling practices, and manufacturer processing techniques [145]. Fresh and fermented cocoa beans contain approximately 10 % flavanols (100 mg/g) prior to processing, while the cocoa powder consumed by the Kuna Indians contains about 3.6 % flavanols [146]. Although little is known about the pharmacokinetic profiles of flavanols in the brain, catechin and epicatechinin can cross the blood–brain barrier to exert their neuroprotective effects [147]. The process is time-dependent and epicatechin was found to reach a peak 2–3 h after ingestion and return to baseline value by 6–8 h after consumption of flavanol-rich chocolate [148]. Thus, it seems plausible that flavanols may beneficially influence the brain, promoting neuroprotection and healthy brain aging. The neuroprotective effects of flavanols are believed to occur through the modulation of several pathways. First, epicatechin can specifically interact with Nrf2-mediated antioxidant response. The administration of epicatechin (30 mg/kg) dose-dependently protects transient ischemia-induced brain injury in both pre- and post-treatment animal studies by activating the Nrf2/HO1 pathway [149]. In addition, it was recently demonstrated in mice that epicatechin (15 mg/kg) protects the brain against injury after traumatic brain injury via Nrf2-dependent and -independent pathways, improving neurologic function, cognitive performance and depression-like behaviours [150]. Pretreatment with 50 or 100 μM of epicatechin also protected primary neurons from oxygen glucose deprivation by increasing neuronal viability and reducing protein oxidation. This effects occurred concomitantly with increased Nrf2-responsive antioxidant protein expression. In the same study, the neuroprotective effect elicited by epicathechin (15 mg/kg) in an animal model of focal brain ischemia was associated with reduced microglia/macrophage activation/recruitment [151]. Further data indicate that catechin exhibits anti-inflammatory effects in LPS-induced BV-2 microglial cells by suppressing the production of pro-inflammatory mediators and attenuating NF-κB activation through regulation of ERK and p38 MAPK pathways [152]. The protective effects of catechin were also demonstrated in experimental models of AD where inflammatory mediators like TNF-α, IL-1β levels and expression of iNOS were significantly attenuated by catechin pretreatment (20 mg/kg) [153]. A recent study revealed that oral administration of cocoa extract (22.9 mg/kg) protects the diabetic retina from glial reaction through SIRT1 activity, providing further evidence that epicatechin can cross the blood retinal barrier and be found in the retinal tissues (4.42 μg of epicatechin/mg of retinal tissue) of animals treated with cocoa [154].

Oleuropein and hydroxytyrosol

Virgin olive oil (VOO) and extra-virgin olive oil (EVOO) are extracted from olive fruits of *Olea europea* and their health beneficial effects are well established. An extensive literature has demonstrated that these effects can be attributed to many different substances belonging to the phenolic fraction of VOO and EVOO. However, the concentration of these compounds in VOO and EVOO is strongly affected by the particular olive cultivar, by agronomic and environmental factors, and by the extraction and storage conditions [155]. In particular, oleuropein and hydroxytyrosol are the most investigated bioactive phytochemicals and may open new avenues for the development of neuroprotective and/or neurorestorative strategies [156, 157]. Oleuropein and hydroxytyrosol have shown neuroprotective activity by acting against oxidation and inflammation and interfering with amyloid Aβ and tau protein aggregation. Indeed, St-Laurent-Thibault et al. found that these compounds (100 μg/mL) can reduce Aβ-induced toxicity in cultured neuroblastoma cells through involvement of NF-κB signaling [158]. Furthermore, it was recently demonstrated that hydroxytyrosol and oleuropein may be effective as tau aggregation inhibitors at low concentrations (10 μM) in vitro [159]. Mechanistic studies in human neuroblastoma cells reveal that an effective concentration of 5 μM hydroxytyrosol can protect against methylmercury (MeHg)-induced neurotoxicity, causing upregulation of pro-survival proteins including Nrf2 [160]. More interestingly, hydroxytyrosol given to rats at doses of 10 and 50 mg/kg/day improves neurogenesis and cognitive function in prenatally stressed offspring. In this study, hydroxytyrosol supplementation increased transcription factors FoxO1 and FoxO3, as well as phase II enzyme-related proteins, including Nrf2 and HO-1, which may contribute to the decreased oxidative stress and increased mitochondrial function [161]. The neuroprotective effect of hydroxytyrosol was investigated in a model of hypoxia-reoxygenation in rat brain slices after in vitro incubation of this compound or after 7 days of oral treatment with 5 or 10 mg/kg per day. Hydroxytyrosol significantly inhibited the efflux of lactate dehydrogenase (LDH), a marker of brain cell death. Other well-known antioxidants such as vitamin E and N-acetyl-cysteine had no neuroprotective effect in this experimental model [162]. Further observations demonstrate that 100 μM of phenolic compounds (tyrosol, hydroxytyrosol, and oleuropein) from olive oil can inhibit the effect of the chronic inflammatory microenvironment on glioblastoma through regulation of TNF-α, COX-2, JNK, ERK and NF-κB [163]. Hydroxytyrosol also improves neuronal survival, mitochondrial function and reduces oxidative stress in the brain cortex of db/db mice. After 8 weeks of hydroxytyrosol administration at doses of 10 and 50 mg/kg, this compound induced phase II antioxidant systems regulated by Nrf2, activated SIRT1 and the energy-sensing protein network known to regulate mitochondrial function and oxidative stress responses [164].

Human studies

The link between diet and health is extremely complex and the efficacy of phytochemicals to improve aspects of human brain function during aging is somewhat equivocal. However, over the past decade one of the preventative strategies that has been increasingly accepted is promoting the brain's endogenous defenses through supplementation with phytochemical-rich foods. The molecular bases for the use of phytochemicals as nutraceutical intervention to prevent cognitive decline are of crucial importance. Animal and in vitro studies have contributed significantly to our understanding, showing a dose-dependent neuroprotective effects. Despite difficulties associated with absorption, bioavailability, and biomarkers, as well as length of the trial and realistic doses, encouraging signs are emerging from intervention and observational studies with improved formulations and appropriate cohorts [165, 166]. Moreover, in order to assess the cause-effect relationship between the consumption of phytochemicals and the beneficial outcome on neuroinflammatory responses, an appropriate study design should always take into account the challenging and controversial regulatory framework of the corresponding authorities worldwide (FDA in USA; EFSA in Europe; FOSHU-Ministry of Health Labour and Welfare in Japan, etc.). In designing human intervention studies and provide high-quality evidence for brain health benefits of phytochemicals, the following factors need to be considered: 1) the phytochemical needs to be sufficiently characterised, 2) optimal physiologic dose, 3) characteristics of targeted populations including their nutritional status, health condition, and genetic background, 4) selection of clinically relevant, sensitive, reproducible, and feasible endpoints, and 5) length of the intervention [167–170]. Moreover, it should be always considered that a phytochemical functional food has a beneficial effect on the health status, thus, the study population should be composed of healthy subjects. However, to date, several human studies have investigated the cognitive enhancing effects of phytochemicals in subjects with both normal cognitive function and people with mild cognitive impairment. The neuroprotective actions of phytochemicals on cognitive function have been attributed to a number of different mechanisms, including antioxidant and anti-inflammatory activities, and increased neurogenesis in the areas of the brain associated with cognition [42]. The lack of specific health claims related to neuroinflammation and brain aging is probably due to the fact that a cluster of clinically relevant markers that reflect the neuroinflammatory state is not well-established. The intake levels and the optimal timing of consumption to prevent age-related cognitive decline in humans have yet to be determined. Despite this, completed human studies on phytochemicals mentioned here are discussed below. The efficacy of curcumin in patients with cognitive decline has been debated, however, Ringman et al. conducted the first 24-week, randomised, double-blind, placebo-controlled study measuring cerebrospinal fluid (CSF) biomarkers and evaluating the efficacy of two dosages of curcumin (2 g/d or 4 g/d) in 36 subjects with mild-to-moderate AD. Bioavailability was reported as a limitation and the results showed no significant differences in cognitive function, in CSF Aβ or tau, between placebo and intervention groups [171]. DiSilvestro et al. evaluated the health promoting effect of curcumin under normal physiological conditions in healthy middle-aged subjects (n 38, 40–60 years). In this placebo-controlled study 80 mg of curcumin (400 mg of Longvida-optimised curcumin) was given orally for 4 weeks, investigating several blood and saliva biomarkers associated with lipids, inflammation, immunity and stress, as well as Aβ levels. Cognitive measures were not included in the study design. Significant changes were shown for several of these markers including increased catalase, NO and antioxidant status, with lowered plasma alanine amino transferase and Aβ levels [172]. Cox et al. randomised 60 healthy adults aged 60–85 using the same curcumin formulation and doses used by DiSilvestro. The authors investigated acute (1 h post dose) and chronic (1-month duration) effects of curcumin intake on mood, blood, and cognition biomarkers. Attention and working memory tasks were improved one hour after administration of curcumin but also after chronic treatment [173]. Age-related cognitive decline is often accompanied by depression. A recent exploratory study provided a partial support of the efficacy of curcumin (500 mg, twice daily) given to 50 participants diagnosed with major depressive disorder. This study demonstrated that curcumin supplementation influences several peripheral biomarkers from salivary, urinary and blood samples and may be associated with its antidepressant mechanisms of action [174].

There is also mounting evidence that dietary supplementation with anthocyanins improve aspects of memory and cognition in older adults. First, supplementation with anthocyanins (300 mg/d) to healthy adults (n 120, 40–74 years) for 3 weeks decreased the plasma concentrations of several NF-κB-regulated pro-inflammatory mediators [175]. Furthermore, a dietary intervention with an anthocyanin-maqui berry extract (486 mg/d) improve oxidative status (Oxidised LDL and F2-isoprostanes) in healthy, overweight, and smoker subjects (n 42 participants, 45–65 years) after 4 weeks of supplementation [176]. Daily consumption of blueberry juice for 12 weeks containing anthocyanins at 877 mg/L improved memory function in older adults with early memory decline (n 9, mean age 76.2) [177]. Anthocyanins comprise 46 % of detected polyphenols in samples of Concord grape juice. Subjects (n 21, mean age 76 years) who received this grape juice for 16 weeks showed increased neural activation in cortical regions along with improved memory function [178]. A recent randomised clinical trial was conducted to assess changes in cognitive function of older adults (n 49, +70 years) with mild-to-moderate dementia after daily consumption of an anthocyanin-rich juice (200 ml/d) over 12 weeks. Secondary outcomes included also blood anti-inflammatory markers (CRP and IL-6). Improvements in verbal fluency, short-term memory and long-term memory were found in the intervention arm but markers of inflammation were not altered [179].

The neurobiological impact of flavanols occurs in two major ways: 1) enhancement of cerebral blood flow throughout the central and peripheral nervous system; 2) interactions with brain signaling cascades increasing expression of neuroprotective and neuromodulatory proteins [180]. To date, evidence for antioxidative and anti-inflammatory properties of flavanols on cognitive decline in human aging is rather limited. However, the known benefits on cerebral blood flow may represent a promising approach in treating cerebrovascular disorders in the elderly. The first dietary intervention study to demonstrate the efficacy of consumption of flavanols on cognitive function was conducted by Desideri et al. in 90 elderly individuals with mild cognitive impairment (mean age, 71 years). In this study, formally known as Cocoa, Cognition, and Aging (CoCoA) study, the subjects were randomised to consume once daily for 8 weeks a drink containing 990 mg (high flavanols), 520 mg (intermediate flavanols), or 45 mg (low flavanols) of cocoa flavanols. The improvement of cognitive performance was recorded in the high- and moderate-flavanol groups, suggesting also a possible role of glucose metabolism in modulating cognitive function [181]. More recently, a parallel-arm of CoCoA study involved 90 elderly individuals without clinical evidence of cognitive dysfunction who were randomly assigned to consume daily for 8 weeks a drink containing 993 mg (high flavanol), 520 mg (intermediate flavanol), or 48 mg (low flavanol) of cocoa flavanols. The results of this study indicate that the regular intake of cocoa flavanols can improve aspects of cognitive performance and these effects appear to be dependent on the amount of flavanols intake [182]. Furthermore, the dentate gyrus (DG) is a key factor in age-related cognitive decline and 3 months of high cocoa flavanol (900-mg daily dose) consumption in healthy 50-69-year-old subjects enhanced DG function in the aging human hippocampal circuit [183]. Finally, high cocoa flavanol drink (494 mg total flavanols; epicatechin 89 mg) improves regional cerebral perfusion in 18 healthy older adults (mean age 61 years), providing additional evidence that cocoa flavanols are associated with benefits for cognitive performance [184]. All these results support the crucial role of flavanols as human dietary supplements in slowing down cognitive decline during brain aging.

Several health claims for olive oil and its derivatives have been assessed in recent years. The only authorized health claim in Europe, relates the impact of olive phenolic compounds on the protection of blood lipids from oxidative stress. "A daily intake of 20 g of olive oil, which contains at least 5 mg of hydroxytyrosol and its derivatives (e.g. oleuropein and tyrosol) provides the expected beneficial effects" [185]. Although the direct cognitive benefits of olive oil require further confirmation and clinical evidence is still lacking, neuropsychological tests in a PREDIMED subcohort of cognitively healthy individuals (n 447, mean age, 66.9 years) demonstrated that adherence to the Mediterranean diet supplemented with EVOO (1 L/week) or nuts (30 g/d) was associated with improved cognitive functions at 4-year follow-up. The authors also measured urinary hydroxytyrosol reporting that the Mediterranean diet plus EVOO group had increased levels of hydroxytyrosol (49.6 μg/L), indicating good adherence with the supplemental foods [186]. However, Crespo et al. recently reported in a double-blind, randomized, placebo-controlled 1-week study that two hydroxytyrosol doses (5 and 25 mg/d) did not modify Phase II enzyme expression in peripheral blood mononuclear cells (PBMCs) of 22 young healthy volunteers [187]. Another study investigated plasma hydroxytyrosol concentration in 62 healthy elderly subjects aged 65–96 years, showing a significant increase after a 6-week daily intake of polyphenol-rich EVOO with high oleuropein contents. The results also show a significant increase of CAT in erythrocytes and a decrease of SOD and glutathione peroxidase activity after EVOO intake [188]. Although several other human studies are still underway, few clinical trials have been conducted thus far. Therefore, it is not possible to make any conclusions concerning the clinical significance of phytochemicals in counteracting neuroinflammation associated with aging and their potential in enhancing cognition. Importantly, even though the concept of hormesis has been explored extensively in terms of its applicability in aging, solid human confirmations are required by future trials.

Conclusions

Current nutrition recommendations are also directed to prevent neurodegenerative pathologies. Recent evidence suggests that dietary phytochemicals may be particularly attractive for preventing dementia and geriatric cognitive disorders. Brain aging predisposes to neurodegeneration via several mechanisms that in part converge on dysregulation of redox-state and inflammatory pathways. From the topics discussed above, light and shade rise on the effects of phytochemicals on human brain health. However, even though experimental findings have not always translated to a definitive clinical effect, the antioxidant and anti-inflammatory properties of phytochemicals have been widely accepted. Despite the abundance of the literature in this field, a clearer understanding of the mechanisms of action of phytochemicals as modulators of cell signalling pathways involved in neuro-inflammaging play a pivotal role for the evaluation of these molecules in short-term or long-term nutritional intervention trials. Furthermore, the preventive effects of phytochemicals on the onset of neurodegenerative conditions still needs to be critically explored. Many dietary supplements containing phytochemicals are already commercially available and marketed to prevent or ameliorate specific diseases, including age-related cognitive decline. The majority of these products are not substantiated by solid scientific evidence and have not yet been approved by the EFSA and/or FDA. For instance, it is unclear the concentrations of phytochemicals that enter the bloodstream and cross the blood-brain barrier. Although delivery systems, such as nanoparticles, might represent a successful strategy for drug delivery into CNS, the bioavailability continues to be highlighted as a major concern in human intervention studies. The quality of the compounds is another major source of variability and conflicting results. A further challenge is to understand whether dietary phytochemicals have appropriate effects on specific epigenetic mechanisms in specific genes or sets of genes. Brain aging is indeed associated with substantial changes in epigenetic profiles and several preclinical studies have revealed that bioactive phytochemicals play an important role in the modulation of overall epigenetic modifications (histone modifications, DNA methylations and microRNA). Another limitation to the clinical application of these compounds is the lack of knowledge on questions concerning the complex metabolic fate of dietary phytochemicals, the role of the gut microbiota in the bioconversion of phytochemicals, and whether the bacterial transformations produce metabolites with increased biological activity. Future studies addressing these issues are needed. Observational studies and dietary intervention trials in large cohorts of healthy subjects are essential to evaluate whether these phytochemicals can help to prevent age-related neurodegenerative disorders.

Competing interests
The authors declare that they have no competing interests.

Authors' contributions
All the authors drafted the manuscript and approved the final version.

Acknowledgements
The authors are grateful to the Department of Medicine and Health Sciences, University of Molise, Italy for the support.

Author details
[1]Department of Medicine and Health Sciences, School of Medicine, University of Molise, Campobasso, Italy. [2]IMPACT Research Center, Deakin University, Geelong, Australia. [3]Department of Psychiatry, Faculty of Medicine, Chulalongkorn University, Bangkok, Thailand. [4]Department of Chemical Sciences, University of Naples "Federico II", Complesso Universitario Monte S. Angelo, Naples, Italy. [5]Department of Human Welfare, Okinawa International University, Okinawa, Japan. [6]Department of Geriatric Medicine, John A. Burns School of Medicine, University of Hawaii, Honolulu, USA.

References
1. Esiri MM. Ageing and the brain. J Pathol. 2007;211:181–7.
2. de Oliveira DM, Ferreira Lima RM, El-Bachá RS. Brain rust: recent discoveries on the role of oxidative stress in neurodegenerative diseases. Nutr Neurosci. 2012;15:94–102.
3. Wang X, Michaelis EK. Selective neuronal vulnerability to oxidative stress in the brain. Front Aging Neurosci. 2010;2:12.
4. Fischer R, Maier O. Interrelation of oxidative stress and inflammation in neurodegenerative disease: role of TNF. Oxid Med Cell Longev. 2015;2015: 610813.
5. Hsieh HL, Yang CM. Role of redox signaling in neuroinflammation and neurodegenerative diseases. Biomed Res Int. 2013;2013:484613.
6. Franceschi C, Capri M, Monti D, Giunta S, Olivieri F, Sevini F, Panourgia MP, Invidia L, Celani L, Scurti M, Cevenini E, Castellani GC, Salvioli S. Inflammaging and anti-inflammaging: a systemic perspective on aging and longevity emerged from studies in humans. Mech Ageing Dev. 2007;128:92–105.
7. De la Fuente M, Miquel J. An update of the oxidation-inflammation theory of aging: the involvement of the immune system in oxi-inflamm-aging. Curr Pharm Des. 2009;15:3003–26.
8. Zipp F, Aktas O. The brain as a target of inflammation: common pathways linkinflammatory and neurodegenerative diseases. Trends Neurosci. 2006;29:518–27.
9. Rosano C, Marsland AL, Gianaros PJ. Maintaining brain health by monitoring inflammatory processes: a mechanism to promote successful aging. Aging Dis. 2012;3:16–33.
10. Taylor JM, Main BS, Crack PJ. Neuroinflammation and oxidative stress: co-conspirators in the pathology of Parkinson's disease. Neurochem Int. 2013;62:803–19.
11. Agostinho P, Cunha RA, Oliveira C. Neuroinflammation, oxidative stress and the pathogenesis of Alzheimer's disease. Curr Pharm Des. 2010;16:2766–78.
12. Quintanilla RA, Orellana JA, von Bernhardi R. Understanding risk factors for Alzheimer's disease: interplay of neuroinflammation, connexin-based communication and oxidative stress. Arch Med Res. 2012;43:632–44.
13. Lau FC, Shukitt-Hale B, Joseph JA. Nutritional intervention in brain aging: reducing the effects of inflammation and oxidative stress. Subcell Biochem. 2007;42:299–318.
14. Davinelli S, Sapere N, Zella D, Bracale R, Intrieri M, Scapagnini G. Pleiotropic protective effects of phytochemicals in Alzheimer's disease. Oxid Med Cell Longev. 2012;2012:386527.
15. Scapagnini G, Vasto S, Abraham NG, Caruso C, Zella D, Fabio G. Modulation of Nrf2/ARE pathway by food polyphenols: a nutritional neuroprotective strategy for cognitive and neurodegenerative disorders. Mol Neurobiol. 2011;44:192–201.
16. Davinelli S, Calabrese V, Zella D, Scapagnini G. Epigenetic nutraceutical diets in Alzheimer's disease. J Nutr Health Aging. 2014;18:800–5.
17. Yang Y, Jiang S, Yan J, Li Y, Xin Z, Lin Y, Qu Y. An overview of the molecular mechanisms and novel roles of Nrf2 in neurodegenerative disorders. Cytokine Growth Factor Rev. 2015;26:47–57.
18. Mennen LI, Walker R, Bennetau-Pelissero C, Scalbert A. Risks and safety of polyphenol consumption. Am J Clin Nutr. 2005;81:326S–9.
19. Wang X, Wang W, Li L, Perry G, Lee HG, Zhu X. Oxidative stress and mitochondrial dysfunction in Alzheimer's disease. Biochim Biophys Acta. 1842;2014:1240–7.
20. Moylan S, Berk M, Dean OM, Samuni Y, Williams LJ, O'Neil A, Hayley AC, Pasco JA, Anderson G, Jacka FN, Maes M. Oxidative & nitrosative stress in depression: why so much stress? Neurosci Biobehav Rev. 2014;45:46–62.
21. Ljubuncic P, Gochman E, Reznick AZ. Nitrosative stress in aging-its importance and biological implications in NF-kB signalling, in Aging and Age-Related Disorders, Bondy S and Maiese K, Eds., vol. 3 of Oxidative Stress in Applied Basic Research and Clinical Practice, Springer Science + Business Media LLC: New York, 2010.
22. Salminen LE, Paul RH. Oxidative stress and genetic markers of suboptimal antioxidant defense in the aging brain: a theoretical review. Rev Neurosci. 2014;25:805–19.
23. Nunomura A, Moreira PI, Castellani RJ, Lee HG, Zhu X, Smith MA, Perry G. Oxidative damage to RNA in aging and neurodegenerative disorders. Neurotox Res. 2012;22:231–48.
24. Klein JA, Ackerman SL. Oxidative stress, cell cycle, and neurodegeneration. J Clin Invest. 2003;111:785–93.
25. Petursdottir AL, Farr SA, Morley JE, Banks WA, Skuladottir GV. Lipid peroxidation in brain during aging in the senescence-accelerated mouse (SAM). Neurobiol Aging. 2007;28:1170–8.
26. Helenius M, Hänninen M, Lehtinen SK, Salminen A. Changes associated with aging and replicative senescence in the regulation of transcription factor nuclear factor-kappa B. Biochem J. 1996;318:603–8.
27. Kim CH, Zou Y, Kim DH, Kim ND, Yu BP, Chung HY. Proteomic analysis of nitrated and 4-hydroxy-2-nonenal-modified serum proteins during aging. J Gerontol A Biol Sci Med Sci. 2006;61:332–8.
28. Franceschi C, Campisi J. Chronic inflammation (inflammaging) and its potential contribution to age-associated diseases. J Gerontol A Biol Sci Med Sci. 2014;69 Suppl 1:S4–9.
29. Nimmerjahn A, Kirchhoff F, Helmchen F. Resting microglial cells are highly dynamic surveillants of brain parenchyma in vivo. Science. 2005; 308:1314–8.
30. von Bernhardi R, Eugenín-von Bernhardi L, Eugenín J. Microglial cell dysregulation in brain aging and neurodegeneration. Front Aging Neurosci. 2015;7:124.
31. Norden DM, Muccigrosso MM, Godbout JP. Microglial priming and enhanced reactivity to secondary insult in aging, and traumatic CNS injury, and neurodegenerative disease. Neuropharmacology. 2015;96:29–41.
32. Perry VH, Holmes C. Microglial priming in neurodegenerative disease. Nat Rev Neurol. 2014;10:217–24.
33. Urrutia PJ, Mena NP, Núñez MT. The interplay between iron accumulation, mitochondrial dysfunction, and inflammation during the execution step of neurodegenerative disorders. Front Pharmacol. 2014;10:5–38.
34. Niranjan R. The role of inflammatory and oxidative stress mechanisms in the pathogenesis of Parkinson's disease: focus on astrocytes. Mol Neurobiol. 2014;49(1):28–38.
35. Okun E, Griffioen KJ, Lathia JD, Tang SC, Mattson MP, Arumugam TV. Toll-like receptors in neurodegeneration. Brain Res Rev. 2009;59:278–92.
36. Glass CK, Saijo K, Winner B, Marchetto MC, Gage FH. Mechanisms underlying inflammation in neurodegeneration. Cell. 2010;140:918–34.
37. Lucas K, Maes M. Role of the Toll Like receptor (TLR) radical cycle in chronic inflammation: possible treatments targeting the TLR4 pathway. Mol Neurobiol. 2013;48:190–204.
38. Rojo AI, McBean G, Cindric M, Egea J, López MG, Rada P, Zarkovic N, Cuadrado A. Redox control of microglial function: molecular mechanisms and functional significance. Antioxid Redox Signal. 2014;21:1766–801.
39. Godbout JP, Johnson RW. Interleukin-6 in the aging brain. J Neuroimmunol. 2004;147:141–4.
40. Weaver JD, Huang MH, Albert M, Harris T, Rowe JW, Seeman TE. Interleukin-6 and risk of cognitive decline: MacArthur studies of successful aging. Neurology. 2002;59:371–8.
41. Chung HY, Cesari M, Anton S, Marzetti E, Giovannini S, Seo AY, Carter C, Yu BP, Leeuwenburgh C. Molecular inflammation: underpinnings of aging and age-related diseases. Ageing Res Rev. 2009;8:18–30.
42. Lee J, Jo DG, Park D, Chung HY, Mattson MP. Adaptive cellular stress pathways as therapeutic targets of dietary phytochemicals: focus on the nervous system. Pharmacol Rev. 2014;66:815–68.
43. Mattson MP, Son TG, Camandola S. Viewpoint: mechanisms of action and therapeutic potential of neurohormetic phytochemicals. Dose Response. 2007;5:174–86.

44. Sandberg M, Patil J, D'Angelo B, Weber SG, Mallard C. NRF2-regulation in brain health and disease: implication of cerebral inflammation. Neuropharmacology. 2014;79:298–306.

45. Sykiotis GP, Bohmann D. Stress-activated cap'n'collar transcription factors in aging and human disease. Sci Signal. 2010;3:re3.

46. Niture SK, Khatri R, Jaiswal AK. Regulation of Nrf2-an update. Free Radic Biol Med. 2014;66:36–44.

47. Joshi G, Johnson JA. The Nrf2-ARE pathway: a valuable therapeutic target for the treatment of neurodegenerative diseases. Recent Pat CNS Drug Discov. 2012;7:218–29.

48. Huang Y, Li W, Su ZY, Kong AT. The complexity of the Nrf2 pathway: beyond the antioxidant response. J Nutr Biochem. 2015;26:1401–13.

49. Davinelli S, Scapagnini G, Denaro F, Calabrese V, Benedetti F, Krishnan S, Curreli S, Bryant J, Zella D. Altered expression pattern of Nrf2/HO-1 axis during accelerated-senescence in HIV-1 transgenic rat. Biogerontology. 2014;15:449–61.

50. Innamorato NG, Rojo AI, García-Yagüe AJ, Yamamoto M, de Ceballos ML, Cuadrado A. The transcription factor Nrf2 is a therapeutic target against brain inflammation. J Immunol. 2008;181:680–9.

51. Zhang H, Davies KJ, Forman HJ. Oxidative stress response and Nrf2 signaling in aging. Free Radic Biol Med. 2015;88:314–36.

52. Gan L, Johnson JA. Oxidative damage and the Nrf2-ARE pathway in neurodegenerative diseases. Biochim Biophys Acta. 1842;2014:1208–18.

53. Johnson DA, Johnson JA. Nrf2-a therapeutic target for the treatment of neurodegenerative diseases. Free Radic Biol Med. 2015;88:253–67.

54. Mattson MP. NF-kappaB in the survival and plasticity of neurons. Neurochem Res. 2005;30:883–93.

55. Snow WM, Stoesz BM, Kelly DM, Albensi BC. Roles for NF-κB and gene targets of NF-κB in synaptic plasticity, memory, and navigation. Mol Neurobiol. 2014;49:757–70.

56. Meffert MK, Chang JM, Wiltgen BJ, Fanselow MS, Baltimore D. NF-kappa B functions in synaptic signaling and behavior. Nat Neurosci. 2003;6:1072–8.

57. O'Neill LA, Kaltschmidt C. NF-kappa B: a crucial transcription factor for glial and neuronal cell function. Trends Neurosci. 1997;20:252–8.

58. Hayden MS, Ghosh S. NF-κB, the first quarter-century: remarkable progress and outstanding questions. Genes Dev. 2012;26:203–34.

59. Yang L, Tao LY, Chen XP. Roles of NF-kappaB in central nervous system damage and repair. Neurosci Bul. 2007;23:307–13.

60. Kaltschmidt B, Widera D, Kaltschmidt C. Signaling via NF-kappaB in the nervous system. Biochim Biophys Acta. 1745;2005:287–99.

61. Gutierrez H, Davies AM. Regulation of neural process growth, elaboration and structural plasticity by NF-κB. Trends Neurosci. 2011;34:316–25.

62. Mattson MP. Pathways towards and away from Alzheimer's disease. Nature. 2004;430:631–9.

63. Mattson MP, Camandola S. NF-kappaB in neuronal plasticity and neurodegenerative disorders. J Clin Invest. 2001;107:247–54.

64. Chang YC, Huang CC. Perinatal brain injury and regulation of transcription. Curr Opin Neurol. 2006;19:141–7.

65. Ravati A, Ahlemeyer B, Becker A, Klumpp S, Krieglstein J. Preconditioning-induced neuroprotection is mediated by reactive oxygen species and activation of the transcription factor nuclear factor-kappaB. J Neurochem. 2001;78:909–19.

66. Kaltschmidt B, Uherek M, Wellmann H, Volk B, Kaltschmidt C. Inhibition of NF-kappaB potentiates amyloid beta-mediated neuronal apoptosis. Proc Natl Acad Sci U S A. 1999;96:9409–14.

67. Son TG, Camandola S, Mattson MP. Hormetic dietary phytochemicals. Neuromolecular Med. 2008;10:236–46.

68. Janssen-Heininger YM, Poynter ME, Baeuerle PA. Recent advances towards understanding redox mechanisms in the activation of nuclear factor kappaB. Free Radic Biol Med. 2000;28:1317–27.

69. Kaltschmidt B, Kaltschmidt C. NF-kappaB in the nervous system. Cold Spring Harb Perspect Biol. 2009;1:a001271.

70. Nair S, Doh ST, Chan JY, Kong AN, Cai L. Regulatory potential for concerted modulation of Nrf2- and Nfkb1-mediated gene expression in inflammation and carcinogenesis. Br J Cancer. 2008;99:2070–82.

71. Soares MP, Seldon MP, Gregoire IP, Vassilevskaia T, Berberat PO, Yu J, Tsui TY, Bach FH. Heme oxygenase-1 modulates the expression of adhesion molecules associated with endothelial cell activation. J Immunol. 2004;172:3553–63.

72. Chang L, Karin M. Mammalian MAP kinase signalling cascades. Nature. 2001;410:37–40.

73. Murugaiyah V, Mattson MP. Neurohormetic phytochemicals: An evolutionary-bioenergetic perspective. Neurochem Int. 2015;89:271–80.

74. Vauzour D. Dietary polyphenols as modulators of brain functions: biological actions and molecular mechanisms underpinning their beneficial effects. Oxid Med Cell Longev. 2012;2012:914273.

75. Kelly A, Laroche S, Davis S. Activation of mitogen-activated protein kinase/extracellular signal-regulated kinase in hippocampal circuitry is required for consolidation and reconsolidation of recognition memory. J Neurosci. 2003;23:5354–60.

76. Kyosseva SV, Elbein AD, Griffin WS, Mrak RE, Lyon M, Karson CN. Mitogen-activated protein kinases in schizophrenia. Biol Psychiatry. 1999;46:689–96.

77. Bowles KR, Jones L. Kinase signalling in Huntington's disease. J Huntingtons Dis. 2014;3:89–123.

78. Subramaniam S, Unsicker K. ERK and cell death: ERK1/2 in neuronal death. FEBS J. 2010;277:22–9.

79. Coffey ET. Nuclear and cytosolic JNK signalling in neurons. Nat Rev Neurosci. 2014;15:285–99.

80. Mehan S, Meena H, Sharma D, Sankhla R. JNK: a stress-activated protein kinase therapeutic strategies and involvement in Alzheimer's and various neurodegenerative abnormalities. J Mol Neurosci. 2011;43:376–90.

81. Yin F, Jiang T, Cadenas E. Metabolic triad in brain aging: mitochondria, insulin/IGF-1 signalling and JNK signalling. Biochem Soc Trans. 2013;41:101–5.

82. Coulthard LR, White DE, Jones DL, McDermott MF, Burchill SA. p38(MAPK): stress responses from molecular mechanisms to therapeutics. Trends Mol Med. 2009;15:369–79.

83. Choi WS, Eom DS, Han BS, Kim WK, Han BH, Choi EJ, Oh TH, Markelonis GJ, Cho JW, Oh YJ. Phosphorylation of p38 MAPK induced by oxidative stress is linked to activation of both caspase-8- and –9-mediated apoptotic pathways in dopaminergic neurons. J Biol Chem. 2004;279:20451–60.

84. Munoz L, Ammit AJ. Targeting p38 MAPK pathway for the treatment of Alzheimer's disease. Neuropharmacology. 2010;58:561–8.

85. Cuny GD. Kinase inhibitors as potential therapeutics for acute and chronic neurodegenerative conditions. Curr Pharm Des. 2009;15:3919–39.

86. Finkel T, Deng CX, Mostoslavsky R. Recent progress in the biology and physiology of sirtuins. Nature. 2009;460:587–91.

87. Braidy N, Jayasena T, Poljak A, Sachdev PS. Sirtuins in cognitive ageing and Alzheimer's disease. Curr Opin Psychiatry. 2012;25:226–30.

88. Ng F, Wijaya L, Tang BL. SIRT1 in the brain-connections with aging-associated disorders and lifespan. Front Cell Neurosci. 2015;9:64.

89. Brunet A, Sweeney LB, Sturgill JF, Chua KF, Greer PL, Lin Y, Tran H, Ross SE, Mostoslavsky R, Cohen HY, Hu LS, Cheng HL, Jedrychowski MP, Gygi SP, Sinclair DA, Alt FW, Greenberg ME. Stress-dependent regulation of FOXO transcription factors by the SIRT1 deacetylase. Science. 2004;303:2011–5.

90. Morris BJ, Willcox DC, Donlon TA, Willcox BJ. FOXO3:A major gene for human longevity-A mini-review. Gerontology. 2015;61:515–25.

91. Parker JA, Vazquez-Manrique RP, Tourette C, Farina F, Offner N, Mukhopadhyay A, Orfila AM, Darbois A, Menet S, Tissenbaum HA, Neri C. Integration of β-catenin, sirtuin, and FOXO signaling protects from mutant huntingtin toxicity. J Neurosci. 2012;32:12630–40.

92. Hori YS, Kuno A, Hosoda R, Horio Y. Regulation of FOXOs and p53 by SIRT1 modulators under oxidative stress. PLoS One. 2013;8:e73875.

93. Salih DA, Rashid AJ, Colas D, de la Torre-Ubieta L, Zhu RP, Morgan AA, Santo EE, Ucar D, Devarajan K, Cole CJ, Madison DV, Shamloo M, Butte AJ, Bonni A, Josselyn SA, Brunet A. FoxO6 regulates memory consolidation and synaptic function. Genes Dev. 2012;26:2780–801.

94. Willcox BJ, Donlon TA, He Q, Chen R, Grove JS, Yano K, Masaki KH, Willcox DC, Rodriguez B, Curb JD. FOXO3A genotype is strongly associated with human longevity. Proc Natl Acad Sci U S A. 2008;105:13987–92.

95. Motta MC, Divecha N, Lemieux M, Kamel C, Chen D, Gu W, Bultsma Y, McBurney M, Guarente L. Mammalian SIRT1 represses forkhead transcription factors. Cell. 2004;116:551–63.

96. Daitoku H, Hatta M, Matsuzaki H, Aratani S, Ohshima T, Miyagishi M, Nakajima T, Fukamizu A. Silent information regulator 2 potentiates Foxo1-mediated transcription through its deacetylase activity. Proc Natl Acad Sci U S A. 2004;101:10042–7.

97. Daitoku H, Fukamizu A. FOXO transcription factors in the regulatory networks of longevity. J Biochem. 2007;14:769–74.

98. Daitoku H, Sakamaki J, Fukamizu A. Regulation of FoxO transcription factors by acetylation and protein-protein interactions. Biochim Biophys Acta. 1813;2011:1954–60.

99. Ferguson D, Shao N, Heller E, Feng J, Neve R, Kim HD, Call T, Magazu S, Shen L, Nestler EJ. SIRT1-FOXO3a regulate cocaine actions in the nucleus accumbens. J Neurosci. 2015;35:3100–11.

100. Sidorova-Darmos E, Wither RG, Shulyakova N, Fisher C, Ratnam M, Aarts M, Lilge L, Monnier PP, Eubanks JH. Differential expression of sirtuin family members in the developing, adult, and aged rat brain. Front Aging Neurosci. 2014;6:333.

101. Sundaresan NR, Gupta M, Kim G, Rajamohan SB, Isbatan A, Gupta MP. Sirt3 blocks the cardiac hypertrophic response by augmenting Foxo3a-dependent antioxidant defense mechanisms in mice. J Clin Invest. 2009;119:2758–71.

102. Rangarajan P, Karthikeyan A, Lu J, Ling EA, Dheen ST. Sirtuin 3 regulates Foxo3a-mediated antioxidant pathway in microglia. Neuroscience. 2015;311:398–414.

103. Faria A, Pestana D, Teixeira D, Couraud PO, Romero I, Weksler B, de Freitas V, Mateus N, Calhau C. Insights into the putative catechin and epicatechin transport across blood–brain barrier. Food Funct. 2011;2:39–44.

104. Ghosh S, Banerjee S, Sil PC. The beneficial role of curcumin on inflammation, diabetes and neurodegenerative disease: A recent update. Food Chem Toxicol. 2015;83:111–24.

105. Jagetia GC, Aggarwal BB. "Spicing up" of the immune system by curcumin. J Clin Immunol. 2007;27:19–35.

106. He LF, Chen HJ, Qian LH, Chen GY, Buzby JS. Curcumin protects pre-oligodendrocytes from activated microglia in vitro and in vivo. Brain Res. 2010;1339:60–9.

107. Yang S, Zhang D, Yang Z, Hu X, Qian S, Liu J, Wilson B, Block M, Hong JS. Curcumin protects dopaminergic neuron against LPS induced neurotoxicity in primary rat neuron/glia culture. Neurochem Res. 2008;33:2044–53.

108. Lee WH, Loo CY, Bebawy M, Luk F, Mason RS, Rohanizadeh R. Curcumin and its derivatives: their application in neuropharmacology and neuroscience in the 21st century. Curr Neuropharmacol. 2013;11:338–78.

109. Boyanapalli SS, Tony Kong AN. "Curcumin, the King of Spices": Epigenetic Regulatory Mechanisms in the Prevention of Cancer, Neurological, and Inflammatory Diseases. Curr Pharmacol Rep. 2015;1:129–39.

110. Jung KK, Lee HS, Cho JY, Shin WC, Rhee MH, Kim TG, Kang JH, Kim SH, Hong S, Kang SY. Inhibitory effect of curcumin on nitric oxide production from lipopolysaccharide-activated primary microglia. Life Sci. 2006;79:2022–31.

111. Jin CY, Lee JD, Park C, Choi YH, Kim GY. Curcumin attenuates the release of pro-inflammatory cytokines in lipopolysaccharide-stimulated BV2 microglia. Acta Pharmacol Sin. 2007;28:1645–51.

112. Kang G, Kong PJ, Yuh YJ, Lim SY, Yim SV, Chun W, Kim SS. Curcumin suppresses lipopolysaccharide-induced cyclooxygenase-2 expression by inhibiting activator protein 1 and nuclear factor kappab bindings in BV2 microglial cells. J Pharmacol Sci. 2004;94:325–8.

113. Kim HY, Park EJ, Joe EH, Jou I. Curcumin suppresses Janus kinase-STAT inflammatory signaling through activation of Src homology 2 domain-containing tyrosine phosphatase 2 in brain microglia. J Immunol. 2003;171:6072–9.

114. Karlstetter M, Lippe E, Walczak Y, Moehle C, Aslanidis A, Mirza M, Langmann T. Curcumin is a potent modulator of microglial gene expression and migration. J Neuroinflammation. 2011;8:125.

115. Lim GP, Chu T, Yang F, Beech W, Frautschy SA, Cole GM. The curry spice curcumin reduces oxidative damage and amyloid pathology in an Alzheimer transgenic mouse. J Neurosci. 2001;21:8370–7.

116. Begum AN, Jones MR, Lim GP, Morihara T, Kim P, Heath DD, Rock CL, Pruitt MA, Yang F, Hudspeth B, Hu S, Faull KF, Teter B, Cole GM, Frautschy SA. Curcumin structure-function, bioavailability, and efficacy in models of neuroinflammation and Alzheimer's disease. J Pharmacol Exp Ther. 2008;326:196–208.

117. Pan MH, Huang TM, Lin JK. Biotransformation of curcumin through reduction and glucuronidation in mice. Drug Metab Dispos. 1999;27:486–94.

118. Kaur H, Patro I, Tikoo K, Sandhir R. Curcumin attenuates inflammatory response and cognitive deficits in experimental model of chronic epilepsy. Neurochem Int. 2015;89:40–50.

119. Sarada SK, Titto M, Himadri P, Saumya S, Vijayalakshmi V. Curcumin prophylaxis mitigates the incidence of hypobaric hypoxia-induced altered ion channels expression and impaired tight junction proteins integrity in rat brain. J Neuroinflammation. 2015;6:12–113.

120. Chen JJ, Dai L, Zhao LX, Zhu X, Cao S, Gao YJ. Intrathecal curcumin attenuates pain hypersensitivity and decreases spinal neuroinflammation in rat model of monoarthritis. Sci Rep. 2015;5:10278.

121. Zhu HT, Bian C, Yuan JC, Chu WH, Xiang X, Chen F, Wang CS, Feng H, Lin JK. Curcumin attenuates acute inflammatory injury by inhibiting the TLR4/MyD88/NF-κB signaling pathway in experimental traumatic brain injury. J Neuroinflammation. 2014;11:59.

122. Wu J, Li Q, Wang X, Yu S, Li L, Wu X, Chen Y, Zhao J, Zhao Y. Neuroprotection by curcumin in ischemic brain injury involves the Akt/Nrf2 pathway. PLoS One. 2013;8:e59843.

123. Wu JX, Zhang LY, Chen YL, Yu SS, Zhao Y, Zhao J. Curcumin pretreatment and post-treatment both improve the antioxidative ability of neurons with oxygen-glucose deprivation. Neural Regen Res. 2015;10:481–9.

124. González-Reyes S, Guzmán-Beltrán S, Medina-Campos ON, Pedraza-Chaverri J. Curcumin pretreatment induces Nrf2 and an antioxidant response and prevents hemin-induced toxicity in primary cultures of cerebellar granule neurons of rats. Oxid Med Cell Longev. 2013;2013:801418.

125. Tegenge MA, Rajbhandari L, Shrestha S, Mithal A, Hosmane S, Venkatesan A. Curcumin protects axons from degeneration in the setting of local neuroinflammation. Exp Neurol. 2014;253:102–10.

126. Miao Y, Zhao S, Gao Y, Wang R, Wu Q, Wu H, Luo T. Curcumin pretreatment attenuates inflammation and mitochondrial dysfunction in experimental stroke: The possible role of Sirt1 signaling. Brain Res Bull. 2015;121:9–15.

127. Zingg JM, Hasan ST, Cowan D, Ricciarelli R, Azzi A, Meydani M. Regulatory effects of curcumin on lipid accumulation in monocytes/macrophages. J Cell Biochem. 2012;113:833–40.

128. Zafra-Stone S, Yasmin T, Bagchi M, Chatterjee A, Vinson JA, Bagchi D. Berry anthocyanins as novel antioxidants in human health and disease prevention. Mol Nutr Food Res. 2007;51:675–83.

129. McGhie TK, Walton MC. The bioavailability and absorption of anthocyanins: towards a better understanding. Mol Nutr Food Res. 2007;51:702–13.

130. Joseph JA, Shukitt-Hale B, Willis LM. Grape juice, berries, and walnuts affect brain aging and behavior. J Nutr. 2009;139:1813S–7.

131. Poulose SM, Carey AN, Shukitt-Hale B. Improving brain signaling in aging: Could berries be the answer? Expert Rev Neurother. 2012;12:887–9.

132. Carvalho FB, Gutierres JM, Bohnert C, Zago AM, Abdalla FH, Vieira JM, Palma HE, Oliveira SM, Spanevello RM, Duarte MM, Lopes ST, Aiello G, Amaral MG, Pippi NL, Andrade CM. Anthocyanins suppress the secretion of proinflammatory mediators and oxidative stress, and restore ion pump activities in demyelination. J Nutr Biochem. 2015;26:378–90.

133. Meireles M, Marques C, Norberto S, Fernandes I, Mateus N, Rendeiro C, Spencer JP, Faria A, Calhau C. The impact of chronic blackberry intake on the neuroinflammatory status of rats fed a standard or high-fat diet. J Nutr Biochem. 2015;26:1166–73.

134. de Pascual-Teresa S. Molecular mechanisms involved in the cardiovascular and neuroprotective effects of anthocyanins. Arch Biochem Biophys. 2014;559:68–74.

135. da Silva Santos V, Bisen-Hersh E, Yu Y, Cabral IS, Nardini V, Culbreth M, Teixeira da Rocha JB, Barbosa F Jr, Aschner M. Anthocyanin-rich açaí (Euterpe oleracea Mart.) extract attenuates manganese-induced oxidative stress in rat primary astrocyte cultures. J Toxicol Environ Health A. 2014;77:390–404.

136. Aboonabi A, Singh I. Chemopreventive role of anthocyanins in atherosclerosis via activation of Nrf2-ARE as an indicator and modulator of redox. Biomed Pharmacother. 2015;72:30–6.

137. Lee SG, Kim B, Yang Y, Pham TX, Park YK, Manatou J, Koo SI, Chun OK, Lee JY. Berry anthocyanins suppress the expression and secretion of proinflammatory mediators in macrophages by inhibiting nuclear translocation of NF-κB independent of NRF2-mediated mechanism. J Nutr Biochem. 2014;25:404–11.

138. Shah SA, Yoon GH, Kim MO. Protection of the developing brain with anthocyanins against ethanol-induced oxidative stress and neurodegeneration. Mol Neurobiol. 2015;51:1278–91.

139. Lau FC, Joseph JA, McDonald JE, Kalt W. Attenuation of iNOS and COX2 by blueberry polyphenols is mediated through the suppression of NF-[kappa]B activation. J Funct Foods. 2009;1:274–83.

140. Joseph JA, Shukitt-Hale B, Brewer GJ, Weikel KA, Kalt W, Fisher DR. Differential protection among fractionated blueberry polyphenolic families against DA-, Abeta(42)- and LPS-induced decrements in Ca(2+) buffering in primary hippocampal cells. J Agric Food Chem. 2010;58:8196–204.

141. Ogawa K, Kuse Y, Tsuruma K, Kobayashi S, Shimazawa M, Hara H. Protective effects of bilberry and lingonberry extracts against blue light-emitting diode light-induced retinal photoreceptor cell damage in vitro. BMC Complement Altern Med. 2014;14:120.

142. Tan L, Yang HP, Pang W, Lu H, Hu YD, Li J, Lu SJ, Zhang WQ, Jiang YG. Cyanidin-3-O-galactoside and blueberry extracts supplementation improves spatial memory and regulates hippocampal ERK expression in senescence-accelerated mice. Biomed Environ Sci. 2014;27:186–96.

143. Stettner M, Wolffram K, Mausberg AK, Albrecht P, Derksen A, Methner A, Dehmel T, Hartung HP, Dietrich H, Kieseier BC. Promoting myelination in an in vitro mouse model of the peripheral nervous system: the effect of wine ingredients. PLoS One. 2013;7(8):e66079.

144. Chen W, Müller D, Richling E, Wink M. Anthocyanin-rich purple wheat prolongs the life span of Caenorhabditis elegans probably by activating the DAF-16/FOXO transcription factor. J Agric Food Chem. 2013;61:3047–53.

145. Scapagnini G, Davinelli S, Di Renzo L, De Lorenzo A, Olarte HH, Micali G, Cicero AF, Gonzalez S. Cocoa bioactive compounds: significance and potential for the maintenance of skin health. Nutrients. 2014;6:3202–13.

146. Latham LS, Hensen ZK, Minor DS. Chocolate–guilty pleasure or healthy supplement? J Clin Hypertens (Greenwich). 2014;16:101–6.

147. Wu L, Zhang QL, Zhang XY, Lv C, Li J, Yuan Y, Yin FX. Pharmacokinetics and blood–brain barrier penetration of (+)-catechin and (–)-epicatechin in rats by microdialysis sampling coupled to high-performance liquid chromatography with chemiluminescence detection. J Agric Food Chem. 2012;60:9377–83.

148. Nehlig A. The neuroprotective effects of cocoa flavanol and its influence on cognitive performance. Br J Clin Pharmacol. 2013;75:716–27.

149. Shah ZA, Li RC, Ahmad AS, Kensler TW, Yamamoto M, Biswal S, Doré S. The flavanol (–)-epicatechin prevents stroke damage through the Nrf2/HO1 pathway. J Cereb Blood Flow Metab. 2010;30:1951–61.

150. Cheng T, Wang W, Li Q, Han X, Xing J, Qi C, Lan X, Wan J, Potts A, Guan F, Wang J. Cerebroprotection of flavanol (–)-epicatechin after traumatic brain injury via Nrf2-dependent and -independent pathways. Free Radic Biol Med. 2016;92:15–28.

151. Leonardo CC, Agrawal M, Singh N, Moore JR, Biswal S, Doré S. Oral administration of the flavanol (–)-epicatechin bolsters endogenous protection against focal ischemia through the Nrf2 cytoprotective pathway. Eur J Neurosci. 2013;38:3659–68.

152. Syed Hussein SS, Kamarudin MN, Kadir HA. (+)-Catechin Attenuates NF-κB Activation Through Regulation of Akt, MAPK, and AMPK Signaling Pathways in LPS-Induced BV-2 Microglial Cells. Am J Chin Med. 2015;43:927–52.

153. Ejaz Ahmed M, Khan MM, Javed H, Vaibhav K, Khan A, Tabassum R, Ashafaq M, Islam F, Safhi MM, Islam F. Amelioration of cognitive impairment and neurodegeneration by catechin hydrate in rat model of streptozotocin-induced experimental dementia of Alzheimer's type. Neurochem Int. 2013;62:492–501.

154. Duarte DA, Rosales MA, Papadimitriou A, Silva KC, Amancio VH, Mendonça JN, Lopes NP, de Faria JB, de Faria JM. Polyphenol-enriched cocoa protects the diabetic retina from glial reaction through the sirtuin pathway. J Nutr Biochem. 2015;26:64–74.

155. Martín-Peláez S, Covas MI, Fitó M, Kušar A, Pravst I. Health effects of olive oil polyphenols: Recent advances and possibilities for the use of health claims. Mol Nutr Food Res. 2013;57:760–71.

156. Rodríguez-Morató J, Xicota L, Fitó M, Farré M, Dierssen M, de la Torre R. Potential role of olive oil phenolic compounds in the prevention of neurodegenerative diseases. Molecules. 2015;20:4655–80.

157. Khalatbary AR. Olive oil phenols and neuroprotection. Nutr Neurosci. 2013;16:243–9.

158. St-Laurent-Thibault C, Arseneault M, Longpré F, Ramassamy C. Tyrosol and hydroxytyrosol, two main components of olive oil, protect N2a cells against amyloid-β-induced toxicity. Involvement of the NF-κB signaling. Curr Alzheimer Res. 2011;8:543–51.

159. Daccache A, Lion C, Sibille N, Gerard M, Slomianny C, Lippens G, Cotelle P. Oleuropein and derivatives from olives as Tau aggregation inhibitors. Neurochem Int. 2011;58:700–7.

160. Mohan V, Das S, Rao SB. Hydroxytyrosol, a dietary phenolic compound forestalls the toxic effects of methylmercury-induced toxicity in IMR-32 human neuroblastoma cells. Environ Toxicol. 2015; [Epub ahead of print.

161. Zheng A, Li H, Cao K, Xu J, Zou X, Li Y, Chen C, Liu J, Feng Z. Maternal hydroxytyrosol administration improves neurogenesis and cognitive function in prenatally stressed offspring. J Nutr Biochem. 2015;26:190–9.

162. González-Correa JA, Navas MD, Lopez-Villodres JA, Trujillo M, Espartero JL, De La Cruz JP. Neuroprotective effect of hydroxytyrosol and hydroxytyrosol acetate in rat brain slices subjected to hypoxia-reoxygenation. Neurosci Lett. 2008;446:143–6.

163. Lamy S, Ben Saad A, Zgheib A, Annabi B. Olive oil compounds inhibit the paracrine regulation of TNF-α-induced endothelial cell migration through reduced glioblastoma cell cyclooxygenase-2 expression. J Nutr Biochem. 2016;27:136–45.

164. Zheng A, Li H, Xu J, Cao K, Li H, Pu W, Yang Z, Peng Y, Long J, Liu J, Feng Z. Hydroxytyrosol improves mitochondrial function and reduces oxidative

165. stress in the brain of db/db mice: role of AMP-activated protein kinase activation. Br J Nutr. 2015;113:1667–76.

165. Rigacci S, Stefani M. Nutraceuticals and amyloid neurodegenerative diseases: a focus on natural phenols. Expert Rev Neurother. 2015;15:41-52.

166. Rabassa M, Cherubini A, Zamora-Ros R, Urpi-Sarda M, Bandinelli S, Ferrucci L, Andres-Lacueva C. Low Levels of a Urinary Biomarker of Dietary Polyphenol Are Associated with Substantial Cognitive Decline over a 3-Year Period in Older Adults: The Invecchiare in Chianti Study. J Am Geriatr Soc. 2015;63:938–46.

167. Navas-Carretero S, Martinez JA. Cause-effect relationships in nutritional intervention studies for health claims substantiation: guidance for trial design. Int J Food Sci Nutr. 2015;66 Suppl 1:S53–61.

168. Pae M, Meydani SN, Wu D. The role of nutrition in enhancing immunity in aging. Aging Dis. 2012;3:91–129.

169. EFSA Panel on Dietetic Products. Nutrition and Allergies (NDA) (2011) Guidance on the scientific requirements for health claims related to gut health and immune function. EFSA J. 2011;9:1984–96.

170. Albers R, Bourdet-Sicard R, Braun D, Calder PC, Herz U, Lambert C, Lenoir-Wijnkoop I, Méheust A, Ouwehand A, Phothirath P, Sako T, Salminen S, Siemensma A, van Loveren H, Sack U. Monitoring immune modulation by nutrition in the general population: identifying and substantiating effects on human health. Br J Nutr. 2013;110:S1–30.

171. Ringman JM, Frautschy SA, Teng E, Begum AN, Bardens J, Beigi M, Gylys KH, Badmaev V, Heath DD, Apostolova LG, Porter V, Vanek Z, Marshall GA, Hellemann G, Sugar C, Masterman DL, Montine TJ, Cummings JL, Cole GM. Oral curcumin for Alzheimer's disease: tolerability and efficacy in a 24-week randomized, double blind, placebo-controlled study. Alzheimers Res Ther. 2012;4:43.

172. DiSilvestro RA, Joseph E, Zhao S, Bomser J. Diverse effects of a low dose supplement of lipidated curcumin in healthy middle aged people. Nutr J. 2012;11:79.

173. Cox KH, Pipingas A, Scholey AB. Investigation of the effects of solid lipid curcumin on cognition and mood in a healthy older population. J Psychopharmacol. 2015;29:642–51.

174. Lopresti AL, Maes M, Meddens MJ, Maker GL, Arnoldussen E, Drummond PD. Curcumin and major depression: a randomised, double-blind, placebo-controlled trial investigating the potential of peripheral biomarkers to predict treatment response and antidepressant mechanisms of change. Eur Neuropsychopharmacol. 2015;25:38–50.

175. Karlsen A, Retterstøl L, Laake P, Paur I, Bøhn SK, Sandvik L, Blomhoff R. Anthocyanins inhibit nuclear factor-kappaB activation in monocytes and reduce plasma concentrations of pro inflammatory mediators in healthy adults. J Nutr. 2007;137:1951–4.

176. Davinelli S, Bertoglio JC, Zarrelli A, Pina R, Scapagnini G. A Randomized Clinical Trial Evaluating the Efficacy of an Anthocyanin-Maqui Berry Extract (Delphinol®) on Oxidative Stress Biomarkers. J Am Coll Nutr. 2015;34 Suppl 1:28–33.

177. Krikorian R, Shidler MD, Nash TA, Kalt W, Vinqvist-Tymchuk MR, Shukitt-Hale B, Joseph JA. Blueberry supplementation improves memory in older adults. J Agric Food Chem. 2010;58:3996–4000.

178. Krikorian R, Boespflug EL, Fleck DE, Stein AL, Wightman JD, Shidler MD, Sadat-Hossieny S. Concord grape juice supplementation and neurocognitive function in human aging. J Agric Food Chem. 2012;60:5736–42.

179. Kent K, Charlton K, Roodenrys S, Batterham M, Potter J, Traynor V, Gilbert H, Morgan O, Richards R. Consumption of anthocyanin-rich cherry juice for 12 weeks improves memory and cognition in older adults with mild-to-moderate dementia. Eur J Nutr. 2015; [Epub ahead of print].

180. Sokolov AN, Pavlova MA, Klosterhalfen S, Enck P. Chocolate and the brain: neurobiological impact of cocoa flavanols on cognition and behavior. Neurosci Biobehav Rev. 2013;37:2445–53.

181. Desideri G, Kwik-Uribe C, Grassi D, Necozione S, Ghiadoni L, Mastroiacovo D, Raffaele A, Ferri L, Bocale R, Lechiara MC, Marini C, Ferri C. Benefits in cognitive function, blood pressure, and insulin resistance through cocoa flavanol consumption in elderly subjects with mild cognitive impairment: the Cocoa, Cognition, and Aging (CoCoA) study. Hypertension. 2012;60:794–801.

182. Mastroiacovo D, Kwik-Uribe C, Grassi D, Necozione S, Raffaele A, Pistacchio L, Righetti R, Bocale R, Lechiara MC, Marini C, Ferri C, Desideri G. Cocoa flavanol consumption improves cognitive function, blood pressure control, and metabolic profile in elderly subjects: the Cocoa, Cognition, and Aging (CoCoA) Study–a randomized controlled trial. Am J Clin Nutr. 2015;101:538–48.

183. Brickman AM, Khan UA, Provenzano FA, Yeung LK, Suzuki W, Schroeter H, Wall M, Sloan RP, Small SA. Enhancing dentate gyrus function with

dietary flavanols improves cognition in older adults. Nat Neurosci. 2014;17:1798–803.

184. Lamport DJ, Pal D, Moutsiana C, Field DT, Williams CM, Spencer JP, Butler LT. The effect of flavanol-rich cocoa on cerebral perfusion in healthy older adults during conscious resting state: a placebo controlled, crossover, acute trial. Psychopharmacology (Berl). 2015;232:3227–34.

185. European Community. Council Regulation No. 432/2012 of 16 May 2012 establishing a list of permitted health claims made on foods, other than those referring to the reduction of disease risk, to children's development, health. Off J Eur Union. 2012;L136:1–40.

186. Valls-Pedret C, Sala-Vila A, Serra-Mir M, Corella D, de la Torre R, Martínez-González MÁ, Martínez-Lapiscina EH, Fitó M, Pérez-Heras A, Salas-Salvadó J, Estruch R, Ros E. Mediterranean Diet and Age-Related Cognitive Decline: A Randomized Clinical Trial. JAMA Intern Med. 2015;175:1094–103.

187. Crespo MC, Tomé-Carneiro J, Burgos-Ramos E, Loria Kohen V, Espinosa MI, Herranz J, Visioli F. One-week administration of hydroxytyrosol to humans does not activate Phase II enzymes. Pharmacol Res. 2015;95-96:132–7.

188. Oliveras-López MJ, Molina JJ, Mir MV, Rey EF, Martín F, de la Serrana HL. Extra virgin olive oil (EVOO) consumption and antioxidant status in healthy institutionalized elderly humans. Arch Gerontol Geriatr. 2013;57:234–42.

Efforts of the human immune system to maintain the peripheral CD8+ T cell compartment after childhood thymectomy

Manuela Zlamy[1], Giovanni Almanzar[2], Walther Parson[3,4], Christian Schmidt[5], Johannes Leierer[6], Birgit Weinberger[7], Verena Jeller[1], Karin Unsinn[8], Matthias Eyrich[2], Reinhard Würzner[9] and Martina Prelog[2*]

Abstract

Background: Homeostatic mechanisms to maintain the T cell compartment diversity indicate an ongoing process of thymic activity and peripheral T cell renewal during human life. These processes are expected to be accelerated after childhood thymectomy and by the influence of cytomegalovirus (CMV) inducing a prematurely aged immune system.

The study aimed to investigate proportional changes and replicative history of CD8+ T cells, of recent thymic emigrants (RTEs) and CD103+ T cells (mostly gut-experienced) and the role of Interleukin-(IL)-7 and IL-7 receptor (CD127)-expressing T cells in thymectomized patients compared to young and old healthy controls.

Results: Decreased proportions of naive and CD31 + CD8+ T cells were demonstrated after thymectomy, with higher proliferative activity of CD127-expressing T cells and significantly shorter relative telomere lengths (RTLs) and lower T cell receptor excision circles (TRECs). Increased circulating CD103+ T cells and a skewed T cell receptor (TCR) repertoire were found after thymectomy similar to elderly persons. Naive T cells were influenced by age at thymectomy and further decreased by CMV.

Conclusions: After childhood thymectomy, the immune system demonstrated constant efforts of the peripheral CD8+ T cell compartment to maintain homeostasis. Supposedly it tries to fill the void of RTEs by peripheral T cell proliferation, by at least partly IL-7-mediated mechanisms and by proportional increase of circulating CD103+ T cells, reminiscent of immune aging in elderly. Although other findings were less significant compared to healthy elderly, early thymectomy demonstrated immunological alterations of CD8+ T cells which mimic features of premature immunosenescence in humans.

Keywords: Thymectomy, Naive T cells, CD8, TRECs, Telomeres, TCR diversity, CMV

Background

The thymus plays an essential role in the differentiation of T cells, which are necessary for an effective cellular immune response against pathogens and tumor cells and for control of self-reactive T cell clones. TCR rearrangement within the thymus generates the basis for a wide TCR repertoire. The thymus is fully developed at birth and reaches its largest size during childhood with subsequent structural changes. The decline of *de novo* T cell production accelerates with puberty with a decreasing rate of approximately 3 % per year during adulthood [1]. Although proportionally declining with age, the number of naive T cells is maintained by peripheral proliferation of pre-existing naive T cells which results in a dilution of T cell receptor excision circles (TRECs) within thymus-derived naive T cells [2–4] and in shortening of the relative telomere lengths (RTLs) by increased replication rounds [5]. IL-7 is known as an essential factor involved in maintenance of the peripheral naive T cell pool, in regulation of T cell homeostasis and in preservation of the TCR repertoire [6]. IL-7 may also participate in the

* Correspondence: Prelog_M@ukw.de
[2]Department of Pediatrics, University Hospital Wuerzburg, University of Wuerzburg, Josef-Schneider-Str. 2, 97080 Wuerzburg, Germany
Full list of author information is available at the end of the article

reconstitution of peripheral T cell subpopulations in conditions of low thymic output [7, 8].

In patients who were partly or totally thymectomized in early childhood due to surgery for congenital heart defects [1, 9, 10], several studies have revealed multiple immune alterations within the peripheral T cell compartments [11–21] and a delayed humoral immune response to new antigens later in life [22, 23]. Cytomegalovirus (CMV) is known to drive the T cell differentiation towards abundance of terminally differentiated CD28- effector T cells and towards a restricted TCR repertoire [24] which was also seen in a subgroup of young adults thymectomized during early childhood (YATEC) similar to elderly individuals [17]. These exacerbated alterations were seen as the likely consequence of the chronic stimulation of the T cell immune system caused by the life-long persistence of CMV in the absence of an adequate T cell renewal capacity [1, 17].

The present study aimed to perform an in-depth analysis of proportional changes of CD8+ T cell subpopulations with inclusion of recent thymic emigrants (RTE) [25, 26] and gut-experienced CD103+ T cells [27]. The role of IL-7 and IL-7 receptor (CD127)-expressing T cells, as well as the proportion of cells that are outside the G0 stage at the time point of blood withdrawal (Ki67 expression) and replicative history of peripheral CD8+ T cells by TRECs and RTLs were studied in order to assess possible mechanisms of maintenance of the peripheral naive T cell compartment under lack of sufficient thymic output as expected in thymectomized individuals. Differentiation of CD8+ T cells and TCR diversity were investigated under the light of peripheral T cell exhaustion by chronic stimulation caused by CMV which is known to influence a prematurely aged immune system and was thought to underline the hypothesis of premature T cell immunosenscence in thymectomized humans. We could demonstrate that

immunological alterations associated with thymectomy particularly affected the CD8+ T cell pool.

Methods
Study population
Peripheral blood mononuclear cells (PBMCs) were collected from young adults or adolescents thymectomized in early childhood at ≤24 months of age (YATEC), from young adults or adolescents thymectomized in childhood at >24 months of age (YAT), from young healthy controls (YHC) as a control group for YATEC and YAT and from older healthy controls (OHC) aged >65 years as a control group for immunosenescence parameters (Table 1). Thymectomy was performed during open heart surgery by total resection of both lobes for surgical reasons with inclusion and exclusion criteria described in detail previously [16]. Reconstitution of the thymus was excluded by magnetic resonance imaging. The study was performed according to the Declaration of Helsinki with approval by the local Ethics Committee, Medical University Innsbruck. All participants or their legal representatives gave written informed consent.

Definition and quantification of T cell subpopulations
PBMCs were incubated with fluorochrome-labeled monoclonal antibodies (mAbs) (BD Pharmingen, San Jose, CA, USA) and analyzed by FACS Calibur flow cytometer (Becton Dickinson, Oxford, United Kingdom) and CELL-Quest software (BD Pharmingen), as described previously [16]. A minimum of 3,000 events was counted for each panel in FACS analysis with results expressed as percentages of gated lymphocytes. For technical limitations regarding available blood volumes, subgroup analysis could not be performed in all subjects. CD45RA, CD27 and CCR7 were used to differentiate between naive (CD45RA + CD27 + CCR7+), early memory (CD45RA-CD27 + CCR7+), late memory (CD45RA-CD27-CCR7-)

Table 1 Demographics of study populations and proportions of lymphocytes

	YATEC	YAT	YHC	OHC
Number (female/male)	23 (5/18)	12 (7/5)	17 (11/6)	9 (4/5)
CMV (positive/negative)[a]	10/13	3/8	5/12	5/2
Age (years)[b]	19.7 ± 8.1 (17.9; 9.0–35.8)	18.4 ± 7.2 (17.4; 9.2–31.3)	23.5 ± 7.9 (25.3; 8.0–33.0)	72.8 ± 4.4 (73.4; 67.0–80.0)
Age at thymectomy (years)[b]	0.5 ± 0.5 (0.2; 0.01–1.7)	7.6 ± 5.0 (5.1; 2.1–16.8)	n. a.	n. a
Time post thymectomy (years)[b]	19.7 ± 7.6 (19.7; 8.8–34.2)[c]	14.4 ± 6.1 (14.6; 3.9–26.1)[c]	n. a.	n. a.
Lymphocytes absolute/μl[b]	1.8 ± 0.5 (1.7; 1.3–2.7)	2.1 ± 0.5 (2.1; 1.7–2.5)	2.0 ± 0.4 (2.1; 1.3–2.7)	1.6 ± 0.7 (1.3; 0.9–2.7)
CD3+ (% of lymphocytes)[b]	70.8 ± 11.9 (75.0; 48.0–85.0)	79.2 ± 2.2 (77.9; 78.0–82.0)	79.0 ± 7.6 (80.9; 62.0–89.0)	69.8 ± 11.8 (70.8; 50.0–85.0)
CD4+ (% of lymphocytes)[b]	44.6 ± 13.7 (43.0; 35.1–61.4)	51.5 ± 6.8 (48.5; 46.7–59.3)	51.8 ± 6.6 (54.2; 36.5–61.6)	43.2 ± 12.2 (43.6; 28.5–65.9)
CD8+ (% of lymphocytes)[b]	24.7 ± 7.5 (22.3; 15.4–39.9)	25.7 ± 7.1 (26.3; 16.3–32.4)	25.8 ± 6.9 (26.0; 12.3–38.2)	25.2 ± 8.2 (23.4; 14.3–39.0)

Abbreviations: young adults/adolescents thymectomized in early childhood at ≤24 months of age, *YATEC*; young adults/adolescents thymectomized in childhood at >24 months of age, *YAT*; young healthy controls, *YHC*; old healthy controls, *OHC*; not applicable, n. a
[a]CMV serology was unknown in 2 cases of the OHC
[b]Values are given in mean ± standard deviation (median; range)
[c]Chronological age significantly correlated with time post thymectomy in YATEC (R^2–0.958; *p* = 0.0001) and in YAT (R^2 = 0.853; *p* = 0.0001)

and terminally differentiated effector (CD45RA + CD27-CCR7-) T cells re-expressing CD45RA [28]. CD31 was previously used to identify RTE in CD4+ T cells [26]. For CD8+ RTEs, CD31 is less well established, but was used as a naive CD8+ T cell marker [25]. CD127, the IL-7 receptor α chain, is generally expressed on T cells susceptible to auto-proliferative mechanisms by IL-7, and, thus, was used mainly in combination with naive T cell markers [28]. Ki67 was used to label the proportion of cells that are outside the G0 stage of their existence [16, 18], reflecting the immune activation status of the individuals at the time point of blood withdrawal. CD103 has been described as a marker of mucosa-derived T cells [19, 27] and of CD8+ T cells which have entered the gut [29].

ELISA tests

Serum IgG directed against CMV (Enzygnost, Dade Behring, Vienna, Austria) and serum IL-7 concentrations were measured by ELISA (BD Pharmingen, San Jose, CA, USA) according to standard laboratory methods.

TCR spectratyping

In order to analyze the clonal composition of the TCR repertoire total RNA was extracted from PBMCs and reverse-transcribed. TCR Vβ transcripts were amplified by PCR using different primers for each of the 24 Vβ families and a specific primer for the constant region of the β chain labeled with the fluorescent dye marker 6-FAM [30]. Aliquots of the PCR product were analyzed on CE 3100 Genetic Analyzer (Perkin Elmer, Norwalk, CT). Raw data were analyzed using GeneScan 3.7 and Gentyper 3.6 software packages (Applied Biosystems, Foster City, CA) using the Local Southern method for fragment size estimation [31]. Scores for clonality were assigned based on the occurrence of dominant clonal expansions for each Vβ family. Clonality score 1 was used for peaks showing Gaussian distribution, 2 for several peaks and 3 for one peak, as described previously [32, 33].

Quantification of TRECs and relative telomere length

DNA was extracted from separated CD8 + CD45RA+ T cells after magnetic activated cell sorting (MACS) (Milteny Biotec, Bergisch-Gladbach, Germany) using QIAamp DNA Mini Kit (Qiagen, Chatsworth, CA, USA) as described previously [22]. Signal-joint TREC concentrations were determined by real-time PCR as described in detail previously [26, 34]. To avoid bias by different numbers of naive T cells, TRECs were calculated in relation to CD8 + CD45RA+ T cell numbers [3]. Determination of relative telomere length (RTL) was performed by calculating the ratio of a quantitative PCR reaction product from the same sample using specific primers for telomeres and a single copy gene as described previously [35–37]. In absence of DNA samples from our OHC

cohort, TRECs and telomeres were analyzed in samples of leucocytes from 10 healthy donors (5 female, 5 male) aged 71 to 78 years as an internal control for aged individuals and measured with the method described above.

Statistical analysis

Shapiro-Wilks test was used to test for normal distribution. Non-parametric Mann–Whitney-U was applied for not normally-distributed independent variables. To avoid bias by multiple testing, a p-value ≤0.05 was considered statistically significant using the less conservative Benjamini-Hochberg-correction to reduce false-positive results by the following assumption: A p-value was considered statistically significant in the case that a p-value was below the highest p-value fulfilling the following requirement that $p(i) \leq (i{*}q)/m$. An arbitrarily set q-value indicates the tolerance for false-significant results (in this case q = 0.1), with i indicating the rank in a step-up ranking of p-values and m indicating the total number of executed tests. X^2 test was used to compare dichotome variables. Correlations between variables were identified by Spearman's rank correlation coefficient. A generalized linear model was generated by step-to-step regression to infer the influence of the time post thymectomy, the age at thymectomy or CMV positivity on the immunological system, adjusted for the chronological age (age at blood withdrawal) of the patient. All statistical analyses were performed with SPSS Version 22.0 (Chicago, IL, USA).

Results

Lower proportions of naive CD8+ T cells after thymectomy

By guiding cells to and within lymphoid organs, CCR7 contributes to immunity and tolerance and is a characteristic marker of naive, regulatory and memory T cells [38]. Together with CD27 it is used to define peripheral naive T cells [28]. YAT showed significantly lower proportions of naive CD8+ T cells compared to YHC (Fig. 1, Fig. 2a).

Lower proportions of CD31-expressing CD8+ T cells after thymectomy

CD31 has been reported as characteristic marker of RTE decreasing with age [26, 39]. For the purpose to evaluate the peripheral existence of CD31+ T cells in the condition of expected low production of RTE in thymectomized patients, we assessed the proportions of CD31-expressing T cells within the CD8+ T cell pool. Significant lower proportions of CD31+ in CD8+ T cells were found in YATEC compared to YHC (Fig. 1, Fig. 2b). In contrast to YATEC, only YHC showed a negative correlation of CD31+ naive CD8+ T cells with chronological age (Fig. 2c, d). In YATEC patients, CD31+ naive CD8 + T cells negatively correlated with age at thymectomy,

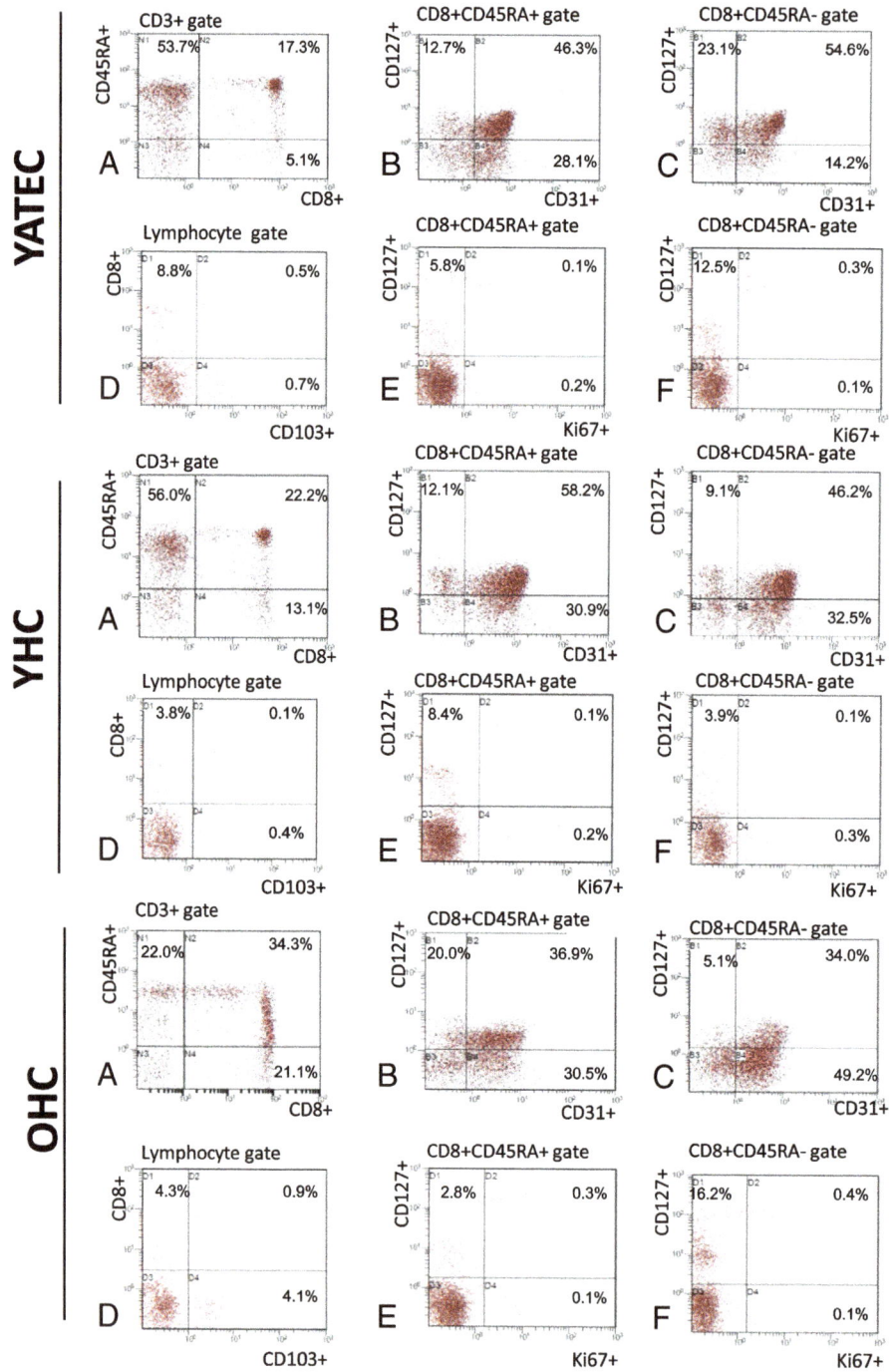

Fig. 1 Analysis of CD127+, CD31+ and CD103+ CD8+ T cell proportions. Representative examples of flow cytometric analysis of CD8+ T cells of one YATEC patient, one YHC and one OHC are shown. Gating strategies were as follows: First, CD8+ T cells were analyzed within the CD3+ lymphocyte gate. Percentages of CD45RA+ and CD45RA- were analyzed in CD8+ within the CD3+ T cell gate (**a**). CD127+ was determined within CD45RA+ (**b**) and CD45RA- CD8+ T cells (**c**) together with CD31, percentages indicating positive events in the CD45RA+ or CD45RA- CD8+ T cell gate, respectively. Due to low percentages of circulating CD103+ CD8+, these cells were determined in the total lymphocyte gate (**d**). Percentages of Ki67+ were determined together with CD127+ in the CD45RA+ (**e**) and CD45RA- CD8+ gate (**f**), respectively

with a trend towards lower proportions when being thymectomized in the second year of life (Fig.2e). This finding was also confirmed by linear regression ($R^2 = 0.445$)

including chronological age, CMV and age at thymectomy, which revealed age at thymectomy as an independent factor for reduction of CD31+ naive CD8 + T cells ($p = 0.04$).

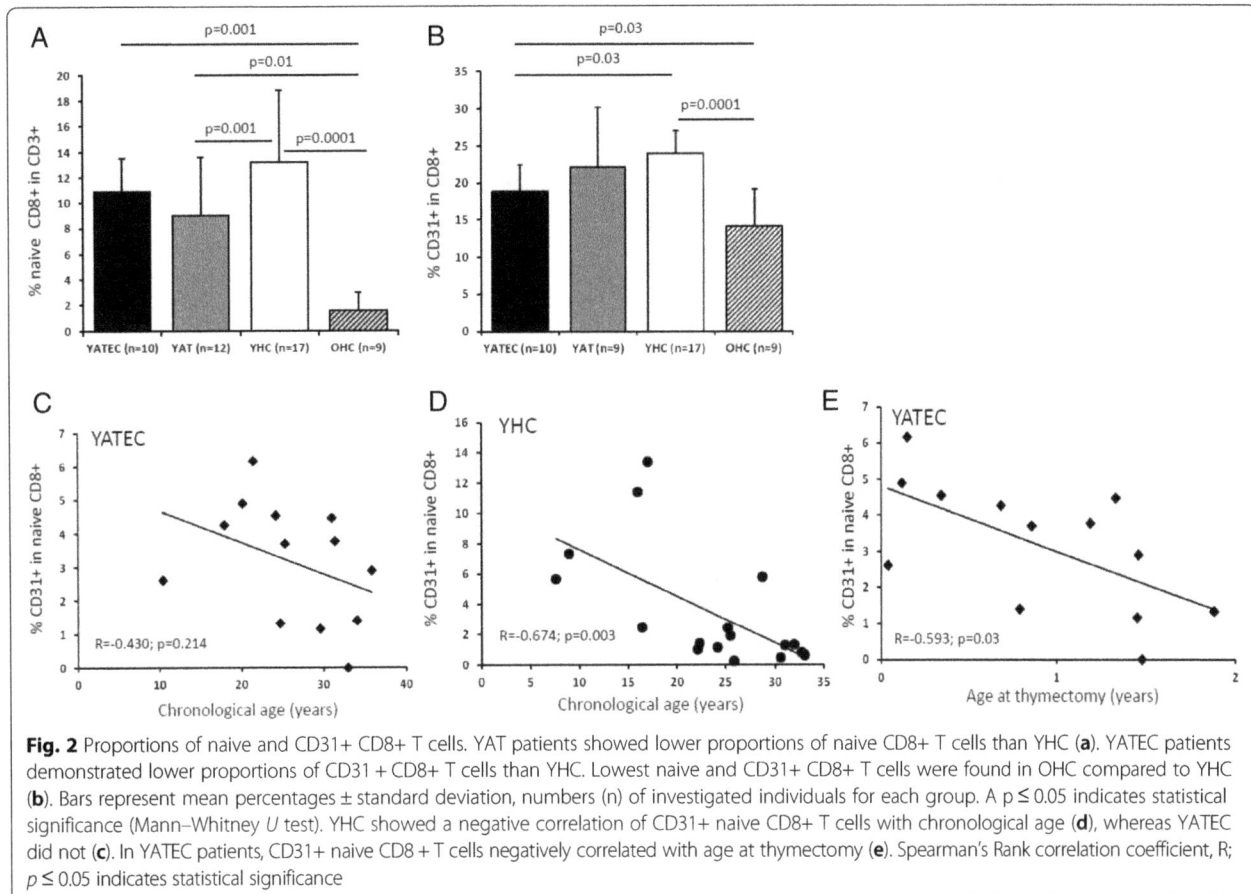

Fig. 2 Proportions of naive and CD31+ CD8+ T cells. YAT patients showed lower proportions of naive CD8+ T cells than YHC (**a**). YATEC patients demonstrated lower proportions of CD31 + CD8+ T cells than YHC. Lowest naive and CD31+ CD8+ T cells were found in OHC compared to YHC (**b**). Bars represent mean percentages ± standard deviation, numbers (n) of investigated individuals for each group. A p ≤ 0.05 indicates statistical significance (Mann–Whitney *U* test). YHC showed a negative correlation of CD31+ naive CD8+ T cells with chronological age (**d**), whereas YATEC did not (**c**). In YATEC patients, CD31+ naive CD8 + T cells negatively correlated with age at thymectomy (**e**). Spearman's Rank correlation coefficient, R; $p \leq 0.05$ indicates statistical significance

Increased Ki67+ expression of CD127-expressing T cells and lower IL-7 serum concentrations after thymectomy

We next aimed to study the potential role of IL-7 and CD127-expressing T cells in their contribution to the peripheral naive T cell compartment in thymectomized individuals (Fig. 3a). IL-7 concentrations positively correlated with time post thymectomy in YATEC (Fig. 3e). YATEC thymectomized more than 25 years ago and over 30 years of age (YATEC > 30a) showed a trend towards higher IL-7 concentrations compared to YHC > 30a (Fig. 5c). As higher concentrations of IL-7 were known from lymphopenic conditions [7, 8], IL-7 concentrations were set in relation to lymphocyte counts. IL-7 concentrations positively correlated with lymphocyte counts only in YHC but not in YATEC (Fig. 3f, g).

For further investigation of naive CD8+ T cells, CD127 was included into the analysis due to its function as IL-7 receptor α chain. A trend to lower proportions of CD127+ cells within naive CD8+ T cells were seen in YATEC and YAT compared to YHC (Fig. 1, Fig. 3b).

In search for the proliferative activation of peripheral CD45RA+ naive or CD45RA- memory CD8+ T cells expressing CD127+ and, thus, expected to be susceptible to IL-7 activity, higher Ki67-expression was found in CD127+ memory CD8+ T cells in YATEC compared to

YHC but not in CD127+ naive CD8+ T cells (Fig. 1, Fig. 3c, d). No correlations were seen between IL-7 concentrations, proportions of CD127-expressing T cells and Ki67 expression in any groups.

Replicative history of naive T cells

TRECs were detectable in only 5 YATEC patients (14.7 %) compared to 14 YHC (82.4 %) ($p = 0.001$). In YATEC, TRECs were significantly lower compared to YHC (Fig. 4a). Telomeres were significantly shorter in YATEC than in YHC (Fig. 4b). These findings were also significant in the comparison between YATEC > 30a and YHC > 30a (Fig. 5d, e).

Proportions of CD103+ T cells

CD103, an α E integrin, necessary for T cell homing and retention in the gut or other epithelia, is highly expressed in gut-derived or mucosa-experienced T cells, particularly in CD8+ T cells [29, 40]. To search for possible extra-thymic T cell generation or increased homing activity of CD8+ T cells to gut mucosa, expression of CD103 was analyzed in YATEC. Higher proportions of CD103+ CD8+ T cells within the total lymphocyte gate were found in YAT compared to YHC (Fig. 1, Fig. 4c),

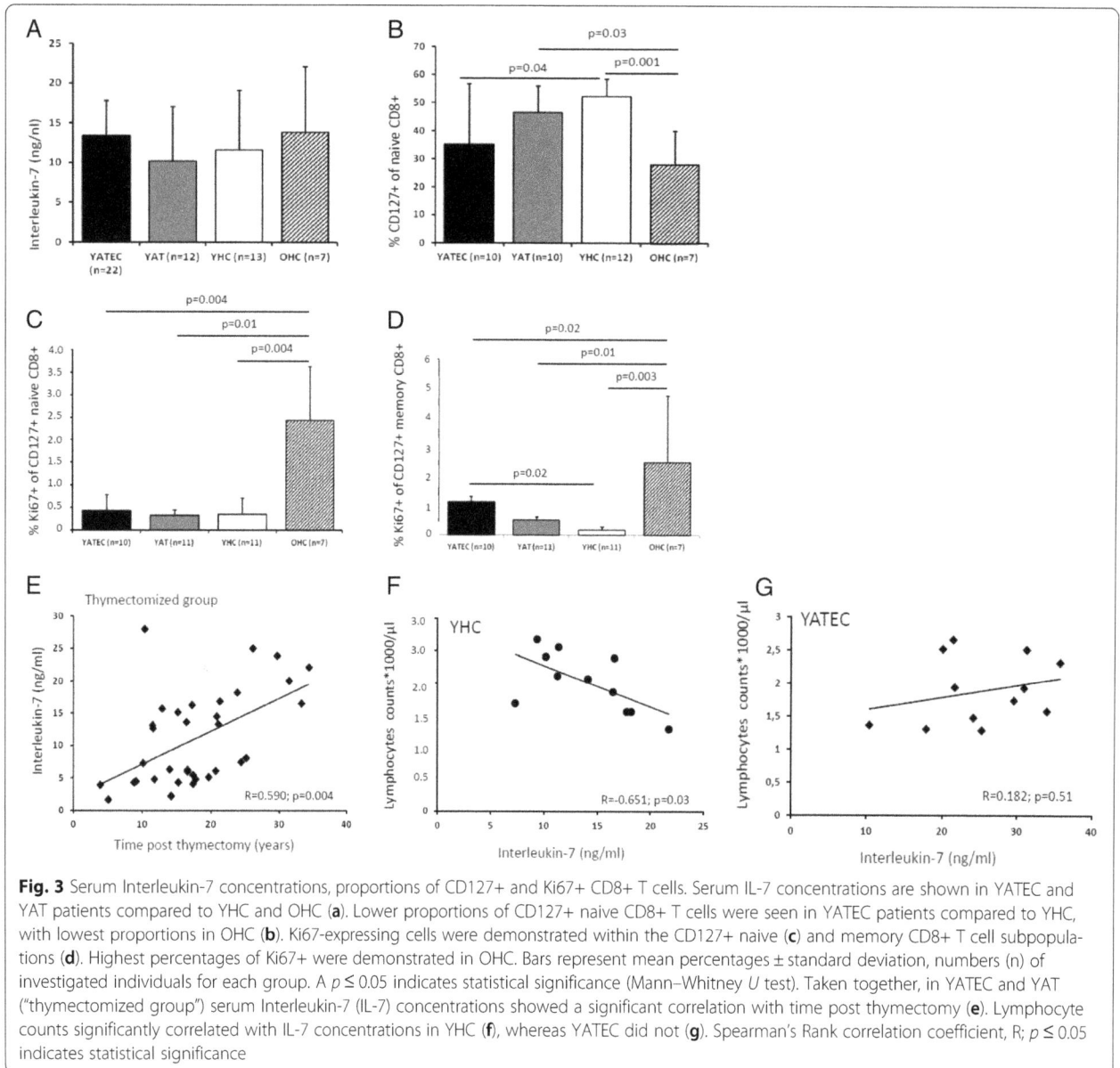

Fig. 3 Serum Interleukin-7 concentrations, proportions of CD127+ and Ki67+ CD8+ T cells. Serum IL-7 concentrations are shown in YATEC and YAT patients compared to YHC and OHC (**a**). Lower proportions of CD127+ naive CD8+ T cells were seen in YATEC patients compared to YHC, with lowest proportions in OHC (**b**). Ki67-expressing cells were demonstrated within the CD127+ naive (**c**) and memory CD8+ T cell subpopulations (**d**). Highest percentages of Ki67+ were demonstrated in OHC. Bars represent mean percentages ± standard deviation, numbers (n) of investigated individuals for each group. A $p \leq 0.05$ indicates statistical significance (Mann–Whitney U test). Taken together, in YATEC and YAT ("thymectomized group") serum Interleukin-7 (IL-7) concentrations showed a significant correlation with time post thymectomy (**e**). Lymphocyte counts significantly correlated with IL-7 concentrations in YHC (**f**), whereas YATEC did not (**g**). Spearman's Rank correlation coefficient, R; $p \leq 0.05$ indicates statistical significance

which could be also shown for YATEC > 30a compared to YHC > 30a (Fig. 5b).

Influence of CMV on lymphocyte subpopulations

CMV may drive T cell differentiation by chronic stimulation [24] and accelerate peripheral T cell exhaustion in the case of low thymic ouput as known from elderly persons [41] and, thus, may influence our results in thymectomized patients. To answer the question whether latent CMV infection may have an impact on proportions of naive T cells in thymectomized patients, groups were separated into CMV positive and negative subgroups. Due to small group size, thymectomized patients were not separated into YATEC and YAT for analysis of associations between CMV positive and negative subgroups. Despite a trend to lower naive CD8+ T cells in CMV positive thymectomized patients, no significant differences between CMV positive and negative individuals were found within each group regarding naive T cells (Fig. 6a), CD31+, early and late memory T cells, CD103+ T cells or effector T cells (data not shown). The proportions of CD127-expressing T cell subpopulations were not affected by CMV positivity. Ki67-expressing T cells were not influenced either (data not shown). Performing multiple regression analysis ($R^2 = 0.622$) including chronological age, age at thymectomy and CMV seropositivity, CMV ($p = 0.009$) and age at thymectomy ($p = 0.035$) were significantly influencing factors for reduced proportions of naive CD8+ T cells.

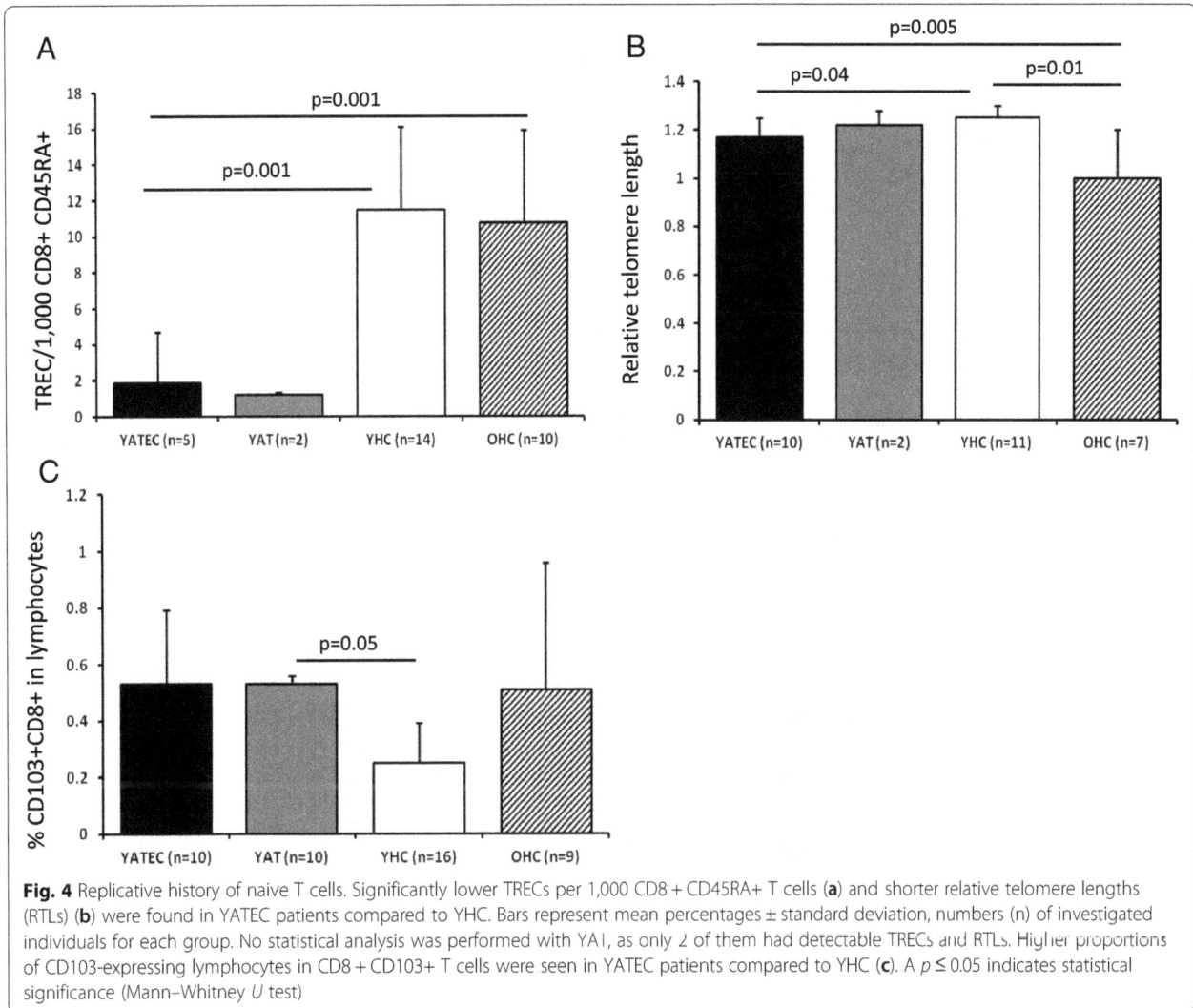

Fig. 4 Replicative history of naive T cells. Significantly lower TRECs per 1,000 CD8 + CD45RA+ T cells (**a**) and shorter relative telomere lengths (RTLs) (**b**) were found in YATEC patients compared to YHC. Bars represent mean percentages ± standard deviation, numbers (n) of investigated individuals for each group. No statistical analysis was performed with YAT, as only 2 of them had detectable TRECs and RTLs. Higher proportions of CD103-expressing lymphocytes in CD8 + CD103+ T cells were seen in YATEC patients compared to YHC (**c**). A *p* ≤ 0.05 indicates statistical significance (Mann–Whitney *U* test)

TCR diversity

Physiological involution of the thymus results in a marked loss of TCR diversity which can be accelerated by CMV positivity [32, 33]. Thus, clonality of the TCR was investigated in YATEC, YHC and OHC by TCR Vβ spectratype analysis (Fig. 6b–g). Mild to strong alterations were seen in diversity compared to healthy controls, with fewer polyclonal distributions among the 24 Vβ gene regions in the YATEC group compared to YHC (Fig. 6f). CMV positivity resulted in higher monoclonal patterns which was more pronounced in YATEC patients but did not reach statistical significance (Fig. 6g).

Discussion

The present study demonstrated that after childhood thymectomy, the peripheral T cells undergo characteristic proportional alterations, particularly of the CD8+ T cell compartment, with increased CD127 cell surface expression and proliferative activity and accumulation of circulating CD103+ T cells. These changes were interpreted as efforts of the peripheral T cell system to maintain homeostasis under the condition of thymic depletion. Together with these features, a skewed TCR repertoire and lower proportions of naive CD8+ T cells in some CMV positive YATEC patients were reminiscent of findings from aged individuals.

Naive T cells seem to be greatly afflicted by childhood thymectomy, as demonstrated by the present study and shown by our previous studies [16, 22] and others [12, 19]. Proportional changes of naive and CD31-expressing T cells were evident in the CD8+ T cell compartment and lack correlation with age in YATEC patients. The well known almost linearly decrease of CD31+ naive T cells with age was confirmed only in YHC [26, 28, 39, 42–44]. The loss of age correlation in YATEC patients may point to other factors than chronological age influencing naive T cell proportions, such as time post thymectomy, as shown in our previous study by assessment

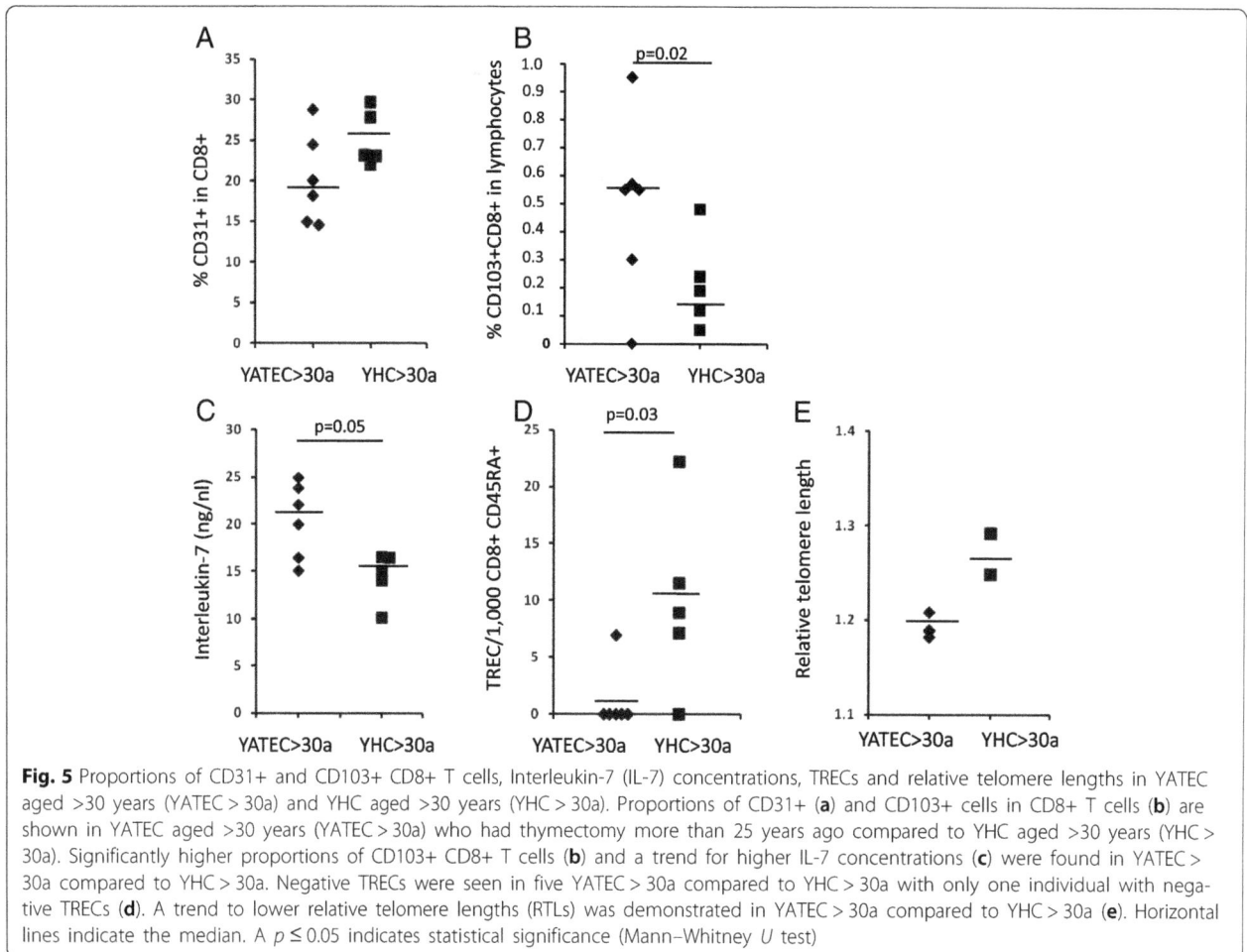

Fig. 5 Proportions of CD31+ and CD103+ CD8+ T cells, Interleukin-7 (IL-7) concentrations, TRECs and relative telomere lengths in YATEC aged >30 years (YATEC > 30a) and YHC aged >30 years (YHC > 30a). Proportions of CD31+ (**a**) and CD103+ cells in CD8+ T cells (**b**) are shown in YATEC aged >30 years (YATEC > 30a) who had thymectomy more than 25 years ago compared to YHC aged >30 years (YHC > 30a). Significantly higher proportions of CD103+ CD8+ T cells (**b**) and a trend for higher IL-7 concentrations (**c**) were found in YATEC > 30a compared to YHC > 30a. Negative TRECs were seen in five YATEC > 30a compared to YHC > 30a with only one individual with negative TRECs (**d**). A trend to lower relative telomere lengths (RTLs) was demonstrated in YATEC > 30a compared to YHC > 30a (**e**). Horizontal lines indicate the median. A $p \leq 0.05$ indicates statistical significance (Mann–Whitney U test)

of T cell receptor excision circles [16], age at acquiring chronic viral infections, such as CMV, and age at thymectomy. Proportions of CD31+ naive CD8 + T cells were independently influenced by age at thymectomy with lower proportions in those patients who had thymectomy later. Significantly lower naive CD8+ T cells were also found in YAT compared to YHC. This fits well to the speculation that removal of thymic tissue in the first months of life may have less influence on the alterations of the T cell pool than the long-term effects of thymectomy during later childhood due to higher regenerative potential in younger children [12, 20, 23].

Homeostatic proliferation of naive T cells is closely related to IL-7 concentrations, with CD127 expression being critical in regulating IL-7 functions [20, 45–49]. On separated subsets of human peripheral CD8+ T cells, almost 100 % of naive (CD45RA + CCR7+) and central memory (CD45R0 + CCR7+) T cells and 60–70 % of effector memory (CD45R0 + CCR7-), but only <20 % of terminally differentiated (CD45RA + CCR7-) T cells express CD127 [50–52] which agrees with our results. Higher Ki67 expression was measured in CD127+ memory CD8+ T cells in YATEC patients, indicating also

compensatory expansion of CD45R0+ memory phenotype T cells probably to fill the void of CD45RA+ naive T cells, as observed previously by our group [16] and by others [12, 15]. This is in agreement with findings, that IL-7 signaling is not only exclusively responsible for the homeostatic proliferation of naive T cells but also of CD8+ memory T cells [53–55], with CD127+ T cells being the population to survive and to develop into long-lived CD8+ memory T cells [55]. Higher proliferative activity in CD127-expressing T cells and a trend towards higher serum IL-7 concentrations in thymectomized patients with increasing age after thymectomy may indicate a role of IL-7 and its receptor in peripheral T cell renewal after thymectomy. The lack of any correlation between serum IL-7 concentrations, CD127 expression and proliferative activity of peripheral T cells in our cohort may be explained by the findings described by others that responsiveness to IL-7 and IL-7-induced down-regulation of CD127 depends very much on cellular activation and additional stimulatory signals and displays to be a dynamic process [56–60]. Studies reported the regulation of T cell homeostasis by IL-7 and the improvement of the long-term survival of RTE by

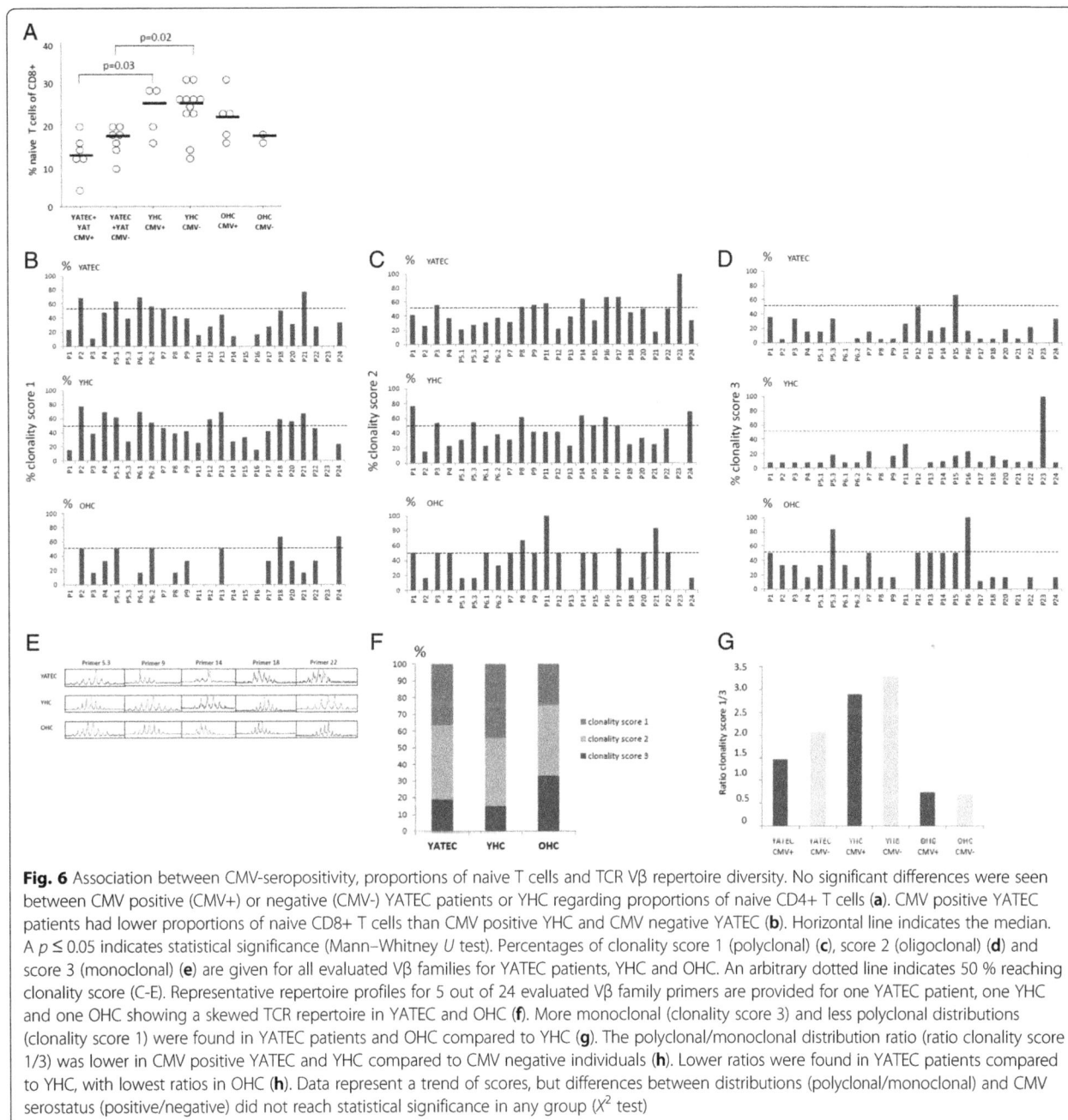

Fig. 6 Association between CMV-seropositivity, proportions of naive T cells and TCR Vβ repertoire diversity. No significant differences were seen between CMV positive (CMV+) or negative (CMV-) YATEC patients or YHC regarding proportions of naive CD4+ T cells (**a**). CMV positive YATEC patients had lower proportions of naive CD8+ T cells than CMV positive YHC and CMV negative YATEC (**b**). Horizontal line indicates the median. A $p \leq 0.05$ indicates statistical significance (Mann–Whitney U test). Percentages of clonality score 1 (polyclonal) (**c**), score 2 (oligoclonal) (**d**) and score 3 (monoclonal) (**e**) are given for all evaluated Vβ families for YATEC patients, YHC and OHC. An arbitrary dotted line indicates 50 % reaching clonality score (C-E). Representative repertoire profiles for 5 out of 24 evaluated Vβ family primers are provided for one YATEC patient, one YHC and one OHC showing a skewed TCR repertoire in YATEC and OHC (**f**). More monoclonal (clonality score 3) and less polyclonal distributions (clonality score 1) were found in YATEC patients and OHC compared to YHC (**g**). The polyclonal/monoclonal distribution ratio (ratio clonality score 1/3) was lower in CMV positive YATEC and YHC compared to CMV negative individuals (**h**). Lower ratios were found in YATEC patients compared to YHC, with lowest ratios in OHC (**h**). Data represent a trend of scores, but differences between distributions (polyclonal/monoclonal) and CMV serostatus (positive/negative) did not reach statistical significance in any group (X^2 test)

overexpression of CD127 in lymphoreplete or lymphopenic conditions [20, 49, 60–67]. In our cohort, IL-7-depend mechanisms of peripheral T cell renewal may be less predominating, as our YATEC patients showed no lymphopenic situation at the time of evaluation of immune parameters. However, significantly decreased TRECs and shortened telomeres as markers of the replicative history of individual cells indicate for an increased peripheral naive T cell turnover.

In order to assess a possible role of gut-derived or even mucosa-experienced T cells [68], CD103, which is necessary for T cell homing and retention in the gut and

other epithelia [69] was included into the analysis. YAT patients showed significantly higher proportions of circulating CD103+ CD8+ T cells. Moreover, despite der relatively young age of YATEC and YAT compared to OHC, proportions of CD103+ CD8+ T cells in thymectomized patients were similar to OHC. Peripheral CD8 + CD103+ memory T cells have been described as non-migratory T cell subpopulations that are maintained as tissue-resident memory T cells without replenishment from the circulating memory T cell pool [29, 70, 71], but CD103+ T cells also contribute to T cells with effector functions [38, 69, 72]. Increased total CD3 + CD103+

numbers were also found in one study investigating children who had thymectomy at least 5 years ago [11] suggesting extra-thymic T cell maturation [27]. We could demonstrate that this effect persists also in our thymectomized patients who had thymectomy more than 25 years ago. The increase of CD103 + CD3+ T cells was previously postulated to reflect extra-thymic T cell generation [27], however, in peripheral blood it is difficult to distinguish between newly generated T cells in the gut versus expansion of previously existing CD8+ memory T cells.

CMV was suggested as a chronic stimulating factor for peripheral T cells [24, 41] and was therefore investigated in thymectomized patients. One hypothesis is that an immune system exposed to the strong pressure by CMV [41] prematurely exhausts its resources in the context of diminished thymic output [17]. A potential risk of early thymectomy was seen for the development of premature immunosenescence and of an immune-risk-phenotype [1, 17, 23] which is defined as a cluster of immune features (e. g., decreased numbers of naive T cells, abundance of highly differentiated memory T cells, increased inflammatory markers, reduction in TCR diversity and CMV seropositivity), which were predictive of early all-cause mortality in one elderly cohort [73]. CMV positive thymectomized patients of our cohort demonstrated lower proportions of CD8 + CD45RA + CD27 + CCR7+ T cells which were independently influenced by CMV and associated with an accelerating effect of CMV on proportional reductions of naive T cells as seen in elderly. However, our results were hampered by low numbers of CMV positive subjects in each group and by the examination of relatively young thymectomized patients which may display less pronounced effects than older ones [17]. In addition, usually the effect of CMV is time-dependent and heterogeneity in age of primary CMV acquisition may vary from study to study.

Considering low thymic output and regenerative peripheral mechanisms, we hypothesized that thymectomized patients may have a restricted TCR repertoire. In fact, a skewed TCR diversity could be found in thymectomized patients. Thus, we could confirm the results of a study investigating the TCR repertoire in YATEC patients compared to young adults and elderly controls which showed mild to strong alterations of the TCR patterns [17]. In that study, strong alterations could be reported in the CD8+ T cell Vβ families, whereas only a few CD4+ T cell Vβ families were affected [17]. The high variability in our thymectomized cohort may be induced by investigating Vβ families in CD3+ T cells without differentiation into CD4+ and CD8+ T cells. However, also at this level and despite small subgroups, changes were evident with a trend towards monoclonal patterns in patients infected with CMV. Variety of results and

existence of outliers may result from regeneration of remaining thymic tissue [12, 20]. Additionally, CMV may also not be the sole factor influencing the TCR repertoire in our thymectomized patients [17, 74–76].

Age plays a crucial role in homeostatic mechanisms. All alterations expected in the elderly [26, 42, 44], were found in our OHC control group, such as low proportions of CD31-expressing RTE, increased Ki67 expression of peripheral T cells and higher proportions of CD103-expressing circulating T cells. CD127 expression was lower in OHC and a great variability was found for IL-7 concentrations in OHC, suggesting an inverse relationship between IL-7 receptor signaling function and age [77] with ongoing controversy as to whether IL-7 concentrations are altered with age [77–80]. Despite decreased proportions of CD127-expressing T cells with age [65], higher proliferative activity in CD127+ T cells of OHC was found in our study. This trend was similar between YATEC and OHC regarding proportions of CD127+ in naive CD8+ T cells and the Ki67+ expression in CD127+ memory CD8+ T cells.

Conclusion

In conclusion, thymectomized patients demonstrated the outstanding situation of artificial depletion of thymic output in an otherwise healthy immune system. We could show that thymectomy is associated with an impairment of the peripheral CD8+ T cell pool. To guarantee renewal of the pre-existing naive T cells, the human immune system seems to struggle in order to fill the void of RTEs after childhood thymectomy by peripheral T cell proliferation, IL-7-mediated mechanisms, and release of CD103+ T cells into circulation. But it cannot avoid skewing of the TCR repertoire and has to deal with chronic viral infections. Despite the moderate changes in T cell proportions, proliferation rates and TCR diversity, no clinical relevant immunodeficiency seems to result from thymectomy in early childhood. However, as many of these findings in adolescents and young adults were reminiscent of immune alterations after thymic involution in the elderly, thymectomized patients may mimic premature immunosenescence [1, 9, 23]. However, not all immunological parameters investigated in thymectomized individuals in this study resemble the findings of elderly persons and in some cases, only trends could be shown. The relatively small immunological alterations found in young adults thymectomized at early infancy or childhood may precede more substantial alterations in later life as suggested by our previous investigations and clinical studies [9, 10, 16, 22, 23]. There is still the possibility that these patients are at risk to suffer from age-related diseases, such as autoimmunity, cancer, atherosclerosis or neurodegeneration, in older age. Also, latent herpes virus infections usually acquired during childhood may have a more pronounced impact on an immune system compensating for thymic loss. Delayed antibody responses to new antigens, such as tick-borne-encephalitis vaccination [22], have suggested that an intact thymus is also necessary for antibody production and affinity maturation [81]. Thus, ongoing follow-up of immunological activity of thymectomized patients is mandatory as they advance into old age to timely recognize age-associated diseases and premature impairments of immune function.

Competing interest
There are no financial and commercial conflicts of interest.

Authors' contributions
MZ carried out the flow cytometric studies, participated in the design of the study and recruited the study population. GA performed the flow cytometric subgroup analysis, organized the TREC and RTL assays and performed the ELISA assays. WP performed the TCR spectratyping. CS carried out the analysis of TRECs. JL performed the analysis of RTLs. BW allocated the samples of OHC and participated in flow cytometric studies of OHC. VJ carried out the preparation of blood samples and performed the MACS separation of T cells and the DNA preparation. KU interpreted the thoracic magnetic resonance imaging of thymectomized individuals to control for residual thymic tissue. ME helped to design the TCR spectratyping and critically discussed the manuscript. RW performed the CMV serology and critically discussed the manuscript. MP designed and coordinated the study and drafted the manuscript. All authors read and approved the final manuscript.

Acknowledgements
We thank Dr. Juliane Kilo, Department of Cardiac Surgery, Prof. Dr. Ralf Geiger and Prof. Dr. Jörg Stein, Department of Pediatrics III, Pediatric Cardiology, Medical University Innsbruck, for support in patient recruitment and Prof. Dr. Beatrix Grubeck-Loebenstein, Institute for Biomedical Aging Research, University of Innsbruck, for providing samples of aged individuals. Daniela Niederwieser, Institute of Legal Medicine, Medical University Innsbruck, is greatly acknowledged for technical assistance. We thank PD Dr. Anita Kloss-Brandstaetter, Institute of Epidemiological Genetics, Medical University Innsbruck, for statistical support. The study was funded by the Medical Science Fund Innsbruck (MFI, project number 6168) donated to Martina Prelog.

Author details
[1]Department of Pediatrics, Medical University Innsbruck, Innsbruck, Austria. [2]Department of Pediatrics, University Hospital Wuerzburg, University of Wuerzburg, Josef-Schneider-Str. 2, 97080 Wuerzburg, Germany. [3]Institute of Legal Medicine, Medical University Innsbruck, Innsbruck, Austria. [4]Penn State Eberly College of Science, University Park, PA, USA. [5]Department of Haematology and Oncology, University of Greifswald, Greifswald, Germany. [6]Department of Internal Medicine, Medical University Innsbruck, Innsbruck, Austria. [7]Institute for Biomedical Aging Research, University of Innsbruck, Innsbruck, Austria. [8]Department of Radiology, Medical University Innsbruck, Innsbruck, Austria. [9]Department of Hygiene and Medical Microbiology, Medical University Innsbruck, Innsbruck, Austria.

References
1. Sauce D, Appay V. Altered thymic activity in early life: how does it affect the immune system in young adults? Curr Opin Immunol. 2011;23:543–8.
2. Douek DC, McFarland RD, Keiser PH, Gage EA, Massey JM, Haynes BF, et al. Changes in thymic function with age and during the treatment of HIV infection. Nature. 1998;396:690–5.
3. Harris JM, Hazenberg MD, Poulin JF, Higuera-Alhino D, Schmidt D, Gotway M, et al. Multiparameter evaluation of human thymic function: interpretations and caveats. Clin Immunol. 2005;115:138–46.

4. Hazenberg MD, Verschuren MC, Hamann D, Miedema F, van Dongen JJ. T cell receptor excision circles as markers for recent thymic emigrants: basic aspects, technical approach, and guidelines for interpretation. J Mol Med (Berl). 2001;79:631–40.
5. Blackburn EH. Structure and function of telomeres. Nature. 1991;350:569–73.
6. Bradley LM, Haynes L, Swain SL. IL-7: maintaining T-cell memory and achieving homeostasis. Trends Immunol. 2005;26:172–6.
7. Crawley AM, Angel JB. The influence of HIV on CD127 expression and its potential implications for IL-7 therapy. Semin Immunol. 2012;24:231–40.
8. Morre M, Beq S. Interleukin-7 and immune reconstitution in cancer patients: a new paradigm for dramatically increasing overall survival. Target Oncol. 2012;7:55–68.
9. Appay V, Sauce D, Prelog M. The role of the thymus in immunosenescence: lessons from the study of thymectomized individuals. Aging (Albany NY). 2010;2:78–81.
10. Zlamy M, Prelog M. Thymectomy in early childhood: a model for premature T cell immunosenescence? Rejuvenation Res. 2009;12:249–58.
11. Eysteinsdottir JH, Freysdottir J, Haraldsson A, Stefansdottir J, Skaftadottir I, Helgason H, et al. The influence of partial or total thymectomy during open heart surgery in infants on the immune function later in life. Clin Exp Immunol. 2004;136:349–55.
12. Halnon NJ, Jamieson B, Plunkett M, Kitchen CM, Pham T, Krogstad P. Thymic function and impaired maintenance of peripheral T cell populations in children with congenital heart disease and surgical thymectomy. Pediatr Res. 2005;57:42–8.
13. Madhok AB, Chandrasekran A, Parnell V, Gandhi M, Chowdhury D, Pahwa S. Levels of recent thymic emigrant cells decrease in children undergoing partial thymectomy during cardiac surgery. Clin Diagn Lab Immunol. 2005;12:563–5.
14. Mancebo E, Clemente J, Sanchez J, Ruiz-Contreras J, De Pablos P, Cortezon S. Longitudinal analysis of immune function in the first 3 years of life in thymectomized neonates during cardiac surgery. Clin Exp Immunol. 2008;154:375–83.
15. Ogle BM, West LJ, Driscoll DJ, Strome SE, Razonable RR, Paya CV, et al. Effacing of the T cell compartment by cardiac transplantation in infancy. J Immunol. 2006;176:1962–7.
16. Prelog M, Keller M, Geiger R, Brandstätter A, Würzner R, Schweigmann U, et al. Thymectomy in early childhood: significant alterations of the CD4(+)CD45RA(+)CD62L(+) T cell compartment in later life. Clin Immunol. 2009;130:123–32.
17. Sauce D, Larsen M, Fastenackels S, Duperrier A, Keller M, Grubeck Loebenstein B, et al. Evidence of premature immune aging in patients thymectomized during early childhood. J Clin Invest. 2009;119:3070–8.
18. Sauce D, Larsen M, Fastenackels S, Roux A, Gorochov G, Katlama C, et al. Lymphopenia-driven homeostatic regulation of naive T cells in elderly and thymectomized young adults. J Immunol. 2012;189:5541–8.
19. Torfadottir H, Freysdottir J, Skaftadottir I, Haraldsson A, Sigfusson G, Ogmundsdottir HM. Evidence for extrathymic T cell maturation after thymectomy in infancy. Clin Exp Immunol. 2006;145:407–12.
20. van Gent R, Schadenberg AW, Otto SA, Nievelstein RA, Sieswerda GT, Haas F, et al. Long-term restoration of the human T-cell compartment after thymectomy during infancy: a role for thymic regeneration? Blood. 2011;118:627–34.
21. Wells WJ, Parkman R, Smogorzewska E, Barr M. Neonatal thymectomy: does it affect immune function? J Thorac Cardiovasc Surg. 1998;115:1041–6.
22. Prelog M, Wilk C, Keller M, Karall T, Orth D, Geiger R, et al. Diminished response to tick-borne encephalitis vaccination in thymectomized children. Vaccine. 2008;26:595–600.
23. Zlamy M, Wurzner R, Holzmann H, Brandstatter A, Jeller V, Zimmerhackl LB, et al. Antibody dynamics after tick-borne encephalitis and measles-mumps-rubella vaccination in children post early thymectomy. Vaccine. 2010;28:8053–60.
24. Almanzar G, Schwaiger S, Jenewein B, Keller M, Herndler-Brandstetter D, Wurzner R, et al. Long-term cytomegalovirus infection leads to significant changes in the composition of the CD8+ T-cell repertoire, which may be the basis for an imbalance in the cytokine production profile in elderly persons. J Virol. 2005;79:3675–83.
25. Fink PJ. The biology of recent thymic emigrants. Annu Rev Immunol. 2013;31:31–50.
26. Kimmig S, Przybylski GK, Schmidt CA, Laurisch K, Mowes B, Radbruch A, et al. Two subsets of naive T helper cells with distinct T cell receptor excision circle content in human adult peripheral blood. J Exp Med. 2002; 195:789–94.

27. Howie D, Spencer J, DeLord D, Pitzalis C, Wathen NC, Dogan A, et al. Extrathymic T cell differentiation in the human intestine early in life. J Immunol. 1998;161:5862–72.

28. Appay V, van Lier RA, Sallusto F, Roederer M. Phenotype and function of human T lymphocyte subsets: consensus and issues. Cytometry A. 2008;73: 975–83.

29. Sheridan BS, Lefrancois L. Regional and mucosal memory T cells. Nat Immunol. 2011;12:485–91.

30. Pfister G, Weiskopf D, Lazuardi L, Kovaiou RD, Cioca DP, Keller M, et al. Naïve T cells in the elderly: are they still there? Ann N Y Acad Sci. 2006;1067:152–7.

31. Herndler-Brandstetter D, Schwaiger S, Veel E, Fehrer C, Cioca DP, Almanzar G, et al. CD25-expressing CD8+ T cells are potent memory cells in old age. J Immunol. 2005;175:1566–74.

32. Day EK, Carmichael AJ, ten Berge IJ, Waller EC, Sissons JG, Wills MR. Rapid CD8+ T cell repertoire focusing and selection of high-affinity clones into memory following primary infection with a persistent human virus: human cytomegalovirus. J Immunol. 2007;179:3203–13.

33. Schwanninger A, Weinberger B, Weiskopf D, Herndler-Brandstetter D, Reitinger S, Gassner C, et al. Age-related appearance of a CMV-specific high-avidity CD8+ T cell clonotype which does not occur in young adults. Immun Ageing. 2008;5:14.

34. Thiel A, Alexander T, Schmidt CA, Przybylski GK, Kimmig S, Kohler S, et al. Direct assessment of thymic reactivation after autologous stem cell transplantation. Acta Haematol. 2008;119:22–7.

35. Almanzar G, Eberle G, Lassacher A, Specht C, Koppelstaetter C, Heinz-Erian P, et al. Maternal cigarette smoking and its effect on neonatal lymphocyte subpopulations and replication. BMC Pediatr. 2013;13:57.

36. Cawthon RM. Telomere measurement by quantitative PCR. Nucleic Acids Res. 2002;30:e47.

37. Koppelstaetter C, Jennings P, Hochegger K, Perco P, Ischia R, Karkoszka H, et al. Effect of tissue fixatives on telomere length determination by quantitative PCR. Mech Ageing Dev. 2005;126:1331–3.

38. Forster R, Davalos-Misslitz AC, Rot A. CCR7 and its ligands: balancing immunity and tolerance. Nat Rev Immunol. 2008;8:362–71.

39. Kohler S, Thiel A. Life after the thymus: CD31+ and CD31– human naïve CD4 + T-cell subsets. Blood. 2009;113:769–74.

40. Casey KA, Fraser KA, Schenkel JM, Moran A, Abt MC, Beura LK, et al. Antigen-independent differentiation and maintenance of effector-like resident memory T cells in tissues. J Immunol. 2012;188:4866–75.

41. Pawelec G, Koch S, Franceschi C, Wikby A. Human immunosenescence: does it have an infectious component? Ann N Y Acad Sci. 2006;1067:56–65.

42. Kilpatrick RD, Rickabaugh T, Hultin LE, Hultin P, Hausner MA, Detels R, et al. Homeostasis of the naïve CD4+ T cell compartment during aging. J Immunol. 2008;180:1499–507.

43. Kohler S, Wagner U, Pierer M, Kimmig S, Oppmann B, Möwes B, et al. Post-thymic in vivo proliferation of naïve CD4+ T cells constrains the TCR repertoire in healthy human adults. Eur J Immunol. 2005;35:1987–94.

44. Wikby A, Mansson IA, Johansson B, Strindhall J, Nilsson SE. The immune risk profile is associated with age and gender: findings from three Swedish population studies of individuals 20-100 years of age. Biogerontology. 2008;9:299–308.

45. Bains I, Antia R, Callard R, Yates AJ. Quantifying the development of the peripheral naïve CD4+ T-cell pool in humans. Blood. 2009;113:5480–7.

46. den Braber I, Mugwagwa T, Vrisekoop N, Westera L, Mögling R, de Boer AB, et al. Maintenance of peripheral naïve T cells is sustained by thymus output in mice but not humans. Immunity. 2012;36:288–97.

47. Hazenberg MD, Otto SA, Cohen Stuart JW, Verschuren MC, Borleffs JC, Boucher CA, et al. Increased cell division but not thymic dysfunction rapidly affects the T-cell receptor excision circle content of the naïve T cell population in HIV-1 infection. Nat Med. 2000;6:1036–42.

48. Hazenberg MD, Otto SA, van Rossum AM, Scherpbier HJ, de Groot R, Kuijpers TW, et al. Establishment of the CD4+ T-cell pool in healthy children and untreated children infected with HIV-1. Blood. 2004;104:3513–9.

49. Le Campion A, Pommier A, Delpoux A, Stouvenel L, Auffray C, Martin B, et al. IL-2 and IL-7 determine the homeostatic balance between the regulatory and conventional CD4+ T cell compartments during peripheral T cell reconstitution. J Immunol. 2012;189:3339–46.

50. Paiardini M, Cervasi B, Albrecht H, Muthukumar A, Dunham R, Gordon S, et al. Loss of CD127 expression defines an expansion of effector CD8+ T cells in HIV-infected individuals. J Immunol. 2005;174:2900–9.

51. Sauce D, Larsen M, Leese AM, Millar D, Khan N, Hislop AD, et al. IL-7R alpha versus CCR7 and CD45 as markers of virus-specific CD8+ T cell differentiation: contrasting pictures in blood and tonsillar lymphoid tissue. J Infect Dis. 2007;195:268–78.

52. Seddiki N, Santner-Nanan B, Martinson J, Zaunders J, Sasson S, Landay A, et al. Expression of interleukin (IL)-2 and IL-7 receptors discriminates between human regulatory and activated T cells. J Exp Med. 2006;203:1693–700.

53. Kieper WC, Tan JT, Bondi-Boyd B, Gapin L, Sprent J, Ceredig R, et al. Overexpression of interleukin (IL)-7 leads to IL-15-independent generation of memory phenotype CD8+ T cells. J Exp Med. 2002;195:1533–9.

54. Schluns KS, Kieper WC, Jameson SC, Lefrancois L. Interleukin-7 mediates the homeostasis of naïve and memory CD8 T cells in vivo. Nat Immunol. 2000;1:426–32.

55. van Leeuwen EM, de Bree GJ, Remmerswaal EB, Yong SL, Tesselaar K, ten Berge IJ, et al. IL-7 receptor alpha chain expression distinguishes functional subsets of virus-specific human CD8+ T cells. Blood. 2005;106:2091–8.

56. Alves NL, van Leeuwen EM, Derks IA, van Lier RA. Differential regulation of human IL-7 receptor alpha expression by IL-7 and TCR signaling. J Immunol. 2008;180:5201–10.

57. Gamadia LE, van Leeuwen EM, Remmerswaal EB, Yong SL, Surachno S, Wertheim-van Dillen PM, et al. The size and phenotype of virus-specific T cell populations is determined by repetitive antigenic stimulation and environmental cytokines. J Immunol. 2004;172:6107–14.

58. Laakso SM, Kekäläinen E, Rossi LH, Laurinolli TT, Mannerström H, Heikkilä N, et al. IL-7 dysregulation and loss of CD8+ T cell homeostasis in the monogenic human disease autoimmune polyendocrinopathy-candidiasis-ectodermal dystrophy. J Immunol. 2011;187:2023–30.

59. Park JH, Yu Q, Erman B, Appelbaum JS, Montoya-Durango D, Grimes HL, et al. Suppression of IL7Ralpha transcription by IL-7 and other prosurvival cytokines: a novel mechanism for maximizing IL-7-dependent T cell survival. Immunity. 2004;21:289–302.

60. Pearson C, Silva A, Saini M, Seddon B. IL-7 determines the homeostatic fitness of T cells by distinct mechanisms at different signalling thresholds in vivo. Eur J Immunol. 2011;41:3656–66.

61. Houston Jr EG, Boursalian TE, Fink PJ. Homeostatic signals do not drive post-thymic T cell maturation. Cell Immunol. 2012;274:39–45.

62. Kimura MY, Pobezinsky LA, Guinter TI, Thomas J, Adams A, Park JH, et al. IL-7 signaling must be intermittent, not continuous, during CD8(+) T cell homeostasis to promote cell survival instead of cell death. Nat Immunol. 2013;14:143–51.

63. Libri V, Azevedo RI, Jackson SE, Di Mitri D, Lachmann R, Fuhrmann S, et al. Cytomegalovirus infection induces the accumulation of short-lived, multifunctional CD4 + CD45RA + CD27+ cells: the potential involvement of interleukin-7 in this process. Immunology. 2011;132:326–39.

64. Mackall CL, Fry TJ, Gress RE. Harnessing the biology of IL-7 for therapeutic application. Nat Rev Immunol. 2011;11:330–42.

65. Schonland SO, Zimmer JK, Lopez-Benitez CM, Widmann T, Ramin KD, Goronzy JJ, et al. Homeostatic control of T-cell generation in neonates. Blood. 2003;102:1428–34.

66. Seddon B, Tomlinson P, Zamoyska R. Interleukin 7 and T cell receptor signals regulate homeostasis of CD4 memory cells. Nat Immunol. 2003;4:680–6.

67. Surh CD, Sprent J. Homeostasis of naïve and memory T cells. Immunity. 2008;29:848–62.

68. Fink PJ, Hendricks DW. Post-thymic maturation: young T cells assert their individuality. Nat Rev Immunol. 2011;11:544–9.

69. Fousteri G, Dave A, Juntti T, Morin B, McClure M, Von Herrath M. Minimal effect of CD103 expression on the control of a chronic antiviral immune response. Viral Immunol. 2010;23:285–94.

70. Ariotti S, Haanen JB, Schumacher TN. Behavior and function of tissue-resident memory T cells. Adv Immunol. 2012;114:203–16.

71. Gebhardt T, Whitney PG, Zaid A, Mackay LK, Brooks AG, Heath WR, et al. Different patterns of peripheral migration by memory CD4+ and CD8+ T cells. Nature. 2011;477:216–9.

72. Bromley SK, Yan S, Tomura M, Kanagawa O, Luster AD. Recirculating memory T cells are a unique subset of CD4+ T cells with a distinct phenotype and migratory pattern. J Immunol. 2013;190:970–6.

73. Koch S, Solana R, Dela Rosa O, Pawelec G. Human cytomegalovirus infection and T cell immunosenescence: a mini review. Mech Ageing Dev. 2006;127: 538–43.

74. Bourgeois C, Hao Z, Rajewsky K, Potocnik AJ, Stockinger B. Ablation of thymic export causes accelerated decay of naive CD4 T cells in the periphery because of activation by environmental antigen. Proc Natl Acad Sci U S A. 2008;105:8691–6.

75. Lee WW, Shin MS, Kang Y, Lee N, Jeon S, Kang I. The relationship of cytomegalovirus (CMV) infection with circulatory IFN-alpha levels and IL-7 receptor alpha expression on CD8+ T cells in human aging. Cytokine. 2012;58:332–5.

76. Miller NE, Bonczyk JR, Nakayama Y, Suresh M. Role of thymic output in regulating CD8 T-cell homeostasis during acute and chronic viral infection. J Virol. 2005;79:9419–29.

77. Bazdar DA, Kalinowska M, Sieg SF. Interleukin-7 receptor signaling is deficient in CD4+ T cells from HIV-infected persons and is inversely associated with aging. J Infect Dis. 2009;199:1019–28.

78. Ferrando-Martinez S, Franco JM, Hernandez A, Ordonez A, Gutierrez E, Abad A, et al. Thymopoiesis in elderly human is associated with systemic inflammatory status. Age (Dordr). 2009;31:87–97.

79. Ferrando-Martinez S, Ruiz-Mateos E, Hernandez A, Gutierrez E, Rodriguez-Mendez Mdel M, Ordonez A, et al. Age-related deregulation of naive T cell homeostasis in elderly humans. Age (Dordr). 2011;33:197–207.

80. Lynch HE, Goldberg GL, Chidgey A, Van den Brink MR, Boyd R, Sempowski GD. Thymic involution and immune reconstitution. Trends Immunol. 2009;30:366–73.

81. AbuAttieh M, Bender D, Liu E, Wettstein P, Platt JL, Cascalho M. Affinity maturation of antibodies requires integrity of the adult thymus. Eur J Immunol. 2012;42:500–10.

Immunosenescence in persons with spinal cord injury in relation to urinary tract infections

David Pavlicek[1], Jörg Krebs[2], Simona Capossela[1], Alessandro Bertolo[1], Britta Engelhardt[3], Jürgen Pannek[2] and Jivko Stoyanov[1*]

Abstract

Background: Individuals with a spinal cord injury (SCI), despite specialized rehabilitation and good health care, have a reduced life expectancy. Infectious diseases, such as pneumonias, infected pressure sores and urinary tract infections (UTI) have been identified as the leading causes of mortality. We hypothesise that a premature onset of immune frailty occurs in SCI, possibly caused also by recurrent urinary tract infections.
A cross sectional study was performed comparing blood and urine samples between able bodied controls ($n = 84$) and persons with spinal cord injury ($n = 85$). The results were grouped according to age (below and above 60 years). Assessed were the abundancies of immune cells, the concentration of soluble biomarkers, the in vitro functioning of lymphocytes as well as phenotypic exhaustion of T-cells in blood and urine. Further, the leucocyte telomere length and the cytomegalovirus (CMV) serological status were compared between the groups.

Results: We observed in people with SCI lower proportions of naïve T-cells, more memory T-cells, reduced T-cell proliferation and higher CMV prevalence compared to age-matched controls. SCI participants older than 60 years had a higher prevalence of UTI compared with SCI persons younger than 60 years.

Conclusion: The immune system of people with SCI shows traits of an increased immunological strain and a premature onset of immune frailty. The role of UTI in the onset of immune frailty remains to be elucidated as we did not see significantly higher abundancies of circulating UTI-bacteria specific T-cell clones in persons with SCI. We assume that any impact of UTI on the immune system might be compartmentalized and locally restricted to the urinary tract.

Keywords: Immunosenescence, Immune frailty, Urinary tract infection, Spinal cord injury, Cytomegalovirus, Memory T-cell

Background

Persons suffering from a spinal cord injury (SCI) face a broad variety of challenges, SCI linked health issues and biological changes. Even with improved early medical health care, specialized rehabilitation and regular follow up visits today, the longevity of persons with SCI still remains below that of the general population [1, 2]. The leading cause of death are infectious diseases such as pneumonia, infected pressure sores and urinary tract infections (UTI) [3]. The reason for the increased infection rate is still a matter of debate. It has been discussed that the reduced physical activity, the elevated prevalence of depression or the exposure to selected medications in SCI persons have a negative impact on immunological health [4, 5]. There is evidence that the decentralisation of the autologous nervous system causes an acute SCI induced immune deficiency syndrome (SCI-IDS) [6] which manifests as significantly decreased immune cell concentration shortly after a traumatic event. However, a study in humans [7] demonstrated that 4–5 months after the traumatic event, the white blood cell concentration has mostly normalized, but nonetheless infection rates among people with SCI remain high. Monahan et al. [8] could show that individuals with chronic SCI still had reduced CD4 T-cell concentrations but increased numbers of activated (HLA-DR+) CD4 T-cells. Otherwise there is

* Correspondence: jivko.stoyanov@paraplegie.ch
[1]Biomedical Laboratories, Swiss Paraplegic Research, Guido A. Zäch Strasse 4, 6207, Nottwil, Switzerland
Full list of author information is available at the end of the article

limited data available on the function of the immune system in people with SCI in the chronic phase of the injury and on the precise interplay between cell types and soluble biomarkers of immunity.

Immune frailty (also referred to as immunosenescence), manifests as a decline in immune function, a higher susceptibility to infectious diseases and a reduced response to vaccines [9, 10]. The age related changes affect both the innate- and the adaptive immune system but are most pronounced in the T-cell compartment [11, 12]. Major changes are the phenotypic shift from naïve- to memory T-cells [13] and the decrease in T cell receptor diversity [14]. In addition to the alternations in the composition and diversity of the T-cell pool, the function of the cells is also affected by age. T-lymphocytes from frail persons have typically a reduced in vitro proliferative and signalling response to mitogens compared to their younger counterparts [15]. Paradoxically and in contrast to the reduced function of the immune system a chronic low grade inflammation, termed inflamm–ageing is observed in frail elderly people [16]. Often described are age-dependant elevated basal levels of interleukine-6 (IL-6), C-reactive protein (CRP) and tumour necrosis factor α (TNF-α) [17].

There is growing evidence that a chronic cytomegalovirus (CMV) infection is a major driving force behind immunosenescence [18]. The recurrent stimulation with the CMV antigen leads to several expansion and reduction cycles of the CMV-specific memory T-cells, eventually leading to an accumulation of DNA mutations, shortened telomeres and an exhausted T-cell phenotype [19].

The incidence of SCI peaks in young adults [2] and therefore their immune system is exposed to UTI over the majority of their life. A further complication is that the affected persons often lack sensory function which increases the risk of a prolonged and undetected bacterial infection.

With this study we aim to investigate if there is a premature onset of immunosenescence among persons with SCI which may be partly responsible for the increased infection rates in the chronic phase of a SCI (>1 year after incidence). We further hypothesize, that chronic and recurrent UTI, as they often occur in SCI persons, could have a similar - CMV- like - effect on the immune system. We speculate that due to the increased exposure to UTI causing bacteria the immune system of SCI persons is changed towards a more exhausted and senescent phenotype.

Methods
Study design and sampling
A cross-sectional study with a total of 169 participants was performed. Included were men with chronic (since at least one year) SCI and able bodied men who were not on an drug regimen influencing the immune system.

Only men were recruited in order to avoid bias through gender specific differences and the inevitable differences in group sizes due to the greater proportion of males among SCI patients. Study participants were divided into four groups: persons with SCI younger than 60 years (ySCI, n = 42), persons with SCI aged 60 or older (oSCI, n = 43), and as a control, able bodied persons younger than 60 years (yCtr, n = 42) and aged 60 or older (oCtr, n = 42). After written informed consent had been obtained, venous blood and urine samples were collected during a routine medical check-up.

Blood processing and differential blood count
Venous blood (27 ml) was collected in 2×9 ml K3E S-Monovettes containing EDTA for white blood cell and plasma isolation, 1×4 ml K3E S-Monovette containing EDTA for differential blood count and 1×4.5 ml S-Monovette for serum isolation (all from Sarstedt). The obtained blood was stored at room temperature and the serum at 4 °C for maximum 5 h after phlebotomy.

Peripheral blood mononuclear cells (PBMC) were isolated by H-Lympholyte Cell Separation Media (Cedarlane, Bioconcept) in a Leucosep tube (Greiner, Sigma-Aldrich) by gradient centrifugation at 800 g and room temperature (21 °C air conditioned room) for 20 min. The plasma fraction was collected without disturbing the beneath lying buffy coat and stored in aliquots at –80 °C. In a next step the PBMC containing buffy coat was carefully retrieved and washed with isotonic phosphate buffered saline (PBS), followed by a centrifugation at 210 g and room temperature for 10 min. The obtained pellet was resuspended in freezing media - 10% dimethyl sulfoxide, 35% RPMI-1640 medium (Amimed; Bio Concept) and 55% fetal bovine serum (FBS, Amimed; Bio Concept) - adjusted to a concentration of $5*10^6$ cells/ml and immediately transferred to –80 °C in a CoolCell (Biocision) container ensuring a cooling rate of –1 °C/min. The next day, the frozen cell suspension was transferred to a long term cryogenic storage (–150 °C Ultra-low Temperature freezer MDF-C2156VAN, Panasonic).

Simultaneously, a differential white blood cell count and a total serum protein, albumin, C reactive protein (CRP) and creatinine quantification were performed at a certified diagnostic laboratory (at the Swiss Paraplegic Centre in Nottwil, Switzerland).

Urine processing and analysis
Approximately 30 ml of midstream urine were collected from the controls and the study participants with SCI either using a sterile urine cup and a urine monovette (Sarstedt) or directly from a catheter (intermittent, indwelling or suprapubic). Urine was kept at 4 °C for a maximum of 5 h before being processed. A urine sample was analyzed in a certified clinical laboratory (at the

Swiss Paraplegic Centre in Nottwil, Switzerland) for creatinine concentration and tested with a urine-Stix test (Combur 10 Test, Roche) with automated result acquisition (cobas u 4111). In case of a positive urine-Stix signal, a leucocyte and microbial quantification of the urine sediment was performed. If more than 90 leucocytes/ μl or an elevated microorganism count (> $1*10^5$ /ml was detected, a subsequent bacteriological analysis was conducted to identify and characterize the infection causing bacteria. The remaining urine was centrifuged at 4 °C and 1'800 g for 10 min. The supernatant was aliquoted and stored at –80 °C until further usage. The urine sediment pellet was resuspended in 1 ml of residual urine and also frozen at –80 °C.

Immunoglobulins ELISA assays

Plasma IgG concentration:

An indirect ELISA was done to measure the concentration of total IgG antibody in plasma as follows: a 96-well plate (Nunc MaxiSorp, Sigma-Aldrich) was coated with 100 μl of 1 ng/μL Protein A (LuBioScience) in PBS and incubated overnight at 4 °C, then washed three times with 100 μl of PBS with a plate washer (Beckman-Coulter, Nyon, Switzerland). Non-specific binding sites were blocked for 2 h at room temperature with blocking solution containing 5% TopBlock (LuBioScience) in PBS. After washing the wells with PBS, thawed plasma aliquots - cleared of cell debris by centrifugation and diluted 20'000 fold in PBS - were incubated for 2 h at room temperature. Supernatants were then removed and the wells washed with PBS. Anti-human-IgG HRP-conjugated secondary antibody (A80-119P, Bethyl) diluted 1:5'000 in blocking buffer was incubated for 1 h at room temperature followed by another washing step with PBS. IgG was determined by colorimetric measurement of the product of the enzymatic reaction mediated by HRP and 100 μl/well of o-phenylenediamine (OPD) solution (15.3 mg/mL in citrate buffer, pH 5.0, Applichem – Axonlab). The reaction was, immediately after the appearance of color (ca. 1–2 min after OPD addition), stopped with 10% sulfuric acid. Absorbance was measured at 450 nm by DTX 880 Multimode Detector (Beckman-Coulter) and IgG concentration (ng/mL) was determined by standard curve made by dilutions of purified human IgG (Bethyl – LuBioScience).

In vitro assays:

IgG quantification in the supernatants of stimulated peripheral white blood cells was done with the same ELISA method as described above. Samples were diluted 10 fold in PBS before loading to the plate.

Urine IgA concentration:

IgA$_{total}$ concentrations in thawed urine aliquots were assessed by a standard indirect ELISA as follows: a 96-well plate (Nunc MaxiSorp, Sigma-Aldrich) was coated with capture antibody (Goat F(ab')2 anti-human IgA-UNLAB, Southern Biotech) 1:500 diluted in diluent (0.05% Tween20 + 0.1% bovine serum albumin (BSA) (Albumin fraction V, Applichem Panreac) in PBS). The plate was subsequently incubated overnight at 4 °C, and then washed with 0.05% Tween20 in PBS with a plate washer (Beckman-Coulter). Non-specific binding sites were blocked for 2 h at room temperature with blocking solution containing 1% BSA in PBS. After washing, thawed urine aliquots - cleared of cell debris by centrifugation and diluted 200 fold in diluent - were incubated for 2 h at room temperature. Following another washing step, IgA$_{total}$ (Goat (F(ab')2 anti-human IgA-biot, Southern Biotech) detection antibodies were added 1:10'000 fold diluted in diluent for 2 h at room temperature. Followed another washing, a 1:8'000 diluted Streptavidin-HRP (Sigma-Aldrich) solution was added to the wells and incubated for 45 min at room temperature. IgA was determined by colorimetric measurement of the product of the enzymatic reaction mediated by HRP and o-phenylenediamine solution and the reaction was stopped with 10% sulfuric acid. Absorbance was measured at 450 nm by DTX 880 Multimode Detector and IgA concentrations (ng/mL) were determined from dilutions of purified human IgA (human IgA kappa-unlab, Southern Biotech).

Plasma cytokine measurements

The concentrations of cytokines and chemokines were analyzed in the thawed plasma aliquot by Bio-Plex Pro Cytokine, Chemokine and Growth Factor Assay (Bio-Rad Laboratories AG) following the manufacturers protocol: 40 μl of plasma were diluted fourfold in sample dilution buffer. The standard curve concentration was expanded 16-fold in the lower range which still resulted in quantifiable amounts of standards and allowed the measurements of lower cytokine levels. Data were collected and analyzed using a Bio-Rad Bio-Plex 200 instrument equipped with Bio-Plex Manager software (Bio-Rad). We measured the concentrations of interleukin-2 (IL-2), interleukin-4 (IL-4), interleukin-6 (IL-6), interleukin-10 (IL-10), granulocyte-colony stimulating factor (G-CSF), granulocyte-macrophage colony-stimulating factor (GM-CSF), monocyte chemoattractant protein 1 (MCP1) and tumor necrosis factor-alpha (TNF-α).

CMV serological status

Thawed plasma samples were tested for anti-cytomegalovirus (CMV) IgG with a commercially available ELISA kit (Cusabio Biotech Co.) according to producers manual using 100 μl of plasma. A sample was considered CMV positive when the measured absorption had a value more than 2.1-fold increase compared to the provided negative control.

T-lymphocyte phenotyping

Peripheral blood lymphocytes (PBL) were thawed in a water bath at 37 °C and immediately diluted 8-fold with PBS containing 10% FBS. The suspension was centrifuged at 210 g for 10 min and the supernatant was discarded. After resuspension in 200 µl of PBS flow cytometric analysis of 200'000 cells/ tube was done for the following surface markers: CD3-PerCP (clone SK7, BD biosciences), CD4-APC (clone RPA-T4, BD bioscience), CD8-PE (clone RPA-T8, BD biosciences) and the senescence associated killer cell lectin-like receptor G1 (KLRG1-FITC, clone SA231A2, BioLegend). Cells were incubated with 5 µl of antibodies for 15 min at room temperature, centrifuged at 500 g for 5 min and the supernatant was removed. And the cell pellet was resuspended in 200 µl PBS. Cell fluorescence was evaluated with FACScalibur flow cytometer (BD Biosciences) and data were analyzed using FlowJo, 10.0 software (Tree star Inc., USA).

The discrimination of the different memory phenotypes was also done with flow cytometry on freshly thawed cells using the phenotypic subsetting of memory T cells based on the work of Mahnke et al. [20] including the following surface markers: CD4-APC (clone RPA-T4, BD bioscience), CD8-APC (clone RPA-T8, BD bioscience), CD28-FITC (clone CD38.2, BD bioscience), CD45Ro-PE (clone UCHL1, BD bioscience) and CD95-PerCP-Cy5.5 (DX2, BD bioscience). This analysis enables the discrimination between naïve T cells (T_n: CD4 or $CD8^+$, $CD45Ro^-$, $CD28^+$, $CD95^-$), stem cell memory T cells (T_{scm}: CD4 or $CD8^+$, $CD45Ro^-$, $CD28^+$, $CD95^+$), central memory and transitional memory T cells (T_{cm} + T_{tm}: CD4 or $CD8^+$, $CD45Ro^+$, $CD28^+$, $CD95^+$), effector memory (T_{em}: CD4 or $CD8^+$, $CD45Ro^+$, $CD28^-$, $CD95^+$) and terminally differentiated effector memory T cells (T_{te}: CD4 or $CD8^+$, $CD45Ro^-$, $CD28^-$, $CD95^+$).

In vitro stimulation of IgG production and quantification

Frozen PBL were thawed in a water bath at 37 °C and then directly diluted 8-fold with PBS + 10% FBS. The suspension was centrifuged at 210 g for 10 min, the supernatant was discarded and the pellet resuspended in control medium - RPMI-1640 medium (Amimed; Bio Concept) supplemented with 10% FBS, penicillin–streptomycin (100 units/ml) and amphotericin B (2.5 µg/ml - to reach a concentration of 4 million cells/ml. This cell suspension was kept overnight in a polypropylene Falcon tube allowing gas exchange at humid 37 °C. The next morning a new cell count was performed and 300'000 cells were plated per well of a 96 U-bottom well plate (TTP, Switzerland) in 270 µl of either control (RPMI-1640 + 10% FBS) or stimulating medium, all in duplicates. The used stimulation medium is adapted from a previous work [21] and consisted of 60 ng/ml human recombinant interleukin-2, 25 ng/ml Interleukin-10, 100 ng/ml Interleukin-21 (all from BioBasic Inc.; Stephan Klee Trading and Consulting,

Switzerland), the synthetic unmethylated oligodeoxynucleotide deoxycytosine-deoxyguanosine (CpG2429: tcgtcgttttcg gcggccgccg, 360 nM [22]; Microsynth AG, Switzerland) and 2.5 µg/ml pokeweed mitogen (Sigma-Aldrich, Switzerland). The cell suspensions were incubated for 7 days at 37 °C in a humid atmosphere and 5% CO_2 before measuring the IgG concentrations in the supernatants as described above.

In vitro leucocyte proliferation assay

The thawed PBL, allowed to rest overnight as described above, were used for an in vitro proliferation assay using the fluorescent cell proliferation indicator CytoTell green (AAT Bioquest; LuBioScience), according to the manufactures protocol (20 min incubation at room temperature in 1:600 diluted dye). Cells (150'000 in 270 µl per well) were plated in duplicates in a 96 U-bottom well plate (TTP, Switzerland) either in control medium or in stimulation medium with 2.5 µg/ml pokeweed mitogen or in stimulation medium with 0.1% phytohaemagglutinin (PHA-M, Sigma-Aldrich, Switzerland). The plates were incubated at 37 °C and 5% CO_2 in humid atmosphere. Proliferative responses of the stimulated PBL and the controls were measured after 7 days of incubation by flow cytometry using the intracellular dye dilution method and following surface marker antibodies: CD3-PerCP (clone SK7, BD biosciences), CD4-APC (clone RPA-T4, BD bioscience), CD8-PE (clone RPA-T8, BD biosciences). Cells were incubated with 5 µl of antibodies for 15 min at room temperature, washed and resuspended in 200 µl PBS. Cell fluorescence was assessed with FACScalibur flow cytometer and data were analyzed using the proliferation tool of the FlowJo, 9.0 software.

Preparation of a medium containing killed bacteria for in vitro PBL stimulation

Five of the most common urinary tract infection causing bacterial strains from the clinical laboratory at Swiss Paraplegic Centre, (*Klebsiella pneumoniae, Proteus vulgaris, Enterococcus sp., Staphylococcus aureus Rosenbach*, ATCC 29213, and *Escherichia coli*) were isolated from urine sediment of SCI-patients. The bacteria were grown overnight in thioglycolate broth at 37 °C. Inactivation was achieved by addition of formaldehyde to a final concentration of 2.5% and an additional overnight incubation at room temperature. Inactivated bacteria were washed three times with PBS to get rid of residual formaldehyde. A spectrophotometric (Diode array spectrophotometer, WPA S2100, Biowave) semi-quantification of the inactivated bacteria was done and the suspensions were normalized to OD_{600} 0.8. The five bacterial strains were pooled together in an equal ratio and diluted 1'000 fold in RPMI-1640 medium supplemented with 10%

FBS, penicillin–streptomycin (100 units/ml) and ampho-tericin B (2.5 µg/ml) for final use.

Detection of bacteria-specific T-cells

Thawed PBL which were allowed to rest overnight, as described above, were used for the in vitro bacterial stimulation assay. 150′000 cells/well of a 96 U-bottom well plate (TTP, Switzerland) were plated in duplicates in 270 µl of either control medium or medium containing inactivated bacteria (as described above). The plate was incubated at 37 °C and 5% CO_2 in humid atmosphere. Flow cytometry was used to identify activated T-lymphocytes at day four after plating. Analyzed were the early activation induced surface antigens CD69 and CD137. The measurement of CD69 and CD137 increases the sensitivity and optical discrimination of rare antigen specific T-cells [23, 24]. PBL were stained with the following antibodies: CD4-FITC (clone RPA-T4, BD bioscience), CD8-APC (clone RPA-T8, BD bioscience), CD69-PerCP-Cy5–5 (clone FN50, BD bioscience) and CD137-PE (clone 4B4–1, BioLegend). Cells were incubated with antibodies for 15 min at room temperature, washed and resuspended in PBS. Cell fluorescence was evaluated with FACScalibur flow cytometer and data were analyzed using FlowJo, 10.0 software. Activated cells were characterized as being $CD69^+CD137^+$ and the percentage of bacteria-specific T-cells was calculated by subtracting percentage of the activated unstimulated T-cells from the percentage of the activated bacterial stimulated T-cells.

Telomere length analysis by PCR

Genomic DNA of freshly thawed PBL was extracted using a commercial kit (Gentra Puregene Cell Kit Qiagen) following manufacturer's instructions. Telomere length was assessed using a quantitative PCR method as already described elsewhere [25]. Briefly: Standard curves for the telomeres and the reference gene 36B4 were done using synthesized oligonucleotides. The DNA plasmid pBR322 (Sigma-Aldrich, Switzerland) was used to increase the DNA content in the standards reaction mix to match the DNA concentration of the isolated samples. Real-time (RT)-PCR reactions were carried out in duplicates with, 4 ng/µL DNA template, and IQ SYBR Green Supermix (Bio Rad). Specific products were amplified by a quantitative PCR system (CFX96™ Real Time System, Bio Rad). Real-time PCR was carried out with the following settings: denaturation 95 °C, 5 min; followed by 30 amplification cycles of 95 °C, 10 s; 60 °C, 30 s PCR reactions were carried out in a final volume of 20 µL in 96-well PCR plates (Bio Rad). Melting curve analysis was performed after the amplification. Telomere and reference gene 36B4 starting quantities were calculated using the standard curves.

Statistic tests

A sample size of 42 in each group was determined to be sufficient to detect a one-fold difference in IgA antibody concentration between the groups in the presence of a 100% variance with a power of 90% and a significance level of 5%.

Data are presented as the mean and standard deviation (SD) or the median and the interquartile range (IQR). The data were tested for normal distribution using visual interpretation of QQ-plots and the Kolmogorov-Smirnov test. According to the distribution of the data, parametric or non-parametric tests (Mann-Whitney U test) were used. Statistics were computed using the SPSS Statistics, 24.0 software (IBM, Somers, USA).

Results

Demographics, UTI and CMV status of study participants

Table 1 summarizes the demographics and results of blood and urine parameters of the four investigated groups.

A total of 169 volunteers participated in the study and the mean age was similar between the SCI and control groups (Table 1). Individuals of the oSCI group had sustained SCI an average 16.2 years later in life than those of the ySCI group, but the mean time of living with a SCI was similar between the two groups. As expected, no case of UTI, was found in the control groups. The laboratory definition of UTI used in our investigation (> $1*10^5$ bacterial colony forming units/ml urine and >90 leucocytes/µl urine) allows the discrimination from bacteriuria without the assessment of clinical UTI symptoms which are difficult to measure in people with a SCI [26]. The UTI prevalence of persons with SCI aged ≥60 years was about 50% higher compared to their younger counterparts. The prevalence of past and current CMV infections, defined as the presence of circulating anti-CMV IgG antibodies, was greater in the older groups and was substantially higher in the SCI population.

Blood biochemistry and peripheral blood leucocyte (PBL) telomere length in the study participants

The measurements of a variety of parameters – including immunoglobulins, cytokines and T-cell ratios (Table 2) - revealed that serum total protein levels were significantly lower in the ySCI group compared to the age matched control group. No significant difference was observed in the total plasma IgG levels between the four groups. We measured the plasma levels of six immune related cytokines interleukin (IL-) 2, IL-4, IL-10, granulocyte colony stimulating factor (G-CSF), granulocyte macrophage colony stimulating factor (GM-CSF) and monocyte chemotactic protein 1 (MCP-1) and compared them between the four groups (Table 2).

Table 1 Demographics and prevalence of infections in study participants

	yCtr (±SD)	ySCI (±SD)	oCtr (±SD)	oSCI (±SD)	yCtr-oCtr (p-value)	ySCI-oSCI (p-value)	yCtr-ySCI (p-value)	oCtr-oSCI (p-value)
N	42	42	42	43	N/A	N/A	N/A	N/A
Age ± SD	42.8 ± 11	44.1 ± 9	67.6 ± 3	66.9 ± 6	<.001	0.68	<0.001	0.27
Time with SCI (y)	N/A	15.7 ± 11	N/A	21.7 ± 19	N/A	0.26	N/A	N/A
Age at SCI incident	N/A	28.5 ± 11	N/A	44.7 ± 20	N/A	<.001 ↑	N/A	N/A
Para- / Tetraplegic ratio	N/A	1.1	N/A	2.6	N/A	N/A	N/A	N/A
UTI	0%	33%	0%	45%	N/A	N/A ↑	N/A	N/A
CMV+	52%	64%	69%	86%	N/A ↑	N/A ↑	N/A	N/A

Mean values are shown unless otherwise stated

SD standard deviation, *N/A* not applicable, *SCI* spinal cord injury, *UTI* urinary tract infections, *CMV+* IgG anti cytomegalovirus present in plasma, ↑ ↓ increasing or decreasing trend with age

Comparison between the age groups:

Generally, cytokine concentrations were more changing with age in the able bodied group than in the SCI group. The IL-2 plasma levels, a cytokine which is mostly produced by T-cells and promotes their growth, were similar in all four groups. In the controls only, the anti-inflammatory IL-4 and IL-10 were both significantly increased with age. The chemoattractant protein MCP-1 showed a similar pattern: in the controls, it was significantly increased with age, but there was no age effect in the SCI population. Age independent levels of the granulocyte inducing GM-CSF were found in the controls, but the SCI individuals showed a significant reduction in GM-CSF plasma concentration with age. The neutrophil inducing G-CSF was significantly higher in both older groups.

Comparison between SCI and controls:

People with SCI had a tendency to lower cytokine concentrations compared with the able bodied controls. IL-2 was significantly higher in the ySCI group compared to the yCtr but there was no statistical difference between oCtr and oSCI. G-CSF and MCP-1 had reduced plasma concentrations in both age categories (younger and older than 60 years). The difference of G-CSF levels was significant between yCtr and ySCI, whereas the difference of MCP-1 was significant between oCtr and oSCI. IL-4 plasma concentrations were significantly lower in ySCI and oSCI groups compared to their age matched able bodied counterparts. No difference between controls and SCI groups was observed in the IL-10 plasma concentrations. GM-CSF was significantly elevated in the ySCI group compared with the yCtr group. However, differences in GM-CSF concentrations between oSCI and oCtr were insignificant.

PBL telomere length in study participants

Telomere length of peripheral blood mononuclear cells (PBMC) and the CD4/CD8 ratio was measured and compared between the groups (Table 2). Significant differences in telomere length were found between the yCtr and oCtr group. Differences between ySCI and oSCI, or controls and SCI groups were insignificant.

Table 2 Blood biochemistry, CD4/8 cell ratio and PBL telomere length in study participants

	yCtr (IQR)	ySCI (IQR)	oCtr (IQR)	oSCI (IQR)	yCtr-oCtr (p-value)	ySCI-oSCI (p-value)	yCtr-ySCI (p-value)	oCtr-oSCI (p-value)
Total prot. (mg/ml)	71.0 (4)	66.5 (7)	70.0 (5)	68.0 (7)	0.06 ↓	0.16 ↔	<.001	0.30
pIgG (mg/ml)	10.7 (4)	9.8 (3)	10.2 (4)	9.7 (4)	0.28 ↔	0.85 ↔	0.30	0.82
IL-2 (pg/ml)	5.5 (3)	6.2 (5)	6.0 (2)	6.1 (2)	0.12 ↔	0.27 ↔	<.01	0.70
IL-4 (pg/ml)	1.5 (0.6)	1.3 (0.2)	2.0 (1.1)	1.4 (0.5)	<.01 ↑	0.14 ↔	<.01	<.001
IL-10 (pg/ml)	3.6 (3)	2.9 (3)	5.0 (4)	3.9 (3)	<.05 ↑	0.12 ↔	0.25	0.19
G-CSF (pg/ml)	26.3 (7)	25.0 (5)	31.0 (10)	26.9 (7)	<.05 ↑	<.05 ↑	<.05	0.05
GM-CSF (pg/ml)	67 (25)	97 (50)	71 (30)	72 (35)	0.14 ↔	<.01 ↓	<.001	0.44
MCP-1 (pg/ml)	138 (28)	131 (20)	153 (43)	134 (27)	<.05 ↑	0.29 ↔	0.10	<.01
CD4/8 (ratio)	2.4 (1.4)	2.1 (2.2)	3.0 (2.7)	2.9 (2.7)	<.05 ↑	0.08 ↑	0.69	0.71
Telomere length PBL (Norm. to yCtr)	1 (0.5)	1.0 (0.4)	0.8 (0.3)	0.9 (0.3)	<.05 ↓	0.09 ↓	0.44	0.07

Median values are shown

IQR inter quartile range is shown in brackets, *N/A* not applicable, *SCI* spinal cord injury, *PBL* peripheral blood leucocyte, ↑ ↓ ↔ increasing, decreasing or no trend (p > 0.1) with age

CD4/CD8 ratio in study participants

A CD4/CD8 ratio below 1 is an immune risk phenotype criterion. Healthy ratio values are reported to be between 1 and 5. We observed that the ratio was increased in the oCtr group compared with yCtr (Table 2). Statistical differences was observed neither between oSCI and ySCI nor between SCI and control groups. In total, only 6 study participants out of 169 had a CD4/CD8 ratio below 1 (2× ySCI, 2× yCtr, 1× oSCI and 1× oCtr).

Inflamm-ageing in study participants

Figure 1 shows the plasma concentration of three pro inflammatory cytokines IL-6 (Fig. 1a), TNF-α (Fig. 1b) and CRP (Fig. 1c) which were measured to assess the inflamm-ageing status in the study participants. Controls aged 60+ years had on average higher CRP and IL-6 concentrations compared to the young controls, whereas in the SCI groups there was no difference between those two cytokines. In average the oSCI group had significant higher TNF-α levels compared with the ySCI. However the difference in TNF- α concentrations was not significant between the two control groups. The SCI population had, independent of age, higher CRP, but lower TNF-α levels compared with the able bodied control.

Urine IgA concentrations in study participants

The local secretion of IgA in the bladder was measured by detection of IgA in the urine, shown on Fig. 2a. While the mean values of urine IgA concentrations seemed unaffected by age, they were strongly increased in SCI persons, and some participants in the ySCI had very high values (depicted as outliers) compared to the oSCI group. The comparison of urine IgA concentrations in SCI persons with and without an ongoing UTI is depicted in Fig. 2b and shows that persons with an UTI in both age categories have significantly higher IgA levels. While the median difference in the concentration

of IgA levels between the young and old SCI groups with an UTI was statistically insignificant, again there was a large shift of mean IgA concentrations with a few very high values observed in the ySCI whereas the oSCI had more homogenous IgA urine levels.

White blood cell distribution among study participants

The abundancies of total leucocytes, neutrophils, lymphocytes, monocytes, eosinophils and basophils were measured, and the results of the complete white blood cell counts (WBC) are shown in Fig. 3. Total leucocytes (Fig. 3a) concentration did not differ between oSCI and ySCI but was reduced in the oCtr group compared to yCtr. The observed difference in the total white blood cells concentrations can be attributed to the lower concentrations of lymphocytes (Fig. 3c), and eosinophils (Fig. 3e). In the SCI groups only the concentration of the monocytes (Fig. 3d) is different between the two age groups with higher levels in the oSCI cohort. The ySCI group had lower lymphocyte concentrations compared to the yCtr. No difference in cell concentrations of all other leucocyte subtypes was observed between ySCI and yCtr. In the 60+ years groups, the SCI group had significantly higher neutrophil (Fig. 3b), lymphocyte and monocyte counts compared to the controls.

Abundancy of memory T-cells

In the lymphocytes compartment, we measured T-cells in five different stages of differentiation as shown in Table 3. Flow cytometric analysis of T-cell surface markers such as the co-stimulatory antigen CD28, the Fas receptor CD95, the phosphatase receptor CD45ro and CD4 or CD8 was used to gate on naïve- (Tn), stem cell memory- (Tscm), central memory and transitional memory- (Tcm + Ttm), effector memory- (Tem), and terminally differentiated effector memory T-cells (Tte).

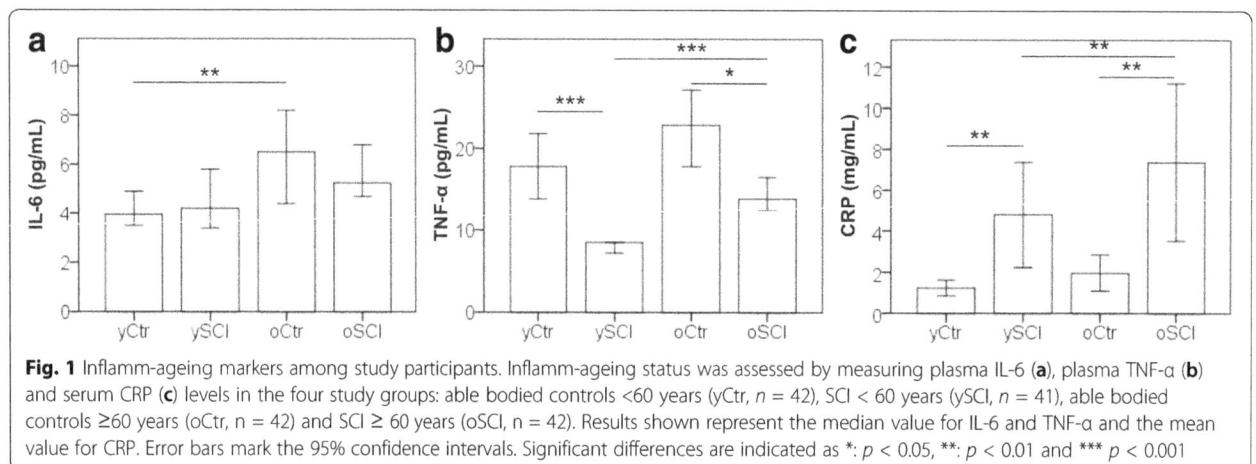

Fig. 1 Inflamm-ageing markers among study participants. Inflamm-ageing status was assessed by measuring plasma IL-6 (**a**), plasma TNF-α (**b**) and serum CRP (**c**) levels in the four study groups: able bodied controls <60 years (yCtr, n = 42), SCI < 60 years (ySCI, n = 41), able bodied controls ≥60 years (oCtr, n = 42) and SCI ≥ 60 years (oSCI, n = 42). Results shown represent the median value for IL-6 and TNF-α and the mean value for CRP. Error bars mark the 95% confidence intervals. Significant differences are indicated as *: $p < 0.05$, **: $p < 0.01$ and *** $p < 0.001$

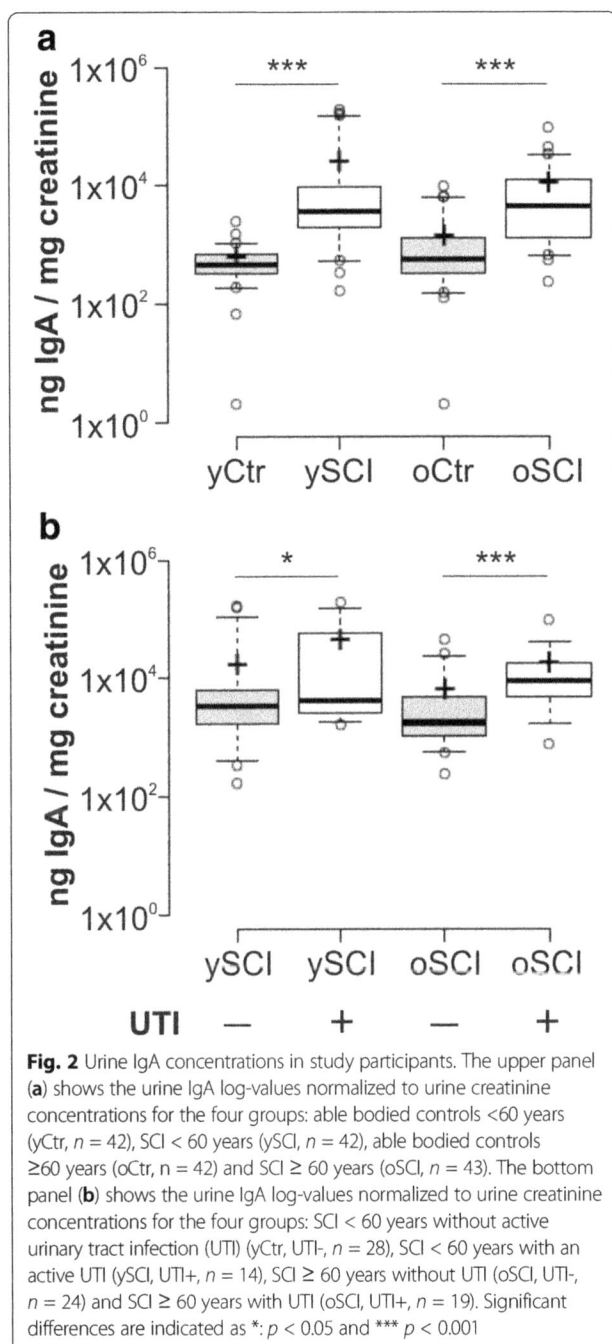

Fig. 2 Urine IgA concentrations in study participants. The upper panel (**a**) shows the urine IgA log-values normalized to urine creatinine concentrations for the four groups: able bodied controls <60 years (yCtr, n = 42), SCI < 60 years (ySCI, n = 42), able bodied controls ≥60 years (oCtr, n = 42) and SCI ≥ 60 years (oSCI, n = 43). The bottom panel (**b**) shows the urine IgA log-values normalized to urine creatinine concentrations for the four groups: SCI < 60 years without active urinary tract infection (UTI) (yCtr, UTI-, n = 28), SCI < 60 years with an active UTI (ySCI, UTI+, n = 14), SCI ≥ 60 years without UTI (oSCI, UTI-, n = 24) and SCI ≥ 60 years with UTI (oSCI, UTI+, n = 19). Significant differences are indicated as *: $p < 0.05$ and *** $p < 0.001$

Comparison between the age groups

While there was no significant difference in the CD4 T-cell subtypes between the age groups in able bodied controls, the oSCI group had, compared to ySCI, higher proportions of effector- and terminally- differentiated memory T-cells. CD8 T-cells, seemed to be more affected by age as seen in the decline of naïve cells. Similar findings were observed in the SCI population with the decline of naïve T-cells and the increase in effector- and terminally differentiated memory T-cells.

Comparison between SCI and control

The comparison between the control and the SCI group in the CD4 compartment revealed significant differences in the cell memory phenotype abundancies. In both age categories, the SCI group had less naïve- and higher central memory T-cells than the control. In contrast to CD4, the CD8 memory T-cell phenotype distributions were more comparable between the control and SCI groups. As a difference, ySCI individuals had less effector memory CD8 T-cells than the age matched control. However, the oSCI group had less naïve T-cells than the oCtr group.

In vitro stimulation assays, B-cells, T-cells and UTI burden

In vitro stimulation assays allow the assessment of the immune cell function in a controlled setting. Figure 4 summarizes the results of the IgG production potential and the T-cell specificity of in vitro stimulated PBL mixtures. IgG concentrations were measured at day 7 in the supernatants of totally stimulated- (Fig. 4a) and with UTI bacteria antigen stimulated PBL (Fig. 4b). The total stimulation (cocktail of IL-2, IL-10, IL-21, pokeweed mitogen and CpG rich DNA sequence) was considered to be the maximum IgG production capacity. The maximum IgG production capacity was lower in the oSCI group compared with ySCI. No significant difference was observed between oCtr and yCtr. When PBL were specifically stimulated with antigens from UTI bacteria, (mix *of Escherichia coli, Staphylococcus aureus, Klebsiella pneumonia, Enterococcus sp.* and *Proteus vulgaris*), the opposite was observed with significant lower IgG concentrations in the oCtr group compared to the yCtr and no difference in the SCI groups between ySCI and oSCI.

The abundancies of antigen specific CD4 (Fig. 4c) and CD8 (Fig. 4d) T-cells were analysed in PBL stimulated for four days with the UTI bacteria antigen mix. No statistical difference was found between the groups in antigen specific CD4 or CD8 T-cell abundancies.

In vitro T cell exhaustion and proliferation

The results of the phenotypic exhaustion, defined as poor effector function, loss of high proliferative capacity and the sustained expression of inhibitory receptors [27], are shown in Fig. 5. The expression of the co-inhibitory "killer cell lectin-like receptor G1" (KLRG-1) surface marker has been postulated to be a marker of senescence and exhaustion on T-cells [28] and was determined by flow cytometry for the CD4-positive (Fig. 5a) and the CD8-positive (Fig. 5b) T-cells. The results indicate a large inter-individual variance in the KLRG expression for both CD4 and CD8 T-cells. No statistical difference in KLRG expression on CD4 T-cells was found between the four groups. CD8 T-cells seemed to be more affected by age, as both elder groups (oCtr and oSCI) had significant higher proportions of KLRG+ cells

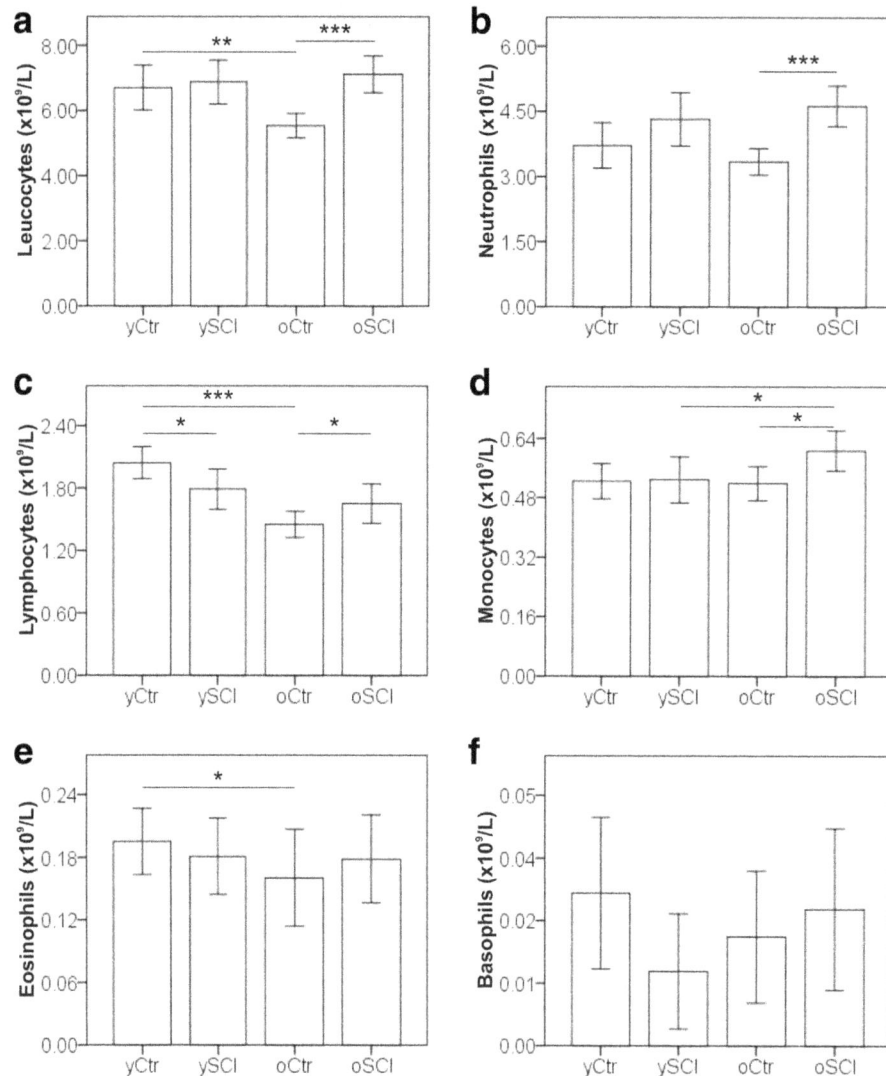

Fig. 3 Leucocyte differential counts in study participants. Mean cell concentrations for leucocytes (**a**), neutrophils (**b**), lymphocytes (**c**), monocytes (**d**), eosinophils (**e**) and basophils (**f**) are shown for the four groups: able bodied controls <60 years (yCtr, n = 42), SCI < 60 years (ySCI, n = 42), able bodied controls ≥60 years (oCtr, n = 42) and SCI ≥ 60 years (oSCI, n = 43). Error bars mark the 95% confidence intervals. Significant differences are indicated as *: $p < 0.05$, **: $p < 0.01$ and *** $p < 0.001$

compared to the young. No difference in KLRG+ cell ratios was observed between the SCI and the control groups.

The proliferation potential as measured by the in vitro cell division in response to the mitogen phytohaemagglutinin (PHA) was determined with flow cytometry at day 7 by the rate of signal reduction of an intracellular dye (Fig. 5c-f). The number of responsive cells, defined as the percent of cells which divided at least once, observed between the four groups was neither different for the CD4-positive (Fig. 5c) nor for the CD8-positive (Fig. 5d) T-cells. However, cells from SCI study participants divided in average fewer times compared the ones from the controls. The number of divisions for CD4 T-

cells (Fig. 5e) was significantly reduced between control and SCI in both age categories whereas in the CD8 T-cell compartment (Fig. 5f) the difference was only significant between the oSCI and oCtr group. On the other hand, age did not have an impact on the number of divisions.

Impact of SCI duration on immunosenescence parameters
An alternative analysis of data was performed in order to see the impact of SCI duration on the immune frailty parameters. The study participants were grouped according to the duration of SCI in the more recent (≤13.8 years with injury) and long-term (>13.8 years with injury) SCI groups (Additional file 1: Table S1). The

Table 3 Subtype abundancies of memory T-cells

		yCtr (SD)	ySCI (SD)	oCtr (SD)	oSCI (SD)	yCtr-oCtr (p-value)	ySCI-oSCI (p-value)	yCtr-ySCI (p-value)	oCtr-oSCI (p-value)
	N	41	42	42	41	N/A	N/A	N/A	N/A
CD4	Tn % of CD4	47 (16)	39 (14)	49 (15)	39 (16)	0.66 ↔	0.81 ↔	<0.05	<0.01
	Tscm % of CD4	8.5 (3)	8.5 (3)	9.0 (4)	8.7 (3)	0.71 ↔	0.73 ↔	0.74	0.76
	Tcm + tm % of CD4	42 (14)	50 (13)	39 (14)	48 (17)	0.27 ↔	0.53 ↔	<0.01	<0.01
	Tem % of CD4	2.0 (3)	1.4 (2)	1.9 (3)	2.3 (3)	0.94 ↔	<0.05 ↑	0.57	0.23
	Tte % of CD4	1.0 (1)	0.6 (1)	1.3 (4)	1.3 (2)	0.16 ↔	<0.01 ↑	<0.01	0.32
CD8	Tn % of CD8	32 (18)	34 (17)	19 (12)	14 (13)	<0.001 ↓	<0.001 ↓	0.48	<0.05
	Tscm % of CD8	13 (7)	14 (8)	15 (10)	12 (6)	0.57 ↔	0.52 ↔	0.80	0.44
	Tcm + tm % of CD8	28 (10)	32 (13)	32 (14)	39 (18)	0.21 ↔	0.08 ↑	0.21	0.12
	Tem % of CD8	8.4 (6)	5.8 (4)	8.1 (6)	9.8 (10)	0.73 ↔	<0.05 ↑	<0.05	0.58
	Tte % of CD8	19 (14)	14 (10)	26 (18)	25 (19)	0.11 ↔	<0.05 ↑	0.19	0.83

Mean values are shown as percentage of total CD4 or CD8 T-cells

SD standard deviation is shown in brackets, N/A not applicable, Tn naïve-, Tscm central-, Tcm + tm central and transitional-, Tem effector-, Tte terminally differentiated memory T-cell, ↑ ↓ ↔ increasing, decreasing or no trend (p > 0.1) with age

threshold of 13.8 years is the median value of SCI duration among participants. Out of 39 compared parameters only 2 differed significantly. People who lived longer with a SCI (>13.8 years) had higher GM-CSF plasma concentrations and lower percentage of CD4 T-cells which responded to an in vitro PHA stimulation assay as described in section 2.9.

Discussion

The results of the study indicate that the immune system in spinal cord injured (SCI) persons is altered towards a more senescent phenotype, possibly due to a higher antigen exposure of microbial origin - either bacterial or viral. The role of UTI in the onset of premature immunosenescence remains unclear.

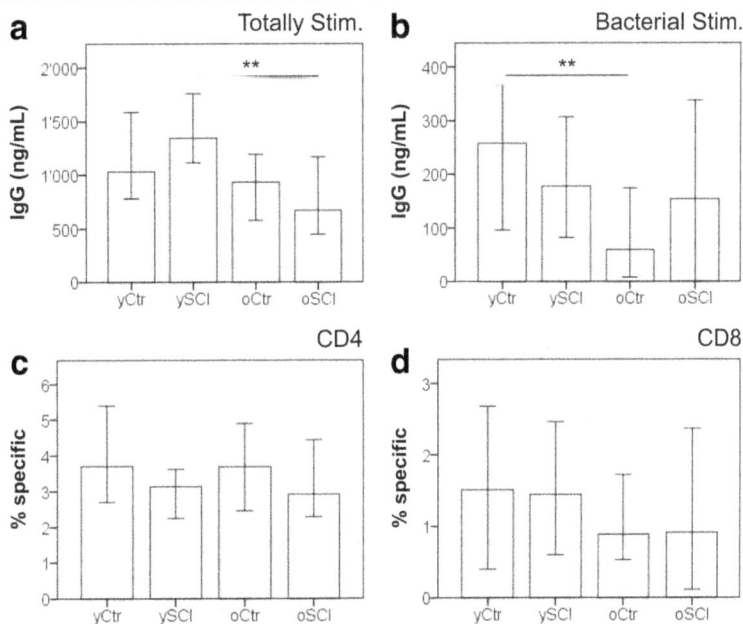

Fig. 4 In vitro functional assays of B-cells, T-cells and UTI burden. Median IgG concentrations were measured at day 7 in the supernatants of (**a**) totally stimulated PBL (cultured with IL-2, IL-10, IL-21, pokeweed mitogen and CpG rich DNA sequence) and (**b**) stimulated, with antigens from UTI bacteria (mix of inactivated E.coli, Staph. aureus, Klebsiella pneumonia, Enterococcus spec. And Proteus vulgaris). The bottom panels depict the median abundancies of antigen specific CD4 (**c**) and CD8 (**d**) T-cells as measured as cells with upregulated surface activation markers (CD69 and CD137) after four days of stimulation with UTI bacteria antigens. Participants were split into four groups: able bodied controls <60 years (yCtr, n = 41), SCI < 60 years (ySCI, n = 42), able bodied controls ≥60 years (oCtr, n = 42) and SCI ≥ 60 years (oSCI, n = 41). Error bars mark the 95% confidence interval. Significant differences are indicated as **: p < 0.01

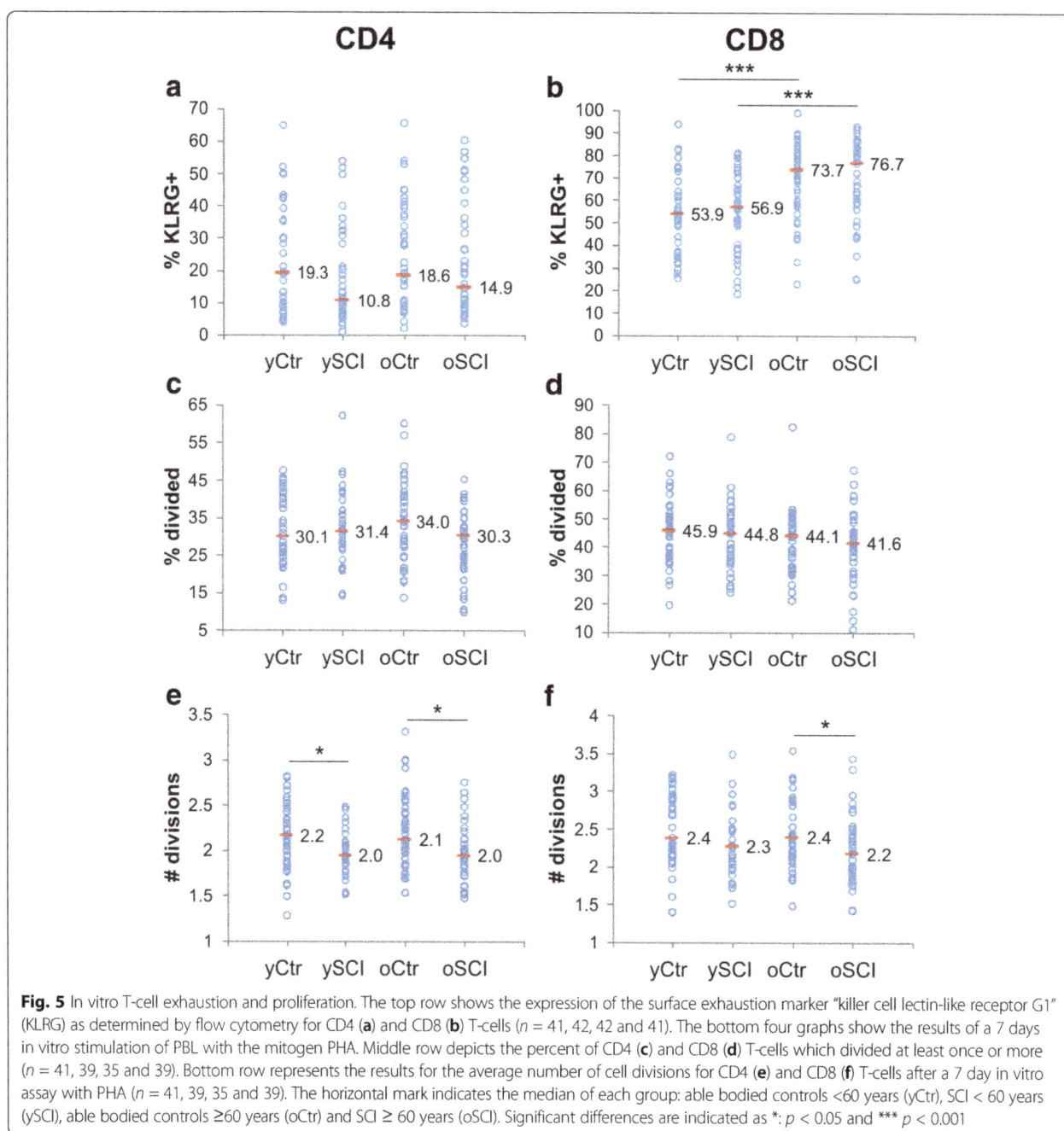

Fig. 5 In vitro T-cell exhaustion and proliferation. The top row shows the expression of the surface exhaustion marker "killer cell lectin-like receptor G1" (KLRG) as determined by flow cytometry for CD4 (**a**) and CD8 (**b**) T-cells ($n = 41, 42, 42$ and 41). The bottom four graphs show the results of a 7 days in vitro stimulation of PBL with the mitogen PHA. Middle row depicts the percent of CD4 (**c**) and CD8 (**d**) T-cells which divided at least once or more ($n = 41, 39, 35$ and 39). Bottom row represents the results for the average number of cell divisions for CD4 (**e**) and CD8 (**f**) T-cells after a 7 day in vitro assay with PHA ($n = 41, 39, 35$ and 39). The horizontal mark indicates the median of each group: able bodied controls <60 years (yCtr), SCI < 60 years (ySCI), able bodied controls ≥60 years (oCtr) and SCI ≥ 60 years (oSCI). Significant differences are indicated as *: $p < 0.05$ and *** $p < 0.001$

Persons with a SCI had on average lower abundancies of naïve- and higher concentrations of memory T-cells when compared with the able bodied control group. This increased shift from naïve to memory phenotype is one of the few accepted hallmarks of immunosenescence [29]. An interesting finding of our study was that the abundancy of naive CD4 T-cells was already reduced in the ySCI compared with yCtr. This suggests, as also others found [4], that the decreased immune function occurs early after an SCI and is maintained thereafter. Memory CD8 T-cell abundancies differed only between oSCI

and oCtr which suggests that CD8-T-cells from SCI individuals converted faster from naïve to memory phenotype compared with the control.

T-cell exhaustion, the progressive loss of T-cell effector functions - such as cytokine secretion and the ability for high proliferative capacity - is also known to be caused by some chronic infections [30, 31]. We measured lower responses to the stimulation with PHA in individuals with SCI compared to able bodied controls. The CD4 T-cell responses were already reduced in the ySCI group, whereas the CD8 T-cells differed only between oSCI and oCtr groups. This finding strengthens our hypothesis that the function of CD4 T-cells is affected early after SCI whereas CD8 function changes faster with age. It should be noted, that the number of cells starting division was the same and only the number of divisions was different between SCI and controls.

Unexpectedly, we observed an elevated initial concentration of circulating neutrophils and monocytes in individuals with SCI, simultaneous to the advancing senescence of the adaptive immune system and the increased pathogen susceptibility. With age increasing neutrophilia could be a sign of a higher antigen load or chronic infections [32]. Further indications for an increased antigenic load of the SCI population are manifested in the elevated serum CRP, increased urine IgA, the higher CMV prevalence and the high rate of active UTI. Secretory IgA is known to be induced by the presence of pathogens [33] and is an essential part of the mucosal immunity with protective functions against bacteria in the urinary tract. Generally, a SCI is a risk factor for increased pathogenic antigen exposure at different locations. The common necessity of urethral catheters (indwelling or intermittent) to empty the bladder and the impaired innervation of the bladder facilitate the occurrence of UTI [34]. Artificial breathing devices, immobility, accumulation of liquids in the lungs and the reduced ability of coughing, further increase the risk for respiratory infections [35]. Additionally, due to immobility and the loss of sensation, pressure sores or skin infections arise more likely [36]. Also the long hospital stay following the injury increases the exposure to pathogens. In fact, based on our observations we speculate that the prolonged hospitalisation increases the risk of an CMV infection, which in turn might contribute to the observed immune alterations – a hypothesis which we plan to test in a following project.

However, the question if recurrent UTI are causing a premature onset of immunosenescence still remains unanswered. On one hand, we were able to detect an age conserved stable IgG response to bacterial antigens in people with SCI (whereas the general population has a decreasing IgG response), but on the other hand, we did not observe a higher proportion of specifically responding T-cells in circulation. In contrast to chronic CMV infections which can infect multiple cell- and tissue types [37], UTI remain restricted to the urinary tract. Therefore it is possible that the occurrence of UTI bacteria specific memory T-cells is compartmentalized to the urothelial tissue and surrounding lymph nodes. These tissue resident memory T-cells are found in several body compartments as described elsewhere [38]. Longitudinal studies are necessary to investigate the influence of SCI and recurrent UTI on tissue resident memory T-cells and memory B-cells.

Fortunately, although some changes which point towards an increased immunological strain and senescence

were found in persons with SCI, our study could not fully support the hypothesis of a premature onset of immune frailty of the type occurring in octo- and nonagenarians [39]. Typically reported senescence traits as increased inflamm-ageing, shortened PBL telomeres [40] or increased proportions of exhaustions markers (KLRG-1) [41] were similar or even lower in the SCI population compared to the general population.

It is also possible, that the increased medication intake in the SCI group, especially antidepressants and painkillers with anti-inflammatory properties, decreased the plasma concentration of TNF-α [42]. In addition, the observed increase of average PBL telomere length could be a result of the elevated abundancy of innate immune cells in SCI persons as previously seen in other patient populations [43]. Importantly, the higher prevalence of active UTI in the oSCI compared to the ySCI group could be a sign of decreased immune defence in the ageing SCI patients.

Among the limitations of the study are its cross sectional design and the wide range of SCI lesion levels. A major discussion point is if our definition of the groups is suitable to detect age-related changes in the immune system. Given the reduced life expectancy of people with SCI, the old SCI group with individuals ≥60 years was relatively young in order to limit the selective survival bias (Neyman-bias). Despite this precaution, we observed that persons sustaining a SCI early in life were underrepresented in the ≥60 years group. However, the duration of a SCI seems not to affect the immune frailty parameters as observed when analysing our data regarding the time living with a SCI (Additional file 1: Table S1). Out of 39 compared parameters 37 did not differ between more recently injured (≤13.8 years) and longer term injured (>13.8 years) study participants.

Another limitation of the study is that we focused on the adaptive immune system (especially T-cells), while the obtained information on how SCI and aging impacted on the innate immune system or the B-cells beyond antibody production was limited. This gap is planned to be addressed in a following study.

Conclusions

The immune system of people with SCI shows traits of an increased immunological strain and a premature onset of immune frailty as manifested in higher UTI susceptibility in people above 60 years. Further, persons with SCI had lower proportions of naïve- and increased number of memory T-cells, combined with reduced T-cell proliferation and higher CMV prevalence compared to age matched controls.

The question if recurrent UTI are causing a premature onset of immunosenescence still remains unanswered. We observed an age conserved high IgG response to bacterial antigens but the abundancy of UTI bacteria specific T-cells was comparable between the control and SCI groups.

Data suggest that alterations in the CD4 T-cell compartment, as described above, occur early after a SCI, already in people <60 years, whereas CD8-T cells changes are observed in ≥60 years old individuals.

Further studies - preferably longitudinal - are necessary to investigate signs of immunosenescence in both the adaptive immune system - such as tissue resident memory T-cells, and memory B-cells - as well as in the cells of the innate immune system among the aged SCI persons.

Abbreviations

CMV: Cytomegalovirus; CRP: C-reactive protein; PBMC: Peripheral blood mononuclear cells; SCI: Spinal cord injury; SCI-IDS: SCI induced immune deficiency syndrome; UTI: Urinary tract infection; WBC: White blood cells

Acknowledgments

The authors thank Prof. Dr. H.R.Widmer from the University of Bern and Prof. Dr. F. Sallusto from the Institute for Research in Biomedicine (IRB) in Bellinzona for their inputs and fruitful discussion. Special thanks to Dr. Med. T. Weingand and her team at the blood donation bank of Lucerne for their help in recruiting and sampling of the controls. We also thank Dr. J. Wöllner and colleagues from the department of urology at the Swiss Paraplegic Centre for their help in recruiting and sampling of study participants with a SCI. Much appreciated was the kind help of Dr. W. L. Wong and her team at the University of Zurich for their technical support with the Bio-Plex measurements. Further, we are very thankful for the cooperation with S. Rieser and her team, especially E. Imbach, from the clinical laboratories at the Swiss Paraplegic Centre.

Authors' contribution

DP designed and performed experiments, performed data analysis, and wrote the manuscript. JK blinded the data, assisted with data analysis and critically reviewed the manuscript. SC performed experiments. AB performed data analysis and assisted with data interpretation. BE Assisted with experimental design and data interpretation. JP recruited study participants and assisted with data interpretation. JS designed experiments, assisted with data analysis, manuscript writing and editing and provided administrative support. All authors read and approved the final manuscript.

Funding

This work was supported by the Swiss Paraplegic Foundation.

Competing interests

The authors declare that they have no competing interests.

Author details

[1]Biomedical Laboratories, Swiss Paraplegic Research, Guido A. Zäch Strasse 4, 6207, Nottwil, Switzerland. [2]Swiss Paraplegic Centre, Guido A. Zäch Strasse 1, 6207, Nottwil, Switzerland. [3]Theodor Kocher Institute, University of Bern, Freiestrasse 1, 3012 Bern, Switzerland.

References

1. Savic G, DeVivo MJ, Frankel HL, Jamous MA, Soni BM, Charlifue S. Long-term survival after traumatic spinal cord injury: a 70-year British study. Spinal Cord. 2017;
2. Spinal Cord Injury. Progress, promise, and priorities. In: The National Academies Press; 2005.
3. National Spinal Cord Injury Statistical Center [https://www.nscisc.uab.edu/].
4. Nash MS. Known and plausible modulators of depressed immune functions following spinal cord injuries. J Spinal Cord Med. 2000;23:111–20.
5. Whiteneck GG. Aging with spinal cord injury. New York: Demos Medical Publishing; 1993.
6. Riegger T, Conrad S, Liu K, Schluesener HJ, Adibzahdeh M, Schwab JM. Spinal cord injury-induced immune depression syndrome (SCI-IDS). Eur J Neurosci. 2007;25:1743–7.
7. Riegger T, Conrad S, Schluesener HJ, Kaps HP, Badke A, Baron C, Gerstein J, Dietz K, Abdizahdeh M, Schwab JM. Immune depression syndrome following human spinal cord injury (SCI): a pilot study. Neuroscience. 2009;158:1194–9.
8. Monahan R, Stein A, Gibbs K, Bank M, Bloom O. Circulating T cell subsets are altered in individuals with chronic spinal cord injury. Immunol Res. 2015;63:3–10.
9. Goronzy JJ, Weyand CM. Understanding immunosenescence to improve responses to vaccines. Nat Immunol. 2013;14:428–36.
10. Li H, Manwani B, Leng SX. Frailty, inflammation, and immunity. Aging Dis. 2011;2:466–73.
11. Pawelec G. Immunity and ageing in man. Exp Gerontol. 2006;41:1239–42.
12. Kohler S. Thy(–im)munosenescence: The Ageing of the Thymus and Its Impact on the Immune System. In: Thiel A, editor. Immunosenescence. Basel: Springer; 2012. p. 37–54. Birkhäuser Advances in Infectious Diseases.
13. Tu W, Rao S. Mechanisms underlying T cell Immunosenescence: aging and cytomegalovirus infection. Front Microbiol. 2016;7:2111.
14. Qi Q, Liu Y, Cheng Y, Glanville J, Zhang D, Lee J-Y, Olshen RA, Weyand CM, Boyd SD, Goronzy JJ. Diversity and clonal selection in the human T-cell repertoire. Proc Natl Acad Sci U S A. 2014;111:13139–44.
15. Akbar AN, Henson SM, Lanna A. Senescence of T lymphocytes: implications for enhancing human immunity. Trends Immunol. 2016;37:866–76.
16. Franceschi C, Bonafe M, Valensin S, Olivieri F, De Luca M, Ottaviani E, De Benedictis G. Inflamm-aging. An evolutionary perspective on immunosenescence. Ann N Y Acad Sci. 2000;908:244–54.
17. Baylis D, Bartlett DB, Patel HP, Roberts HC. Understanding how we age: insights into inflammaging. Longev Healthspan. 2013;2:8–8.
18. Fulop T, Larbi A, Pawelec G. Human T cell aging and the impact of persistent viral infections. Front Immunol. 2013;4:271.
19. Booth NJ, Akbar AN, Vukmanovic-Stejic M. Regulation of adaptive immunity in the elderly. In: Thiel A, editor. Immunosenescence. Basel: springer Basel; 2012. p. 1–23.
20. Mahnke YD, Brodie TM, Sallusto F, Roederer M, Lugli E. The who's who of T-cell differentiation: human memory T-cell subsets. Eur J Immunol. 2013;43:2797–809.
21. Heidt S, Hester J, Shankar S, Friend PJ, Wood KJ. B cell repopulation after alemtuzumab induction-transient increase in transitional B cells and long-term dominance of naive B cells. Am J Transplant. 2012;12:1784–92.
22. Jurk M, Schulte B, Kritzler A, Noll B, Uhlmann E, Wader T, Schetter C, Krieg AM, Vollmer J. C-class CpG ODN: sequence requirements and characterization of immunostimulatory activities on mRNA level. Immunobiology. 2004;209:141–54.
23. Bacher P, Scheffold A. Flow-cytometric analysis of rare antigen-specific T cells. Cytometry A. 2013;83:692–701.
24. Litjens NH, de Wit EA, Baan CC, Betjes MG. Activation-induced CD137 is a fast assay for identification and multi-parameter flow cytometric analysis of alloreactive T cells. Clin Exp Immunol. 2013;174:179–91.
25. O'Callaghan NJ, Fenech M. A quantitative PCR method for measuring absolute telomere length. Biol Proced Online. 2011;13:3.
26. Pannek J. Treatment of urinary tract infection in persons with spinal cord injury: guidelines, evidence, and clinical practice: a questionnaire-based survey and review of the literature. J Spinal Cord Med. 2011;34:11–5.
27. Wherry EJ. T cell exhaustion. Nat Immunol. 2011;12:492–9.
28. Henson SM, Akbar AN. KLRG1—more than a marker for T cell senescence. Age. 2009;31:285–91.
29. Pawelec G. Hallmarks of human "immunosenescence": adaptation or dysregulation? Immun Ageing. 2012;9:15–5.
30. Yi JS, Cox MA, Zajac AJ. T-cell exhaustion: characteristics, causes and conversion. Immunology. 2010;129:474–81.
31. Wherry EJ, Kurachi M. Molecular and cellular insights into T cell exhaustion. Nat Rev Immunol. 2015;15:486–99.
32. Soehnlein O, Steffens S, Hidalgo A, Weber C. Neutrophils as protagonists and targets in chronic inflammation. Nat Rev Immunol. 2017;17:248–61.
33. Macpherson AJ, McCoy KD, Johansen FE, Brandtzaeg P. The immune geography of IgA induction and function. Mucosal Immunol. 2008;1:11–22.
34. Wyndaele J-J, Brauner A, Geerlings SE, Bela K, Peter T, Bjerklund-Johanson TE. Clean intermittent catheterization and urinary tract infection: review and guide for future research. BJU Int. 2012;110:E910–7.

Immunosenescence in persons with spinal cord injury in relation to urinary tract...

127

35. Brown R, DiMarco AF, Hoit JD, Garshick E. Respiratory dysfunction and Management in Spinal Cord Injury. Respir Care. 2006;51:853–70.

36. Chen Y, Devivo MJ, Jackson AB. Pressure ulcer prevalence in people with spinal cord injury: age-period-duration effects. Arch Phys Med Rehabil. 2005;86:1208–13.

37. Krishna BA, Spiess K, Poole EL, Lau B, Voigt S, Kledal TN, Rosenkilde MM, Sinclair JH. Targeting the latent cytomegalovirus reservoir with an antiviral fusion toxin protein. Nat Commun. 2017;8:14321.

38. Farber DL, Yudanin NA, Restifo NP. Human memory T cells: generation, compartmentalization and homeostasis. Nat Rev Immunol. 2014;14:24–35.

39. Wikby A, Strindhall J, Johansson B. The immune risk profile and associated parameters in late life: lessons from the OCTO and NONA longitudinal studies. In: Fulop T, Franceschi C, Hirokawa K, Pawelec G, editors. Handbook on Immunosenescence. Netherlands: Springer; 2009. p. 3–28.

40. Malaguarnera L, Ferlito L, Imbesi RM, Gulizia GS, Di Mauro S, Maugeri D, Malaguarnera M, Messina A. Immunosenescence: a review. Arch Gerontol Geriatr. 2001;32:1–14.

41. Weng N-P. aging of the immune system: how much can the adaptive immune system adapt? Immunity. 2006;24:495–9.

42. Gallelli L, Galasso O, Falcone D, Southworth S, Greco M, Ventura V, Romualdi P, Corigliano A, Terracciano R, Savino R, et al. The effects of nonsteroidal anti-inflammatory drugs on clinical outcomes, synovial fluid cytokine concentration and signal transduction pathways in knee osteoarthritis. A randomized open label trial. Osteoarthr Cartil. 2013;21:1400–8.

43. Wong LSM, Huzen J, de Boer RA, van Gilst WH, van Veldhuisen DJ, van der Harst P. Telomere length of circulating leukocyte subpopulations and buccal cells in patients with ischemic heart failure and their offspring. PLoS One. 2011;6:e23118.

Elastic band resistance training influences transforming growth factor-ß receptor I mRNA expression in peripheral mononuclear cells of institutionalised older adults: the Vienna Active Ageing Study (VAAS)

Barbara Schober-Halper[1], Marlene Hofmann[1], Stefan Oesen[1], Bernhard Franzke[1], Thomas Wolf[2], Eva-Maria Strasser[3], Norbert Bachl[2], Michael Quittan[3], Karl-Heinz Wagner[1,4] and Barbara Wessner[1,2*] (iD)

Abstract

Background: Ageing, inactivity and obesity are associated with chronic low-grade inflammation contributing to a variety of lifestyle-related diseases. Transforming growth factor-β (TGF-β) is a multimodal protein with various cellular functions ranging from tissue remodelling to the regulation of inflammation and immune functions. While it is generally accepted that aerobic exercise exerts beneficial effects on several aspects of immune functions, even in older adults, the effect of resistance training remains unclear. The aim of this study was to investigate whether progressive resistance training (6 months) with or without nutritional supplementation (protein and vitamins) would influence circulating C-reactive protein and TGF-β levels as well as TGF-β signalling in peripheral mononuclear cells (PBMCs) of institutionalised adults with a median age of 84.5 (65.0–97.4) years.

Results: Elastic band resistance training significantly improved performance as shown by the arm-lifting test ($p = 0.007$), chair stand test ($p = 0.001$) and 6-min walking test ($p = 0.026$). These results were paralleled by a reduction in TGF-β receptor I (TGF-βRI) mRNA expression in PBMCs ($p = 0.006$), while circulating inflammatory markers were unaffected. Protein and vitamin supplementation did not provoke any additional effects. Interestingly, muscular endurance of upper and lower body and aerobic performance at baseline were negatively associated with changes in circulating TGF-β at the early phase of the study. Furthermore, drop-outs of the study were characterised not only by lower physical performance but also higher TGF-β and TGF-βRI mRNA expression, and lower miRNA-21 expression.

Conclusions: Progressive resistance training with elastic bands did not influence chronic low-grade inflammation but potentially affected TGF-β signalling in PBMCs through altered TGF-βRI mRNA expression. There appears to be an association between physical performance and TGF-β expression in PBMCs of older adults, in which the exact mechanisms need to be clarified.

Keywords: Vienna Active Ageing Study (VAAS), TGF-β pathway, microRNA, Chronic inflammation, Inflammageing, Strength training

* Correspondence: barbara.wessner@univie.ac.at
[1]Research Platform Active Ageing, University of Vienna, Althanstraße 14, 1090 Vienna, Austria
[2]Department of Sports and Exercise Physiology, Centre for Sport Science and University Sports, University of Vienna, Auf der Schmelz 6, 1150 Vienna, Austria
Full list of author information is available at the end of the article

Background

Population ageing resulting from a higher life expectancy concomitant with a decline in fertility will lead to a global increase in the proportion of people over the age of 60 years from 12 % in 2015 to 22 % by 2050 [1]. With higher ages, the prevalence of cardiovascular, metabolic and neurodegenerative disorders and cancer is increased. It has been shown that many of these conditions are related to compromised homeostasis between proper activation of the immune system and its resolution, leading to a limited response to pathogens and vaccines and a chronic inflammatory state [2, 3].

Transforming growth factor-β (TGF-β) is a multifunctional protein involved in the regulation of cell proliferation, extracellular matrix production, inflammation and immune functions [4]. Higher circulating levels of TGF-β are related to obesity with impaired insulin sensitivity [5], cardiovascular diseases among individuals with higher C-reactive protein (CRP) levels [6], type II diabetes [7, 8], and a higher age [9]. TGF-β interacts with several cell types by binding to membrane serine/threonine kinase receptors, TGF-β receptor I (TGF-βRI; also known as ALK5) and TGF-βRII, initiating diverse cellular responses [10]. An approach to modulate TGF-β signalling is to alter the expression of its receptors. It has become evident that microRNAs (miRNAs) regulate thousands of human genes by either mRNA degradation or suppression of mRNA translation [11]. A recent investigation estimated that 84–89 % of miRNA-induced suppression of gene expression is the result of degradation of target mRNAs [12]. Currently, close to 1900 human miRNA precursors are listed in the miRBase registry, which give rise to 2588 mature miRNAs [13, 14]. One of these miRNAs, miRNA-21, plays a crucial role in a plethora of biological functions and diseases including the development of cancer, cardiovascular diseases and inflammation [15]. Interestingly, miRNA-21 targets both TGF-βRI and TGF-βRII [16], and overexpression of miRNA-21 is associated with elevated levels of proinflammatory cytokines in a dominant-negative TGF-βRII mouse model [17].

Regular physical activity offers protection against, and may be a useful treatment for, a wide variety of chronic diseases associated with low-grade inflammation [18]. In particular, endurance exercise training combined with dietary weight loss strategies have been shown to decrease the chronic inflammatory state associated with obesity and old age [19, 20]. Resistance training prevents or counteracts age-related loss of muscle mass and functions [21, 22], but there is an ongoing discussion whether this type of exercise alters the chronic inflammatory state associated with ageing [23–25].

In the Vienna Active Ageing Study (VAAS), we previously showed that resistance training using elastic bands for 6 months leads to an increase in functional performance of the lower and upper extremities and improves muscle quality in older people [22, 26]. Furthermore, we detected higher CRP levels and lower TGF-βRI and TGF-βRII expression in peripheral blood mononuclear cells (PBMCs) of older women compared with younger women [27]. Therefore, the aim of this sub-study of the VAAS was to investigate whether progressive resistance training alone or in combination with a nutritional supplement containing protein and vitamins influenced expression of TGF-β, its receptors, and/or miRNA-21 in older institutionalised people.

Results
Subject characteristics

A total of 230 potential participants were screened for eligibility, and 117 participants (89 women and 12 men) agreed to participate in the VAAS. The participants were randomised into intervention groups: cognitive training (CT), resistance training (RT), and resistance training plus nutritional supplementation (RTS) (Fig. 1). Blood samples were available from 95 participants (84 women and 11 men). To prevent any potential interference by acute inflammatory processes, we excluded all subjects with CRP levels above 10 mg/L at any time point as done previously [28, 29]. Finally, data from 88 participants (77 women and 11 men) with a median age of 84.5 (65.2–97.4) years and a median body mass index (BMI) of 28.9 (18.1–50.0) kg/m^2 were included in the current study (Fig. 1). No differences between study groups with respect to age, gender, anthropometric data and health status were detected at baseline, whereas leukocyte numbers differed significantly between intervention groups ($p = 0.002$). Post-hoc analyses revealed that subjects from the RT group had lower leukocyte numbers than those from the CT group (+28 %, $p = 0.002$) and the RTS group (+19 %, $p = 0.039$), which was owing to lower numbers of neutrophils (CT: +51 %, $p < 0.001$; RTS: +33 %, $p = 0.092$). Circulating inflammatory markers (hs-CRP and TGF-β) and mRNA expression of TGF-β, its receptors and miRNA-21 in PBMCs (lymphocytes and monocytes) did not differ between groups at baseline (Table 1).

Dropout analysis

During 6 months of intervention, 18 women and 3 men (27 %) left the study because of several reasons (loss of interest or acute medical reasons such as joint pain or cardiological issues). The dropout rate did not differ between groups. In addition, age, sex, and existing co-morbidities in general were not related to adherence to the study. Only the number of participants diagnosed for hyperlipidaemia was higher in finishers compared with the dropouts ($p = 0.016$). Baseline performance appeared to be related to study adherence because

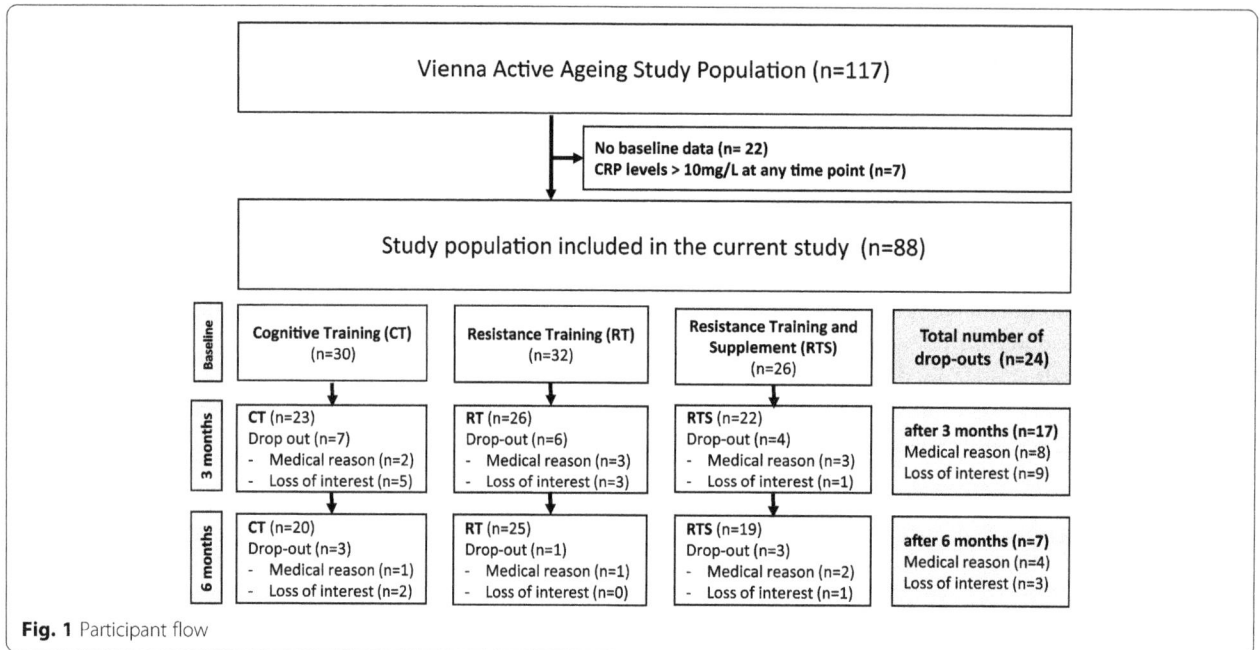

Fig. 1 Participant flow

dropouts had lower aerobic (6MWT: −19 %, p = 0.020) and chair stand (−13 %, p = 0.015) performance than finishers of the study. Strength (p = 0.608) and muscular endurance (p = 0.924) of the upper extremities were not different between finishers and dropouts. The observed differences also became evident in some of the TGF-β-related parameters because TGF-β (+106 %, p = 0.016) and TGF-βRI (+237 %, p < 0.001) mRNA expression was higher in dropouts, while miRNA-21 expression was lower (−65 %, p < 0.001) (Table 2). As a consequence we performed a per-protocol analysis by excluding the dropouts from all subsequent analyses (Tables 3 and 4).

Resistance training improves physical performance of older subjects

We have previously shown that resistance training intervention specifically improved muscular endurance (chair stand and arm-lifting tests), while isometric strength (handgrip test) and aerobic capacity (6-min walking test; 6MWT) increased similarly in CT, RT and RTS groups [22]. Because the current study included just a subset of the original study population, the data on physical performance were re-analysed. At baseline, no differences in any of the physical fitness parameters were observed between intervention groups (p > 0.05). Similar to the previous results, chair stand performance was increased in the RT group (3 months: +18 %, p = 0.041; 6 months: +27 %, p = 0.001) and RTS group (6 months: +15 %, p = 0.017). Arm-lifting performance was enhanced in RT and RTS groups only after 6 months (RT: +24 %, p = 0.007; RTS +61 %, p = 0.007). While handgrip strength was unaltered over time in all intervention groups (CT: p = 0.454;

RT: p = 0.238, RTS: p = 0.810), aerobic performance during the 6MWT was slightly improved in the RT group after 6 months (+9 %, p = 0.026) but not in the CT or RTS groups (CT: p = 0.959, RTS: p = 0.080) (data not shown).

Effects of interventions on leukocyte subpopulations and circulating inflammatory markers

Except for an adaptation of the leukocyte numbers in the RT group (overall: p = 0.001; 3 months: p = 0.166; 6 months: p = 0.001; +7 %) caused by an increase in neutrophils (overall: p = 0.011; 3 months: p = 0.166; 6 months: p = 0.010 + 22 %), we did not detect any other alterations in leukocyte, lymphocyte, monocyte or granulocyte counts. Similarly, the circulating levels of TGF-β and hs-CRP remained unchanged (Table 3).

Influence of interventions on intracellular TGF-β and TGF-β receptor mRNA expression, and miRNA-21 expression

The mRNA expression of TGF-β, TGF-βRI, TGF-βRII and miRNA-21 in PBMCs did not differ between groups at any time point. Resistance training led to a significant decrease in TGF-βRI mRNA levels (p = 0.006). Post-hoc analyses revealed that the initial decrease at 3 months (−27 %, p = 0.015) was reversed at 6 months (p = 0.117). Interestingly, this decrease could not be confirmed in the RTS group, although the median level decreased similarly to the RT group. Intracellular TGF-β and TGF-βRII mRNA expression, and miRNA-21 expression, were not influenced by any of the interventions (Table 4).

Because resistance training only led to marginal changes in the TGF-β signalling pathway, we examined whether

Table 1 Baseline characteristics

	All (n = 88)	CT (n = 30)	RT (n = 32)	RTS (n = 26)	P-value
Gender [female/male]	77/11	25/5	28/4	24/2	0.602
Age [years]	84.5 (65.0–97.4)	84.5 (69.4–97.4)	84.4 (71.7–93.2)	84.3 (65.0–92.2)	0.864
BMI [kg/m^2]	28.9 (18.1–50.0)	29.8 (18.1–36.9)	28.2 (22.7–40.2)	27.9 (22.9–50.0)	0.741
Obesity [n (%)]	32 (36.8 %)	14 (46.7 %)	8 (25.0 %)	10 (35.7 %)	0.235
Hyperlipidaemia [n (%)]	32 (36.4 %)	9 (30.0 %)	10 (31.3 %)	13 (46.4 %)	0.226
Diabetes Type II [n (%)]	14 (15.9 %)	6 (20 %)	7 (21.9 %)	1 (3.6 %)	0.132
Hypertension [n (%)]	70 (79.5 %)	26 (86.7 %)	27 (84.4 %)	17 (60.7 %)	0.100
Cardiac diseases [n (%)]	27 (30.7 %)	12 (40.0 %)	9 (28.1 %)	6 (21.4 %)	0.362
Osteoporosis [n (%)]	35 (39.8 %)	12 (40.0 %)	12 (37.5 %)	11 (39.3 %)	0.933
History of cancer [n (%)]	12 (13.6 %)	5 (16.7 %)	4 (12.5 %)	3 (10.7 %)	0.833
Leukocyte subpopulations and circulating biomarkers					
Leukocytes [x10^9 cells/L]	6.6 (3.3–13.0)	7.4 (4.9–10.3)*	5.8 (3.1–9.8)	6.9 (4.4–13.3)*	**0.002**
Lymphocytes [cells/µl]	1990 (930–4930)	1985 (910–3510)	1835 (830–3330)	2200 (1460–4700)	0.085
Neutrophils [cells/µl]	3695 (1530–9860)	4414 (2410–6630)*	2931 (1530–6800)	3889 (2370–9860)	**<0.001**
Eosinophils [cells/µl]	200 (10–740)	225 (36–620)	160 (10–740)	220 (10–470)	0.135
Basophils [cells/µl]	40 (10–111)	45 (10–111)	35 (10–190)	35 (10–90)	0.397
Monocytes [cells/µl]	560 (250–910)	587 (72–950)	520 (260–860)	545 (320–960)	0.189
hs-CRP [mg/L]	1.95 (0.3–7.9)	2.1 (0.5–7.9)	1.9 (0.3–7.6)	1.9 (0.6–6.7)	0.918
TGF-β [µg/L]	33.3 (16.7–73.7)	38.2 (18.7–73.7)	32.8 (16.7–55.4)	32.1 (21.0–51.2)	0.083
PBMC gene expression					
TGF-β/GAPDH [-]	0.85 (0.06–3.36)	0.48 (0.23–2.66)	0.60 (0.21–2.52)	0.58 (0.06–3.36)	0.725
TGF-βRI/GAPDH [-]	2.05 (0.14–28.82)	1.99 (0.14–22.39)	2.04 (0.69–19.25)	2.11 (0.29–28.81)	0.990
TGF-βRII/GAPDH [-]	1.67 (0.51–15.85)	1.54 (0.66–7.79)	1.60 (0.66–14.85)	1.79 (0.51–10.80)	0.714
miRNA-21 [copies/pg]	2400 (57–4720)	2920 (343–4500)	2120 (57–4720)	2350 (550–4590)	0.765

Data are expressed as medians (min–max); Group differences were detected using X^2 or Kruskal Wallis tests and if significant, followed by Bonferroni-corrected post-hoc analyses (*$p < 0.05$ vs. RT); significant differences are marked in bold

Abbreviations: *CT* cognitive training, *RT* resistance training, *RTS* resistance training plus supplement, *PBMC* peripheral blood mononuclear cell, *hs-CRP* high sensitive C-reactive protein, *TGF-β* transforming growth factor-β, *TGF-βR* TGF-β receptor, *GAPDH* glyceraldehyde 3-phosphate dehydrogenase, *miR-21* microRNA-21

different components of physical fitness (strength, muscular endurance and aerobic performance) at baseline influenced the TGF-β signalling response (difference between 3 or 6 months and baseline values). While isometric handgrip strength was not associated with alterations in TGF-β-related parameters, muscular endurance and aerobic performance at baseline were negatively associated with changes in circulating TGF-β levels after 3 months (chair rise test: $\rho = -0.349$, $p = 0.003$, arm-lifting test: $\rho = -0.352$, $p = 0.024$; 6MWT: $\rho = -0.308$, $p = 0.009$), but chair stand performance was positively associated with changes in TGF-βRII mRNA expression ($\rho = 0.254$, $p = 0.033$) (Table 5).

Discussion

The aim of the current study was to investigate the effects of progressive resistance training alone and in combination with a nutritional supplement enriched with protein and vitamins on systemic inflammation and TGF-β signalling in PBMCs of institutionalised, but independent older people. Circulating TGF-β and hs-CRP levels as well as intracellular TGF-β gene expression were not influenced by elastic band resistance training. Interestingly, TGF-βRI, but not TGF-βRII, gene expression was reduced in the RT group after 3 months and returned to baseline levels thereafter.

It is well known that regular endurance training reduces the chronic proinflammatory state caused by ageing and physical inactivity [30, 31]. Adipose tissue appears to play a substantial role in this scenario because it is a major source of several hormones and cytokines [32]. In particular, visceral fat depots and the macrophages within these depots release proinflammatory cytokines such as interleukin-6 (IL-6), tumour necrosis factor-α (TNF-α) and TGF-β1 [33]. The increase in energy expenditure caused by enhanced physical activity reduces body fat, thereby influencing the capacity to produce and release proinflammatory mediators [33]. Recommended strategies to lose weight and body fat include aerobic exercise training combined with

Table 2 Baseline differences between drop-outs and finishers

	Total ($n = 88$)	Dropouts ($n = 21$)	Non-Dropouts ($n = 67$)	p-value
Gender [female/male]	77/11	18/3	59/8	0.777
Age [years]	84.5 (65.0–97.4)	85.2 (69.4–92.2)	84.2 (65.0–97.4)	0.282
BMI [kg/m^2]	28.9 (18.1–50.0)	28.3 (18.1–43.7)	30.7 (23.4–50.0)	0.094
hs-CRP [mg/L]	1.9 (0.3–7.9)	2.0 (0.8–7.9)	1.9 (0.3–7.6)	0.413
TGF-β signalling				
TGF-β [µg/L]	33.3 (16.7–73.7)	39.3 (22.5–58.0)	32.8 (16.7–73.7)	0.178
TGF-β/GAPDH [-]	0.53 (0.06–3.36)	1.07 (0.21–3.36)	0.52 (0.06–2.66)	**0.016**
TGF-β RI/GAPDH [-]	2.05 (0.14–28.81)	6.41 (1.31–28.81)	1.90 (0.14–22.39)	**<0.001**
TGF-β RII/GAPDH [-]	1.67 (0.51–14.85)	3.00 (0.91–10.80)	1.59 (0.51–14.85)	0.099
miR–21 [copies/pg RNA]	2400 (57–5720)	979 (498–3640)	2815 (57–4720)	**<0.001**
Co-morbidities				
Obesity [n (%)]	32 (36.4 %)	10 (47.6 %)	22 (32.8 %)	0.162
Hyperlipidemia [n (%)]	32 (36.4 %)	3 (14.2 %)	29 (43.3 %)	**0.016**
Diabetes Type II [n (%)]	14 (15.9 %)	3 (14.3 %)	11 (16.4 %)	0.816
Hypertension [n (%)]	70 (79.5 %)	17 (81.0 %)	53 (79.1 %)	0.855
Cardiac diseases [n (%)]	27 (30.7 %)	7 (33.3 %)	20 (29.9 %)	0.763
Osteoporosis [n (%)]	35 (39.8 %)	9 (42.9 %)	26 (38.8 %)	0.741
History of cancer [n (%)]	12 (13.6 %)	3 (14.3 %)	9 (13.4 %)	0.921

Data for continuous variables are shown as medians (min–max). For co-morbidities, the respective numbers of affected participants were determined at the medical entrance examination. Obesity was defined as a BMI of >30 kg/m^2. Differences between groups were determined by Mann–Whitney U or X^2 tests; significant differences are marked in bold

caloric reduction. Although it is known that resistance training does not promote clinically significant weight loss, it influences body composition by increasing muscle mass and decreasing body fat [34, 35]. Thus, it has been hypothesised that muscle-strengthening exercises also exert anti-inflammatory effects. Based on intervention studies investigating the effects of strength training on inflammatory markers such as CRP, TNF-α and IL-6, the data are ambiguous because some studies have revealed a positive effect [23, 36], whereas others did not observe any amelioration in the inflammatory state [24, 25, 37]. While the TGF-β superfamily has been studied extensively in the adaptation of muscles and tendons to exercise [38], investigations into the context of exercise immunology are scarce. Our data are in line with a previous study showing that strength training does not alter the level of circulating TGF-β [39]. Another study, investigating the influence of a combined strength and endurance exercise programme in type 2 diabetic patients revealed an increase in circulating TGF-β [36], but study population and training programme were different making a direct comparison difficult. Nevertheless, in our study, parameters measuring aerobic fitness and muscular endurance, but not handgrip strength, correlated negatively with TGF-β alterations. This could hint to the fact that endurance training is an important component of an exercise intervention to target circulating TGF-β levels, but further

studies are needed to clearly identify the underlying associations.

While circulating levels of TGF-β were unaffected, our data revealed that resistance training seems to lower the TGF-βRI mRNA expression in PBMCs of older adults, potentially leading to decreased signalling through the type I receptor. Furthermore, higher levels of TGF-βR1 mRNA were detected in the less fit dropouts. As the mRNA was extracted from isolated PBMCs which include lymphocytes and monocytes, but not neutrophils or erythrocytes, it is very unlikely that the observed alterations in TGF-βRI mRNA are directly caused by varying neutrophil counts between groups. However, due to the pleiotropic effects of TGF-β, it is difficult to interpret the clinical implication of these findings. While TGF-β signalling is essential for regulatory T (T_{reg}) cell maturation and immune homeostasis [40, 41], excessive signalling may lead to dysregulated T_{Reg} cell activity and may underlie a diverse range of allergic diseases in humans [42, 43]. Drugs which aim to block the TGF-β signalling are under investigation in connection with several disorders such as hypertrophic cardiomyopathy [44], hypertension [45] or the Marfan syndrome [46] and are suggested to be valuable for treating food allergies [42]. Therefore, the observed alterations in TGF-βRI mRNA expression caused by resistance training could be beneficial in these situations, whereby future studies need to clarify whether lower mRNA levels de facto lead

Table 3 Intervention effects on leukocyte subpopulations and circulating inflammatory markers

	Baseline ($n = 67$)	3 months ($n = 67$)	6 months ($n = 67$)	P-value (time)
Leukocytes [x10^9 cells/L]				
CT ($n = 26$)	7.2 (4.9–10.3)**	7.2 (4.1–11.9)	7.1 (5.4–9.4)	0.440
RT ($n = 20$)	5.6 (3.1–9.1)	6.0 (3.2–8.9)	6.0 (3.3–9.8)*	**0.001**
RTS ($n = 21$)	7.0 (4.4–13.3)**	7.2 (4.5–11.7)**	7.1 (4.7–13.0)	0.586
Lymphocytes [cells/μl]				
CT ($n = 26$)	1985 (910–3510)	2090 (890–3980)	2250 (930–3540)	0.387
RT ($n = 20$)	1675 (830–3330)	1765 (912–3190)	1720 (1010–3430)	0.651
RTS ($n = 21$)	2255 (1460–4700)	2340 (1570–4680)	2190 (1640–4930)	0.810
Monocytes [cells/μl]				
CT ($n = 26$)	610 (72–950)	550 (300–780)	590 (400–910)	0.534
RT ($n = 20$)	520 (260–790)	475 (250–960)	510 (250–880)	0.104
RTS ($n = 21$)	585 (320–960)	490 (300–840)	545 (330–900)	0.404
Neutrophils [cells/μl]				
CT ($n = 26$)	4300 (2410–6630)**	4010 (1990–7420)	3910 (3110–5880)	0.247
RT ($n = 20$)	2876 (1530–6800)	3390 (1720–5880)	3520 (1800–7330)*	**0.011**
RTS ($n = 21$)	4030 (2430–9860)	3930 (1720–8730)	4290 (1664–8680)	0.368
Basophils [cells/μl]				
CT ($n = 26$)	40 (20–111)	30 (10–90)	30 (20–100)	**0.027**
RT ($n = 20$)	35 (10–90)	30 (10–100)	30 (10–80)	0.878
RTS ($n = 21$)	40 (10–90)	40 (10–90)	40 (10–80)	0.344
Eosinophils [cells/μl]				
CT ($n = 26$)	210 (36–448)	170 (80–470)	220 (90–330)	0.911
RT ($n = 20$)	160 (10–690)	186 (40–530)	200 (80–570)	0.381
RTS ($n = 21$)	248 (90–470)	195 (20–630)	260 (90–650)	0.137
hs-CRP [mg/L]				
CT ($n = 26$)	2.0 (0.5–4.8)	2.4 (0.2–5.5)	1.8 (0.3–8.5)	0.424
RT ($n = 20$)	1.9 (0.3–7.6)	2.4 (0.5–7.7)	2.0 (0.6–9.6)	0.645
RTS ($n = 21$)	1.8 (0.6–5.4)	2.1 (0.6–8.5)	1.6 (0.4–5.5)	0.135
TGF-β [μg/L]				
CT ($n = 26$)	36.0 (18.7–73.7)	39.8 (18.4–67.8)	40.8 (21.9–67.9)	0.953
RT ($n = 20$)	31.5 (16.7–50.0)	34.5 (18.3–59.7)	34.6 (12.7–57.3)	0.075
RTS ($n = 21$)	33.7 (21.0–51.2)	38.0 (22.9–50.5)	35.5 (22.1–52.1)	0.431

Data are expressed as medians (min–max); Differences over the time course were detected using the Friedman test and if significant, followed by Bonferroni-corrected post-hoc analyses (*$p < 0.05$ vs. baseline within respective study group). Differences between groups were analysed by Kruskal Wallis test, followed by Bonferroni-corrected post-hoc analyses (**$p < 0.05$ vs. RT group within respective time point; significant differences are marked in bold) *Abbreviations*: *CT* cognitive training, *RT* resistance training, *RTS* resistance training plus supplement, *hs-CRP* high sensitive C-reactive protein, *TGF-β* transforming growth factor-β

to a lower expression of the receptor on the surface of the respective cells and whether these changes are clinically relevant.

It has to be mentioned that the median TGF-βR1 mRNA expression was slightly lower in both, the RT and the RTS group (-14 % and -16 %, respectively), but reached significance only in the RT group. For physical performance (chair stand and arm lifting performance) similar gains could be detected in both groups. A recent systematic review demonstrated that combining protein supplementation with resistance training is effective for eliciting gains in fat-free mass among older adults, but does not appear to further increase muscle mass or strength, which was similar to our study [47]. In addition to proteins, the supplement in this study contained several vitamins. Based on previous analyses, this supplement aids to increase the uptake of vitamin D and folic acid as well as the plasma levels of vitamin B$_{12}$ and folic acid in erythrocytes [48, 49]. As some of the variables in this study (TGF-βRI mRNA expression, leukocyte

Table 4 Intervention effects on TGF-β signalling gene expression

	Baseline ($n = 67$)	3 months ($n = 67$)	6 months ($n = 67$)	P-value (time)
TGF-β/GAPDH [-]				
CT ($n = 21$)	0.47 (0.23–2.66)	0.47 (0.27–4.10)	0.44 (0.25–1.93)	0.772
RT ($n = 26$)	0.54 (0.26–2.30)	0.52 (0.16–2.63)	0.52 (0.23–2.30)	0.568
RTS ($n = 20$)	0.55 (0.06–1.63)	0.45 (0.15–2.20)	0.56 (0.09–1.32)	0.692
TGF-βRI/GAPDH [-]				
CT ($n = 21$)	1.99 (0.14–22.39)	1.62 (0.46–29.89)	1.97 (0.11–9.24)	0.717
RT ($n = 26$)	1.87 (0.69–9.54)	1.61 (0.34–9.21)*	1.77 (0.54–15.91)	**0.006**
RTS ($n = 20$)	1.95 (0.30–8.63)	1.63 (0.28–8.59)	2.38 (0.52–6.73)	0.801
TGF-βRII/GAPDH [-]				
CT ($n = 21$)	1.54 (0.66–7.79)	1.39 (0.68–9.17)	1.48 (0.67–6.32)	0.827
RT ($n = 26$)	1.60 (0.66–14.86)	1.59 (0.57–13.50)	1.67 (0.63–8.79)	0.296
RTS ($n = 20$)	1.58 (0.51–5.13)	1.73 (0.44–3.98)	1.95 (0.69–4.73)	0.331
miRNA-21 [copies/pg RNA]				
CT ($n = 21$)	3163 (343–4500)	2840 (276–5120)	2460 (1050–4700)	0.861
RT ($n = 26$)	2602 (57–4720)	2340 (758–5600)	2540 (330–5020)	0.368
RTS ($n = 20$)	2536 (845–4590)	2535 (353–4780)	2810 (1600–4630)	0.854

Data are expressed as medians (min–max); Differences were detected using the Friedman test and if significant, followed by Bonferroni-corrected post-hoc analyses (* $p < 0.05$ vs. baseline; significant differences are marked in bold)
Abbreviations: *CT* cognitive training, *RT* resistance training, *RTS* resistance training plus supplement, *TGF-β* transforming growth factor-β, *TGF-βR* TGF-β receptor, *GAPDH* glyceraldehyde 3-phosphate dehydrogenase, *miR-21* microRNA-21

numbers, 6MWT) were altered in the RT but not in the RTS group, it seems that the supplement prevented some of the responses to exercise. There is an ongoing discussion whether antioxidant supplementation may even blunt an exercise-induced training effect [50]. Evidence indicates that reactive oxygen species modulate TGF-β signalling. In turn, TGF-β increases the production of reactive oxygen species and suppresses antioxidant enzymes [51]. Therefore, it cannot be excluded that rigorous scavenging of free radicals impaired the TGF-β pathway response in the RTS group.

A reduction in TGF-βRI expression can be caused by either lower production or an increase in degradation of its mRNA. Post-transcriptional degradation of mRNAs often involves miRNAs specific for the respective target gene [12]. We have investigated miRNA-21 that has been shown to suppress TGF-βRI and TGF-βRII [16]. Additionally, circulating miRNA-21 levels are increased

in men with a low aerobic capacity as measured by maximal oxygen uptake [52]. However, its levels were not enhanced in RT or RTS groups, suggesting that other mechanisms and/or other miRNAs are involved in the down-regulation of TGF-βRI in PBMCs by strength training [53].

One striking secondary outcome of this study is that TGF-β, TGF-βRI and potentially TGF-βRII mRNA expression at the beginning of the study were higher in drop-outs compared with finishers, while miRNA-21 expression was lower. Drop-outs were less physically fit than finishers. We confirmed that age, sex, body composition and the presence of several co-morbidities might not contribute to this effect, but the proportion of subjects with hyperlipidaemia was higher among finishers.

Although this study provides interesting data on TGF-β-related parameters in the context of inflammaging and

Table 5 Association between physical performance at baseline and the response of TGF-β-related parameters

		Baseline performance			
		Handgrip strength	Chair stand test	Arm lifting test	6-MWT
Change (difference between 3 months and baseline)	Circulating TGF-β	-0.039	**-0.349***	**-0.352***	**-0.308***
	TGF-β/GAPDH	0.103	0.220	-0.051	0.199
	TGF-β RI/GAPDH	0.222	0.222	-0.148	0.148
	TGF-β RII/GAPDH	0.142	**0.254***	-0.027	0.204
	miRNA-21	0.201	0.143	-0.029	0.038

Data indicate Spearman-Rho correlation coefficients. * $p < 0.05$ (significant correlations are marked in bold)

Elastic band resistance training influences transforming growth factor-ß receptor I mRNA...

135

exercise training, we also have to highlight some of its limitations. Because the study is a secondary analysis of a previously conducted trial [22], it is obvious that the data need to be confirmed in a future prospective study. Similar to other studies, we were interested in additive effects of the nutritional supplement to strength training rather than investigating the effects of the supplement alone. While this approach represents a best practice model in exercise nutrition, this study design has a limited explanatory power in describing the observed differences between the RT and RTS groups. Finally, the number of female participants outnumbered the male participants by a significant degree. It also has to be mentioned that the proportion of community-dwelling men at an age of 85 years in Vienna is 34 % [54], but the proportion of male individuals in Viennese retirement homes is 19 % for this age group [55] making our study population representative in terms of sex distribution of institutionalised older individuals in Austria. Although it was not possible to perform sub-group analyses because of the low numbers of men, their exclusion led to the same conclusion, indicating that the data are reliable at least for older women.

Conclusions

Resistance training is beneficial, even in very old subjects, and potentially influences TGF-β signalling through altered receptor mRNA expression. Furthermore, adherence to the intervention was significantly related to alterations in the TGF-β pathway at baseline, but further information is needed to clearly understand the role of TGF-β in the context of inflammaging, resistance training and nutritional supplementation.

Methods

Participants and study design

The study was conducted using a randomised observer-blind design with three parallel groups, RT, RTS and CT. Briefly, participants were untrained, over 65 years of age with a Mini-Mental State Examination score of ≥23 and free of any medical conditions that would impair their participation in a resistance training study [56]. From a total of 117 participants in the VAAS, only those with available blood samples and a hs-CRP level below 10 mg/L at any time point were included in the current study (n = 88). A detailed description of the study design has been published previously [22].

Interventions

Interventions were conducted for 6 months, and measurements were obtained at baseline, after 3 and 6 months. Twice a week, RT and RTS groups performed supervised progressive resistance training without using any equipment other than elastic bands and their own body weight.

Each exercise session consisted of a general warm-up of 10 min, followed by a resistance training session (35–40 min) incorporating one to two exercises for each of the six main muscle groups (legs, back, abdomen, chest, shoulder and arms), and was completed by a cool-down routine. Following an adaptation phase of 4 weeks using low external resistance (yellow Thera-Band®, 1 set of 15 repetitions per exercise with a higher resistance only if the subject was obviously unchallenged) exercise intensity was progressively increased by changing the Thera-Band® from yellow to red and further to black. Additionally, the exercise volume was enhanced by increasing the number of sets from one to two. Rate of progression was based on individual improvements (band colour was changed if participant would have been able to perform two more repetitions in the second set. A detailed description has been provided previously [22]. Additionally to the exercises, participants from the RTS group were encouraged to drink a supplement that was distributed every morning as well as directly after the resistance training (in total nine times per week). One portion consisted of 20.7 g protein (55 En %; 19.7 g whey protein containing more than 10 g essential amino acids including 3 g leucine), 9.4 g carbohydrates (25 En %), 3.0 g fat (18 En %), 1.2 g fibre (2 En %), various vitamins such as 800 IU (20 µg) vitamin D, minerals and trace elements (FortiFit; Nutricia GmbH, Vienna, Austria). Total energy per drink was 150 kcal. Intake of the nutritional supplement was controlled at breakfast as well as after each training session. The CT group served as a control group and performed activities based on cognitive tasks (memory training) and coordinative tasks (such as manual dexterity) twice weekly to provide a timely effort which was equal to those of the RT and RTS groups, respectively [22, 57].

Determination of body composition, physical fitness and health

Standing height was assessed using a commercial stadiometer (Seca, Hamburg, Germany), Body mass was evaluated with a digital scale (BWB 700; Tanita, Amsterdam, Netherlands) to the nearest 0.1 kg with subjects lightly dressed and barefoot. BMI was calculated by dividing the body mass in kilograms by height in meters squared. To measure strength of the upper extremities, participants performed two trials of an isometric handgrip strength test (kg) using a dynamometer (JAMAR compatible handgrip dynamometer adapted to handle various hand sizes) in a sitting position with an angle of 90° in the elbow [58]. Functional performance of the lower extremities was measured by a chair stand test, and that of the upper extremities by an arm-lifting test as described previously [22, 59]. Aerobic capacity was assessed by the 6MWT conducted on a 30-m shuttle track [60].

Global cognitive function was determined by the Mini-Mental State Examination [61]. Co-morbidities (hyperlipidaemia, hypertension, osteoporosis, cardiac diseases, history of cancer and diabetes mellitus) were determined at the medical entrance examination. Adiposity was defined by a BMI of >30 kg/m^2 according to the World Health Organization criteria.

Blood sampling and analyses

After overnight fasting, venous blood samples were obtained in a resting state between 06:30 and 08:00 using Z serum Clot Activator collection tubes (Vacuette®; Greiner Bio-One GmbH, Kremsmünster, Austria) to analyse circulating TGF-β and hs-CRP, EDTA tubes (Vacuette®; Greiner Bio-One GmbH) to determine leukocyte subpopulations and BD Vacutainer® CPT Tubes (Becton, Dickenson and Company, Schwechat, Austria) containing ~130 IU Na-Heparin and 2 mL Ficoll™ to isolate PBMCs.

Hs-CRP was quantified on a Cobas 8000 (Roche Diagnostics, Vienna, Austria). Leukocyte subpopulations were determined by flow cytometric analyses on a XE-2100 automated hematology system (Sysmex Austria GmbH, Vienna, Austria). TGF-β was analysed using a commercially available DuoSet development kit to perform an enzyme-linked immunosorbent assay (DY240; R&D Systems, Abingdon, UK) following the manufacturer's instructions including plasma activation by acidification (pH 2) by adding hydrochloric acid (final concentration: 0.1 mmol/L) and neutralisation with sodium hydroxide (final concentration: 0.12 mmol/L) before measurement.

PBMCs were separated from red blood cells and neutrophils using BD Vacutainer® CPT Tubes (Becton Dickinson Austria, Vienna, Austria). The obtained pellet was carefully resuspended in 700 μL QIAzol Lysis Reagent (Qiagen, Hilden, Germany) and stored at −80 °C until analysis.

Total RNA including small RNAs was isolated using a miRNeasy Mini Kit (Qiagen, Hilden, Germany) following the supplier's protocol. To prepare a miRNA-enriched fraction separated from the larger RNAs (>200 nt), we used an RNeasy MinElute Cleanup Kit (Qiagen). Reverse transcription of the miRNA-enriched fraction was performed using a miScript II RT Kit (Qiagen), whereas larger RNAs were reverse transcribed using a QuantiTect Reverse Transcription Kit (Qiagen).

TGF-β, TGF-βRI and TGF-βRII mRNA levels were determined using the respective primer pairs [Hs_TGFB1_1 (QT00000728), Hs_TGFBR1_1 (QT00083412) and Hs_TGFBR2_1 (QT00014350); Qiagen] in conjunction with a QuantiTect SYBR Green PCR kit (Qiagen). In addition, glyceraldehyde-3-phosphate dehydrogenase [Hs_GAPDH_2 (QT01192646)] served as the endogenous control to normalise the data. Quantification was performed on an Applied Biosystems® 7500 Real-Time PCR System.

MiRNA-21 expression levels were detected using a miScript Primer Assay specific for miRNA-21 [hs_miR-21_2 (MS00009079); Qiagen]. Quantification was performed on the Applied Biosystems® 7500 Real-Time PCR System.

Statistical analyses

Data acquisition and processing were performed using commercial software (IBM SPSS 20). The Shapiro–Wilk test was used to test for a normal distribution. Because most of the variables were not distributed normally, the non-parametric Mann-Whitney U-test or the Kruskal-Wallis test were used to compare two or more independent groups, whereas the Friedman test was applied to detect changes over time in different intervention groups. To avoid bias by multiple testing, the results were Bonferroni-corrected for post-hoc analyses. Correlations between variables were identified by Spearman's rank correlation coefficient. Data are shown as the median (minimum–maximum). Statistical significance was set at $p < 0.05$.

Abbreviations
BMI, body mass index; CT, cognitive training; GAPDH, glyceraldehyde 3-phosphate dehydrogenase; hs-CRP, high sensitive C-reactive protein; IL-6, interleukin-6; miRNA, microRNAv; PBMCs, peripheral mononuclear cells; RT, resistance training; RTS, resistance training plus nutritional supplementation; TGF-β, transforming growth factor-β; TGF-βR, TGF-β receptor; TNF-α, tumour necrosis factor-α; T$_{reg}$, regulatory T cells; VAAS, Vienna Active Ageing Study

Acknowledgements
Not applicable.

Funding
The study was conducted with internal financial support from the University of Vienna, which enabled the establishment of the Research Platform "Active Ageing" as a means to foster interdisciplinary research. The University of Vienna was neither involved in designing the study nor in collecting, analysing and interpreting the data.

Authors' contributions
BSH, MH, SO, BF and TW were responsible for data acquisition, data analysis and interpretation of the data. BSH drafted the manuscript. EMS, MQ and NB were responsible for all medical aspects in the study. BW and KHW were involved in the conception and design of the study. BW supervised all aspects of laboratory analyses. All authors were involved in revising the manuscript and approved the final version.

Competing interests
The authors declare that they have no competing interests.

Author details
[1]Research Platform Active Ageing, University of Vienna, Althanstraße 14, 1090 Vienna, Austria. [2]Department of Sports and Exercise Physiology, Centre for Sport Science and University Sports, University of Vienna, Auf der Schmelz 6, 1150 Vienna, Austria. [3]Karl Landsteiner Institute for Remobilization and Functional Health/Institute for Physical Medicine and Rehabilitation, Kaiser Franz Joseph Hospital, Social Medical Centre - South, Kundratstrasse 3, 1100 Vienna, Austria. [4]Department of Nutritional Sciences, Faculty of Life Sciences, University of Vienna, Althanstraße 14, 1090 Vienna, Austria.

References

1. World Health Organization. World report on ageing and health. Luxembourg. 2015. http://apps.who.int/iris/bitstream/10665/186463/1/9789240694811_eng.pdf?ua=1. Accessed 29 June 2016.
2. Pera A, Campos C, Lopez N, Hassouneh F, Alonso C, Tarazona R, et al. Immunosenescence: Implications for response to infection and vaccination in older people. Maturitas. 2015;82(1):50–5. doi:10.1016/j.maturitas.2015.05.004.
3. Pawelec G, Goldeck D, Derhovanessian E. Inflammation, ageing and chronic disease. Curr Opin Immunol. 2014;29:23–8. doi:10.1016/j.coi.2014.03.007.
4. Ceco E, McNally EM. Modifying muscular dystrophy through transforming growth factor-beta. FEBS J. 2013;280(17):4198–209. doi:10.1111/febs.12266.
5. Romano M, Guagnano MT, Pacini G, Vigneri S, Falco A, Marinopiccoli M, et al. Association of inflammation markers with impaired insulin sensitivity and coagulative activation in obese healthy women. J Clin Endocrinol Metab. 2003;88(11):5321–6. doi:10.1210/jc.2003-030508.
6. Agarwal I, Glazer NL, Barasch E, Biggs ML, Djousse L, Fitzpatrick AL, et al. Fibrosis-related biomarkers and incident cardiovascular disease in older adults: the cardiovascular health study. Circ Arrhythm Electrophysiol. 2014;7(4):583–9. doi:10.1161/CIRCEP.114.001610.
7. Pfeiffer A, Middelberg-Bisping K, Drewes C, Schatz H. Elevated plasma levels of transforming growth factor-beta 1 in NIDDM. Diabetes Care. 1996;19(10):1113–7.
8. Esmatjes E, Flores L, Lario S, Claria J, Cases A, Inigo P, et al. Smoking increases serum levels of transforming growth factor-beta in diabetic patients. Diabetes Care. 1999;22(11):1915–6.
9. Lin Y, Nakachi K, Ito Y, Kikuchi S, Tamakoshi A, Yagyu K, et al. Variations in serum transforming growth factor-beta1 levels with gender, age and lifestyle factors of healthy Japanese adults. Dis Markers. 2009;27(1):23–8. doi:10.3233/DMA-2009-0643.
10. Blank U, Karlsson S. TGF-beta signaling in the control of hematopoietic stem cells. Blood. 2015;125(23):3542–50. doi:10.1182/blood-2014-12-618090.
11. Lewis BP, Burge CB, Bartel DP. Conserved seed pairing, often flanked by adenosines, indicates that thousands of human genes are microRNA targets. Cell. 2005;120(1):15–20. doi:10.1016/j.cell.2004.12.035.
12. Guo H, Ingolia NT, Weissman JS, Bartel DP. Mammalian microRNAs predominantly act to decrease target mRNA levels. Nature. 2010;466(7308):835–40. doi:10.1038/nature09267.
13. Griffiths-Jones S. miRBase: the microRNA sequence database. Methods Mol Biol. 2006;342:129–38. doi:10.1385/1-59745-123-1:129.
14. Kozomara A, Griffiths-Jones S. miRBase: annotating high confidence microRNAs using deep sequencing data. Nucleic Acids Res. 2014;42(Database issue):D68–73. doi:10.1093/nar/gkt1181.
15. Kumarswamy R, Volkmann I, Thum T. Regulation and function of miRNA-21 in health and disease. RNA Biol. 2011;8(5):706–13. doi:10.4161/rna.8.5.16154.
16. Olivieri F, Spazzafumo L, Santini G, Lazzarini R, Albertini MC, Rippo MR, et al. Age-related differences in the expression of circulating microRNAs: miR-21 as a new circulating marker of inflammaging. Mech Ageing Dev. 2012;133(11-12):675–85. doi:10.1016/j.mad.2012.09.004.
17. Ando Y, Yang GX, Kenny TP, Kawata K, Zhang W, Huang W, et al. Overexpression of microRNA-21 is associated with elevated pro-inflammatory cytokines in dominant-negative TGF-beta receptor type II mouse. J Autoimmun. 2013;41:111–9. doi:10.1016/j.jaut.2012.12.013.
18. Mathur N, Pedersen BK. Exercise as a mean to control low-grade systemic inflammation. Mediators Inflamm. 2008;2008:109502. doi:10.1155/2008/109502.
19. Ryan AS, Ge S, Blumenthal JB, Serra MC, Prior SJ, Goldberg AP. Aerobic exercise and weight loss reduce vascular markers of inflammation and improve insulin sensitivity in obese women. J Am Geriatr Soc. 2014;62(4):607–14. doi:10.1111/jgs.12749.
20. Mikkelsen UR, Couppe C, Karlsen A, Grosset JF, Schjerling P, Mackey AL, et al. Life-long endurance exercise in humans: circulating levels of inflammatory markers and leg muscle size. Mech Ageing Dev. 2013;134(11-12):531–40. doi:10.1016/j.mad.2013.11.004.
21. Peterson MD, Sen A, Gordon PM. Influence of resistance exercise on lean body mass in aging adults: a meta-analysis. Med Sci Sports Exerc. 2011;43(2):249–58. doi:10.1249/MSS.0b013e3181eb6265.
22. Oesen S, Halper B, Hofmann M, Jandrasits W, Franzke B, Strasser EM, et al. Effects of elastic band resistance training and nutritional supplementation on physical performance of institutionalised elderly - A randomized controlled trial. Exp Gerontol. 2015;72:99–108. doi:10.1016/j.exger.2015.08.013.
23. Phillips MD, Patrizi RM, Cheek DJ, Wooten JS, Barbee JJ, Mitchell JB. Resistance training reduces subclinical inflammation in obese, postmenopausal women. Med Sci Sports Exerc. 2012;44(11):2099–110. doi:10.1249/MSS.0b013e3182644984.
24. Bruunsgaard H, Bjerregaard E, Schroll M, Pedersen BK. Muscle strength after resistance training is inversely correlated with baseline levels of soluble tumor necrosis factor receptors in the oldest old. J Am Geriatr Soc. 2004;52(2):237–41.
25. Wanderley FA, Moreira A, Sokhatska O, Palmares C, Moreira P, Sandercock G, et al. Differential responses of adiposity, inflammation and autonomic function to aerobic versus resistance training in older adults. Exp Gerontol. 2013;48(3):326–33. doi:10.1016/j.exger.2013.01.002.
26. Hofmann M, Schober-Halper B, Oesen S, Franzke B, Tschan H, Bachl N, et al. Effects of elastic band resistance training and nutritional supplementation on muscle quality and circulating muscle growth and degradation factors of institutionalized elderly women - the Vienna Active Ageing Study (VAAS). Eur J Appl Physiol. 2016. doi:10.1007/s00421-016-3344-8.
27. Halper B, Hofmann M, Oesen S, Franzke B, Stuparits P, Vidotto C, et al. Influence of age and physical fitness on miRNA-21, TGF-beta and its receptors in leukocytes of healthy women. Exerc Immunol Rev. 2015;21:154–63.
28. Brinkley TE, Leng X, Miller ME, Kitzman DW, Pahor M, Berry MJ, et al. Chronic inflammation is associated with low physical function in older adults across multiple comorbidities. J Gerontol Ser A, Biol Sci Med Sci. 2009;64(4):455–61. doi:10.1093/gerona/gln038.
29. Mavros Y, Kay S, Simpson KA, Baker MK, Wang Y, Zhao RR, et al. Reductions in C-reactive protein in older adults with type 2 diabetes are related to improvements in body composition following a randomized controlled trial of resistance training. J Cachex Sarcopenia Muscle. 2014;5(2):111–20. doi:10.1007/s13539-014-0134-1.
30. Jahromi AS, Zar A, Ahmadi F, Krustrup P, Ebrahim K, Hovanloo F, et al. Effects of Endurance Training on the Serum Levels of Tumour Necrosis Factor-alpha and Interferon-gamma in Sedentary Men. Immune Netw. 2014;14(5):255–9. doi:10.4110/in.2014.14.5.255.
31. Wang CH, Chung MH, Chan P, Tsai JC, Chen FC. Effects of endurance exercise training on risk components for metabolic syndrome, interleukin-6, and the exercise capacity of postmenopausal women. Geriatr Nurs. 2014;35(3):212–8. doi:10.1016/j.gerinurse.2014.02.001.
32. Czarkowska-Paczek B, Zendzian-Piotrowska M, Bartlomiejczyk I, Przybylski J, Gorski J. The influence of physical exercise on the generation of TGF-beta1, PDGF-AA, and VEGF-A in adipose tissue. Eur J Appl Physiol. 2011;111(5):875–81. doi:10.1007/s00421-010-1693-2.
33. Sallam N, Laher I. Exercise Modulates Oxidative Stress and Inflammation in Aging and Cardiovascular Diseases. Oxid Med Cell Longev. 2016;2016:7239639. doi:10.1155/2016/7239639.
34. Donnelly JE, Blair SN, Jakicic JM, Manore MM, Rankin JW, Smith BK, et al. American College of Sports Medicine Position Stand. Appropriate physical activity intervention strategies for weight loss and prevention of weight regain for adults. Med Sci Sports Exerc. 2009;41(2):459–71. doi:10.1249/MSS.0b013e3181949333.
35. Miller PE, Alexander DD, Perez V. Effects of whey protein and resistance exercise on body composition: a meta-analysis of randomized controlled trials. J Am Coll Nutr. 2014;33(2):163–75. doi:10.1080/07315724.2013.875365.
36. Touvra AM, Volaklis KA, Spassis AT, Zois CE, Douda HD, Kotsa K, et al. Combined strength and aerobic training increases transforming growth factor-beta1 in patients with type 2 diabetes. Hormones (Athens). 2011;10(2):125–30.
37. Perreault K, Courchesne-Loyer A, Fortier M, Maltais M, Barsalani R, Riesco E, et al. Sixteen weeks of resistance training decrease plasma heat shock protein 72 (eHSP72) and increase muscle mass without affecting high sensitivity inflammatory markers' levels in sarcopenic men. Aging Clin Exp Res. 2015. doi:10.1007/s40520-015-0411-7.
38. Gumucio JP, Sugg KB, Mendias CL. TGF-beta superfamily signaling in muscle and tendon adaptation to resistance exercise. Exerc Sport Sci Rev. 2015;43(2):93–9. doi:10.1249/JES.0000000000000041.
39. Bautmans I, Njemini R, Vasseur S, Chabert H, Moens L, Demanet C, et al. Biochemical changes in response to intensive resistance exercise training in the elderly. Gerontology. 2005;51(4):253–65. doi:10.1159/000085122.
40. Sledzinska A, Hemmers S, Mair F, Gorka O, Ruland J, Fairbairn L, et al. TGF-beta signalling is required for CD4(+) T cell homeostasis but dispensable for regulatory T cell function. PLoS Biol. 2013;11(10):e1001674. doi:10.1371/journal.pbio.1001674.

41. Li MO, Sanjabi S, Flavell RA. Transforming growth factor-beta controls development, homeostasis, and tolerance of T cells by regulatory T cell-dependent and -independent mechanisms. Immunity. 2006;25(3):455–71. doi:10.1016/j.immuni.2006.07.011.

42. Frischmeyer-Guerrerio PA, Guerrerio AL, Oswald G, Chichester K, Myers L, Halushka MK, et al. TGFbeta receptor mutations impose a strong predisposition for human allergic disease. Sci Transl Med. 2013;5(195): 195ra94. doi:10.1126/scitranslmed.3006448.

43. Bordon Y. Asthma and allergy: TGFbeta–too much of a good thing? Nat Rev Immunol. 2013;13(9):618–9. doi:10.1038/nri3519.

44. Lim DS, Lutucuta S, Bachireddy P, Youker K, Evans A, Entman M, et al. Angiotensin II blockade reverses myocardial fibrosis in a transgenic mouse model of human hypertrophic cardiomyopathy. Circulation. 2001;103(6):789–91.

45. Lavoie P, Robitaille G, Agharazii M, Ledbetter S, Lebel M, Lariviere R. Neutralization of transforming growth factor-beta attenuates hypertension and prevents renal injury in uremic rats. J Hypertens. 2005;23(10):1895–903.

46. Habashi JP, Judge DP, Holm TM, Cohn RD, Loeys BL, Cooper TK, et al. Losartan, an AT1 antagonist, prevents aortic aneurysm in a mouse model of Marfan syndrome. Science. 2006;312(5770):117–21. doi:10.1126/science.1124287.

47. Finger D, Goltz FR, Umpierre D, Meyer E, Rosa LH, Schneider CD. Effects of protein supplementation in older adults undergoing resistance training: a systematic review and meta-analysis. Sports Med. 2015;45(2):245–55. doi:10.1007/s40279-014-0269-4.

48. Franzke B, Halper B, Hofmann M, Oesen S, Jandrasits W, Baierl A, et al. The impact of six months strength training, nutritional supplementation or cognitive training on DNA damage in institutionalised elderly. Mutagenesis. 2015;30(1):147–53. doi:10.1093/mutage/geu074.

49. Franzke B, Halper B, Hofmann M, Oesen S, Pierson B, Cremer A, et al. The effect of six months of elastic band resistance training, nutritional supplementation or cognitive training on chromosomal damage in institutionalized elderly. Exp Gerontol. 2015;65:16–22. doi:10.1016/j.exger.2015.03.001.

50. Peternelj TT, Coombes JS. Antioxidant supplementation during exercise training: beneficial or detrimental? Sports Med. 2011;41(12):1043–69. doi:10.2165/11594400-000000000-00000.

51. Liu RM, Desai LP. Reciprocal regulation of TGF-beta and reactive oxygen species: A perverse cycle for fibrosis. Redox Biol. 2015;6:565–77. doi:10.1016/j.redox.2015.09.009.

52. Bye A, Rosjo H, Aspenes ST, Condorelli G, Omland T, Wisloff U. Circulating microRNAs and aerobic fitness–the HUNT-Study. PLoS One. 2013;8(2):e57496. doi:10.1371/journal.pone.0057496.

53. Stolzenburg LR, Wachtel S, Dang H, Harris A. miR-1343 attenuates pathways of fibrosis by targeting the TGF-beta receptors. Biochem J. 2016;473(3):245–56. doi:10.1042/BJ20150821.

54. Statistik Austria. 2015. Statistik des Bevölkerungsstandes. http://www.statistik.at/web_de/statistiken/menschen_und_gesellschaft/bevoelkerung/bevoelkerungsstruktur/bevoelkerung_nach_alter_geschlecht/023468.html. Accessed 29 June 2016.

55. Bader E, Graumann G, Hacker M, Heissenberger C, Honeder M, Koblinger N, Krb W, Nutz W, Redolfi T, Scheidl A, Schlöss R, Stieb H, Warmuth H. Geschäftsbericht der Häuser zum Leben. 2013. http://www.kwp.at/pics/web/Dokumente/KWP_gesamt_web_low.pdf. Accessed 29 June 2016.

56. Williams MA, Haskell WL, Ades PA, Amsterdam EA, Bittner V, Franklin BA, et al. Resistance exercise in individuals with and without cardiovascular disease: 2007 update: a scientific statement from the American Heart Association Council on Clinical Cardiology and Council on Nutrition, Physical Activity, and Metabolism. Circulation. 2007;116(5):572–84. doi:10.1161/CIRCULATIONAHA.107.185214.

57. Gatterer G, Croy A. Geistig fit ins Alter. Vienna: Springer; 2004.

58. Mijnarends DM, Meijers JM, Halfens RJ, ter Borg S, Luiking YC, Verlaan S, et al. Validity and reliability of tools to measure muscle mass, strength, and physical performance in community-dwelling older people: a systematic review. J Am Med Dir Assoc. 2013;14(3):170–8. doi:10.1016/j.jamda.2012.10.009.

59. Jones CJ, Rikli RE, Beam WC. A 30-s chair-stand test as a measure of lower body strength in community-residing older adults. Res Q Exerc Sport. 1999; 70(2):113–9. doi:10.1080/02701367.1999.10608028.

60. Steffen TM, Hacker TA, Mollinger L. Age- and gender-related test performance in community-dwelling elderly people: Six-Minute Walk Test, Berg Balance Scale, Timed Up & Go Test, and gait speeds. Phys Ther. 2002;82(2):128–37.

61. Folstein MF, Folstein SE, McHugh PR. "Mini-mental state". A practical method for grading the cognitive state of patients for the clinician. J Psychiatr Res. 1975;12(3):189–98.

TLR-6 SNP P249S is associated with healthy aging in nonsmoking Eastern European Caucasians - A cohort study

Lutz Hamann[1*], Jasmin Bustami[1], Leonid Iakoubov[2], Malgorzata Szwed[3], Malgorzata Mossakowska[4], Ralf R. Schumann[1] and Monika Puzianowska-Kuznicka[3,5]

Abstract

Background: To investigate mechanisms that determine healthy aging is of major interest in the modern world marked by longer life expectancies. In addition to lifestyle and environmental factors genetic factors also play an important role in aging phenotypes. The aged immune system is characterized by a chronic micro-inflammation, known as *inflamm-aging*, that is suspected to trigger the onset of age-related diseases such as cardiovascular disease, Alzheimer's disease, cancer, and Diabetes Mellitus Type 2 (DMT2). We have recently shown that a Toll-like receptor 6 variant (P249S) is associated with susceptibility to cardiovascular disease and speculated that this variant may also be associated with healthy aging in general by decreasing the process of *inflamm-aging*.

Results: Analyzing the PolSenior cohort we show here that nonsmoking S allele carriers are significantly protected from age-related diseases ($P = 0.008$, OR: 0.654). This association depends not only on the association with cardiovascular diseases ($P = 0.018$, OR: 0.483) for homozygous S allele carriers, but is also driven by a protection from Diabetes Mellitus type 2 ($P = 0.010$, OR: 0.486) for S allele carriers. In addition we detect a trend but no significant association of this allele with inflamm-aging in terms of baseline IL-6 levels.

Conclusion: We confirm our previous finding of the TLR-6 249S variant to be protective regarding cardiovascular diseases. Furthermore, we present first evidence of TLR-6 249S being involved in DMT2 susceptibility and may be in general associated with healthy aging possibly by reducing the process of inflamm-aging.

Keywords: Healthy aging, *Inflamm-aging*, Toll-like receptor 6, Polymorphism

Background

The process of successful aging and longevity is complex and far from being understood. Lifestyle, environment, and a limited aging-related impairment of the immune system (termed *immunosenescence*) are among the most important factors contributing to the healthy aging phenotype. The aged adaptive immune system is characterized by a decreased effectiveness due to decreased T- and B-cell responses and accumulation of functionally impaired memory lymphocytes [1]. Furthermore, the aged adaptive immune system is characterized by a dysregulation of T-cell subtypes, with a relative increase

of Th2 lymphocytes resulting in increased levels of Th2 cytokines [2]. The aged innate immune system is characterized by reduced functions of neutrophils, macrophages, NK cells, and dendritic cells [3]. In addition, an important feature of the aged immune system is a chronic low grade inflammatory state, also known as micro-inflammation or inflamm-aging, which has been suspected to trigger aging-associated diseases such as cardiovascular disease (CVD), diabetes mellitus type 2 (DMT 2), metabolic syndrome, and neurodegeneration [4]. The mechanisms inducing the process of inflamm-aging are multifactorial and not completely understood. One reason may be the dysregulation of T lymphocyte subtypes. An enhanced translocation of gut bacteria as well as an enhanced DNA-damage in the elderly, which both trigger the innate pro-inflammatory immune response, are also discussed [5–7]. Furthermore,

* Correspondence: lutz.hamann@charite.de
[1]Institute for Microbiology and Hygiene, Charité University Medical Center Berlin, Rahel-Hirsch-Weg 3, 10117 Berlin, Germany
Full list of author information is available at the end of the article

epigenetic changes in innate immune cells are discussed to be involved in inflamm-aging [8].

However, numerous genetic factors have also been proposed to influence aging. Several studies show that healthy aging and particularly longevity are highly heritable. For example, siblings of centenarians also have an enhanced probability for a longer healthy life [9, 10]. Genetic variations associated with the onset of age-related diseases such as atherosclerosis resulting in CVD, DMT 2, Alzheimer's Disease, and cancer may play a pivotal role in determining successful aging [11]. Among aging-associated diseases, CVD plays a crucial role regarding mortality in the middle-aged population of the Western world [12, 13]. Recently, we have shown that the Toll-like receptor (TLR)-6 SNP P249S is associated with the risk for CVD with the homozygous S/S variant protecting from CVD. We also speculated whether this SNP may influence successful aging in general [14].

It has been shown that aging is associated with the dysregulation of expression and signal transduction of a variety of innate immune receptors, among them TLRs [15]. TLRs are important receptors of the innate immune system recognizing "pathogen associated molecular patterns (PAMPs)" followed by the activation of the innate immune response [16]. Although the process of inflammation is fundamental for survival in terms of combating infections or coping with damaging agents, it is also an important cause of many aging-associated diseases such as atherosclerosis, DMT 2, cognitive decline, and cancer, since these diseases are all associated with chronic inflammation [17]. The inflammatory response is driven by a variety of signaling pathways, however, the transcription factor NFκB has been considered to be the master regulator of inflammation [18], and is also a central part of TLR signaling [16].

Since inflamm-aging seems to be one of the reasons for the development of aging-related diseases, we postulated previously that variations within the TLR-system that decrease the inflammatory response may lead to a decreased process of inflamm-aging and may be, therefore, beneficial in terms of healthy aging. First evidence for this hypothesis was given by the finding that such variations are overrepresented in healthy elderly subjects in comparison to healthy younger subjects [19]. Following this discovery, we here investigated a cohort of elderly Caucasians and show that in nonsmoking elderly subjects the TLR-6 SNP P249S is associated with healthy aging. Analysis of certain aging related diseases revealed a significant protective effect on CVD and DMT 2.

Methods
Study subjects
A sub-group of 1544 participants of the PolSenior program, the first ones for whom the complete medical records (including, among others, data on cardio-vascular and respiratory diseases, cancer, diabetes, stroke and cognitive impairment) and DNA samples were available at the beginning of current study, was analyzed. PolSenior was a multicenter, interdisciplinary project, designed to assess health and socio-economic status of the Polish Caucasians aged ≥65 years. Details of the PolSenior recruitment are described elsewhere [20]. Project participants completed a detailed questionnaire regarding their medical, social, and economic past and current health status, underwent an examination including elements of comprehensive geriatric assessment, and donated blood for biochemical and genetic analyses. Steady state IL-6 level were measured using ELISA method (R&D System, Minneapolis, MN, USA, sensitivity 0.04 pg/mL). Blood pressure was measured three times during the first and second visit using validated, automatic blood pressure measuring device (A&D UA 787, A&D Company Limited, Tokyo, Japan) in a seated position. The study subject was diagnosed as suffering from hypertension if his/her average blood pressure from these measurements was ≥ 140/90 mmHg, or the disease has been previously diagnosed and the patient was taking hypotensive drugs over the past two weeks. The study was approved by the Bioethics Commission of the Medical University of Silesia in Katowice. All participants gave a written, informed consent for participation in the study. All investigations were carried out in accordance with the ethical guidelines of the 1975 Declaration of Helsinki. Subjects with MMSE < 24, determined according to the Polish version of the Mini-Mental State Examination test, were classified as subjects with cognitive impairment. According to Akbaraly et al. we set IL-6 levels ≤1.0 ng/L as low, 1.1–2.0 ng/L as intermediate, and >2 ng/L as high [21]. Low IL-6 levels were used as reference in logistic regression analysis.

Genotyping
Genomic DNA was prepared by standard procedures from whole blood. Genotyping for TLR-6 SNP P249S (rs5743810) was performed by melting curve analysis as described previously [14]. Melting curve analysis was carried out employing primers gaaagactctgaccagg cat (forward), ctagtttattcgctatccaagtg (reverse), and FRET-hybridization probes: accagaggtccaaccttactgaa-FL and LC-red 640-ttaccctcaaccacatagaaacgacttgga resulting in melting points of 61, and 52 °C for the wild-type and the mutated allele, respectively.

Statistics
Binary logistic regression analyses, Mann–Whitney U-test, Kruskal-Wallis, and T-test have been performed employing the IBM SPSS Statistics software package (version 20.0, IBM, Munich, Germany).

Results

Association of common risk factors with age related diseases

First we analyzed whether common risk factors such as age, BMI, micro-inflammation (presented as IL-6 levels), smoking, and hypertension are associated with aging-related diseases in our cohort of elderly Caucasians by comparison of healthy subjects without any aging-related disease ($n = 517$), and subjects suffering from one or more aging-related diseases ($n = 1027$), e.g. CVD ($n = 496$), cancer ($n = 93$), lung disease ($n = 254$), DMT 2 ($n = 122$), and cognitive impairment ($n = 406$). Baseline characteristics of the cohort are shown in Table 1. As expected, increased age and BMI were strongly associated with the occurrence of aging-related diseases ($P < 0.001$ for both). Also inflamm-aging, determined by baseline IL-6 levels with levels ≤ 1 ng/L serving as reference and 1.1–2.0 ng/L as intermediate or >2 ng/L as high levels, could be shown to be a strong risk factor ($P = 0.016$ and $P < 0.001$, respectively). Hypertension, interestingly, failed to be a significant risk factor in our cohort. Surprisingly, current smoking revealed a significant "protective" effect ($P = 0.003$, OR: 0.586), whereas past smoking showed no association (Table 2). However, further analysis of the distribution of age and BMI in nonsmokers, past smokers, and current smokers revealed current smokers to be significantly younger and having a significantly lower BMI, which might account for the "protective" effect of current smoking (data not shown). Indeed, performing a multivariate analysis with inflamm-aging, age, BMI and smoking as risk factors revealed that micro-inflammation - presented as intermediate or high IL-6 levels -, age and BMI remained significant independent risk factors in our elderly cohort,

with P-values of 0.034, 0.001, 0.001, and 0.008, respectively. Past smoking and current smoking in a multivariate analysis failed to be significantly associated with aging-related diseases (Table 3).

The TLR-6 variant 249S/S is significantly associated with protection from aging-related diseases in non-smoking subjects

Having shown that common risk factors (with the exception of smoking) exhibited the expected association with aging-related diseases in our cohort, we next analyzed whether the TLR-6 P249S variation is also associated with such diseases. Analyzing the whole cohort by logistic regression, using the wild-type genotype as reference we failed to find any significant association. Correction for age, BMI and inflamm-aging was done by adding these factors as co-factors in the regression analysis (Table 4). Since in this population smokers are significantly younger and exhibit a significantly lower BMI the pattern of association of smoking with diseases could not be analyzed in detail, and in order to avoid further statistical problems, only non-smokers were selected for

Table 1 Baseline characteristic of the study subjects

PolSenior group	
N	1544
Age range	61–92
Mean age (SD)	76.76 (6.44)
Males/females	811/733
Mean BMI (SD)	28.46 (4.87)
Smoking: never/past/current (%)	849 (55.0)/534 (34.6)/152 (9.8)
Hypertension yes/no (%)	1167/372 (75.6/24.1)
Baseline IL-6 (ng/L)	3.21 (2.98)
Disease-free	517 (33.5)
CVD (%)	496 (32.1)
Cancer (%)	93 (6.0)
Lung disease (%)	254 (16.5)
DMT 2 (%)	122 (7.9)
Cognitive impairment (%)	406 (26.3)
TLR-6 PP/PS/SS (%)	615 (39.8)/718 (46.5)/211 (13.7)

Table 2 Association of common risk factors with aging-related diseases in the PolSenior group. Univariate analysis of common risk factors and aging related diseases

Risk factor		P-value	Mean (SD)
Age		<0.001	75.7 (6.6)/77.3 (6.3)
BMI		<0.001	27.9(4.8)/28.6 (4.9)
		P-value	OR (95 % CI)
IL-6	Intermediate	0.016	1.578 (1.088–2.289)
	High	<0.001	2.108 (1.472–3.020)
Smoking	Past	0.619	1.061 (0.841–1.338)
	Current	0.003	0.586 (0.413–0.831)
Hypertension		0.175	1.184 (0.928–1.512)

Age was analyzed by T-test and BMI was analyzed by Mann–Whitney U test. Micro-inflammation (IL-6), smoking and hypertension were analyzed by logistic regression with IL-6 levels ≤1 ng/L as reference and 1.1–2.0 ng/L (intermediate) and >2 ng/L (high) as predictors, as well as no smoking or no hypertension as reference

Table 3 Association of common risk factors with aging-related diseases in the PolSenior group. Multivariate analysis of common risk factors and aging-related diseases

Risk factor		P-value	OR (95 % CI)
Age		0.001	1.033 (1.014–1.052)
BMI		0.008	1.033 (1.009–1.058)
IL-6	Intermediate	0.034	1.507 (1.031–2.202)
	High	0.001	1.863 (1.286–2.700)
Smoking	Past	0.310	1.134 (0.890–1.446)
	Current	0.052	0.683 (0.465–1.003)

Analysis was done by logistic regression with IL-6 levels ≤1 ng/L as reference and 1.1–2.0 ng/L (intermediate) and >2 ng/L (high) as predictors for inflamm-aging, and no smoking as reference

Table 4 TLR-6 P249S is associated with healthy aging in non-smokers

Disease	Variant	P-value	OR (95 % CI)
All subjects			
Combined aging related diseases	P/P	-	-
	P/S	0.281	0.876 (0.689–1.114)
	S/S	0.273	0.825 (0.585–1.163)
	P/S + S/S	0.208	0.864 (0.689–1.085)
Non smokers			
Combined aging related diseases	P/P	-	-
	P/S	0.024	0.682 (0.489–0.951)
	S/S	0.018	0.566 (0.353–0.909)
	P/S + S/S	0.008	0.654 (0.477–0.897)

P-values and OR were determined by logistic regression using the wild type genotype as reference, and micro-inflammation (IL-6 level), age and BMI as co-factors. Subjects with a white blood cell count above 10.000/μl were excluded

Table 5 TLR-6 P249S is associated with CVD and DMT 2 in non-smokers

Disease	Variant	P-value	OR (95 % CI)
All subjects			
CVD	P/P	-	-
	P/S	0.188	0.770 (0.522–1.136)
	S/S	0.018	0.483 (0.265–0.882)
	P/S + S/S	0.061	0.702 (0.484–1.017)
Cancer	P/P	-	-
	P/S	0.416	0.745 (0.367–1.513)
	S/S	0.353	0.602 (0.207–1.756)
	P/S + S/S	0.318	0.710 (0.363–1.390)
Lung disease	P/P	-	-
	P/S	0.216	0.732 (0.446–1.201)
	S/S	0.509	0.793 (0.399–1.577)
	P/S + S/S	0.219	0.746 (0.467–1.191)
DMT 2	P/P	-	-
	P/S	0.007	0.443 (0.244–0.804)
	S/S	0.230	0.617 (0.281–1.356)
	P/S + S/S	0.010	0.486 (0.281–0.839)
Cognitive impairment	P/P	-	-
	P/S	0.284	0.794 (0.522–1.210)
	S/S	0.345	0.751 (0.415–1.360)
	P/S + S/S	0.232	0.784 (0.526–1.1168)
Combined aging related diseases, CVD excluded	P/P	-	-
	P/S	0.016	0.628 (0.431–0.915)
	S/S	0.116	0.656 (0.388–1.109)
	P/S + S/S	0.012	0.635 (0.445–0.906)

P-values and OR were determined by logistic regression using the wild type genotype as reference, and micro-inflammation (IL-6 level), age and BMI as co-factors. Subjects with a white blood cell count above 10.000/μl were excluded

association studies of TLR-6 polymorphism with aging-related diseases.

Comparing non-smoking healthy subjects ($n = 278$) with non-smoking diseased subjects ($n = 571$) we found a significant protective association of the TLR-6 P/S and TLR-6 S/S variants with aging-related diseases in general, $P = 0.024$, OR: 0.682 (95 % CI: 0.489–0.951) and $P = 0.018$, OR: 0.566 (95 % CI: 0.353–0.909), respectively. The protective effect for mutated allele carriers was still in effect when heterozygous and homozygous genotypes were combined, $P = 0.008$, OR: 0.654 (95 % CI: 0.477–0.897) (Table 4), which is compatible with the dominant model. No significant effects were found in formerly or currently smoking subjects, which, as stated above, may be due to the different age-distribution of these groups (data not shown). As shown in Table 5, a subgroup analysis of individual diseases revealed a significant protective effect of the TLR-6 S/S variant regarding CVD ($n = 255$), $P = 0.018$, OR: 0.483 (95 % CI: 0.265–0.882). Correction for age, BMI and inflamm-aging was done by adding these factors as co-factors in the regression analysis. Interestingly, the heterozygous P/S variant as well as the combined heterozygous and homozygous genotypes exhibited a significant protection regarding DMT 2 ($n = 79$), $P = 0.007$ OR: 0.443 (95 % CI: 0.244–0.804) and $P = 0.010$ OR: 0.486 (95 % CI: 0.281–0.839), respectively. For cancer ($n = 42$), lung disease ($n = 116$), and cognitive impairment ($n = 250$), no significant associations were found. Analysis of combined aging-related diseases with exclusion of CVD ($n = 309$) revealed significant protection for the TLR-6 P/S variant, $P = 0.016$ OR. 0.628 (95 % CI: 0.431–0.915) and the combined heterozygous and homozygous genotypes, $P = 0.012$, OR: 0.635 (95 % CI: 0.445–0.906) indicating a protective effect independent of the protection against CVD.

No association of TLR-6 6 P249S variation with baseline IL-6 levels

Since we have speculated previously that a beneficial effect of TLR SNPs may rely on a decreased process of inflamm-aging due to a reduced sensitivity of the innate immune system, we analyzed whether the TLR-6 P249S variant was associated with baseline levels of IL-6. To exclude current infections that could affect the level of IL-6, we excluded subjects with a white blood cell count above 10.000/μl. As shown in Table 6, baseline IL-6 levels are significantly higher in subjects suffering from one or more aging-related diseases in comparison to healthy subjects: 3.33 ng/L vs. 2.75 ng/L, $P > 0.000$. Although there is a trend for decreased IL-6 baseline levels in S allele carriers, P/P: 3.23 ng/L, P/S: 3.08 ng/L and S/S: 3.05 ng/L, this association is not significant, $P = 0.850$.

Table 6 TLR-6 P249S is not associated with baseline levels of IL-6

	IL-6 (ng/L, mean, SD)	P-value
Disease free	2.75 (2.60)	<0.001
Aging related diseases	3.33 (3.01)	
TLR-6 genotype		
P/P	3.23 (3.05)	0.850
P/S	3.08 (2.73)	
S/S	3.05 (2.93)	

P-values were determined by Mann–Whitney U test or Kruskal-Wallis test, subjects with white blood cells above 10.000/μl were excluded

Discussion

We have recently shown that TLR-6 P249S is associated with coronary artery disease, one of the most important aging-related diseases, and have speculated that this genetic variation may be also associated with healthy aging in general by decreasing the process of inflamm-aging due to decreased sensitivity of the innate immune response [14, 19]. Healthy, or successful aging is affected by a variety of factors including environmental factors, life style, micro-inflammation, and genetic factors that determine the occurrence, onset and course of aging-related diseases. Since most age-related diseases are associated with chronic inflammation [21], a sensitive immune system may be an example of antagonistic pleiotropy with beneficial effects at early age but adverse effects in later life since evolution optimizes for fitness, not for longevity [22]. By analyzing a middle-aged population-based cohort, exhibiting the typical distribution of aging-related diseases, we here confirmed our previous finding of TLR-6 P249S being associated with CVD and showed that this SNP is associated with healthy aging in non-smoking subjects of the PolSenior cohort. This positive association with healthy aging remains significant after exclusion of subjects suffering from CVD indicating a more general effect, not only restricted to CVD. Furthermore we present first evidence of this SNP to be also involved in DMT-2 and the process of inflamm-aging in non-smoking subjects.

We have currently no conclusive explanation why this effect could not be shown in smoking subjects. Although our study does not show smoking to be one of the strongest risk factors for aging-related diseases in individuals 65 years old and older, the effect of TLR-6 variants on healthy aging may nevertheless be masked by smoking. Such modifying effect of smoking has recently been reported for several genetic associations in age-related macular degeneration which are largely restricted to non-smokers [23]. One possible explanation could be that in our cohort smoking is associated with both, lower ager and lower BMI which in turn are associated

with the absence of aging-related diseases. The association of TLR-6 P249S with DMT 2 has not been shown before. However, since the number of non-smoking subjects with DMT 2 was rather low in our cohort ($n = 79$), and TLR-6 has not been found by GWAs for DMT 2, these findings have to be confirmed in larger studies [24].

Analyzing the whole cohort for common risk factors by multivariate regression analysis showed, as expected, increased age, BMI, and inflamm-aging to be strongly associated with the occurrence of aging-related diseases. Since we have previously speculated that less functional TLR variants decreasing the sensitivity of the innate immune system may dampen the process of inflamm-aging, we analyzed the association of TLR-6 P249S with baseline IL-6 levels. Although the S allele at position 249 of TLR-6 has been shown to decrease TLR-6 signaling [25], we could not find a significant effect on inflamm-aging. However, we could show a trend towards decreased IL-6 levels in S allele carriers. The failure of finding significant changes may potentially be explained by the fact that other pro-inflammatory cytokines such as TNF-α and IL-1β, the serum-levels of which were not available to us, may be more involved in the process of inflamm-aging as compared to IL-6. Recent data show that inflamm-aging is not simply the chronic increase of pro-inflammatory markers such as IL-6 and CRP. Inflamm-aging seem to be much more complex and is characterized by the simultaneous change in both pro- and anti- inflammatory markers [26]. Furthermore, repeated measurements of IL-6 levels, which were not available to us in this cohort are known to be more accurate in determining inflamm-aging [2]. Finally, the SNPs investigated by us may lead to changes in cytokines in certain tissues, which cannot be monitored by measuring serum levels.

On the other hand, comparing healthy subjects with diseased subjects, a strong correlation of increased IL-6 baseline levels and aging-related diseases was shown. This may be evidence for the fact that inflamm-aging is driven mainly by a dysregulated T lymphocyte subpopulation [2] and chronic stimulation of the innate immune system via TLRs does not play the dominant role.

Since the limitation of our study is relatively small sample number, especially in disease subgroups, our results require further investigation by independent studies.

Conclusion

In conclusion we confirm here our previous results of less functional TLR-6 variant 249S to protect from CVD. In addition we show here that this variant protects also from DMT-2 and is in general associated with healthy aging in the PolSenior cohort. Furthermore, we could show a trend for a decreased process of inflamm-aging by the TLR-6 249S allele as measured by IL-6 levels. However, the effect of TLR variants on the process of *inflamm-aging* needs to be confirmed by further studies.

Competing interests
The authors declare that they have no competing interests.

Authors' contributions
LH: Study design, statistic, writing the manuscript; JB: genotyping, LI: Study design; MS: DNA sampling; MM: DNA sampling; RS: critical reading and discussion of the manuscript, MP-K: Study design, writing and discussion of the manuscript, DNA sampling. All authors read and approved the final manuscript.

Acknowledgments
Financial support was provided by Charité - Universitätsmedizin Berlin (grant 2007-486), the Berliner Krebsgesellschaft e.V. (all to R.R.S), and by the Polish Ministry of Science and Higher Education grant PBZ-MEiN-9/2/2006 – K143/ P01/2007/1 (to M.P.K., M.S. and M.M.). We thank Inga Wyroslak for outstanding technical assistance.

Author details
[1]Institute for Microbiology and Hygiene, Charité University Medical Center Berlin, Rahel-Hirsch-Weg 3, 10117 Berlin, Germany. [2]Cellecta Inc, Mountain View, CA, USA. [3]Department of Human Epigenetics, Mossakowski Medical Research Centre, Polish Academy of Sciences, Warsaw, Poland. [4]Polsenior Project, International Institute of Molecular and Cell Biology, Warsaw, Poland. [5]Department of Geriatrics and Gerontology, Medical Centre of Postgraduate Education, Warsaw, Poland.

References

1. Weng NP. Aging of the immune system: how much can the adaptive immune system adapt? Immunity. 2006;24(5):495–9.
2. Michaud M, Balardy L, Moulis G, Gaudin C, Peyrot C, Vellas B, et al. Proinflammatory cytokines, aging, and age-related diseases. J Am Med Dir Assoc. 2013;14(12):877–82.
3. Shaw AC, Joshi S, Greenwood H, Panda A, Lord JM. Aging of the innate immune system. Curr Opin Immunol. 2010;22(4):507–13.
4. Cevenini E, Monti D, Franceschi C. Inflamm-ageing. Curr Opin Clin Nutr Metab Care. 2013;16(1):14–20.
5. Brenchley JM, Price DA, Schacker TW, Asher TE, Silvestri G, Rao S, et al. Microbial translocation is a cause of systemic immune activation in chronic HIV infection. Nat Med. 2006;12(12):1365–71.
6. Cavanagh MM, Weyand CM, Goronzy JJ. Chronic inflammation and aging: DNA damage tips the balance. Curr Opin Immunol. 2012;24(4):488–93.
7. Kim KA, Jeong JJ, Yoo SY, Kim DH. Gut microbiota lipopolysaccharide accelerates inflamm-aging in mice. BMC Microbiol. 2016;16(1):9.
8. Fulop T, Dupuis G, Baehl S, Le Page A, Bourgade K, Frost E, et al. From inflamm-aging to immune-paralysis: a slippery slope during aging for immune-adaptation. Biogerontology. 2015;17:147–57.
9. Atzmon G, Schechter C, Greiner W, Davidson D, Rennert G, Barzilai N. Clinical phenotype of families with longevity. J Am Geriatr Soc. 2004;52(2):274–7.
10. Perls TT, Wilmoth J, Levenson R, Drinkwater M, Cohen M, Bogan H, et al. Life-long sustained mortality advantage of siblings of centenarians. Proc Natl Acad Sci U S A. 2002;99(12):8442–7.
11. Barzilai N, Shuldiner AR. Searching for human longevity genes: the future history of gerontology in the post-genomic era. J Gerontol A Biol Sci Med Sci. 2001;56(2):M83–7.
12. Lozano R, Naghavi M, Foreman K, Lim S, Shibuya K, Aboyans V, et al. Global and regional mortality from 235 causes of death for 20 age groups in 1990 and 2010: a systematic analysis for the Global Burden of Disease Study 2010. Lancet. 2012;380(9859):2095–128.
13. Niccoli T, Partridge L. Ageing as a risk factor for disease. Curr Biol. 2012; 22(17):R741–52.
14. Hamann L, Koch A, Sur S, Hoefer N, Glaeser C, Schulz S, et al. Association of a common TLR-6 polymorphism with coronary artery disease - implications for healthy ageing? Immun Ageing. 2013;10(1):43.
15. Solana R, Tarazona R, Gayoso I, Lesur O, Dupuis G, Fulop T. Innate immunosenescence: effect of aging on cells and receptors of the innate immune system in humans. Semin Immunol. 2012;24(5):331–41.
16. Beutler B. Microbe sensing, positive feedback loops, and the pathogenesis of inflammatory diseases. Immunol Rev. 2009;227(1):248–63.
17. De Martinis M, Franceschi C, Monti D, Ginaldi L. Inflamm-ageing and lifelong antigenic load as major determinants of ageing rate and longevity. FEBS Lett. 2005;579(10):2035–9.
18. Perkins ND. Integrating cell-signalling pathways with NF-kappaB and IKK function. Nat Rev Mol Cell Biol. 2007;8(1):49–62.
19. Hamann L, Kupcinskas J, Berrocal Almanza LC, Skieceviciene J, Franke A, Nothlings U, et al. Less functional variants of TLR-1/-6/-10 genes are associated with age. Immun Ageing. 2015;12:7.
20. Bledowski P, Mossakowska M, Chudek J, Grodzicki T, Milewicz A, Szybalska A, et al. Medical, psychological and socioeconomic aspects of aging in Poland: assumptions and objectives of the PolSenior project. Exp Gerontol. 2011; 46(12):1003–9.
21. Akbaraly TN, Hamer M, Ferrie JE, Lowe G, Batty GD, Hagger-Johnson G, et al. Chronic inflammation as a determinant of future aging phenotypes. CMAJ. 2013;185(16):E763–70.
22. Vijg, J. and B.K. Kennedy: The Essence of Aging. Gerontology, 2015 [Epub ahead of print].
23. Naj AC, Scott WK, Courtenay MD, Cade WH, Schwartz SG, Kovach JL, et al. Genetic factors in nonsmokers with age-related macular degeneration revealed through genome-wide gene-environment interaction analysis. Ann Hum Genet. 2013;77(3):215–31.
24. McCarthy MI, Zeggini E. Genome-wide association studies in type 2 diabetes. Curr Diab Rep. 2009;9(2):164–71.
25. Shey MS, Randhawa AK, Bowmaker M, Smith E, Scriba TJ, de Kock M, et al. Single nucleotide polymorphisms in toll-like receptor 6 are associated with altered lipopeptide- and mycobacteria-induced interleukin-6 secretion. Genes Immun. 2010;11(7):561–72.
26. Morrisette-Thomas V, Cohen AA, Fulop T, Riesco E, Legault V, Li Q, et al. Inflamm-aging does not simply reflect increases in pro-inflammatory markers. Mech Ageing Dev. 2014;139:49–57.

Expression of cellular protective proteins SIRT1, HSP70 and SOD2 correlates with age and is significantly higher in NK cells of the oldest seniors

Lucyna Kaszubowska[1*], Jerzy Foerster[2], Jan Jacek Kaczor[3], Daria Schetz[4], Tomasz Jerzy Ślebioda[1] and Zbigniew Kmieć[1]

Abstract

Background: NK cells are key effector lymphocytes of innate immunity provided with constitutive cytolytic activity, however, their role in human ageing is not entirely understood. The study aimed to analyze the expression of proteins involved in cellular stress response sirtuin 1 (SIRT1), heat shock protein 70 (HSP70) and manganese superoxide dismutase (SOD2) in non-stimulated NK cells of the oldest seniors (n = 25; aged over 85; mean age 88 years) and compare with NK cells of the old (n = 30; aged under 85; mean age 76 years) and the young (n = 32; mean age 21 years) to find potential relationships between the level of expression of these proteins in NK cells and longevity. The concentration of carbonyl groups and 8-isoprostanes in NK cell lysates reflecting the level of oxidative stress was also measured.

Results: The group of the oldest seniors differed from the other age groups by significantly higher percentage of NK cells expressing SIRT1, HSP70 and SOD2. The concentration of both carbonyl groups and 8-isoprostanes in NK cell extracts remained within the normal range in all age groups. The percentage of NK cells with the expression of, respectively, SIRT1, HSP70 and SOD2 correlated positively with age. Some correlations between expression levels of particular protective proteins SIRT1, HSP70 and SOD2 were observed in the study population.

Conclusions: The increased expression of cellular protective proteins SIRT1, HSP70 and SOD2 in NK cells of the oldest seniors seems to correspond to longevity and the observed correlations may suggest the involvement of these proteins in establishing NK cell homeostasis specific for healthy ageing process.

Keywords: NK cells, Ageing, Immunosenescence, Seniors, SIRT1, HSP70, SOD2, Oxidative stress, Innate immunity

Background

The main function of NK cells is related to immune response against viral infections, tumor cells and intracellular pathogens. These lymphocytes reveal also some regulatory properties to activate other cells of both innate and adaptive immunity by secretion of cytokines and chemokines [20]. NK cells do not act in a constant manner but rather adapt to the temporary conditions of the cellular environment. They can display a form of antigen-specific immunologic memory demonstrating attributes of both innate and adaptive immunity [52]. Human NK cells consist of two functional subsets differing in the cell surface expression of CD56, i.e. immunoregulatory CD56[bright] cells, considered to be precursors to the cytotoxic NK CD56[dim] cells [18, 44]. These NK cell subsets are differentially affected by the process of ageing, i.e. more immature CD56[bright] cells are decreased whereas more differentiated CD56[dim] cells are expanded [18, 20, 31].

Ageing is associated with the up-regulation of the inflammatory responses caused by chronic antigenic stress and dysregulation of cytokine secretion with increased serum levels of pro-inflammatory cytokines IL-6 and

* Correspondence: lkras@gumed.edu.pl
[1]Department of Histology, Medical University of Gdańsk, Dębinki 1, Gdańsk PL-80-211, Poland
Full list of author information is available at the end of the article

TNF, increased level of C reactive protein and decreased concentration of anti-inflammatory cytokine IL-10 [8]. This phenomenon was referred to as "inflamm-aging" [17]. The ageing process is also accompanied by chronic oxidative stress that affects all regulatory body systems, including the immune system, and this phenomenon has been called "oxi-inflamm-aging" [14]. Oxidative stress can cause serious cell damage of cells, counteracted by the development of anti-oxidant protective systems that involve glutathione (GSH), glutathione S-transferase, glutathione peroxidase, glutathione reductase, catalase, and superoxide dismutases (MnSOD, CuZnSOD) [25]. Continuous low-dose oxidative stress during ageing results in adaptive responses based on the activation of NF-κB and subsequently superoxide dismutases (SODs) with a key role played by the mitochondrial manganese dismutase (SOD2). In this process also heat-shock proteins (HSP70) are induced to protect cells from stress-induced molecular damage [9]. HSP70 reveals distinct functions depending on its location. Intracellular HSP70 presents a cytoprotective, anti-apoptotic and anti-inflammatory function while extracellular HSP70 mediates pro-inflammatory immunological response via Toll-like receptors (TLRs) contributing to a link between innate and adaptive immune systems [3].

Sirtuins are evolutionary conserved proteins with deacetylase activity dependent on nicotinamide adenine nucleotide (NAD+) considered as histone deacetylases involved in the control of ageing and longevity, DNA repair, transcriptional silencing, apoptosis and cellular metabolism [47]. SIRT1 acetylates forkhead transcription factor class O (FOXO) upon peroxide stress and that results in the activation of SOD2 and subsequent reduction of the level of reactive oxygen species [21].

There are no literature data concerning changes in expression of SIRT1, SOD2 and HSP70 in NK cells in the process of ageing. Generally, a decline in function of chaperones in aged organisms was reported [2, 30, 40]. This tendency concerned also basal expression of HSP72 in human lymphocytes and monocytes or induced expression after heat shock [55]. Higher basal levels of HSP70 and several other families of HSP proteins in non-stimulated monocytes and lymphocytes of seniors suggested the maintenance of HSP system at activation state in the elderly [41]. Moreover, it was shown that elevated expression of HSPs was associated with longevity and their decreased levels corresponded to increased protein deterioration during ageing, loss of protein quality control, degeneration and cell death [11].

HSP proteins are expressed also on the cell surface and circulate in peripheral blood. PBMCs (Peripheral Blood Mononuclear Cells) are thought to be a main source of these circulating proteins [41]. The previous studies showed an apparent decrease in serum levels of HSP60 and

HSP70 during ageing [45]. Increased serum level of these proteins corresponded to inflammation process and frailty in seniors [42]. However, these data refer to HSP proteins released into plasma in response to a cellular stress by different types of PBMCs.

SIRT1 has been shown to play a major role in the determination of lifespan and stress resistance [6, 9, 49]. In humans levels of SIRT1, SIRT2 and SIRT3 were analyzed in sera of both frail and non-frail seniors and the lower circulating SIRT1 and SIRT3 levels were found to be a distinguishing marker of frailty [29].

SOD2 similarly to SIRT1 seems to play a role in longevity [46]. Experiments on mice with heterozygous deficiency of manganese superoxide dismutase (SOD2) demonstrated that SOD2 was involved in the regulation of "inflamm-aging" of the aged skin immune system. The impairment of SOD2 and reduction of its antioxidative capacities promoted proinflammatory effects through alteration of dendritic cells and T cell functions [50].

Despite the established role of HSP70, SIRT1 and SOD2 proteins in the ageing process [22, 39, 54], little is known about their contribution to healthy ageing of the immune system, and NK cells in particular. There are only few studies concerning this issue and they refer to monocytes [41], lymphocytes [23, 41] and granulocytes [28]. There was observed age-related raise in the basal level of HSP70 in monocytes and lymphocytes [41]. Previous study, however, showed a significant age-related decrease in HSP70 levels in lymphocytes [23]. Studies performed on neutrophils did not expose any significant age-dependent changes in HSP70 basal content in the cells [28]. Since NK cells are associated with the process of healthy ageing, the preservation of NK cell function until very advanced age may contribute to longevity [12, 18, 31]. Therefore, the aim of our study was to analyze the expression of cellular protective proteins in NK cells of the oldest seniors (over 85 years old), the old (aged under 85) and the young subjects (aged 19–24 years).

Methods
Participants
Eighty-seven volunteers aged between 19 and 94 years (63 women and 24 men) participated in this study. The exclusion criteria included: CRP > 5 mg/L, cancer, autoimmune disease, diabetes, infection, use of immunosuppressors, glucocorticoids or non-steroid anti-inflammatory drugs (NSAIDs); moderate to severe dementia assessed using the "Mini Mental State Examination" (MMSE below 23 points) [16]. Senior volunteers were also considered with geriatric conditions. Katz's scale was used to assess "Activities of Daily Living" (ADL) and only seniors with 5–6 points were enrolled to the study [26]. Senior volunteers were recruited among inhabitants of local senior houses

and young volunteers were students of Medical University of Gdańsk, Poland. The participants were subdivided into 3 groups including: 32 young subjects referred to as 'young' (mean age 21.0 ± 0.3 years, range 19–24 years, 23 women and 9 men); 30 seniors aged under 85 referred to as 'old' (mean age 75.6 ± 0.9 years, range 65–84 years, 20 women and 10 men) and 25 seniors at the age over 85 referred to as the 'oldest' (mean age 88.4 ± 0.5 years, range 85–94 years; 20 women and 5 men). All volunteers signed informed consent and the study received approval from Ethical Committee of Medical University of Gdańsk, Poland (225/2010).

Separation of peripheral blood mononuclear cells

Peripheral blood mononuclear cells (PBMCs) were isolated from venous blood samples collected in tubes with EDTA by conventional Ficoll-Uropoline density gradient centrifugation. PBMCs were then washed and resuspended in PBS-1% FBS solution.

Staining of surface and intracellular antigens for flow cytometry

Whole blood samples (0.1 ml) were aliquoted into flow cytometry tubes and CD3-FITC-conjugated (0.125 µg/ml; clone UCHT1) (BD Biosciences, San Jose, CA, USA) or CD3-PE-Cy7-conjugated (0.125 µg/ml; clone SK7) (BD Biosciences, San Jose, CA, USA), CD56-APC-conjugated (0.6 µg/ml; clone NCAM16.2) (BD Biosciences, San Jose, CA, USA) and Hsp70-PE-conjugated (1 µg/ml; clone N27F34) (Abcam, Cambridge, England) monoclonal antibodies were added for cell surface antigen staining. After 30 min of incubation in the dark at room temperature 2 ml of BD FACS Lysing Solution was added and samples were incubated for subsequent 10 min in the same conditions. Then cells were washed twice with 1 ml of BD Staining Buffer (PBS without Ca^{2+} and Mg^{2+}, 1% FBS, 0.09% sodium azide) and resuspended in 0.25 ml of Fixation/Permeabilization Solution for 20 min at 4 °C according to manufacturer's protocol (BD Cytofix/ Cytoperm Fixation/Permeabilization Kit). Cells were washed twice with 1 ml of BD Perm/Wash buffer and appropriate volumes of MnSOD-FITC-conjugated (1 µg/ ml; clone MnS-1) (eBioscience, San Diego, CA, USA), Hsp70-PE-conjugated (1 µg/ml; clone N27F34) (Abcam, Cambridge, England), SIRT1-Alexa Fluor 488 – conjugated (1 µg/ml; clone 19A7AB4) (Abcam, Cambridge, England), TNF-PE-Cy7- conjugated (0.125 µg/ml; clone MAb11) (BD Biosciences, San Jose, CA, USA) and IFN-γ-PE-conjugated (0.125 µg/ml; clone 4S.B3) (BD Biosciences, San Jose, CA, USA) monoclonal antibodies were added for staining of intracellular antigens according to the manufacturer's instructions. After 30 min of incubation in the dark at room temperature cells were washed twice with 1 ml of BD Perm/Wash buffer and resuspeded in Staining Buffer prior

to flow cytometric analysis. Samples were run on a BD FACSCalibur flow cytometer equipped with argon-ion laser (488 nm) and data were analyzed with BD CellQuest Pro software (BD Biosciences, San Jose, CA, USA) after acquiring 10,000 gated events (lymphocytes). NK cells were identified as CD3-CD56+ cells. Appropriate isotype controls for both surface and intracellular staining were also prepared. Staining and fixation procedure were carried out within 4 h after blood sample collection.

NK cell separation for measurement of protein carbonyl groups content and 8-isoprostanes level in cell lysates

NK cells ($CD3^-CD56^+$) were isolated from PBMCs by negative selection with the use of Human NK Cell Enrichment Kit and EasySep Magnet (Stemcell Technologies, Vancouver, Canada). PBMCs were incubated with EasySep Human NK Cell Enrichment Cocktail (a suspension of monoclonal antibodies bound in bispecific Tetrameric Antibody Complexes (TAC) directed against cell surface antigens on human blood cells: CD3, CD4, CD14, CD19, CD20, CD36, CD66b, CD123, HLA-DR, glycophorin A and dextran for 10 min, then vortexed for 30 s and incubated with EasySep D Magnetic Particles (a suspension of magnetic dextran iron particles) for subsequent 5 min. Then cells were resuspended in 2.5 ml of recommended medium (PBS with 2% FBS and 1 mM EDTA, Ca^{2+} and Mg^{2+} free), mixed gently and placed into the magnet. After 2.5 min the desired fraction was poured off into a new tube. Aliquots of the cell fractions were stained with appropriate volumes of CD56-PE- and CD3-PerCP-conjugated monoclonal antibodies (BD Biosciences, San Jose, CA, USA). After 30 min of incubation in the dark at room temperature cells were washed with 2 ml of BD CellWASH solution and finally 0.5 ml of BD CellFIX solution was added. Samples were stored at 4 °C up to 24 h until analyzed by flow cytometry to check the purity of the enriched NK cell fractions and all presented almost 95% purity.

Then, NK cell extracts were prepared with the use of Mammalian Cell & Tissue Extraction Kit (BioVision Research Products, Mountain View, CA, USA) according to the manufacturer's protocol. The total protein concentration of samples was determined with Bradford assay (Sigma - Aldrich, Saint Louis, MO, USA). Cell lysates were stored at -70 °C for further analysis. The content of protein carbonyl groups in NK cell extracts was measured with the BioCell PC Test Kit, an enzyme-linked immunosorbent assay (BioCell, Auckland, New Zealand). Samples were prepared for ELISA procedure according to the manufacturer's protocol. Absorbances were measured at 450 nm with Bio-Rad plate reader. A standard curve reflecting absorbances of the increasing concentrations of protein carbonyls in the supplied oxidized protein standards was prepared and used to measure the content of carbonyl groups in experimental samples. Data in the study are presented as nanomoles of carbonyl groups per mg of cellular extract protein (nmol/mg).

The concentration of 8-isoprostanes in NK cell extracts was measured with the 8-Isoprostane ELISA Kit (Cayman Chemical, Ann Arbor, MI, USA). Samples were provided for ELISA procedure according to the manufacturer's protocol. Cell lysates were supplied in the presence of 0.005% BHT. Absorbances were measured at 405 nm with Bio-Rad plate reader. A standard curve was prepared with the use of 8-Isoprostane ELISA Standard supplied with the kit and the concentrations of 8-isoprostanes in experimental samples were estimated. Data in the study show the total 8-isoprostane content in NK cell lysates expressed in pg/ml.

Statistics

All data are expressed as means ± SEM. Normality of data distribution was analyzed by Shapiro-Wilk test. Student's t test for normal distribution and Mann-Whitney U test for nonparametric distribution were applied to compare two groups. ANOVA test for normal distribution and Kruskal-Wallis test for nonparametric distribution were used to compare the three studied age groups. The multiple comparisons were performed with Tukey's post-hoc test for normal distribution and Dunn's post-hoc test for non-parametric distribution. The Spearman correlation coefficient (R) was applied to present the strength of the relationship between variables (Statistica, version 12; Statsoft, Tulsa, OK, USA). Differences or correlations with $p < 0.05$ were considered as statistically significant.

Results

Immunological characteristics of the study population

The study population was divided into 3 age groups: 'young' (32 subjects, mean age 21 years), 'old' (30 seniors at the age under 85, mean age 76 years) and the 'oldest' (25 seniors aged over 85, mean age 88 years). Blood morphology of all participants was analyzed prior to the study. The oldest seniors presented normal white blood cell (WBC) count; however, they had more leukocytes in one microliter of peripheral blood than the old ones and this difference was statistically significant (Table 1). All compared groups did not differ significantly in both the number and percentage of lymphocytes. However, seniors under the age of 85 revealed significantly higher percentage of NK cells in the population of lymphocytes than the young subjects, whereas the oldest did not differ significantly from the other age groups. After merging two groups of seniors into one we still observed that the population of seniors presented significantly higher percentage of NK cells compared to the young (seniors: 12.71% vs young: 9.22%; $p = 0.026$; U-Mann-Whitney test).

The young people had almost two times more CD56^{bright} cells compared to the oldest and the old ones and significantly less CD56^{dim} cells as compared with the oldest and the old. C reactive protein (CRP) values of all the analyzed groups remained within the reference range (0 to 5 mg/dL), although seniors revealed two times higher values compared to the young (Table 1).

Expression of SIRT1, SOD2 and HSP70 in non-stimulated NK cells of the elderly and the young

The gating strategy performed for flow cytometric analysis of NK cells is shown in Fig. 1. The expression of SIRT1 was many times higher in NK cells of the oldest seniors (14.99 ± 4.04%) compared to the old and the young (0.99 ± 0.69% and 0.46 ± 0.17%, respectively) (Fig. 2a) and these significant differences were confirmed by measurement of mean fluorescence intensity (MFI) of the analyzed populations (Fig. 2b).

The expression of SOD2 in NK cells of the oldest seniors (83.22 ± 3.92%) differed significantly from NK cells of the old and the young (60.74 ± 4.66% and 52.91 ± 3.38%, respectively) (Fig. 2c) and these results were supported by MFI values of the studied populations,

Table 1 Hematological parameters and CRP values of peripheral blood in the studied age groups

Parameters\studied group	Seniors > 85 (oldest), age: 88.4 ± 0.5 y	Seniors < 85 (old), age: 75.6 ± 0.9 y	Young, age: 21.0 ± 0.3 y	P value
Total WBC count [k/µl]	6.91 ± 0.34 *	5.92 ± 0.23 *	6.33 ± 0.23	* 0.040
Lymphocyte count [k/µl]	2.17 ± 0.12	2.12 ± 0.12	2.37 ± 0.10	0.246
Lymphocyte percentage [%]	32.22 ± 1.72	36.05 ± 1.87	37.67 ± 1.13	0.059
NK cell percentage [%]	11.06 ± 1.31	14.00 ± 1.49 #	9.22 ± 0.84 #	# 0.034
NK cells CD56^{bright} [%]	4.49 ± 0.78 *	4.15 ± 0.68 #	7.17 ± 0.76 *#	# 0.004 *0.037
NK cells CD56^{dim} [%]	93.67 ± 0.71 *	93.58 ± 0.63 #	90.01 ± 0.74 *#	# 0.001 *0.002
CRP [mg/L]	2.16 ± 0.29 *	1.87 ± 0.27 #	0.81 ± 0.18 *#	# 0.001 *0.00003

All data are presented as means ± SEM. The same symbols *, # in one row denote statistically significant differences between the marked values

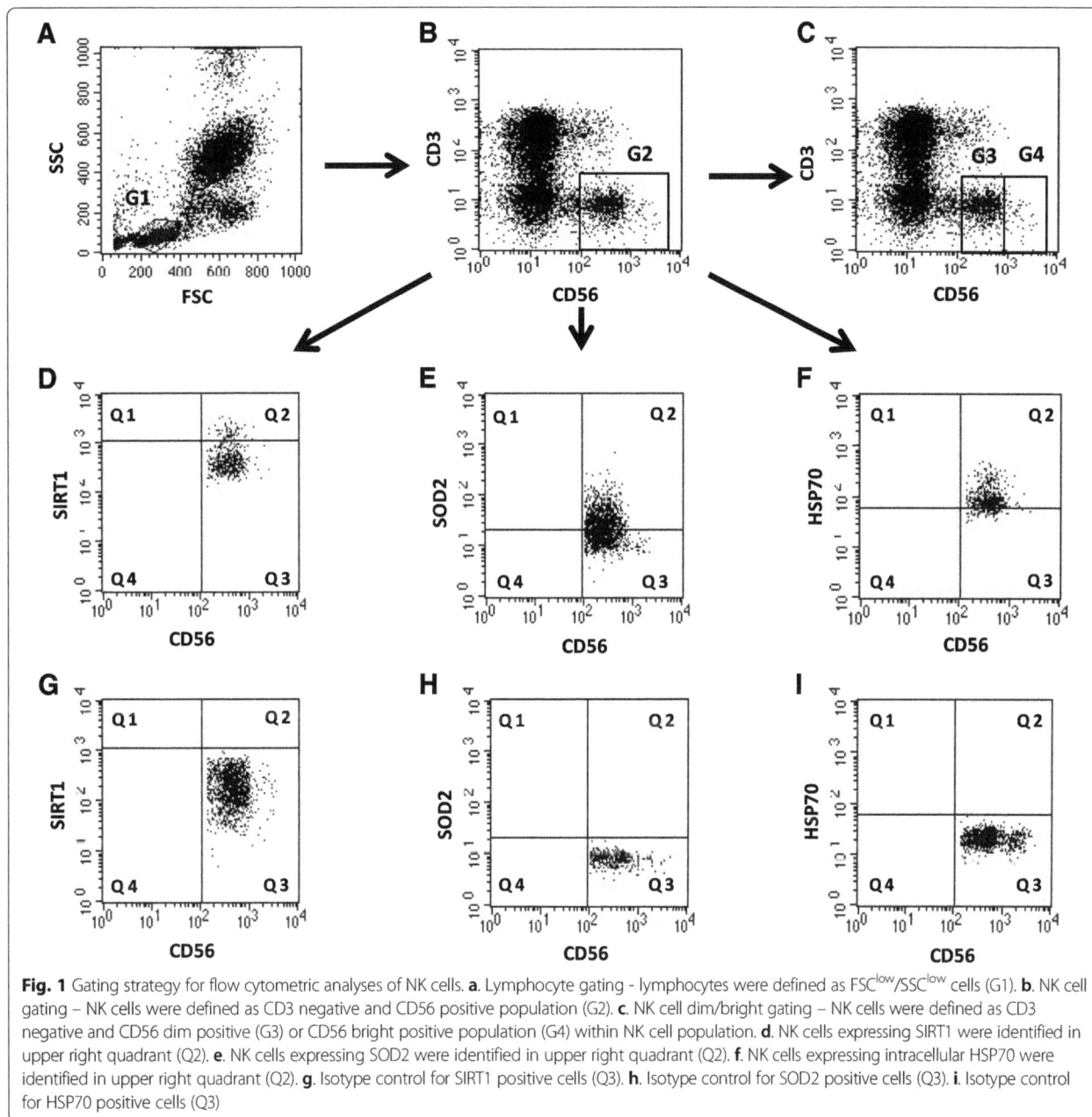

Fig. 1 Gating strategy for flow cytometric analyses of NK cells. **a**. Lymphocyte gating - lymphocytes were defined as FSC^{low}/SSC^{low} cells (G1). **b**. NK cell gating – NK cells were defined as CD3 negative and CD56 positive population (G2). **c**. NK cell dim/bright gating – NK cells were defined as CD3 negative and CD56 dim positive (G3) or CD56 bright positive population (G4) within NK cell population. **d**. NK cells expressing SIRT1 were identified in upper right quadrant (Q2). **e**. NK cells expressing SOD2 were identified in upper right quadrant (Q2). **f**. NK cells expressing intracellular HSP70 were identified in upper right quadrant (Q2). **g**. Isotype control for SIRT1 positive cells (Q3). **h**. Isotype control for SOD2 positive cells (Q3). **i**. Isotype control for HSP70 positive cells (Q3)

although statistically significant difference was observed only between NK cells of the old and the oldest (Fig. 2d).

The expression of intracellular HSP70 in NK cells of the oldest (76.43 ± 5.47%) was significantly higher than in NK cells of the old and the young (34.34 ± 4.98% and 41.22 ± 4.17% respectively) (Fig. 2e). The similar results were obtained for MFI values of the analyzed populations (Fig. 2f). Differences between age groups in the expression of the surface HSP70 protein revealed statistical significance only between the young and the oldest (Fig. 2g). 45% of NK cells (45.14 ± 7.7%) of the oldest seniors expressed this protein on their surface in contrast to significantly lower expression on NK cells of the

young (13.17 ± 1.9%). NK cells of the old also revealed lower expression (16.67 ± 2.98%) but without statistical significance. Results received for MFI values of these populations presented the similar tendency, but the significant difference concerned the old and the oldest (Fig. 2h).

Correlations between levels of expression of the studied cellular protective proteins in NK cells

It was found that percentages of NK cells expressing SIRT1, SOD2, intracellular HSP70 and surface HSP70 correlated positively with the age of participants ($R = 0.455$, $R = 0.520$, $R = 0.402$ and $R = 0.320$, respectively) (Table 2).

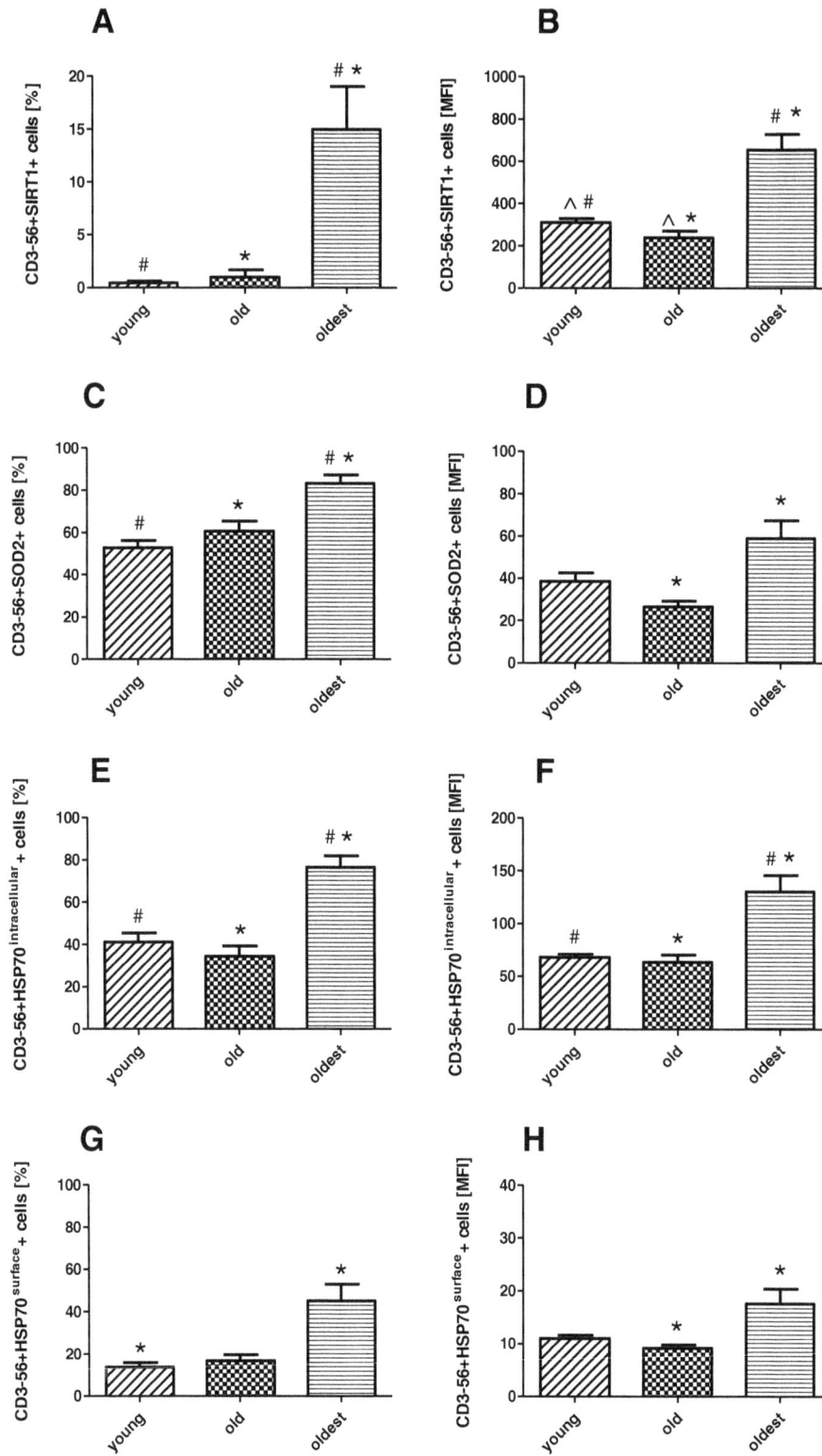

Fig. 2 (See legend on next page.)

(See figure on previous page.)

Fig. 2 Expression of cellular protective proteins in non-stimulated NK cells of the oldest seniors (aged over 85), the old aged under 85 and the young. Data are presented as means ± SEM and concern expression of the studied proteins in NK cells demonstrated as percentages of cells with expression of a particular protein (%) or mean fluorescence intensity (MFI). The same #,*,∧ symbols over bars denote statistically significant differences between NK cells of different age groups. **a**. Expression of SIRT1 (%): #$p = 0.0001$; * $p = 0.000002$. **b**. Expression of SIRT1 (MFI): ∧ $p = 0.022$; #$p = 0.004$; * $p = 0.000001$. **c**. Expression of SOD2 (%): #$p = 0.000009$; * $p = 0.006$. **d**. Expression of SOD2 (MFI): * $p = 0.0003$. **e**. Expression of intracellular HSP70 (%): #$p = 0.0002$; * $p = 0.000005$. **f**. Expression of intracellular HSP70 (MFI): #$p = 0.0023$; * $p = 0.000002$. **g**. Expression of surface HSP70 (%): * $p = 0.02$. **h**. Expression of surface HSP70 (MFI): * $p = 0.045$

Some correlations between the expression of SIRT1 and other protective proteins were observed. The percentage of SIRT1-expressing NK cells correlated with the percentage of NK cells expressing: (i) SOD2 ($R = 0.517$), (ii) intracellular HSP70 ($R = 0.705$), (iii) surface HSP70 ($R = 0.439$) and (iv) TNF ($R = 0.262$) (Table 2).

Moreover, the statistical analysis revealed correlations between the percentage of NK cells expressing SOD2 and the percentage of NK cells expressing: (i) intracellular HSP70 protein ($R = 0.466$), and (ii) surface HSP70 protein ($R = 0.669$). We also noted a correlation between the percentage of NK cells expressing intracellular HSP70 and: (i) surface HSP70 protein ($R = 0.418$), (ii) TNF ($R = 0.263$) (Table 2).

Correlations between serum concentration of CRP and expression of cellular protective proteins in NK cells

The serum concentration of C reactive protein correlated with age ($R = 0.507$). We found also correlations between CRP and percentages of NK cells expressing SOD2, intracellular HSP70 and TNF ($R = 0.274$, $R = 0.292$ and $R = -0.262$, respectively) (Table 2).

Intracellular expression of TNF and IFN-γ in non-stimulated NK cells

Intracellular TNF, a proinflammatory cytokine secreted usually by stimulated NK cells, in our study was detected at a low level also in non-stimulated NK cells of whole blood samples. $2.15 \pm 0.49\%$, $0.97 \pm 0.19\%$ and $1.68 \pm 0.51\%$ of NK cells of the young, the old and the oldest, respectively, revealed its expression. However, the differences between the studied groups were not statistically significant (Fig. 3a). Similarly, MFI values obtained for

the analyzed populations did not show any differences between the age groups (Fig. 3b).

On the contrary, the expression of intracellular IFN-γ in non-stimulated NK cells showed some differences between the age groups. The young had significantly more NK cells expressing intracellular IFN-γ ($3.78 \pm 0.42\%$) than the oldest ($1.52 \pm 0.65\%$) but they did not differ from the old ($3.04 \pm 0.59\%$) (Fig. 3c). The significant differences were not, however, confirmed by MFI values (Fig. 3d).

The percentage of NK cells expressing IFN-γ correlated negatively with age ($R = -0.254$) (Table 2).

Expression of SIRT1, SOD2 and HSP70 in non-stimulated CD56dim and CD56bright NK cells of the elderly and the young

The gating strategy performed for flow cytometric analysis of CD56dim and CD56bright NK cells is shown in Fig. 1. The expression of SIRT1, SOD2 and both HSP70intracellular and HSP70 surface was compared between three age groups (Kruskal-Wallis test) and between CD56dim and CD56bright cells of the same age group (Mann-Whitney U test). Interestingly, the general pattern of SIRT1 and HSP70intracellular expression was similar in both CD56dim and CD56bright NK cells (Fig. 4a and c). There were some statistically significant differences between young vs oldest and old vs oldest observed, similarly to the total population of NK cells (Fig. 2a and c). Moreover, the comparison of CD56dim to CD56bright cells revealed also significantly higher expression of SIRT1 in CD56dim cells in both young and the old population but not in the oldest (respectively 0.51 ± 0.18 vs 0.43 ± 0.19 and 1.14 ± 0.76 vs 0.89 ± 0.57). Some differences between CD56dim and CD56bright

Table 2 Correlation analysis of the study population

Spearman's correlation coefficient (R)	SIRT1	SOD2	HSP70intracellular	HSP70surface	TNF	IFN-γ	CRP
SOD2	0.517						
HSP70intracellular	0.705	0.466					
HSP70surface	0.439	0.669	0.418				
TNF	0.262	ns	0.263	ns			
IFN-γ	ns	ns	ns	ns	ns		
CRP	ns	0.274	0.292	ns	−0.262	ns	
Age	0.455	0.520	0.402	0.320	ns	−0.254	0.507

All values are presented as statistically significant Spearman's correlation coefficients (R). 'ns' denotes statistically not significant

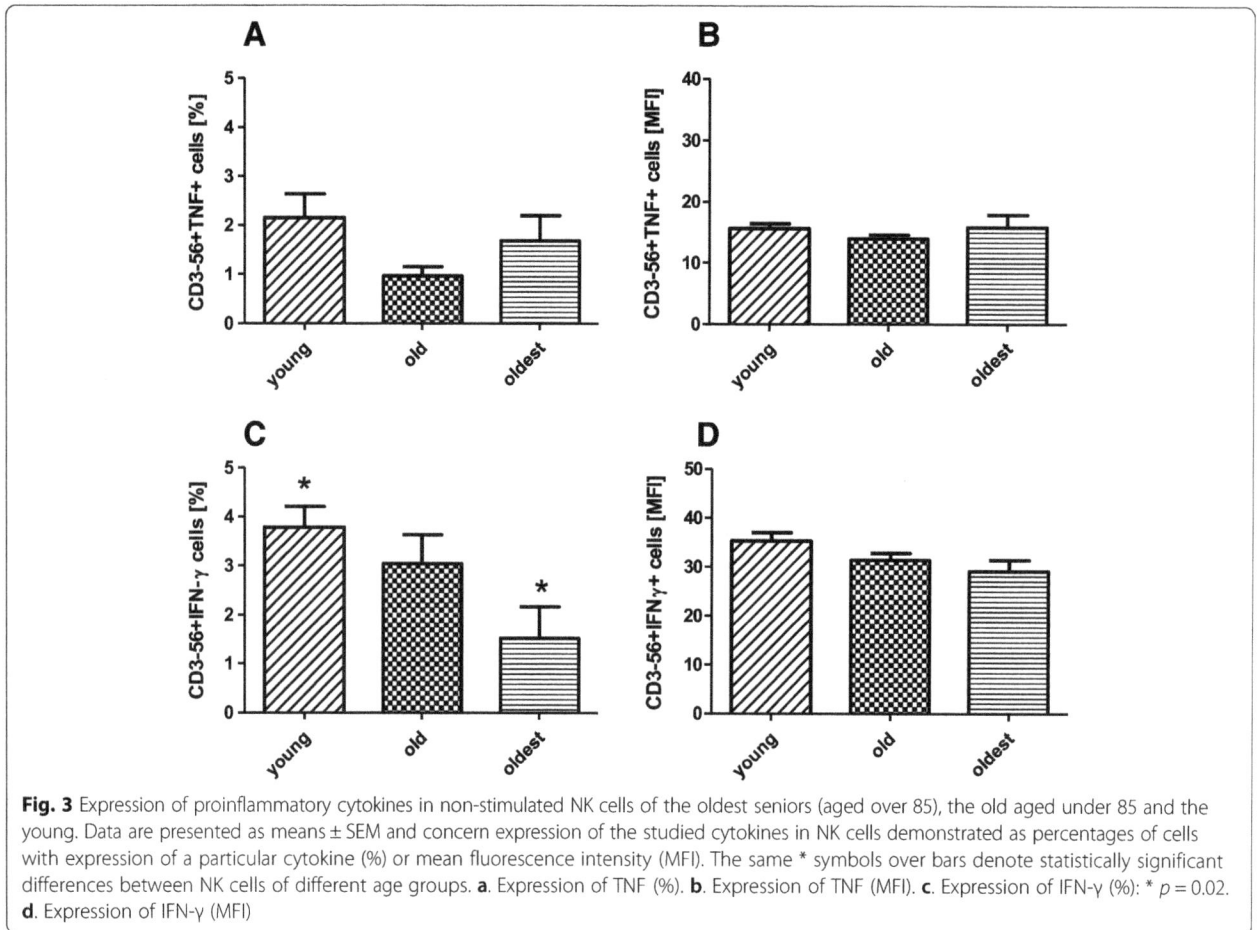

Fig. 3 Expression of proinflammatory cytokines in non-stimulated NK cells of the oldest seniors (aged over 85), the old aged under 85 and the young. Data are presented as means ± SEM and concern expression of the studied cytokines in NK cells demonstrated as percentages of cells with expression of a particular cytokine (%) or mean fluorescence intensity (MFI). The same * symbols over bars denote statistically significant differences between NK cells of different age groups. **a**. Expression of TNF (%). **b**. Expression of TNF (MFI). **c**. Expression of IFN-γ (%): * $p = 0.02$. **d**. Expression of IFN-γ (MFI)

cells were observed also within SOD2-expressing NK cells. Comparably to SIRT1, in the group of the young and the old, but not in the oldest, CD56dim cells presented significantly higher expression of SOD2 compared to CD56bright cells (55.5 ± 3.48% vs 42.32 ± 4.16% and 62.21 ± 4.73 vs 47.99 ± 4.73, respectively) (Fig. 4b). The expression of HSP70^{surface} (Fig. 4d) was comparable to the expression of SIRT1 and HSP70^{intracellular} with the only significant difference between CD56dim of the young and CD56dim of the oldest observed also in the total population of NK cells (Fig. 2g).

Intracellular expression of TNF and IFN-γ in non-stimulated CD56dim and CD56bright NK cells

The gating strategy performed for flow cytometric analysis of CD56dim and CD56bright NK cells is shown in Fig. 1. Some differences between CD56dim and CD56bright cells expressing TNF and IFN-γ were observed in the young, old and the oldest. In the young, significantly more CD56dim cells expressed TNF compared with CD56bright cells (2.33 ± 0.5% vs 1.3 ± 0.44%). On the contrary, in the old significantly more CD56bright cells revealed expression of TNF compared with CD56dim cells (respectively:

1.39 ± 0.6% vs 0.96 ± 0.21%). The tendency similar to the old group was observed also in the oldest one but it was not statistically significant (Fig. 4e). Correspondingly, when the expression of IFN-γ was analyzed, some similar to TNF expression trends were observed between CD56dim and CD56bright cells of all three age groups, however, they were not statistically significant. The only significant difference was observed between CD56dim cells of the young vs CD56dim cells of the oldest (Fig. 4f) comparable to the total population of NK cells (Fig. 3c).

Protein carbonyl groups and 8-isoprostanes content in NK cell lysates

The concentration of carbonyl groups in NK cell extracts of the young (0.36 ± 0.04 nmol/mg of protein) was significantly higher compared to the old (0.22 ± 0.02 nmol/mg) and the oldest (0.21 ± 0.03 nmol/mg) (Fig. 5a). These differences between age groups, however, were not confirmed by changes in concentration of 8-isoprostanes in NK cell extracts of the analyzed populations (Fig. 5b). In these last experiments the highest concentration of 8-isoprostanes was observed in NK cells of the oldest (14.22 ± 4.57 pg/ml) on the contrary to the young (9.26 ±

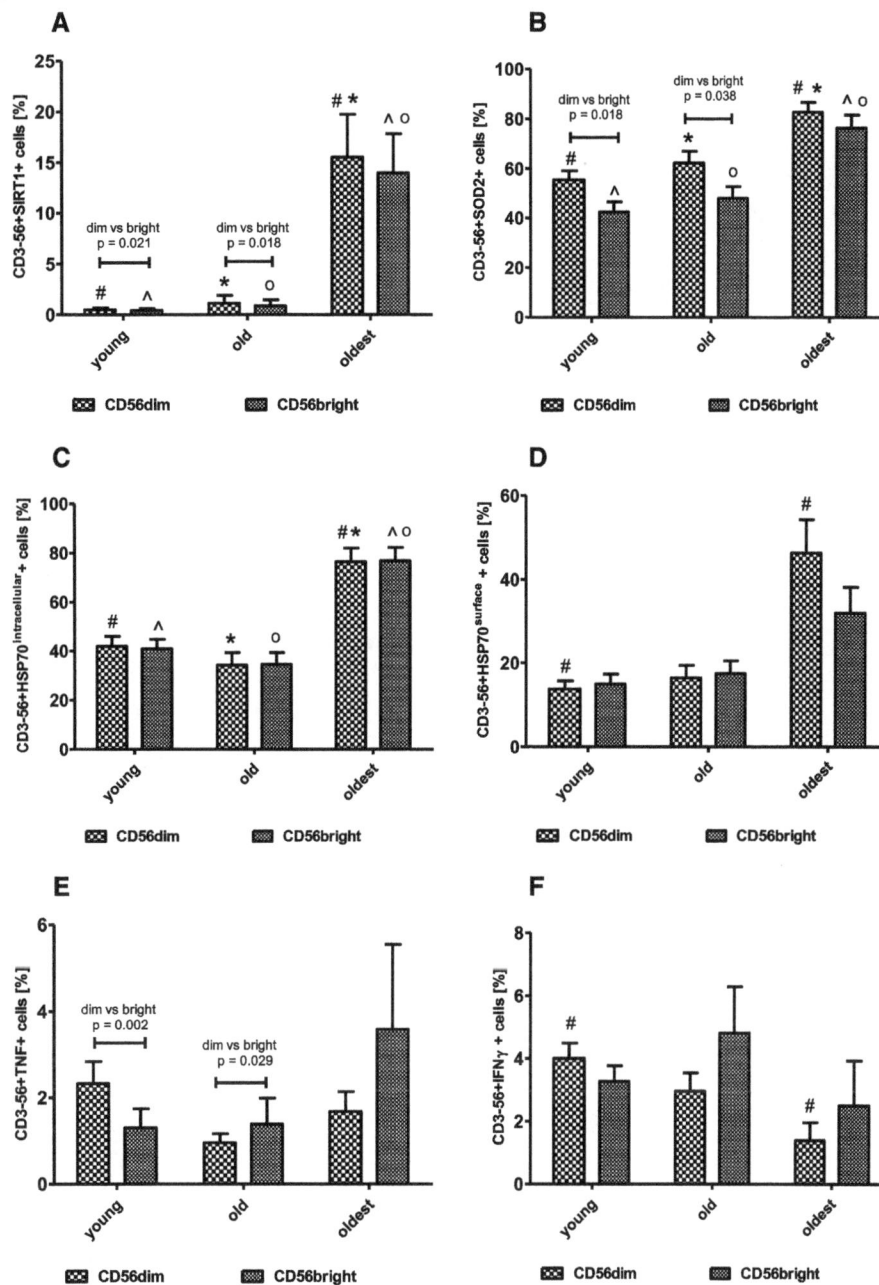

Fig. 4 Expression of cellular protective proteins and proinflammatory cytokines in non-stimulated CD56dim and CD56bright NK cells of the oldest seniors (aged over 85), the old aged under 85 and the young. Data are presented as means ± SEM and concern percentages of CD56dim and CD56bright NK cells expressing the studied proteins (%). The same #,*,^,° symbols over bars denote statistically significant differences between respectively CD56dim or CD56bright NK cells of different age groups. Horizontal lines above paired bars denote differences with statistical significance between CD56dim and CD56bright NK cells of the same age group. **a**. Expression of SIRT1 (%): #$p = 0.0004$; * $p = 0.000008$; ^ $p = 0.003$; °$p = 0.002$. **b**. Expression of SOD2 (%): #$p = 0.00003$; * $p = 0.02$; ^ $p = 0.00007$; °$p = 0.005$. **c**. Expression of intracellular HSP70 (%): #$p = 0.0003$; * $p = 0.000005$; ^ $p = 0.0002$; °$p = 0.000002$. **d**. Expression of surface HSP70 (%): #$p = 0.02$. **e**. Expression of TNF (%). **f**. Expression of IFN-γ (%): #$p = 0.01$

2.06 pg/ml) and the old (7.59 ± 2.14) but these differences were not statistically significant.

Discussion

The main finding of this study is that in the oldest seniors NK cells, a specific group of lymphocytes involved in innate immunity, reveal higher expression of stress response proteins, i.e. SIRT1, HSP70 and SOD2 compared to seniors aged under 85 and the young people. The study shows also for the first time the existing correlations between the expression of these proteins in NK cells and age of the study participants.

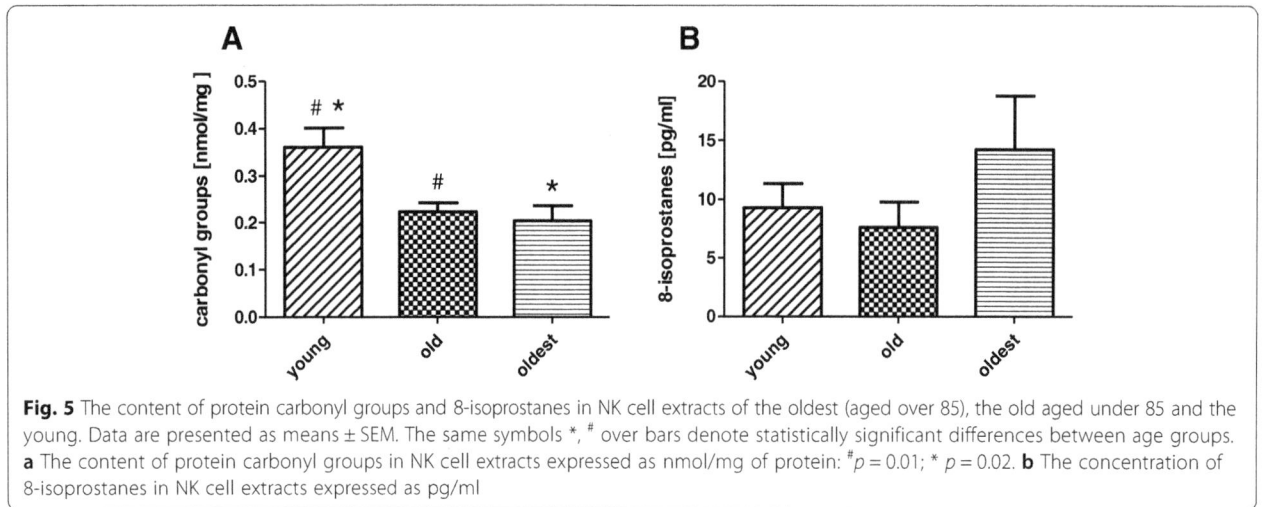

Fig. 5 The content of protein carbonyl groups and 8-isoprostanes in NK cell extracts of the oldest (aged over 85), the old aged under 85 and the young. Data are presented as means ± SEM. The same symbols *, # over bars denote statistically significant differences between age groups. **a** The content of protein carbonyl groups in NK cell extracts expressed as nmol/mg of protein: #$p = 0.01$; * $p = 0.02$. **b** The concentration of 8-isoprostanes in NK cell extracts expressed as pg/ml

The studies of immunosenescence provided various data on the number of leukocytes and lymphocytes in peripheral blood. For instance, similarly to our results, no differences between the elderly and the young were reported [4] whereas an Italian study showed a decrease in the number of both leukocytes and lymphocytes in the process of ageing [48]. Although in our study the oldest seniors had significantly more leukocytes per microliter of peripheral blood than the old ones, the values remained within the reference range (4.0 to 10.0 k/μl). Despite similar numbers and percentages of lymphocytes in all compared groups, we found age-dependent alterations in the number of NK cells. Seniors aged under 85 had significantly higher percentage of NK cells in the population of lymphocytes than the young group but after merging the two groups of seniors, the elderly still presented significantly higher percentage of NK cells, similarly to an earlier study by Sansoni et al. who found the increase in the number of NK cells with advancing age [48]. Although another study did not report changes of the absolute NK cell number during ageing, the decrease by 48% in the number of CD56[bright] NK cells was found in the old compared to the young group [13], similarly to our results. Earlier, Borrego and coworkers found the increase in percentage of NK cells in the elderly due to expansion of CD56dim cells [7]. Thus, immunosenescence is characterized by the expansion of the mature CD56[dim] subset of NK cells at the cost of immature CD56[bright] cells.

The expression of SIRT1, SOD2 and HSP70 in NK cells has yet not been investigated during the process of ageing. In our study the oldest seniors presented significantly higher percentage of SIRT1-expressing NK cells compared to the old and the young. Moreover, the positive correlation between the percentage of NK cells with SIRT1 expression and the age of study participants suggests that high expression of SIRT1 may be associated with human longevity. This observation adds up to the increasing evidence that SIRT1 affects lifespan and stress resistance in yeast, worms, flies and mice [6]. Although SIRT1expression was not studied in peripheral blood cells during ageing, a significant increase in SIRT1 concentration in sera of the older people compared to adults and children, and a significant positive correlation between SIRT1 level and age in the overall studied population were observed by Kilic and coworkers [27].

The increased basal expression of SOD2 in NK cells of the oldest seniors compared to the old and the young and a positive correlation between the percentage of SOD2-expressing NK cells and the age of the participants presented in our study underscore the role of SOD2 in healthy ageing of human NK cells. SOD2, similarly to SIRT1, seems to play a role in longevity, at least in some species, i.e. *Drosophila* [43] and mice [46]. However, studies performed on extensive collection of 1,612 long-lived individuals showed no relationships between the analyzed SNPs (Single Nucleotide Polymorphisms) of the SOD2 gene and the longevity phenotype [19].

Our findings of significantly higher expression of intracellular HSP70 protein in non-stimulated NK cells of the oldest seniors and correlation between the expression of this protein and the age of the study participants are in line with the results of a Belgian group. They reported higher levels of HSP70, HSP32 and HSP90, but not HSP27, assessed by flow cytometry in non-stimulated monocytes and lymphocytes of the elderly (mean age 75.0, $n = 18$) compared to young subjects (mean age 36.4, $n = 17$) [41]. These studies, similarly to our observations concerning NK cells, indicate that the increased expression of HSP70, and some other HSP proteins, may be a general feature of leukocyte ageing.

We observed the enhanced expression of HSP70 protein on NK cell surface in the oldest seniors. The membrane association of HSP70 may come, however in two forms, i.e. integrated within the plasma membrane (in tumor cells) or associated with cell surface receptors (in normal cells) [38]. According to these authors commercially available antibodies are able to detect rather receptor-bound HSP70 than the integrated in the plasma membrane. The latter one need specific antibodies that recognize C terminal domain (aa 450-461) of HSP70 molecule [38]. Thus we might observed no expression of HSP70 on the surface of NK cells but rather binding of extracellular HSPs to TLR receptors on the surface of NK cells but more detailed studies are necessary to explain that clearly.

SIRT1 was found to activate several transcription factors of FOXO family that promote the expression of stress response genes including *SOD2* [21]. SIRT1 was also described to control HSF1 (heat shock factor 1) activity, a transcription factor involved in the regulation of expression of chaperons HSP70 and HSP90 [34]. These already known data may indirectly suggest observed in our study correlations between the expression of SIRT1 and SOD2 or SIRT1 and HSP70 in NK cells.

Our studies provided also some interesting observations concerning significantly higher expression of both SIRT1 and SOD2 in CD56dim cells compared with CD56bright cells in the young and the old but not in the oldest. There were no significant differences between CD56dim and CD56bright cells in the expression of both HSP70^{intracellular} and HSP70^{surface} in all age groups. The observed differences seem to be interesting especially regarding the process of ageing. These data are, however, preliminary and need subsequent studies to explain this phenomenon.

The process of ageing is in general characterized by the increased level of oxidative stress [35]. Numerous studies showed a positive correlation between resistance to oxidative stress and maximal lifespan in a variety of mammals, from hamsters to humans [24, 33]. The detected levels of carbonyl groups in NK cells of the studied population, however, did not exceed the normal ranges found in cell lysates, i.e. MRC-5-fibroblasts, 1.3 nmol/mg [51], human plasma, i.e. 1.83 ± 0.4 nmol/mg [1] or serum, i.e. 0.52 ± 0.34 nmol/mg [32]. Thus we did not observe the raise of oxidative stress level in the process of ageing. These data are in line with the results of 8-isoprostane total content test in the analyzed samples. We did not find any significant increase of concentration of 8-isoprostanes in NK cell extracts, which are similarly to carbonyl groups regarded as markers of oxidative stress [36, 37]. Statistically significant differences between carbonyl groups content in NK cells of the young versus old or the oldest were not observed in 8-isoprostane test. Similarly to carbonyl groups, concentrations of isoprostanes in NK cell extracts remained within the normal range found in human plasma and urine (range from 5–40 pg/ml) [37] or breath condensates of healthy subjects (15.8 ± 1.6 pg/ml) [36].

Concentrations of CRP, the acute-phase protein, which level reflects the presence of acute or chronic inflammation, found in the sera of the analyzed subjects, correspond to many data documenting CRP increase with advancing age in apparently healthy humans [5, 42]. Although all participants in our study presented normal CRP values, some age-related differences were observed also within the normal range. It is noteworthy, that in our study CRP serum level correlated positively with the percentage of NK cells expressing cellular protective proteins SOD2 and intracellular HSP70 [10].

The process of ageing is characterized by the increase of serum concentrations of proinflammatory cytokines, i.e. IL-6 and TNF [25, 41]. To test whether non-stimulated NK cells present in the whole blood may contribute to this process the expression of intracellular TNF and IFN-γ, a cytokine considered as a marker of NK activity, was analyzed by flow cytometry. Our study revealed low expression of both cytokines independent on the age of the study participants with the exception of higher expression of IFN-γ in NK cells of the young. In the whole studied population the percentage of NK cells with the expression of IFN-γ correlated positively with the percentage of CD56^{bright} cells ($R = 0.264$) and negatively with CD56dim cells ($R = -0.321$) (data not shown in Table 2). CD56bright cells are the main source of secreted cytokines in NK cells and their number decreases with age [13, 18]. Moreover, the expression of IFN-γ correlated negatively with age. Our results are in line with earlier reports showing a decreased production of IFN-γ in the elderly, although most studies concerned stimulated NK cells [18, 31]. Together with the normal serum levels of CRP, these data suggest that we have studied apparently healthy groups of the young, old and very old individuals.

Analysis of expression of both TNF and IFN-γ in CD56dim and CD56bright non-stimulated NK cells provided also some interesting observations concerning significantly higher expression of TNF in CD56dim cells compared to CD56bright cells in the young. The similar but not statistically significant tendency regarding expression of IFN- γ was also noted. In the old, however, the significantly higher expression of TNF was observed in CD56bright cells compared to CD56dim cells. Then in the oldest the similar, but not statistically significant results were obtained, comparably to IFN-γ expression in both the old and the oldest seniors. Takahashi and coworkers showed that CD56dim cells could be both highly cytotoxic and produce cytokines, similarly to CD56bright cells which could both secrete cytokines and acquire cytolytic activity in some conditions [53]. De Maria and coworkers showed that CD56^{dim} NK cells can produce IFN-γ at 2-4 h after stimulation, but not later and CD56^{bright} cells secrete IFN-γ only at late intervals (over 16 h after stimulation) [15]. Intracellular staining of cytokines was performed within 4 h from blood sample collection so the described by De Maria et al. phenomenon corresponds in our studies to the young group but it does not fit to the old and the oldest. Further studies are necessary to explain these data, especially in the context of ageing process.

The strength of the presented results is based on the careful recruitment of the oldest seniors as they represent healthy mode of ageing and differ significantly from the group of seniors under 85. This advantage counterbalances the limitation of the study, i.e. not large size of the study group ($n = 87$). The other advantage concerns the choice of the analyzed parameters as they have appeared to be involved in the process of NK cell ageing and expand our understanding of immunosenescence and its contribution to longevity.

Conclusions

Our study provides novel data concerning ageing of the human immune system. The increased expression of cellular protective proteins involved in stress response, i.e. SIRT1, HSP70 and SOD2 in NK cells correlates with the age of study participants and this phenomenon seems to correspond to longevity.

Abbreviations

ADL: activities of daily living; BHT: butylated hydroxytoluene; CRP: C reactive protein; FBS: fetal bovine serum; FOXO: forkhead transcription factor class O; HSF: heat shock factor; HSP: heat shock protein; IFN: interferon; IL: interleukin; MMSE: mini mental state examination; NK cells: natural killer cells; NSAID: nonsteroid anti-inflammatory drug; PBMCs: peripheral blood mononuclear cells; PBS: phosphate-buffered saline; SIRT: sirtuin; SNPs: single nucleotide polymorphisms; SOD: superoxide dismutase; TAC: tetrameric antibody complexes; TLR: toll-like receptor; TNF: tumor necrosis factor; WBC: white blood cell

Acknowledgements
Not applicable.

Funding
This study was supported by grant N N404 597640 from the National Science Centre (NCN, Poland).

Authors' contributions
LK conceived the project, performed flow cytometry experiments, analyzed and interpreted the data and wrote the manuscript, JF qualified young and old subjects to the project and participated with DS and TS in project development, JJK performed measurements of carbonyl groups and isoprostanes, ZK supervised the project performance, analyzed the data and prepared with LK the final version of the article. All authors approved the final version of the manuscript.

Competing interests
The authors declare that they have no competing interests.

Author details
[1]Department of Histology, Medical University of Gdańsk, Dębinki 1, Gdańsk PL-80-211, Poland. [2]Department of Social and Clinical Gerontology, Medical University of Gdańsk, Dębinki 1, Gdańsk PL-80-211, Poland. [3]Department of Physiotherapy, Gdansk University of Physical Education and Sport, Górskiego 1, Gdańsk PL-80-336, Poland. [4]Department of Clinical Toxicology, Medical University of Gdańsk, Kartuska 4/6, Gdańsk PL-80-104, Poland.

References
1. Adams S, Green P, Claxton R, Simcox S, Williams MV, Walsh K, Leeuwenburgh C. Reactive carbonyl formation by oxidative and non-oxidative pathways. Front Biosci. 2001;6:A17–24.
2. Arslan MA, Csermely P, Soti C. Protein homeostasis and molecular chaperones in aging. Biogerontology. 2006;7(5-6):383–9.
3. Asea A. Hsp70: a chaperokine. Novartis Found Symp. 2008;291:173–9. discussion 179-183, 221-174.
4. Aspinall R, Carroll J, Jiang S. Age-related changes in the absolute number of CD95 positive cells in T cell subsets in the blood. Exp Gerontol 1998;33(6):581–91.
5. Ballou SP, Lozanski FB, Hodder S, Rzewnicki DL, Mion LC, Sipe JD, Ford AB, Kushner I. Quantitative and qualitative alterations of acute-phase proteins in healthy elderly persons. Age Ageing. 1996;25(3):224–30.
6. Bishop NA, Guarente L. Genetic links between diet and lifespan: shared mechanisms from yeast to humans. Nat Rev Genet. 2007;8(11):835–44.
7. Borrego F, Alonso MC, Galiani MD, Carracedo J, Ramirez R, Ostos B, Peña J, Solana R. NK phenotypic markers and IL2 response in NK cells from elderly people. Exp Gerontol. 1999;34(2):253–65.
8. Bueno V, Sant'Anna OA, Lord JM. Ageing and myeloid-derived suppressor cells: possible involvement in immunosenescence and age-related disease. Age (Dordr). 2014;36(6):9729.
9. Calabrese V, Cornelius C, Dinkova-Kostova AT, Calabrese EJ, Mattson MP. Cellular stress responses, the hormesis paradigm, and vitagenes: novel targets for therapeutic intervention in neurodegenerative disorders. Antioxid Redox Signal. 2010;13(11):1763–811.
10. Calabrese V, Cornelius C, Dinkova-Kostova AT, Iavicoli I, Di Paola R, Koverech A, Cuzzocrea S, Rizzarelli E, Calabrese EJ. Cellular stress responses, hormetic phytochemicals and vitagenes in aging and longevity. Biochim Biophys Acta. 2012;1822(5):753–83.
11. Calderwood SK, Murshid A, Prince T. The shock of aging: molecular chaperones and the heat shock response in longevity and aging–a mini-review. Gerontology. 2009;55(5):550–8.
12. Campos C, Pera A, Lopez-Fernandez I, Alonso C, Tarazona R, Solana R. Proinflammatory status influences NK cells subsets in the elderly. Immunol Lett. 2014;162(1 Pt B):298–302.
13. Chidrawar SM, Khan N, Chan YL, Nayak L, Moss PA. Ageing is associated with a decline in peripheral blood CD56bright NK cells. Immun Ageing. 2006;310.
14. De la Fuente M, Miquel J. An update of the oxidation-inflammation theory of aging: the involvement of the immune system in oxi-inflamm-aging. Curr Pharm Des. 2009;15(26):3003–26.
15. De Maria A, Bozzano F, Cantoni C, Moretta L. Revisiting human natural killer cell subset function revealed cytolytic CD56dimCD16+ NK cells as rapid producers of abundant IFN-γ on activation. PNAS. 2011;108(2):728–32.
16. Folstein MF, Folstein SE, McHugh PR. "Mini-mental state". A practical method for grading the cognitive state of patients for the clinician. J Psychiatr Res. 1975;12(3):189–98.
17. Franceschi C, Bonafe M, Valensin S, Olivieri F, De Luca M, Ottaviani E, De Benedictis G. Inflamm-aging. An evolutionary perspective on immunosenescence. Ann N Y Acad Sci. 2000;908244–254.
18. Gayoso I, Sanchez-Correa B, Campos C, Alonso C, Pera A, Casado JG, Morgado S, Tarazona R, Solana R. Immunosenescence of human natural killer cells. J Innate Immun. 2011;3(4):337–43.
19. Gentschew L, Flachsbart F, Kleindorp R, Badarinarayan N, Schreiber S, Nebel A. Polymorphisms in the superoxidase dismutase genes reveal no association with human longevity in Germans: a case-control association study. Biogerontology. 2013;14(6):719–27.
20. Hazeldine J, Lord JM. The impact of ageing on natural killer cell function and potential consequences for health in older adults. Ageing Res Rev. 2013;12(4):1069–78.

21. Hori YS, Kuno A, Hosoda R, Horio Y. Regulation of FOXOs and p53 by SIRT1 modulators under oxidative stress. PLoS One. 2013;8(9), e73875.

22. Hwang JW, Yao H, Caito S, Sundar IK, Rahman I. Redox regulation of SIRT1 in inflammation and cellular senescence. Free Radic Biol Med. 2013;6195–110.

23. Jin X, Wang R, Xiao C, Cheng L, Wang F, Yang L, Feng T, Chen M, Chen S, Fu X, Deng J, Tang F, Wei Q, Tanguay RM, Wu T. Serum and lymphocyte levels of heat shock protein 70 in aging: a study in the normal Chinese population. Cell Stress Chaperones. 2004;9(1):69–75.

24. Kapahi P, Boulton ME, Kirkwood TB. Positive correlation between mammalian life span and cellular resistance to stress. Free Radic Biol Med. 1999;26(5-6):495–500.

25. Kaszubowska L, Kaczor JJ, Hak L, Dettlaff-Pokora A, Szarynska M, Kmiec Z. Sensitivity of natural killer cells to activation in the process of ageing is related to the oxidative and inflammatory status of the elderly. J Physiol Pharmacol. 2011;62(1):101–9.

26. Katz S, Ford AB, Moskowitz RW, Jackson BA, Jaffe MW. Studies of Illness in the Aged. The Index of AdI: A Standardized Measure of Biological and Psychosocial Function. JAMA. 1963;185:914–9.

27. Kilic U, Gok O, Erenberk U, Dundaroz MR, Torun E, Kucukardali Y, Elibol-Can B, Uysal O, Dundar T. A remarkable age-related increase in SIRT1 protein expression against oxidative stress in elderly: SIRT1 gene variants and longevity in human. PLoS One. 2015;10(3), e0117954.

28. Kovalenko EI, Boyko AA, Semenkov VF, Lutsenko GV, Grechikhina MV, Kanevskiy LM, Azhikina TL, Telford WG, Sapozhnikov AM. ROS production, intracellular HSP70 levels and their relationship in human neutrophils: effects of age. Oncotarget. 2014;5(23):11800–12.

29. Kumar R, Mohan N, Upadhyay AD, Singh AP, Sahu V, Dwivedi S, Dey AB, Dey S. Identification of serum sirtuins as novel noninvasive protein markers for frailty. Aging Cell. 2014;13(6):975–80.

30. Larbi A, Kempf J, Wistuba-Hamprecht K, Haug C, Pawelec G. The heat shock proteins in cellular aging: is zinc the missing link? Biogerontology. 2006;7(5-6):399–408.

31. Le Garff-Tavernier M, Beziat V, Decocq J, Siguret V, Gandjbakhch F, Pautas E, Debre P, Merle-Beral H, Vieillard V. Human NK cells display major phenotypic and functional changes over the life span. Aging Cell. 2010;9(4):527–35.

32. Lemarechal H, Allanore Y, Chenevier-Gobeaux C, Kahan A, Ekindjian OG, Borderie D. Serum protein oxidation in patients with rheumatoid arthritis and effects of infliximab therapy. Clin Chim Acta. 2006;372(1-2):147–53.

33. Lin YH, Chen YC, Kao TY, Lin YC, Hsu TE, Wu YC, Ja WW, Brummel TJ, Kapahi P, Yuh CH, Yu LK, Lin ZH, You RJ, Jhong YT, Wang HD. Diacylglycerol lipase regulates lifespan and oxidative stress response by inversely modulating TOR signaling in Drosophila and C. elegans. Aging Cell. 2014;13(4):755–64.

34. Martinez de Toda I, De la Fuente M. The role of Hsp70 in oxi-inflamm-aging and its use as a potential biomarker of lifespan. Biogerontology. 2015;16(6):709–21.

35. Maurya PK, Kumar P, Chandra P. Biomarkers of oxidative stress in erythrocytes as a function of human age. World J Methodol. 2015;5(4):216–22.

36. Montuschi P, Corradi M, Ciabattoni G, Nightingale J, Kharitonov SA, Barnes PJ. Increased 8-Isoprostane, a Marker of Oxidative Stress, in Exhaled Condensate of Asthma Patients. Am J Respir Crit Care Med. 1999;160:216–20.

37. Morrow JD, Hill KE, Burk RF, Nammour TM, Badr KF, Roberts LJ. A series of prostaglandin F2-like compounds are produced in vivo in humans by a non-cyclooxygenase, free radical-catalyzed mechanism. PNAS. 1990;87:9383–7.

38. Multhoff G, Hightower LE. Distinguishing integral and receptor-bound heat shock protein 70 (Hsp70) on the cell surface by Hsp70-specific antibodies. Cell Stress Chaperones. 2011;16:251–5.

39. Murshid A, Eguchi T, Calderwood SK. Stress proteins in aging and life span. Int J Hyperthermia. 2013;29(5):442–7.

40. Nardai G, Csermely P, Soti C. Chaperone function and chaperone overload in the aged. A preliminary analysis. Exp Gerontol. 2002;37(10-11):1257–62.

41. Njemini R, Lambert M, Demanet C, Kooijman R, Mets T. Basal and infection-induced levels of heat shock proteins in human aging. Biogerontology. 2007;8(3):353–64.

42. Njemini R, Bautmans I, Onyema OO, Van Puyvelde K, Demanet C, Mets T. Circulating heat shock protein 70 in health, aging and disease. BMC Immunol. 2011;1224.

43. Paul A, Belton A, Nag S, Martin I, Grotewiel MS, Duttaroy A. Reduced mitochondrial SOD displays mortality characteristics reminiscent of natural aging. Mech Ageing Dev. 2007;128(11-12):706–16.

44. Poli A, Michel T, Theresine M, Andres E, Hentges F, Zimmer J. CD56bright natural killer (NK) cells: an important NK cell subset. Immunology. 2009;126(4):458–65.

45. Rea IM, McNerlan S, Pockley AG. Serum heat shock protein and anti-heat shock protein antibody levels in aging. Exp Gerontol. 2001;36:341–52.

46. Rodriguez-Iturbe B, Sepassi L, Quiroz Y, Ni Z, Wallace DC, Vaziri ND. Association of mitochondrial SOD deficiency with salt-sensitive hypertension and accelerated renal senescence. J Appl Physiol (1985). 2007;102(1):255–60.

47. Santos L, Escande C, Denicola A. Potential Modulation of Sirtuins by Oxidative Stress. Oxid Med Cell Longev. 2016;20169831825.

48. Sansoni P, Cossarizza A, Brianti V, Fagnoni F, Snelli G, Monti D, Marcato A, Passeri G, Ortolani C, Forti E, et al. Lymphocyte subsets and natural killer cell activity in healthy old people and centenarians. Blood. 1993;82(9):2767–73.

49. Satoh A, Brace CS, Rensing N, Cliften P, Wozniak DF, Herzog ED, Yamada KA, Imai S. Sirt1 extends life span and delays aging in mice through the regulation of Nk2 homeobox 1 in the DMH and LH. Cell Metab. 2013;18(3):416–30.

50. Scheurmann J, Treiber N, Weber C, Renkl AC, Frenzel D, Trenz-Buback F, Ruess A, Schulz G, Scharffetter-Kochanek K, Weiss JM. Mice with heterozygous deficiency of manganese superoxide dismutase (SOD2) have a skin immune system with features of "inflamm-aging". Arch Dermatol Res. 2014;306(2):143–55.

51. Sitte N, Merker K, Grune T. Proteasome-dependent degradation of oxidized proteins in MRC-5 fibroblasts. FEBS Lett. 1998;440(3):399–402.

52. Sun JC, Ugolini S, Vivier E. Immunological memory within the innate immune system. EMBO J. 2014;33(12):1295–303.

53. Takahashi E, Kuranaga N, Satoh K, Habu Y, Shinomiya N, Asano T, Seki S, Hayakawa M. Induction of CD16+ CD56bright NK Cells with Antitumour Cytotoxicity not only from CD16- CD56bright NK Cells but also from CD16- CD56dim NK Cells. Scand J Immunol. 2007;65:126–38.

54. Velarde MC, Flynn JM, Day NU, Melov S, Campisi J. Mitochondrial oxidative stress caused by Sod2 deficiency promotes cellular senescence and aging phenotypes in the skin. Aging (Albany NY). 2012;4(1):3–12.

55. Visala Rao D, Boyle GM, Parsons PG, Watson K, Jones GL. Influence of ageing, heat shock treatment and in vivo total antioxidant status on gene-expression profile and protein synthesis in human peripheral lymphocytes. Mech Ageing Dev. 2003;124(1):55–69.

Nutraceutical effects of table green olives: a pilot study with *Nocellara del Belice* olives

Giulia Accardi[1][*][†], Anna Aiello[1][*][†], Valeria Gargano[2], Caterina Maria Gambino[1], Santo Caracappa[2], Sandra Marineo[2], Gesualdo Vesco[2], Ciriaco Carru[3], Angelo Zinellu[3], Maurizio Zarcone[4], Calogero Caruso[1] and Giuseppina Candore[1]

Abstract

Background: The aim of this study was to analyse the nutraceutical properties of table green olives *Nocellara del Belice*, a traditional Mediterranean food. The Mediterranean Diet has as key elements olives and extra virgin olive oil, common to all Mediterranean countries. Olive oil is the main source of fat and can modulate oxidative stress and inflammation, whereas little is known about the role of olives. Moreover, emerging evidences underline the association between gut microbiota and food as the basis of many phenomena that affect health and delay or avoid the onset of some age-related chronic diseases.

Methods: In order to show if table green olives have nutraceutical properties and/or probiotic effect, we performed a nutritional intervention, administering to 25 healthy subjects (mean age 38,3), 12 table green olives/day for 30 days. We carried out anthropometric, biochemical, oxidative stress and cytokines analyses at the beginning of the study and at the end. Moreover, we also collected fecal samples to investigate about the possible variation of concentration of *Lactobacilli*, after the olives consumption.

Result: Our results showed a significant variation of one molecule related to oxidative stress, malondialdehyde, confirming that *Nocellara del Belice* green olives could have an anti-oxidant effect. In addition, the level of interleukin-6 decreased significantly, demonstrating how this food could be able to modulate the inflammatory response. Moreover, it is noteworthy the reduction of fat mass with an increase of muscle mass, suggesting a possible effect on long time assumption of table olives on body mass variation. No statistically significant differences were observed in the amount of *Lactobacilli*, although a trend towards an increased concentration of them at the end of the intervention could be related to the nutraceutical effects of olives.

Conclusion: These preliminary results suggest a possible nutraceutical effect of daily consumption of green table olives *Nocellara del Belice*. To best of our knowledge, this is the first study performed to assess nutraceutical properties of this food. Of course, it is necessary to verify the data in a larger sample of individuals to confirm their role as nutraceuticals.

Keywords: Table green olives, Mediterranean Diet, Nutraceuticals, Dietary intervention, Oxidative stress, Inflammatory status

Background

Nowadays, ageing process and the related diseases constitute one of the bigger challenges in Western countries. The general increase of lifespan does not go, hand in hand, with the increase of healthy lifespan, the so-called "healthspan". This constitutes a worldwide problem, in particular due to age-related chronic diseases [1].

It is well known that the pathogenesis of age-related diseases is characterized by a low-grade inflammation. In particular, the visceral adipose tissue is a source of inflammatory mediators produced by adipocytes and infiltrating monocytes [2].

Abdominal obesity with dyslipidaemia, elevated blood pressure and impaired glucose tolerance characterizes metabolic syndrome (MS) that predisposes to the onset of age-related diseases. As many studies demonstrate, a

* Correspondence: giuliabio@gmail.com; anna.aiello2903@gmail.com
[†]Equal contributors
[1]Sezione di Patologia generale del Dipartimento di Biopatologia e Biotecnologie Mediche (DIBIMED), Università di Palermo, Corso Tukory 211, 90134 Palermo, Italy
Full list of author information is available at the end of the article

dietary Mediterranean regimen can positively influence these parameters. Large intervention trials showed, in fact, that Mediterranean Diet (MedDiet) could prevent and or delay the onset of age-related diseases with a great implication in the health social system [3–7].

The traditional MedDiet is a common dietary pattern, adopted by inhabitants of countries within Mediterranean basin where the olive tree, *Olea europaea*, is widely cultivated for the production of table olives and oil. They are the essential components of the MedDiet with a very significant economic value. Besides of the economical contribution to national economies, these are important in terms of nutritional value. Extra virgin olive oil (EVOO) has been claimed to play a key role in the prevention of age-related diseases and in the attainment of longevity. This is due to the high levels of monounsaturated fatty acids, likely responsible for the decreased low density lipoprotein levels, and phenolic compounds claimed to play a role as antioxidants and anti-inflammatories [6, 8, 9].

Foods with bioactive molecules can be considered "nutraceuticals", defined as "Naturally derived bioactive compounds that are found in foods, dietary supplements and herbal products, and have health promoting, disease preventing, or medicinal properties". The term was coined in 1989 by Stephen De Felice and was born from the conjunction between nutrition and pharmaceutics [10].

As reported in a recent review, table olives are extremely rich sources of polyphenols, especially oleuropein and hydroxytyrosol, comprising 1–3 % of the fresh pulp weight. Despite the high levels of hydroxytyrosol in both table olives and EVOO, in humans its bioavailability was proved only in oil. Accordingly, to the best of our knowledge, there are no human studies on health effects of table olives [11]. However, the amount of polyphenols is strongly influenced by the variety and the geographical origin. *Greek Koroneiki* have a very high level of them, while the polypenol content of the *Spanish Arbequina* is low and that of *Sicilian Nocellara* is medium-high [12]. So, a possible anti-inflammatory and anti-oxidant effect of these Sicilian olives is conceivable.

The development of strategies aimed at counterbalancing the frailty in the elderly is a major challenge for the medicine of 21st century [1]. As recently reviewed, ageing affects the gut microbiota composition and its influence in immune response. Age-related gut microbiota changes are associated with immunosenescence and inflamm-ageing. Hence, the gut ecosystem shows the potential to become a promising target for strategies able to contribute to the health status of elderly. In this context, the consumption of pro/prebiotics may be useful in both prevention and treatment of age-related pathophysiological conditions, favouring the attainment of longevity [13].

Probiotics are defined as "Live microorganisms which when administered in adequate amounts confer a health benefit on the host". *Lactobacilli* (*L.*) and *Bifidobacteria* are the most commonly used bacterial probiotics [14]. Nutritional supplementation in aged people might help to maintain good immune-inflammatory responses by re-equilibrating the gut microbiota.

Fermentation is one of the oldest methods to preserve olives. It has applied worldwide for thousands of years. The microbiota of olives during fermentation, that varies somewhat from *cultivar* to *cultivar*, has been recently reviewed, showing that *L.* are the major constituents of *Nocellara del Belice* olives microbiota [15, 16]. So, a possible probiotic-like effect of these olives is feasible.

The aim of this pilot study was to evaluate the effect of green table olives *Nocellara del Belice* on clinical and biological parameters of healthy individuals at baseline (T0) and after the assumption of 12 olives/day for 30 days (T1) (this amount was chosen to assure the administration of $2x10^7$ *L.*/die, see below).

Results and discussion
Hematochemical tests
At the end of the intervention, all hematochemical parameters did not experienced variations, with the exception of alkaline phosphatase that significantly increased (Table 1).

However, the increased values were in normal range. This means that a regular consumption of 12 green olives/day for 30 days does not have a detrimental effect on liver and kidney function and on lipid values.

Anthropometric measurements
At T1, in analysed subjects the fat mass significantly decreased together to an increase of muscle mass (Table 1). The possible explanation could be linked to the capacity of conjugated linoleic acid (CLA) to reduce the body fat levels [17]. This molecule is present both in EVOO and

Table 1 The Table shows the arithmetic average values at T0 and T1, the p-value and the variation in percentage (+ indicates an increase of the variable at T1; - a decrease at T1)

Variable	T0 ± SD	T1 ± SD	p-value	%
Alkaline phosphate (IU/L)	49.95 ± 13.26	53.73 ± 16.81	0.022	+7.57
Fat mass%	29.70 ± 7.92	28 ± 7.24	0.004	−5.72
Muscle mass %	66.97 ± 7.62	68.36 ± 6.85	0.003	+2.09
IL-6 (FI)	31.52 ± 29.37	20.89 ± 11.93	0.027	−33.73
MDA (μmol/L)	2.72 ± 0.64	2.33 ± 0.49	0.005	−14.24
Weight (Kg)	70.44 ± 14.07	69.93 ± 13.77	0.08	−0.72
BMI (Kg/m^2)	24.37 ± 4.19	24.24 ± 4.16	0.22	−0.53

T0 baseline, *T1* the end of the nutritional intervention (30 days), *BMI* Body Mass Index, *IL-6* interleukin-6, *IF* indirect fluorescence, *MDA* malondialdehyde, *SD* standard deviation

table olives, and can also be produced during their digestion. In experimental models, acting as signalling mediators, CLAs inhibit lipogenesis, increase fat oxidation, and reduce adipocytes size [18, 19].

Cytokines analyses

The serological analysis of the levels of the main pro and anti-inflammatory cytokines was conducted. Although it was not possible to evaluate the absolute concentration of interleukin (IL)-6 because it is too low, a significant variation was measured in the indirect fluorescence (IF). In fact, its levels significantly decreased at the end of the dietary intervention (Table 1).

IL-6 is a pleiotropic cytokine capable of regulating proliferation, differentiation and activity in a variety of cell types. In particular, it plays a pivotal role in acute phase responses and in the balancing of the pro and anti-inflammatory pathways. It is involved in impaired lipid metabolism and in the production of triglycerides. Moreover, it decreases lipoprotein lipase activity and monomeric lipoprotein lipase levels in plasma which contributes to increased macrophage uptake of lipids [20]. This datum suggests that a regular consumption of green olives can have anti-inflammatory effects linked to polyphenols, known to have anti-inflammatory properties [6].

Oxidative stress analyses

At the end of intervention, the values of malondialdehyde (MDA) significantly decreased (Table 1), while paraoxonase (PON) plasma levels and reduced glutathione in the red blood cells were not changed (data not shown). MDA is the main product of the polyunsaturated fatty acids peroxidation and is an important index of oxidative stress [21]. So, its reduction should be linked to the increased assumption of mono-unsatured oleic acid by olives.

Microbiological analyses on feces

The amount of *L.*/g of feces was quantified before and after the intervention. No statistically significant differences were observed, although a trend towards an increased amount of *L.* was highlighted in some subjects at T1 (data not shown). Thus, we can speculate that a more durable dietary intervention and a bigger sample of people could give more interesting results.

Conclusions

The traditional MedDiet is a common dietary pattern that identify a lifestyle and a culture. It was proven that it contributes to better health and quality of life. Concerning its healthy effects, low content of animal protein and low glycaemic index may directly modulate the insulin/insulin-like growth factor-1 and the mammalian target of rapamycin pathways, known to be involved in ageing, age-related diseases and longevity. In addition to the influence on nutrient sensing pathways, many single components of MedDiet are known to have positive effects on health, reducing inflammation, oxidative stress and other important risk factors of age-related diseases [6].

This pilot study demonstrates an anti-inflammatory and anti-oxidant effect of daily consumption of green table olives *Nocellara del Belice*. Moreover, it is noteworthy the reduction of fat mass with an increase of muscle mass. Although no statistically significant probiotic effect was observed, the positive trend related to *L.* amount at T1 could represent a starting point for further studies.

It is to note that the study presents limitations. One is strictly related to the intrinsic complexity of human as study model and to the inter/intra-individual variability. These features are more evident in ageing than in younger people. This is the reason why we chose middle age people. So, our choice represented the second limitation of the study because we did not analyze the effects of the intervention in elderly. Thirdly, it is necessary to verify these data in a larger sample of individuals to confirm the role of table green olives as nutraceutical foods. Also the duration of the intervention could be inadequate. In fact, we developed a short-term dietary regimen (30 days). This is a good choice in terms of compliance to the study because the more is the time of intervention the more is the drop out effect. But, a long-term dietary intervention could be stronger in terms of variation of analyzed parameters *(e.g.,* *L.* amount in feces).

However, these new knowledges give an important achievement for the food and farming industry, especially in Sicily, where the olives represent a great potential resource. No approved healthy property and claim exist for them. Therefore, adding such a common product to the class of nutraceuticals could represent a big deal.

In the era of many expansive and mysterious longevity elixirs, the olives could represent a traditional, cheap and accessible to everyone "healthy food".

Methods
Study design

The trial consisted in the assumption of 12 olives/day for 30 days. They belonging to the variety *Nocellara del Belice*, were processed in salt solution without any chemical additives.

See Fig. 1 for the flow chart of the study design.

Study population

Twenty-five randomized volunteers (mean age 38,3), both men and women, were recruited from April 2015 to July 2015. The subjects included were: healthy, with age between 18 and 65 years and Caucasian. The

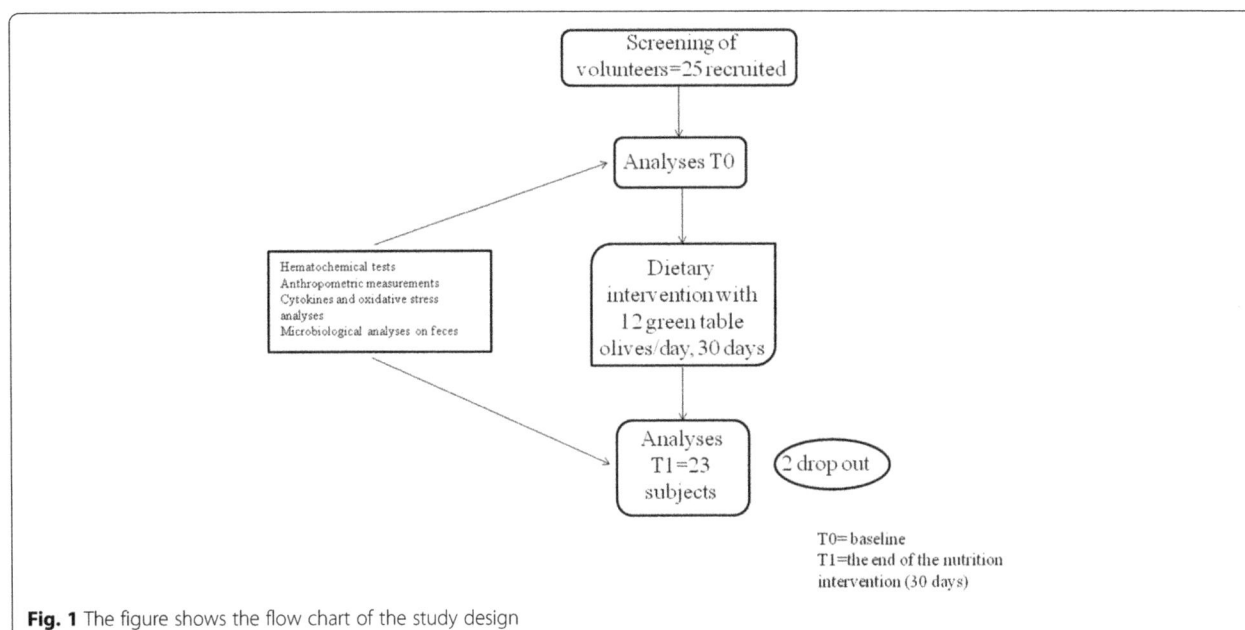

Fig. 1 The figure shows the flow chart of the study design

exclusion criteria provided: a history of the absence of pathologies (obesity, MS); a history of use of any pre or probiotics as dietary supplements within 3 months prior to the study; a history of treatment with statins or similar and with lyposoluble drugs; the onset of gastrointestinal disorders or the use of antibiotics during the nutritional intervention. No restriction related to sex was considered. Two subjects dropped out of the trial. All participants signed an informed consent before the enrolment. To respect the privacy, everyone was identified with an alphanumeric code. Height and weight were measured wearing light clothes and barefoot. The body composition was registered using specific hardware and software. Body mass index was calculated as weight (in kilos) over height squared (in square metre) (Table 1). Dietary habits were assessed through a food frequency questionnaire, officially validate by the EPIC study. Blood tests, oxidative stress and cytokines analyses were carried out for all subjects at T0 and T1. Molecular analyses were conducted on *L.* DNA obtained from fecal samples to measure the variation of its amount. A database was created to insert all participants' data and to handle the collected information.

Hematochemical tests

The recruited people underwent to venipuncture at T0 and at T1. Blood samples were collected in specific blood collection tubes containing ethylenediaminetetraacetic acid (EDTA) for plasma analyses and in serum tubes with no additives. Plasma and sera were separated from whole blood by low-speed centrifugation at 2,500 rpm for 15′ at 4 °C. After separation, the samples were stored at −80 °C for further tests. We also obtained

gruel of red blood cells from blood collected in tubes with EDTA through three washes with physiological solution (centrifugation at 2,500 rpm for 15′ at 4 °C).

Evaluation of parameters of oxidative stress

These analyses were conducted in collaboration with the University of Sassari. Thiobarbituric acid reactive substances (TBARS) were determined according to the method described by Esterbauer and Cheeseman [22]. TBARS methodology measures MDA and other aldehydes produced by lipid peroxidation induced by hydroxyl free radicals. For the measurements, plasma was mixed with 10 % trichloroacetic acid and 0.67 % thiobarbituric acid and heated at 95 °C in thermoblock heater for 25′. TBARS were determined by measuring the absorbance at 535 nm. A calibration curve was obtained using standard MDA and each curve point was subjected to the same treatment as that of the samples.

PON activity was determined by measuring the increase in absorbance at 412 nm (formation of 4-nitrophenol), using paraoxon (O, O diethyl-O-p-nitrophenyl phosphate) as a substrate [22]. The enzyme activity was calculated by using the molar extinction coefficient of 17,100 $M^{-1}cm^{-1}$ and one unit of PON activity was defined as 1 nanomole of 4-nitrophenol formed per minute. For red blood cell glutathione quantification, 200 μl (μL) of thawed packed cells were lysed by adding 600 μL of cold water and keeping the samples at 4 °C for 15′. 200 μL of lysed samples were deproteinized by adding 200 μL acetonitrile and centrifuged at 2,000 × g for 5′. Samples were then derivatized by mixing 100 μL of supernatant with 100 μL of sodium phosphate buffer (60 μmol (mmol)/L, pH 12.5), and 25 μL of 5-

Iodoacetamidofluorescein (4.1 mmol/L). After vortex mixing, samples were incubated for 15′ at room temperature. Derivatized samples were diluted 100-fold in water and analysed by capillary electrophoresis with laser induced fluorescence detection [23].

Pro and anti-inflammatory cytokines analyses

These analyses were conducted using Luminex assays, coupled to Bio-Plex Manager software.

Data obtained have been checked by technical department and quality control parameters. Values of the standard curve were compared to the values provided by the manufacturer of the kits used and must not exceed a CV of 15 %. All of above parameters were applied on, at least, the 90 % of the standard curve values.

Microbiological and molecular analyses of *Lactobacilli*

In order to quantify the amount of *L.* in each olive, 1 g of pulp was suspended in phosphate-buffered saline solution (1 mL), homogenized for 2′ at maximum speed, and then serially diluted. Decimal dilutions were plated and incubated on *de Man, Rogosa and Sharpe* at 30 °C for 48 h to observe the *L.* growth. The colonies' count was performed in triplicate and the *L.* DNA was extracted from them to perform molecular analyses. Moroever, colony suspension were used as a template for Real Time PCR. The primers and probes used to detect *L. species* (*spp*) were based on 16S rRNA gene sequences retrieved from the NCBI databases (Table 2). The amplification reactions were carried out in a total volume of 25 ml containing 1X SSoFast Probe mix (BIORAD), primers (each at 200 nM concentration), 100 nM Taq-Man MGB probe, 60 ng purified target DNA. Amplification (1 cycle of 5′ at 95 °C, 45 cycles of 15″ at 95 °C and 1 cycle of 1′ at 60 °C) and detection were carried out on a CFX Real Time system (BIORAD).

Fluorescent probe was labeled at 5′ end with the reporter dye 6-carboxyfluorescein and at 3′ end with a quencher dye. A negative and a positive control were included on the reaction plate.

In order to perform the quantification of *L.* in each feces sample, the QIAamp DNA Stool Minikit (Qiagen) was used to extract DNA from an appropriate amount of frozen stool sample, according to the manufacturer's instructions. The Real Time PCR was performed as previous described and the cycle threshold of each sample

Table 2 Primer and probe sequences for analyses of *L. spp* in Real Time PCR

	Oligonucleotide sequence 5′-3′
Primer Forward	GAGGCAGCAGTAGGGAATCTTC
Primer Reverse	GGCCAGTTACTACCTCTATCCTTCTTC
Probe	FAM-ATGGAGCAACGCCGC-QUENCER

was compared to a standard curve made by diluting genomic DNA (10-fold serial dilution) from cultures of known concentrations of *L.* (10^6 CFU/ml).

Statistical analyses

The paired comparisons were performed with the Student's *t*-test or the Wilcoxon signed rank test, according to the normality of samples. Statistical analyses were performed with the IDE RStudio for the R (version 3.2.2) software [24, 25].

Competing interests

The authors declare that they have no competing interest.

Authors' contribution

GA, AA, VG, and CC* conceived and designed the study; GA, AA, CMG, VG, SM, SC, GV, AZ, CC* and CC** performed or supervised experiments. MZ executed statistical analysis. GA, AA, VG, CC*, and CC** analyzed and interpreted data; GA and AA drafted the paper. GC, CC* and CC** made critical revisions to the draft. All authors read and approved the final manuscript. CC*: Calogero Caruso. CC**: Ciriaco Carru

Acknowledgments

This work was supported by PON DIMESA (Programma Operativo Nazionale Ricerca e Competitività 2007/2013 - Progetto "DI.ME.Sa." PON02_00451_3361785. Valorisation of typical products of the Mediterranean diet and their nutraceutical use to improve health) to CC. GA is a Post Doc at DiBiMed. AA and CMG are students of the PhD course directed by CC.
We are grateful to Dr. Nicola Locorotondo for his continuous enthusiastic support.

Author details

[1]Sezione di Patologia generale del Dipartimento di Biopatologia e Biotecnologie Mediche (DIBIMED), Università di Palermo, Corso Tukory 211, 90134 Palermo, Italy. [2]Istituto Zooprofilattico Sperimentale della Sicilia, Via Gino Marinuzzi 3, 90129 Palermo, Italy. [3]Dipartimento di Scienze Biomediche, Università di Sassari, Viale San Pietro 43/b, 07100 Sassari, Italy. [4]UOC Epidemiologia Clinica con registro tumori di Palermo e provincia, AOUP "Paolo Giaccone", Palermo, c/o Dipartimento di Scienze per la promozione della salute e materno infantile "G. D'Alessandro", Università di Palermo, Via del Vespro 133, 90131 Palermo, Italy.

References

1. Longo VD, Antebi A, Bartke A, Barzilai N, Brown-Borg HM, Caruso C, Curiel TJ, de Cabo R, Franceschi C, Gems D, Ingram DK, Johnson TE, Kennedy BK, Kenyon C, Klein S, Kopchick JJ, Lepperdinger G, Madeo F, Mirisola MG, Mitchell JR, Passarino G, Rudolph KL, Sedivy JM, Shadel GS, Sinclair DA, Spindler SR, Suh Y, Vijg J, Vinciguerra M, Fontana L. Interventions to Slow Aging in Humans: Are We Ready? Aging Cell. 2015;14:497–510. doi:10.1111/acel.12338.
2. Balistreri CR, Caruso C, Candore G. The role of adipose tissue and adipokines in obesity-related inflammatory diseases. Mediators Inflamm. 2010. doi:10.1155/2010/802078.
3. Estruch R, Martínez-González MA, Corella D, Salas-Salvadó J, Ruiz-Gutiérrez V, Covas MI, Fiol M, Gómez-Gracia E, López-Sabater MC, Vinyoles E, Arós F, Conde M, Lahoz C, Lapetra J, Sáez G, Ros E; PREDIMED Study Investigators. Effects of a Mediterranean-style diet on cardiovascular risk factors: a randomized trial. Ann Intern Med. 2006;145:1–11.
4. Fitó M, Guxens M, Corella D, Sáez G, Estruch R, de la Torre R, Francés F, Cabezas C, López-Sabater Mdel C, Marrugat J, García-Arellano A, Arós F, Ruiz-Gutierrez V, Ros E, Salas-Salvadó J, Fiol M, Solá R, Covas MI; PREDIMED Study Investigators. Effect of a traditional Mediterranean diet on lipoprotein oxidation: a randomized controlled trial. Arch Intern Med. 2007;167:1195–203.

5. Casas R, Sacanella E, Estruch R. The immune protective effect of the Mediterranean diet against chronic low-grade inflammatory diseases. Endocr Metab Immune Disord Drug Targets. 2014;14:245–54.

6. Vasto S, Buscemi S, Barera A, Di Carlo M, Accardi G, Caruso C. Mediterranean diet and healthy ageing: a Sicilian perspective. Gerontology. 2014;60:508–18. doi:10.1159/000363060.

7. Kastorini CM, Milionis HJ, Esposito K, Giugliano D, Goudevenos JA, Panagiotakos DB. The effect of Mediterranean diet on metabolic syndrome and its components: a meta-analysis of 50 studies and 534,906 individuals. J Am Coll Cardiol. 2011;57:1299–313. doi:10.1016/j.jacc.2010.09.073.

8. Uylaşer V, Yildiz G. The historical development and nutritional importance of olive and olive oil constituted an important part of the Mediterranean diet. Crit Rev Food Sci Nutr. 2014;54:1092–101. doi:10.1080/10408398.2011. 626874.

9. Vasto S, Rizzo C, Caruso C. Centenarians and diet: what they eat in the Western part of Sicily. Immun Ageing. 2012;9:10. doi:10.1186/1742-4933-9-10.

10. DeFelice SL. FIM, Rationale and Proposed Guidelines for the Nutraceutical Research & Education Act NREA, Foundation for Innovation in Medicine. 2002. http://www.fimdefelice.org/archives/arc.researchact.html archact.html. Accessed 10 Nov 2002.

11. Hoffman R, Gerber M. Food Processing and the Mediterranean Diet. Nutrients. 2015;7:7925–64. doi:10.3390/nu7095371.

12. Aiello A, Guccione GD, Accardi G, Caruso C. What olive oil for healthy ageing? Maturitas. 2015;80:117–8. doi:10.1016/j.maturitas.2014.10.016.

13. Biagi E, Candela M, Turroni S, Garagnani P, Franceschi C, Brigidi P. Ageing and gut microbes: perspectives for health maintenance and longevity. Pharmacol Res. 2013;69:11–20. doi:10.1016/j.phrs.2012.10.005.

14. Lefevre M, Racedo SM, Ripert G, Housez B, Cazaubiel M, Maudet C, Jüsten P, Marteau P, Urdaci MC. Probiotic strain Bacillus subtilis CU1 stimulates immune system of elderly during common infectious disease period: a randomized, double-blind placebo-controlled study. Immun Ageing. 2015; 12:24. doi:10.1186/s12979-015-0051-y.

15. Heperkan D. Microbiota of table olive fermentations and criteria of selection for their use as starters. Front Microbiol. 2013;4:143. doi:10.3389/fmicb.2013. 00143.

16. Aponte M, Ventorino V, Blaiotta G, Volpe G, Farina V, Avellone G, Lanza CM, Moschetti G. Study of green Sicilian table olive fermentations through microbiological, chemical and sensory analyses. Food Microbiol. 2010;27: 162–70. doi:10.1016/j.fm.2009.09.010.

17. Lehnen TF, da Silva MR, Camacho A, Marcadenti A, Lehnen AM. A review on effects of conjugated linoleic fatty acid (CLA) upon body composition and energetic metabolism. J Int Soc Sports Nutr. 2015;12:36. doi:10.1186/s12970-015-0097-4.

18. Fazzari M, Trostchansky A, Schopfer FJ, Salvatore SR, Sánchez-Calvo B, Vitturi D, Valderrama R, Barroso JB, Radi R, Freeman BA, Rubbo H. Olives and olive oil are sources of electrophilic fatty acid nitroalkenes. PLoS One. 2014;14(9): e84884. doi:10.1371/journal.pone.0084884.

19. Wang Y, Jones PJ. Dietary conjugated linoleic acid and body composition. Am J Clin Nutr. 2004;6 Suppl 79:1153S–8S.

20. Ershler WB, Keller ET. Age-associated increased interleukin-6 gene expression, late-life diseases, and frailty. Annu Rev Med. 2000;51:245–70.

21. Czerska M, Mikołajewska K, Zieliński M, Gromadzińska J, Wąsowicz W. Today's oxidative stress markers. Med Pr. 2015;66:393–405. doi:10.13075/mp. 5893.00137.

22. Gan KN, Smolen A, Eckerson HW, La Du BN. Purification of human serum paraoxonase/arylesterase. Evidence for one esterase catalyzing both activities. Drug Metab Dispos. 1991;19:100–6.

23. Zinellu A, Sotgia S, Usai MF, Chessa R, Deiana L, Carru C. Thiol redox status evaluation in red blood cells by capillary electrophoresis-laser induced fluorescence detection. Electrophoresis. 2005;26:1963–8.

24. RStudio Team. RStudio: Integrated Development for R. Boston, MA: RStudio, Inc.; 2015. http://www.rstudio.com/.

25. R Core Team. R. A language and environment for statistical computing. Vienna, Austria: R Foundation for Statistical Computing; 2015. https://www. R-project.org/.

Immunological and non-immunological mechanisms of allergic diseases in the elderly: biological and clinical characteristics

Gabriele Di Lorenzo[1,3*], Danilo Di Bona[2], Federica Belluzzo[1] and Luigi Macchia[2]

Abstract

A better hygiene, a Westernized diet, air pollution, climate changes, and other factors that influence host microbiota, a key player in the induction and maintenance of immunoregulatory circuits and tolerance, are thought to be responsible for the increase of allergic diseases observed in the last years. The increase of allergic diseases in elderly is related to the presence of other factors as several comorbidities that should interfere with the development and the type of allergic reactions. A central role is played by immunosenescence responsible for modifying response to microbiota and triggering inflamm-ageing. In addition, in elderly there is a shift from Th1 responses vs. Th2, hence favouring allergic responses. Better understanding of the mechanisms of immunosenescence and its effects on allergic inflammation will most certainly lead to improved therapy.

Keywords: Elderly, Immunosenescence, Allergic conjunctivitis, Allergic rhinitis, Asthma, Skin diseases

Background

Immediate hypersensitivity (Type I) is the most common immunological disease. About 25% of the population in industrialized countries is affected by Type I reactions, with manifestations ranging from impairment of quality of life to severely life-threatening. They may include eczema, conjunctivitis, rhinitis, asthma and anaphylaxis. Among the causes of the rapid increase in allergies are climate, pollution, diet, and the resulting microbial colonization patterns. These factors trigger and maintain a low chronic inflammatory state that characterizes allergic diseases. Most of the studies of allergic diseases and their clinical manifestations have been conducted on children or adolescents rather than on adults aged >65 years who will represent about 25% of the population in industrialized countries within the next few years.

The prevalence of allergic diseases in the elderly ranges from 5 to 10% and appears to be rising [1].

Immunosenescence

Immunosenescence is the reduction of the immune system capabilities to face stressing agents and to maintain the homeostasis. This process contributes to the reduced resistance to infectious diseases, increased propensity to develop cancer, and more frequent autoimmune diseases observed in aged individuals. A central role in allergies is played by a compromise of the integrity of epithelial barriers, a sub-clinical chronic inflammatory condition, and an enhanced Th2 (allergic) immune response [2].

Many aspects of immune function decline with ageing, while others become more active. The main hallmarks of immunosenescence are lymphocyte sub-population imbalances (decreased naive and increased memory lymphocytes with accumulation of dysfunctional senescent cells with shortened telomeres), thymus involution with decreased new T-cell generation, hematopoietic stem cell dysfunctions [3], defects in apoptotic cell death, mitochondrial function and stress responses, and malfunctioning of immune regulatory cells. As a consequence, a

* Correspondence: gabriele.dilorenzo@unipa.it
[1]Dipartimento BioMedico di Medicina Interna e Specialistica (Di.Bi.M.I.S.), Università di Palermo, Palermo, Italy
[3]Dipartimento BioMedico di Medicina Interna e Specialistica (Di.Bi.M.I.S), Via del Vespro, 141, 90127 Palermo, Italy
Full list of author information is available at the end of the article

senescent immune system is characterized by impaired interactions between innate and adaptive immune responses, continuous reshaping and shrinkage of the immune repertoire by persistent antigenic challenges, and chronic low-grade inflammation [4].

The most extensively studied component of the immune system with regard to immunosenescence is the T-cell population. The involution of the thymus gland begins shortly after birth, undergoes replacement by fatty tissue, and is nearly complete by 60 years of age. As a consequence, there is a reduction of circulating naive T-cells and an imbalance towards memory T-cells (CD45RO+). Additionally, the T-cell receptor repertoire diversity appears to diminish, and T helper cell activity declines [5]. Other observations of the T-cell population with ageing include reduced proliferation responses [6], a decrease in CD8+ T cell levels, a shift of Th1 to Th2 cytokine profiles upon stimulation with phorbol myristic acid, a decline in FAS-mediated T-cell apoptosis [7], and increased DR expression on T-cells. In addition, an increased proportion of FOXP3+ CD4+ T regulatory cells with intact suppression capabilities has been found in peripheral blood from elderly subjects, which may help explain the decreased T-cell activities described above. Whether any of these age-related changes is more or less pronounced in specific inflammatory disorders, such as allergic diseases or asthma, is not known.

The role of cytokines in the elderly has been debated because ageing is a dynamic process characterized by a continuous remodelling sustained by DNA repair, apoptosis, immune response, oxidation stress and inflammation. In other words, the genetic background of any subject controls immunity and inflammation and influences the chronic antigen load and the inflammation in ageing responsible for immunosenescence and hence age-related disorders.

Immunosenescence is the name given to the global age-associated immune dysfunctions [8–10]. There are several hypotheses to explain the ageing process; the same is true for immunosenescence [11, 12]. Virtually all cells of the immune system can undergo immunosenescence, which can lead to the general erosion of immune capacities. Animal and in vitro models [13] substantiate the existence of immunosenescence in humans [14].

NK cells are cytotoxic cells that play a significant role in innate defence against virus infected cells and possibly cancer. It was speculated that the cytotoxicity of NK cells is directly correlated to a successful ageing; a weaker response in also related to augmented morbidity and mortality due to infective and cardiovascular agents and to a worse response to influenza vaccination. Other aspects of NK cell function, such as the secretion of chemokines or interferon-γ (IFN-γ) in response to IL-2 also decrease in the aged. NK cells have an important role in immune surveillance, and any alterations in their function will influence susceptibility to pathogens and the control of cancer development [15].

The number and phagocyte capacity of neutrophils is well preserved in the elderly. However, certain other functional characteristics of neutrophils from elderly individuals, such as super-oxide anion production, chemotaxis, and apoptosis in response to certain stimuli, are reduced. It has been hypothesized that a reduction of the transduction ability of some receptors could be a decrease in signal transduction of certain receptors could be involved in the defective function of neutrophils with advancing age [16]. In particular, there is triggering of activating receptors such as Toll-like receptor-4 (TLR4), granulocyte macrophage colony stimulating factor (GM-CSF). Similarly, anti-apoptotic signals delivered by GM-CSF failed to rescue neutrophils from apoptosis in the elderly [16].

The number of monocytes in peripheral blood does not change substantially with age, although there is a reduced number of macrophage precursors and bone marrow macrophages. However, ageing demonstrated to affect macrophage phagocytosis, immune cells recruitment ability, ROS production and TLR function response [9]. Finally, the reduction of Class II major histocompatibility (MHC) expression is thought to be responsible for decreased antigen presentation by macrophages with age [17]. Furthermore, the hyperproduction of prostaglandin E2 by activated macrophages at least partly explains the reduced surface expression of Class II MHC [18].

DCs are the major antigen-presenting cells (APC), which are considered the starter of the adaptive immune response. It has been shown that DCs retain their antigen presentation function with healthy ageing [19], whereas DCs from frail elderly people display changes in co-stimulatory molecules. In brief, impaired activation of the immune response, poorer vaccine response, higher susceptibility to infection, higher susceptibility to cancer, and greater morbidity and mortality, are explained by alterations of the NK cells, phagocytes, and DCs. Ageing is correlated with a reduced number of DC descending from myeloid precursors, and have a more efficacy and mature phenotype such as a defecting ability to generate IL-12 with age. [20, 21]. Macropino-cytosis, endocytosis, response to chemokines, and cytokine secretion are also impaired, probably as a consequence of decreased activation of the phosphoinositide-3 kinase pathway [22].

Immune longitudinal studies in octo- and nonagenarians performed to establish predictive factors for longevity [23–25] in the context of function, and also measuring disability parameters, favour the hypothesis that the immune risk profile (IRP) predictive of subsequent mortality seems to depend in part on CD4 < CD8, low B cells, poor proliferation response, high CD8 + CD28 cells, low native cells, cytomegalovirus (CMV) seropositivity, and expansion of CMV-specific clones. Therefore there is an interplay between the IRP, low grade inflammation, and cognitive impairment in mortality. The IRP was constituted by immune subsections consisting of a high count of CD8+ T cells, a reduced number of CD4+ T cells and CD19+ B cells, a reverted CD4-CD8 ratio, and a diminished response to concanavalin A [23]. Extensive analysis to search for associations between this IRP and various psychosocial parameters revealed that the IRP was associated only with evidence of persistent CMV infection, becoming prevalent in the very old. The accumulation of large numbers of CMV-specific CD8+ T cells [24] is found, as well as a majority of clonal expansions. In the very old an association with CMV has provided additional support for the hypothesis that CMV contributes markedly to the development of an IRP and thus constitutes a good biomarker of immunosenescence in the elderly [10]. The increase in circulating inflammatory mediators such as cytokines and acute phase proteins seems to contribute to the low-grade inflammation observed with ageing. Age-related alterations in responses to stimulation also contribute to low-grade inflammation by changing the level of pro-inflammatory mediators such as TNF-α and IL-6. Because of their association with pathological cases and chronic diseases, inflammatory mediators can also act as biomarkers or risk factors for age-associated diseases and predictors of mortality.

Both the IRP and inflammageing demonstrated being independent predictors of successful ageing and survival, suggesting that the physiological immunosenescence of T cells and low-grade inflammation are vital in late-life survival [23]. Major functions known to decrease with age are IL-2 production and T-cell proliferation [5]. This in vitro evidence would suggest an in vivo clonal expansion deficiency following antigen recognition partly explaining age-associated increased susceptibility to infections, auto-immune diseases, and cancers.

The dysfunction age-related of the immune system described above might also influence the efficacy of the vaccination in the old patient [26].

Although efficient in the great percentage of the individuals, only a small percentage of frail elderly is protected after influenza vaccination [27, 28]. This is partly due to the fact that antibodies produced by aged B cells are commonly of low affinity, providing less efficient protection compared to young individuals [29]. B-cell lymphopoiesis is also reduced, which leads to an increase in the percentage of antigen-experienced cells compared to newly produced naive B cells, parallel to the situation with T cells [30].

Recently Minciullo et al. have described the role of IL-1, IL-2, IL-6, IL-12, IL-15, IL-18, IL-22, IL-23, TNF-α, IFN-γ as pro-inflammatory cytokines, and IL-1Ra, IL-4, IL-10, TGF-β1 as anti-inflammatory cytokines, and lipoxin A4 and heat shock proteins as mediators of cytokines. They hypothesize that if inflamm-ageing is a key to understand ageing, anti-inflamm-ageing may be one of the secrets of longevity [31].

Allergic diseases in the elderly
The allergic diseases in the elderly are driven by cell ageing at large, and by immunosenescence and tissue structure modifications typical of advanced age.

Allergic conjunctivitis
Ocular allergy is a disease affecting the entire ocular surface including conjunctiva, lids, cornea, lachrymal gland and tear film. The spectrum of atopic eye diseases encompasses seasonal allergic conjunctivitis (SAC), perennial allergic conjunctivitis (PAC), vernal kerato-conjunctivitis (VKC), atopic kerato-conjunctivitis (AKC), atopic blepharo-conjunctivitis (ABC), and giant papillary conjunctivitis (GPC). A papillary conjunctivitis is common to these diseases, and with the exception of GPC, there is also evidence of a Type I, IgE-mediated, hypersensitivity response [32].

Very few data are available in literature regarding the prevalence, role, and management of allergic conjunctivitis in the aged population [33]. Allergic conjunctivitis affects mainly children and young adults, but an increasing number of cases is being diagnosed in the elderly. Conjunctivitis can be classified as "mild", "moderate," or "severe," depending on the character of disease presentation, or according to onset and duration, it can be classified as "acute," or "chronic," and "recurrent", or as "follicular" and "papillary conjunctivitis," "cicatrising" and "non-cicatrising," emphasizing the predominant clinical presentations. AKC is a chronic conjunctivitis, with progressive corneal vascularization and scarring [34]. The new classification for allergic conjunctivitis divides the conditions into IgE-mediated and non-IgE-mediated conjunctivitis. IgE-mediated conjunctivitis can be further divided into intermittent and persistent conjunctivitis. Persistent allergic conjunctivitis is classified into VKC and AKC. [35] The International Ocular Inflammation Society (IOIS) proposed a more comprehensive classification for conjunctivitis and blepharitis, including ocular allergy in the "non infectious, immuno-mediated" conjunctivitis and including both the "IgE-mediated" SAC and PAC, and "non-IgE-mediated" VKC and AKC. [36].

In Table 1 we report a schematic summary of the mechanisms and cells involved in ocular allergic diseases. The symptoms of allergic conjunctivitis were reported by

Table 1 Immunoglobulin and cells involved in ocular allergic diseases

	IgE	MC	Eos	TH1	TH2	Corneal involvement
SAC	+++	+++	+	−	+	−
PAC	+++	++	+	−	+	−
VKC	+	++	+++	+	+++	+++
AKC	+	++	+++	++	+++	+++
GPC	−	+	−	+	+	+
CDC	−	−	+	+++	−	−

68.6% of subjects with current rhinitis, accounting for a prevalence of rhino-conjunctivitis of 20.5% (95% CI: 19.2%–21.8%) in the studied population [37].

Allergic rhinitis

Allergic rhinitis (AR) is prevalent among older people, affecting around 5.4 to 10.7% of patients over 65 years old [38]. Typical symptoms of allergic rhinitis such as nasal obstruction, postnasal drip or cough may be worsened by the anatomic and physiological changes of the nose that occur with age. The ageing nose undergoes changes in all of its structural components. The fibroelastic attachments between the upper and lower cartilages of the nose fragment undergo ossification with ageing. Because of maxillary alveolar hypoplasia, the columella shortens, resulting in a droopy tip appearance [39].

Information about the effect of ageing on the changes of the nasal ciliated epithelium is very limited. The number of goblet cells decreases, resilient structures atrophy, and the basement membrane gets thicker with ageing. Human respiratory and olfactory mucosa present an age-related decrease in the intensity and extent of immunoreactivity within the nasal cells [40]. However, there is no significant age-related change in gross and electron microscopic examination of the histopathology of the mucosa of either the septum or the turbinates [39].

Few studies have addressed the impact of age on nasal airflow. The ageing mucosa is less soft and less elastic (possibly hormonal effects), which may lead to increased resistance. The results of studies on the effect of ageing on nasal mucociliary clearance (NMCC) and nasal ciliary beat frequency (NCBF) are controversial. However, a decrease in NCBF and an increase in NMCC time could have a negative effect on the efficiency of NMCC [41].

It is well known that the sense of smell diminishes with age. The mean prevalence of disturbance of olfaction on a population of U.S. residents between 53 and 97 years of age is 24.5%. The prevalence increased with age, and 62.5% of 80- to 97-year-old subjects has olfactory impairment [42]. The sense of smell comprises multiple sensations that are predominantly mediated by two independent neural systems—the olfactory and the somatosensory (trigeminal) [43].

These alterations of the nasal anatomy and physiology due directly to the normal ageing process result in symptoms of postnasal dripping, nasal drainage, sneezing, olfactory loss, and gustatory rhinitis. The other common nasal symptoms include nasal obstruction, headache, sinus pain, itching, and epistaxis. Below we report important aetiologies of nasal problems in elderly patients.

Vasomotor rhinitis, atrophic rhinitis, and gustatory rhinitis are common types of nonallergic rhinitis types that occur in older patients [44]. Gastroesophageal reflux has often been associated with vasomotor rhinitis [45]. Primary atrophic rhinitis was commonly associated with infection of *Klebsiella ozaenae*. Currently, it is more commonly seen as a result of aggressive surgery, trauma, granulomatous diseases, and radiation therapy [44].

Gustatory rhinitis is a profuse watery rhinorrhoea that may be exacerbated by eating. It is believed to arise from α-adrenergic activity stimulated by the regular use of antihypertensives. Allergic rhinitis and its severity decrease with age, and there are significantly fewer cases of atopy among elderly subjects (60 years or older) compared to younger individuals [46]. However, the repeatedly claimed global decline in the prevalence of allergic disorders in the elderly might be ascribed to the expected decrease in serum IgE antibodies due to an unbalance of cytokines and soluble factors involved in its production. In the assessment of serum IgE, sCD23 and Th2 type cytokine production, however, IgE serum levels did not differ in a relevant way among all the ages in non allergic subjects [47]. This was confirmed in another, similar study [48] that suggests the Type 2 cytokine pattern is not necessarily defective in old age. Data also confirmed that IL-13, a key cytokine in IgE regulation, is not impaired in old subjects. Although IL-4 has been considered the most critical cytokine linked to allergic responses and immunity against parasites, recent observations indicate that IL-13 has equal or even greater importance in those processes. IL-4 and IL-13 share several functional properties, but IL-13 can independently induce class switching and IgE secretion from human B cells. In addition, IL-13 enhances expression of CD23 and the MHC Class II antigens, and may act as a monocyte chemo-attractant [49]. Rhinitis associated symptoms seems to be milder and allergy-related parameters usually gradually decline in the long run; often, these nasal symptoms appear to be linked to the nasal eosinophils and are independent on SPT and specific IgE [50].

The increase of AR in elderly can be explained on the basis of the general hypothesis that imbalance of gut microbiota, linked to immunosnescence, influences the development of allergic diseases [51].

Asthma

Asthma represents a significant cause of morbidity and mortality in the elderly, while in the past it was regarded as an illness of childhood and youth. Asthma remains under-diagnosed in old people, and the percentage increases when respiratory symptoms are present. There are two kinds of old patients affected by asthma: one who had the onset of the disease in the childhood and one having encountered the symptoms in the sixth decade of life [52]. Current knowledge suggests a phenotype difference of asthma in old and young subjects, and this could potentially impact on diagnosis, assessment, and management of the disease. The same diagnostic tests and clinical findings applied in youth are used to diagnose asthma in the elderly, but interpreting clinical data becomes more difficult [53]. Asthma in the elderly is broadly divided into patients with long-standing disease present from childhood, and late-onset disease describing those developing symptoms following the sixth decade of life. The diagnosis in the second case could be difficult due to the presence of similar diseases with almost few equal symptoms, which have more prevalence in the elderly such as chronic obstructive lung disease (COPD) or heart failure [54].

Although the shortness of breath, chest tightness, cough, and wheezing that characterize asthma in young people are present in the elderly, mimicry by congestive heart failure, chronic obstructive pulmonary disease, ischemic heart disease, gastroesophageal reflux, pulmonary emboli, recurrent aspiration, respiratory track cancer, and laryngeal dysfunction make the diagnosis a challenge. Angiotensin converting enzyme inhibitor-induced cough is also a frequent masquerade. Older individuals often have poorer perception of airway obstructive symptoms and are less likely to report them. They may falsely attribute symptoms to "getting older" and avoid activities, including exercise, that trigger asthma symptoms. For many years asthma in older patients was characterized as non-atopic [55]. However, in the past two decades, data from large populations or from studies incorporating data from multiple sites of asthma care, demonstrate that some older patients with asthma are also atopic (demonstrated either by serum evaluation or skin prick testing). Busse et al., demonstrated a higher allergic sensitization rate among asthmatics, at 62.5%, compared to 38.8% in the general population in subjects ≥55 years of age [56].

Sensitization to indoor allergens alone, rather than indoor and outdoor allergens, has been suggested as potentially more important to asthma in older patients [1]. Distinguishing between asthma and COPD frequently becomes an issue when airway obstruction is evaluated in the elderly. In a study focusing on the lung function and inflammatory differences between asthma and COPD, it was observed that in the asthma subjects there was significantly more allergic sensitivity, higher values for alveolus-capillary diffusion of carbon monoxide,

greater increases in forced expiratory volume in the 1st second, following bronchodilator or corticosteroids, and more eosinophils in peripheral blood, bronchoalveolar lavage and sputum [53]. However, it is also likely that an overlap syndrome exists for some patients in which features of asthma and COPD are both present, but this subset of patients has yet to be carefully examined and is typically excluded from investigation studies. The "Dutch Hypothesis" is an interesting view of asthma and COPD that proposes there is one common obstructive lung disease that includes both asthma and COPD [57]. This hypothesis suggests that a common genetic predisposition for obstructive lung disease exists, and that asthma and COPD differ with respect to the lung exposures (allergen versus tobacco smoke) that trigger and drive the disorder towards airway obstruction. However, this hypothesis remains controversial because it cannot fully explain some of the differences observed between asthma and COPD [58].

Because viral infections of the upper respiratory tract trigger the majority of asthma exacerbations, age-related decline in antiviral responses affects the associated morbidity and mortality [2].

Skin diseases

Ageing contributes progressively to a loss of structural integrity and physiological function of the skin. Although skin is incredibly durable, it is affected by ageing, like all other organ systems [59]. The synergistic effects of biological, environmental, mechanical ageing, and miscellaneous factors including diet, sleep patterns, morbidity, and mental health over the human lifespan combine to cause deterioration of the cutaneous barrier and the structural integrity of the skin. Hormonal changes that also play a role in the ageing of skin, especially in females, lead to earlier signs of ageing for women [60]. However, skin ageing can also produce significant morbidity, pervasive dryness and itching, and increased risk of numerous skin diseases, including cutaneous malignancy. Most people over 65 have at least one skin disorder, and many have two or more. Cell numbers in the epidermis are reduced in older adults [61]. Keratinocytes change shape, becoming shorter and fatter, as skin ages [62], whereas corneocytes in aged skin become bigger as a result of decreased epidermal turnover [61]. Epidermal turnover time increases in aged skin [63].

Since permeability barrier function in ageing epidermis does not appear to be impaired under basal conditions, it has been generally assumed that barrier function does not alter significantly with ageing [64]. Recovery of barrier function in aged subjects was also dramatically different. Only 15% of those older than 80 years had recovered barrier function at 24 h, compared to 50% of the younger group [65]. The findings reveal a profound change in barrier integrity even though barrier function under normal conditions appears normal. A lack of functional reserve is exposed when the epidermal permeability barrier is under stress [65]. Although the lipid composition of aged skin is not significantly altered, the global lipid content of aged skin is reduced [65]. Total lipid content in aged skin decreased as much as 65% [66].

The flattened dermal–epidermal junction, with its reduced interdigitation between layers, results in less resistance to shearing forces and an increased vulnerability to insult [67]. Dermal thickness decreases with age [68], with a decrease in vascularity and cellularity. There is also a decrease in the number of mast cells and fibroblasts [69]. However, ageing is inevitably associated with a decrease in collagen turnover (due to a decrease in fibroblasts and their collagen synthesis) as well as elastin [69]. The loss of molecular integrity of the dermis leads to increased rigidity, decreased torsion extensibility and diminished elasticity (eroding faster in females than in males), with a concomitant increase in vulnerability to tear type injuries [67].

The overall volume of subcutaneous fat typically diminishes with age, although the proportion of body fat increases until approximately age 70 [67]. Contact dermatitis is common in the elderly population (particularly allergy-type reactions) [2]. Reduced ability to mount a delayed-type hypersensitivity reaction in the elderly decreases individual susceptibility to allergic contact sensitivity due to a reduction in numbers of Langerhans cells [70], decreased T-cells, and diminished vascular reactivity [71]. However, decades of potential sensitization [72] and an increased level of exposure maintain a presence of allergic contact sensitivity in the geriatric population [73]. The most common culprit in allergic contact sensitivity is topical medications [74]. As many as 81% of patients being treated for chronic leg ulcers exhibit allergic reactions to topical medications. Patch testing before the use of topical medications may be beneficial, especially within high-risk populations like those being treated for dermatitis or ulceration of the lower extremities [75]. Testing should include medication and dressings, as well as dental prostheses, and medications for ocular disease [76]. In the elderly a generalized allergic rash is far more likely to be due to drugs rather than to be food-related. Occasionally an agent increases the patient's sensitivity to the sun in a phototoxic (photoirritant) reaction, or produces a hypersensitivity reaction upon sun exposure [77].

However, it may be relevant that with ageing, in the skin, total IgE production increases with the decrease in IgE levels towards specific allergens [78].

Conclusion

In the last years the prevalence of allergic diseases in general population is increased because of environmental changes such as the a better hygiene, a Westernized diet, air pollution, climate changes, and other factors that influence host microbiota. Microbiota is a key player in the induction and maintenance of immunoregulatory circuits and tolerance and its changes can determine immune dysregulation, and subsequent low-grade chronic inflammation, which is a common pathogenic mechanism in several diseases including the allergic ones. Additional factors are responsible for the increase of allergic diseases in elderly as the presence of several comorbidities that should interfere with the development and the type of allergic reactions. However, immunosenescence plays a central role by modifying response to microbiota and triggering inflamm-ageing. In addition, in elderly there is a shift from Th1 responses vs. Th2, hence favouring allergic responses. Better understanding of the mechanisms of immunosenescence and its effects on allergic inflammation will most certainly lead to improved therapy [79–81]. Optimal treatment of elderly patients requires an alliance between the patient, geriatrician, and allergist.

Abbreviations

ABC: Atopic blepharoconjunctivitis; AKC: Atopic keratoconjunctivitis; APC: Antigen-presenting cells; AR: Allergic rhinitis; CMV: Cytomegalovirus; COPD: Chronic obstructive pulmonary disease; DC: Dendritic Cell; GM-CSF: Granulocyte-macrophage colony stimulating factor; GPC: Giant papillary conjunctivitis; IFN-γ: Interferon-γ; IOIS: International Ocular Inflammation Society; IRP: Immune risk profile; MCH: Major histocompatibility complex; NCBF: Nasal ciliary beat frequency; NK: Natural Killer; NMCC: Nasal mucociliary clearance; PAC: Perennial allergic conjunctivitis; SAC: Seasonal allergic conjunctivitis; Th: T helper; TLR4: Toll-like receptor-4; VKC: Vernal keratoconjunctivitis

Acknowledgements

None

Funding

This work was entirely supported by the authors' respective institutions.

Authors' contributions

GDL wrote the paper. All the Authors edited the paper and approved its final version.

Competing interests

The authors declare that they have no competing interests.

Author details

[1]Dipartimento BioMedico di Medicina Interna e Specialistica (Di.Bi.M.I.S.), Università di Palermo, Palermo, Italy. [2]Department of Allergy, Clinical Immunology, Emergency Medicine, and Transplants, University of Bari, Bari,

Italy. [3]Dipartimento BioMedico di Medicina Interna e Specialistica (Di.Bi.M.I.S), Via del Vespro, 141, 90127 Palermo, Italy.

References

1. Mathur SK. Allergy and asthma in the elderly. Semin Respir Crit Care Med. 2010;31:587–95.

2. Milgrom H, Huang H. Allergic disorders at a venerable age: a mini-review. Gerontology. 2014;60:99–107.

3. Denkinger MD, Leins H, Schirmbeck R, Florian MC, Geiger H. HSC aging and senescent immune remodeling. Trends Immunol. 2015;36:815–24.

4. Jenny NS. Inflammation in aging: cause effect or both? Discover Med. 2012; 13:451–60.

5. Caruso C, Di Lorenzo G, Modica MA, Candore G, Portelli MR, Crescimanno G, Ingrassia A, Barbagallo Sangiorgi G, Salerno A. Soluble interleukin-2 receptor release defect in vitro in elderly subjects. Mech Aging Dev. 1991;59:27–35.

6. Franceschi C, Valensin S, Bonafè M, Paolisso G, Yashin AI, Monti D, De Benedictis G. The network and the remodeling theories of aging: historical background and new perspectives. Exp Gerontol. 2000;35:879–96.

7. Potestio M, Pawelec G, Di Lorenzo G, Candore G, D'Anna C, Gervasi F, Lio D, Tranchida G, Caruso C, Colonna RG. Age-related changes in the expression of CD95 (APO1/FAS) on blood lymphocytes. Exp Geront. 1999;34:659–73.

8. Effros RB. Genetic alterations in the ageing immune system: impact on infection and cancer. Mech Ageing Dev. 2003;124:71–7.

9. Gomez CR, Boehmer ED, Kovacs EJ. The aging innate immune system. Curr Opin Immunol. 2005;17:457–62.

10. Ouyang Q, Wagner WM, Zheng W, Wikby A, Remarque EJ, Pawelec G. Dysfunctional CMV-specific CD8(+) T cells accumulate in the elderly. Exp Gerontol. 2004;39:607–13.

11. Pawelec G, Akbar A, Caruso C, Solana R, Grubeck-Loebenstein B, Wikby A. Human immunosenescence: is it infectious? Immunol Rev. 2005;205:257–68.

12. Frasca D, Riley RL, Blomberg BB. Humoral immune response and B-cell functions including immunoglobulin class switch are down-regulated in aged mice and humans. Semin Immunol. 2005;17:378–84.

13. Pawelec G, Rehbein A, Haehnel K, Merl A, Adibzadeh M. Human T-cell clones in long-term culture as a model of immunosenescence. Immunol Rev. 1997;160:31–42.

14. Colonna Romano G, Cossarizza A, Aquino A, Scialabba G, Bulati M, Lio D, Candore G, Di Lorenzo G, Fradà G, Caruso C. Age and gender-related values of lymphocyte subsets in subjects from northern and southern Italy. Arch. Gerontol. 2002;35 (suppl 8):99–107.

15. Di Lorenzo G, Balistreri CR, Candore G, Cigna D, Colombo A, Colonna Romano G, Colucci AT, Gervasi F, Listì F, Potestio M, Caruso C. Granulocyte and natural killer activity in the elderly. Mech Ageing Dev. 1999;108:25–38.

16. Fortin CF, Larbi A, Lesur O, Douziech N, Fulop T Jr. Impairment of SHP-1 down-regulation in the lipid rafts of human neutrophils under GM-CSF stimulation contributes to their age-related, altered functions. J Leukoc Biol. 2006;79:1061–72.

17. Villanueva JL, Solana R, Alonso MC, Peña J. Changes in the expression of HLA-class II antigens on peripheral blood monocytes from aged humans. Dis Markers. 1990;8:85–91.

18. Plowden J, Renshaw-Hoelscher M, Engleman C, Katz J, Sambhara S. Innate immunity in aging: impact on macrophage function. Aging Cell. 2004;3:161–7.

19. Lung TL, Saurwein-Teissl M, Parson W, Schönitzer D, Grubeck-Loebenstein B. Unimpaired dendritic cells can be derived from monocytes in old age and can mobilize residual function in senescent T cells. Vaccine. 2000;18:1606–12.

20. De Martinis M, Franceschi C, Monti D, Ginaldi L. Inflammation markers predicting frailty and mortality in the elderly. Exp Mol Pathol. 2006;80:219–27.

21. Lio D, D'Anna C, Scola L, Potestio M, Di Lorenzo G, Candore G, Colombo A, Caruso C. Interleukin-12 release by mitogen-stimulated mononuclear cells in the elderly. Mechanism of ageing and. Development. 1998;102:211–9.

22. Agrawal A. Mechanisms and implications of age-associated impaired innate interferon secretion by dendritic cells: a mini-review. Gerontology. 2013;59(5): 421–16.

23. Wikby A, Ferguson F, Forsey R, Thompson J, Strindhall J, Löfgren S, Nilsson BO, Ernerudh J, Pawelec G, Johansson B. An immune risk phenotype, cognitive impairment, and survival in very late life: impact of allostatic load in Swedish octogenarian and nonagenarian humans. J Gerontol A Biol Sci Med Sci. 2005; 60:556–65.

24. Wikby A, Johansson B, Olsson J, Löfgren S, Nilsson BO, Ferguson F. Expansions of peripheral blood CD8 T-lymphocyte subpopulations and an association with cytomegalovirus seropositivity in the elderly: the Swedish NONA immune study. Exp Gerontol. 2002;37:445–53.

25. Strindhall J, Nilsson BO, Löfgren S, Ernerudh J, Pawelec G, Johansson B, Wikby A. No immune risk profile among individuals who reach 100 years of age: findings from the Swedish NONA immune longitudinal study. Exp Gerontol. 2007;42:753–61.

26. Myśliwska J, Trzonkowski P, Szmit E, Brydak LB, Machała M, Myśliwski A. Immunomodulating effect of influenza vaccination in the elderly differing in health status. Exp Gerontol. 2004;39:1447–58.

27. Intonazzo V, La Rosa G, Di Lorenzo G, Sferlazzo A, Perna AM, Ingrassia A, Crescimanno G. Risposta sierologica indotta da vaccino influenzale trivalente a subunità. L'Igiene Moderna. 1991;96:800–10.

28. Skowronski DM, Tweed SA, De Serres G. Rapid decline of influenza vaccine-induced antibody in the elderly: is it real, or is it relevant? J Infect Dis. 2008; 197:490–502.

29. Listì F, Candore G, Modica MA, Russo M, Di Lorenzo G, Esposito-Pellitteri M, Colonna-Romano G, Aquino A, Bulati M, Lio D, Franceschi C, Caruso C. A study of serum immunoglobulin levels in elderly persons that provides new insights into B cell immunosenescence. Ann N Y Acad Sci. 2006;1089:487–95.

30. Colonna-Romano G, Aquino A, Bulati M, Di Lorenzo G, Listì F, Vitello S, Lio D, Candore G, Clesi G, Caruso C. Memory B cell subpopulations in the aged. Rejuvenation Res. 2006;9:149–52.

31. Minciullo PL, Catalano A, Mandraffino G, Casciaro M, Crucitti A, Maltese G, Morabito N, Lasco A, Gangemi S, Basile G. Inflammaging and anti-Inflammaging: the role of cytokines in extreme longevity. Arch Immunol Ther Exp. 2016;64:111–26.

32. Bonini S, Gramiccioni C, Bonini M, Bresciani M. Practical approach to diagnosis and treatment of ocular allergy: a 1-year systematic review. Curr Opin Allergy Clin Immunol. 2007;7:446–9.

33. Wüthrich B, Schmid-Grendelmeier P, Schindler C, Imboden M, Bircher A, Zemp E, Probst-Hensch N. Prevalence of atopy and respiratory allergic diseases in the elderly SAPALDIA population. Int Arch Allergy Immunol. 2013;162:143–8.

34. Creuzot-Garcher C. Different clinical forms of conjunctival allergy. J Fr Ophtalmol. 2007;30:288–91.

35. Bonini S. Allergic conjunctivitis: the forgotten disease. Chem Immunol Allergy. 2006;91:110–20.

36. BenEzra D. Classification of conjunctivitis and blepharitis. In: BenEzra D, editor. Blepharitis and conjunctivitis: guidelines for diagnosis and treatment. Barcelona: Editorial Glosa; 2006.

37. Morais-Almeida M, Pite H, Pereira AM, Todo-Bom A, Nunes C, Bousquet J, Fonseca J. Prevalence and classification of rhinitis in the elderly: a nationwide survey in Portugal. Allergy. 2013;68:1150–7.

38. Pinto JM, Jeswani S. Rhinitis in the geriatric population. Allergy Asthma Clin Immunol. 2010;6:6.

39. Edelstein DR. Aging of the normal nose in adults. Laryngoscope. 1996; 106:1–25.

40. Getchell ML, Chen Y, Ding X, Sparks DL, Getchell TV. Immunohistochemical localization of a cytochrome P-450 isozyme in human nasal mucosa: age-related trends. Ann Otol Rhinol Laryngol. 1993;102:368–74.

41. Kalmovich LM, Elad D, Zaretsky U, Adunsky A, Chetrit A, Sadetzki S, Segal S, Wolf M. Endonasal geometry changes in elderly people: acoustic rhinometry measurements. J Gerontol A Biol Sci Med Sci. 2005;60:396–8.

42. Murphy C, Schubert CR, Cruickshanks KJ, Klein BE, Klein R, Nondahl DM. Prevalence of olfactory impairment in older adults. JAMA. 2002;288:2307–12.

43. Hummel T, Livermore A. Intranasal chemosensory function of the trigeminal nerve and aspects of its relation to olfaction. Int Arch Occup Environ Health. 2002;75:305–13.

44. Lieberman P, Pattanaik D. Nonallergic rhinitis. Curr Allergy Asthma Rep. 2014;14:439.

45. Berger WE, Schonfeld JE. Nonallergic rhinitis in children. Curr Allergy Asthma Rep. 2007;7:112–6.

46. Bozek A. Pharmacological Management of Allergic Rhinitis in the elderly. Drugs Aging. 2017;34:21–8.

47. Di Lorenzo G, Pacor ML, Esposito Pellitteri M, Listì F, Colombo A, Candore G, Mansueto P, Lo Bianco C, Ditta V, Rini GB, Caruso C. A study of age-related IgE pathophysiological changes. Mech Ageing Dev. 2003;124:445–8.

48. Moro-García MA, Alonso-Arias R, López-Larrea C. Molecular mechanisms involved in the aging of the T-cell immune response. Curr Genomics. 2012;13:589–602.

49. Ridolo E, Anti R, Ventura MT, Martignago I, Incorvaia C, Di Lorenzo G, Passlacqua G. How fit allergen immunotherapy in the elderly. Clin Mol Allergy. 2017;15:17.

50. Di Lorenzo G, Leto-Barone MS, La Piana S, Ditta V, Di Fede G, Rini GB. Clinical course of rhinitis and changes in vivo and in vitro of allergic parameters in elderly patients: a long-term follow-up study. Clin Exp Med. 2013;13:67–73.

51. Kim BJ, Lee SY, Kim HB, Lee E, Hong SJ. Environmental changes, microbiota, and allergic diseases. Allergy Asthma Immunol Res. 2014;6:389–400.

52. Pite H, Pereira AM, Morais-Almeida M, Nunes C, Bousquet J, Fonseca JA. Prevalence of asthma and its association with rhinitis in the elderly. Respir Med. 2014;108:1117–26.

53. Di Lorenzo G, Mansueto P, Ditta V, Esposito-Pellitteri M, Lo Bianco C, Leto-Barone MS, D'Alcamo A, Farina C, Di Fede G, Gervasi F, Caruso C, Rini G. Similarity and differences in elderly patients with fixed airflow obstruction by asthma and by chronic obstructive pulmonary disease. Respir Med. 2008; 102:232–8.

54. Bahadori K, Doyle-Waters MM, Marra C, Lynd L, Alasaly K, Swiston J, FitzGerald JM. Economic burden of asthma: a systematic review. BMC Pulm Med. 2009;9:24.

55. Braman SS, Kaemmerlen JT, Davis SM. Asthma in the elderly. A comparison between patients with recently acquired and long-standing disease. Am Rev Respir Dis. 1991;143:336–40.

56. Busse PJ, Cohn RD, Salo PM, Zeldin DC. Characteristics of allergic sensitization among asthmatic adults older than 55 years: results from the National Health and nutrition examination survey, 2005-2006. Ann Allergy Asthma Immunol. 2013;110:247–52.

57. Kraft M. Asthma and chronic obstructive pulmonary disease exhibit common origins in any country. Am J Respir Crit Care Med. 2006;174(3):238–40.

58. Barnes PJ. Against the Dutch hypothesis: asthma and chronic obstructive pulmonary disease are distinct diseases. Am J Respir Crit Care Med. 2006; 174:240–3.

59. Le Varlet B, Chaudagne C, Saunois A, Barré P, Sauvage C, Berthouloux B, Meybeck A, Dumas M, Bonté F. Age-related functional and structural changes in human dermo-epidermal junction components. J Investig Dermatol Symp Proc. 1998;3:172–9.

60. McCallion R, Li Wan Po A. Dry and photo-aged skin: manifestations and management. J Clin Pharm Ther. 1993;18:15–32.

61. Fenske NA, Lober CW. Structural and functional changes of normal aging skin. J Am Acad Dermatol. 1986;15:571–85.

62. Živicová V, Lacina L, Mateu R, Smetana K Jr, Kavková R, Drobná Krejčí E, Grim M, Kvasilová A, Borský J, Strnad H, Hradilová M, Šáchová J, Kolář M, Dvořánková B. Analysis of dermal fibroblasts isolated from neonatal and child cleft lip and adult skin: developmental implications on reconstructive surgery. Int J Mol Med 2017; 40: 1323-1334.

63. Dos Santos M, Metral E, Boher A, Rousselle P, Thepot A, Damour O. In vitro 3-D model based on extending time of culture for studying chronological epidermis aging. Matrix Biol. 2015 Sep;47:85–97.

64. Parrish AR. The impact of aging on epithelial barriers. Tissue Barriers. 2017: e1343172.

65. Coderch L, López O, de la Maza A, Parra JL. Ceramides and skin function. Am J Clin Dermatol. 2003;4:107–29.

66. Antonov D, Schliemann S, Elsner P. Hand dermatitis: a review of clinical features, prevention and treatment. Am J Clin Dermatol. 2015;16:257–70.

67. Farage MA, Miller KW, Berardesca E, Maibach HI. Clinical implications of aging skin: cutaneous disorders in the elderly. Am J Clin Dermatol. 2009;10:73–86.

68. Waller JM, Maibach HI. Age and skin structure and function, a quantitative approach II: blood flow, pH, thickness, and ultrasound echogenicity. Skin Res Technol. 2005;11:221–35.

69. Audisio RA, Ramesh H, Longo WE, Zbar AP, Pope D. Preoperative assessment of surgical risk in oncogeriatric patients. Oncologist. 2005; 10:262–8.

70. Zegarska B, Pietkun K, Giemza-Kucharska P, Zegarski T, Nowacki MS, Romańska-Gocka K. Changes of Langerhans cells during skin ageing. Postepy Dermatol Alergol. 2017;34:260–7.

71. Negru T, Ghiea V, Diaconu V, Păsărică D. Survey on some aspects of immunologic reactivity in old age. Rom J Physiol. 1995;32:125–36.

72. Na CR, Wang S, Kirsner RS, Federman DG. Elderly adults and skin disorders: common problems for nondermatologists. South Med J. 2012;105:600–6.

73. Jacob SE, Elsaie ML, Castanedo-Tardan MP, Stechschulte S, Kaufman J. Aging and contact dermatitis: a review. Curr Aging Sci. 2009;2:121–6.

74. Uter W, Spiewak R, Cooper SM, Wilkinson M, Sánchez Pérez J, Schnuch A, Schuttelaar ML. Contact allergy to ingredients of topical medications: results of the European surveillance system on contact allergies (ESSCA), 2009-2012. Pharmacoepidemiol Drug Saf. 2016;25:1305–12.

75. Liu DJ, Collaku A, Dosik JS. Skin irritation and sensitization potential of fixed-dose combination of Diclofenac 1% and menthol 3% topical gel: results of two phase I patch studies. Drug Res (Stuttg). 2017;67:119–26.

76. Nedorot ST, Stevens SR. Diagnosis and treatment of allergic skin disorders in the elderly. Drugs Aging. 2001;18:827–35.

77. Dawe RS. Chronic actinic dermatitis in the elderly: recognition and treatment. Drugs Aging. 2005;22:201–7.

78. De Amici M, Ciprandi G. The age impact on serum Total and allergen-specific IgE. Allergy Asthma Immunol Res. 2013;5:170–4.

79. Shreiner A, Huffnagle GB, Noverr MC. The "Microflora Hypothesis" of allergic disease. Adv Exp Med Biol. 2008;635:113–34.

80. Caruso C, Candore G, Cigna D, DiLorenzo G, Sireci G, Dieli F, Salerno A. Cytokine production pathway in the elderly. Immunol Res. 1996;15(1):84–90.

81. De Martinis M, Sirufo MM, Ginaldi L. Allergy and aging: an old/new emerging health issue. Aging Dis. 2017;8:162–75.

Virtual memory cells make a major contribution to the response of aged influenza-naïve mice to influenza virus infection

Kathleen G. Lanzer, Tres Cookenham, William W. Reiley and Marcia A. Blackman[*]

Abstract

Background: A diverse repertoire of naïve T cells is thought to be essential for a robust response to new infections. However, a key aspect of aging of the T cell compartment is a decline in numbers and diversity of peripheral naïve T cells. We have hypothesized that the age-related decline in naïve T cells forces the immune system to respond to new infections using cross-reactive memory T cells generated to previous infections that dominate the aged peripheral T cell repertoire.

Results: Here we confirm that the CD8 T cell response of aged, influenza-naïve mice to primary infection with influenza virus is dominated by T cells that derive from the memory T cell pool. These cells exhibit the phenotypic characteristics of virtual memory cells rather than true memory cells. Furthermore, we find that the repertoire of responding CD8 T cells is constrained compared with that of young mice, and differs significantly between individual aged mice. After infection, these virtual memory CD8 T cells effectively develop into granzyme-producing effector cells, and clear virus with kinetics comparable to naïve CD8 T cells from young mice.

Conclusions: The response of aged, influenza-naive mice to a new influenza infection is mediated largely by memory CD8 T cells. However, unexpectedly, they have the phenotype of VM cells. In response to de novo influenza virus infection, the VM cells develop into granzyme-producing effector cells and clear virus with comparable kinetics to young CD8 T cells.

Keywords: T cell receptor repertoire, Virtual memory (VM) T cells, True memory (TM) T cells, Influenza, Ageing, Mouse model

Background

A diverse repertoire of naïve T cells is thought to be necessary for an optimal response to infections [1–6]. With age, the numbers of naïve T cells decline, such that the ratio of memory-phenotype to naïve T cells in the periphery greatly increases. In addition, the repertoire diversity becomes constrained [7–15]. The decline of the naïve repertoire of CD8 T cells with age is a consequence of reduced thymic output, increasing antigen experience, peripheral homeostatic proliferation and the development of large clonal expansions of cells displaying a memory phenotype [16–21].

The decline in naïve T cells with aging has been correlated with impaired immunity and reduced ability to respond to new infections [3–6, 13, 22, 23]. Consistent with this, our previous studies confirmed that declining numbers of naïve CD8 T cells in aged mice correlated with poor responses to de novo infection with influenza virus [7]. Specifically, the response to an immunodominant nucleoprotein epitope (NP_{366}), but not the co-dominant epitope (PA_{224}), was found to be dramatically reduced in aged mice. We further showed that the naïve precursor frequency of NP-specific CD8 T cells was 10-fold lower than PA-specific CD8 T cells in aged mice, providing an explanation for the selective decline in the immune response to influenza virus NP. This study provided proof of

* Correspondence: mblackman@trudeauinstitute.org
Trudeau Institute, 154 Algonquin Avenue, Saranac Lake, NY 12983, USA

concept that the naïve repertoire to epitopes with a low precursor frequency may become so constrained during aging that "holes" develop in the repertoire [7].

With increasing antigen experience during the lifespan and the decline in numbers and diversity of naïve T cells, we have hypothesized that memory CD8 T cells generated in response to previous antigen exposure and that are fortuitously cross reactive make a major contribution to T cell responses to de novo infections in aged mice [6]. Consistent with this hypothesis, unexpected cross-reactivity has been demonstrated between CD8 T cells specific for distinct epitopes expressed by different viruses [24–31]. It has also been shown that CD4 T cells respond to antigens to which the individual has never been exposed, as a consequence of cross-reactivity [32]. Together, the data show that T cell recognition of antigen/MHC is highly degenerate, and T cell responses exhibit extensive and unexpected cross reactivity [5, 33].

Fortuitously cross-reactive memory CD8 T cells provide a potential explanation of how protection can be maintained within aged mice as the naïve repertoire declines. One prediction of this hypothesis is that the CD8 T cell response to new infections in aged mice would be likely to exhibit reduced repertoire diversity compared to CD8 T cell responses in young mice. In addition, the specific and perhaps unique prior antigenic experience and repertoire of memory cells in each individual would result in heterogeneous responses in individual aged animals. Another prediction of the hypothesis is that the reduced repertoire diversity of the fortuitously cross reactive memory T cell responses would result in impaired immunity and delayed viral clearance in aged mice [6]. The goal of the current study was to test these possibilities.

Conventional memory CD8 T cells can be classified into three distinct types that are distinguished by phenotypic markers and trafficking patterns. One population, effector memory cells (EM), express low levels of CD62L and CCR7, lack the ability to home to lymph nodes, and preferentially localize to peripheral tissues. A second population, central memory cells (CM), express high levels of CD62L and CCR7, and circulate through the blood and secondary lymphoid organs. A third population, resident memory cells (T_{RM}), express CD69 and CD103, reside in the peripheral tissues, and do not circulate [34–37].

Memory cells were originally defined as a population of long-lasting cells generated by exposure to antigen. However, recently it has become apparent that antigen-specific, memory-phenotype T cells can also develop in the absence of antigenic stimulation. For example, antigen-specific memory phenotype T cells can be detected by antigen/MHC tetramers from naïve and germ-free mice. In one study, CD8 T cells specific for three different peptides from ovalbumin, vaccinia virus and herpes simplex virus were isolated from naïve mice and, unexpectedly, a significant percentage

of the cells were of a memory phenotype ($CD44^{High}$) [38]. There are two major subsets of these antigen-inexperienced memory cells, termed innate memory and virtual memory (VM) [39]. These subsets are difficult to distinguish phenotypically, as both populations of antigen-inexperienced memory cells are characterized by their high expression of CD62L and CD122, and low expression of CD49d. However, there are developmental and functional differences between the two subsets of cells [39]. Importantly for this study, there are relatively few innate memory cells in C57BL/6 mice [39, 40], and the frequency of VM cells have been shown to increase with age, such that the majority of CD8 T cells in aged C57BL/6 mice, used in this study, have a VM phenotype [2, 41, 42]. These data raise the possibility that VM cells contribute to the response of aged, influenza-naïve mice to de novo influenza infection.

In this study we have tested the hypothesis that cross-reactive memory T cells not specifically elicited by previous infection play a major role in the response of aged mice to new infections. As predicted, we show that the response of aged, influenza-naive mice to a new influenza infection is mediated largely by memory CD8 T cells that exhibit reduced repertoire diversity that is heterogeneous in individual mice. However, unexpectedly, they have the phenotype of VM cells. In response to de novo influenza virus infection, the VM cells develop into granzyme-producing effector cells and clear virus with comparable kinetics to young CD8 T cells.

Results

Memory CD8 T cells from aged, influenza-naïve mice respond to de novo infection with influenza virus and produce only minimal responses to influenza NP

To demonstrate that memory CD8 T cells from aged mice that had not previously been exposed to influenza virus were capable of responding to influenza virus, we FACS-sorted memory CD8 T cells ($CD44^{High}$) from aged, naïve specific pathogen free mice and adoptively transferred them into young T cell-deficient (TCR $\beta\delta$ $-/-$) mice. The following day the mice were infected with influenza virus and on day 12 post infection (p.i.) the responding CD8 T cells were tested for reactivity to a panel of five MHC class I influenza-specific epitopes from the viral proteins - nucleoprotein (NP_{366}/D^b), acid polymerase (PA_{224}/D^b), basic polymerase I ($PB1_{703}/K^b$), the F2 of PB1 ($PB1\ F2_{62}\ /D^b$) and non-structural protein 2 ($NS2_{114}/K^b$) Fig. 1a. It has previously been shown in young mice that the antigen-specific T cell response to the NP_{366}/D^b and the PA_{224}/D^b epitopes are relatively equi-dominant following primary infection with influenza virus (see a representative control response in Fig. 1b), whereas the secondary antigen-specific T cell response is sharply biased toward the NP_{366}/D^b epitope [43–45]. In contrast, we have demonstrated a dramatically reduced response to NP_{366}/D^b in

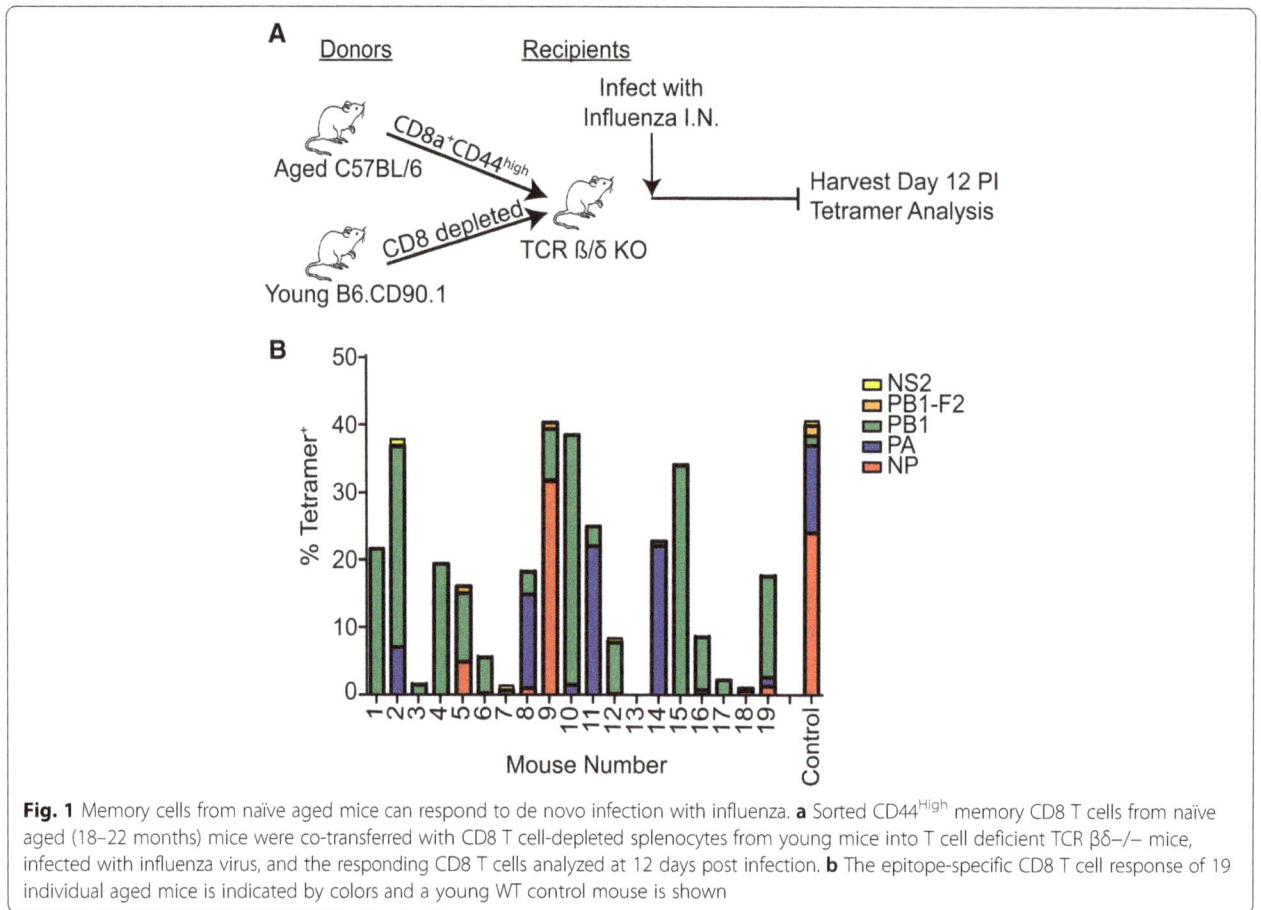

Fig. 1 Memory cells from naïve aged mice can respond to de novo infection with influenza. **a** Sorted CD44^{High} memory CD8 T cells from naïve aged (18–22 months) mice were co-transferred with CD8 T cell-depleted splenocytes from young mice into T cell deficient TCR βδ–/– mice, infected with influenza virus, and the responding CD8 T cells analyzed at 12 days post infection. **b** The epitope-specific CD8 T cell response of 19 individual aged mice is indicated by colors and a young WT control mouse is shown

aged mice [7]. Consistent with this, analysis of adoptive transfers from 19 individual aged mice showed that the pattern of response to the two epitopes was heterogeneous in individual mice and was not consistent with what was typically seen in either primary or recall responses in young mice (Fig. 1b). In only one of the 19 adoptive transfers of aged mouse cells did we observe a dominant NP$_{366}$/D^b response after influenza infection. In three additional mice we observed a PA$_{224}$/D^b dominant response, and in nine mice we observed a PB1$_{703}$/K^b-dominant response (which in a young intact SPF mouse represents a sub-dominant epitope). These adoptive transfer data are consistent with our previous data showing a selective reduction in the ability of aged mice to mediate a response to the immunodominant NP$_{366}$/D^b epitope after influenza infection, which is highly variable in individual mice [7]. In order to ensure that the development of the immunodominant NP$_{366}$/D^b response in the aged mice was not impaired due to lack of some deficiency in the TCR βδ –/– mice, such as CD4 T cell help, we co-transferred CD8-depleted splenocytes from young, congenically disparate mice along with the aged memory CD8 T cells. The number of sorted CD44^{High} memory cells transferred from individual mice was variable,

depending upon the yield of cells from the sort, but this did not correlate with the reduction of the NP$_{366}$/D^b response (Additional file 1).

While these findings demonstrate skewing of the epitope diversity within the aged memory populations of cells, it is important to also take into consideration that T cell clonal expansions increase with aging and can be a contributing factor to the declining ratio of naïve:memory CD8 T cells. These clonal expansions could be a significant component of the transferred CD44^{High} cells [20, 21, 46, 47]. Therefore, to eliminate this complication in the current experiments, we routinely pre-screened aged mice and eliminated those mice with TCE, determined as described in the Materials and Methods.

Competition between memory and naïve CD8 T cells from aged mice responding to de novo influenza virus infection

The previous data show that memory CD8 T cells from influenza-naïve, aged mice could respond to influenza virus infection when they were transferred in isolation and were the only source of CD8 T cells. However, in order to understand whether these cells could dominate the response in the context of the total population of peripheral CD8 T cells from aged mice, it was important to determine the ability of these cells to compete with naïve CD8 T cells. Therefore, we co-transferred naïve (CD44^{Low}) and memory (CD44^{High}) cells from aged mice into TCR βδ –/– mice (as previously) in a 1:1 ratio (Fig. 2a). Cells were isolated from congenically distinct mice (Fig. 2b), to allow for the identification of naïve and memory donor cells during the response. In an additional set of experiments, we co-transferred naïve and memory CD8 T cells in a 1:9 ratio, more typical of the ratio in aged mice. In both cases, as previously, we co-transferred CD8-depleted spleen cells from young mice, distinguished by a third congenic marker (see Figure legend for details).

The data (Fig. 2c) show that memory CD8 T cells made a minor contribution to de novo influenza infection in the bronchoalveolar lavage (BAL), lung tissue and spleen when the naïve and memory cells were transferred in a 1:1 ratio, and a greater contribution to the response when the cells were transferred in a 1:9 ratio, a ratio more reflective of their natural distribution in aged mice. These data show that cross-reactive memory cells in aged, influenza-naive mice can make a major contribution to the response to a de novo influenza virus infection.

We also analyzed the epitope specificity of the response within these competitive transfer experiments (Fig. 2d). The repertoire of naïve CD8 T cells in the 1:1 transfer was

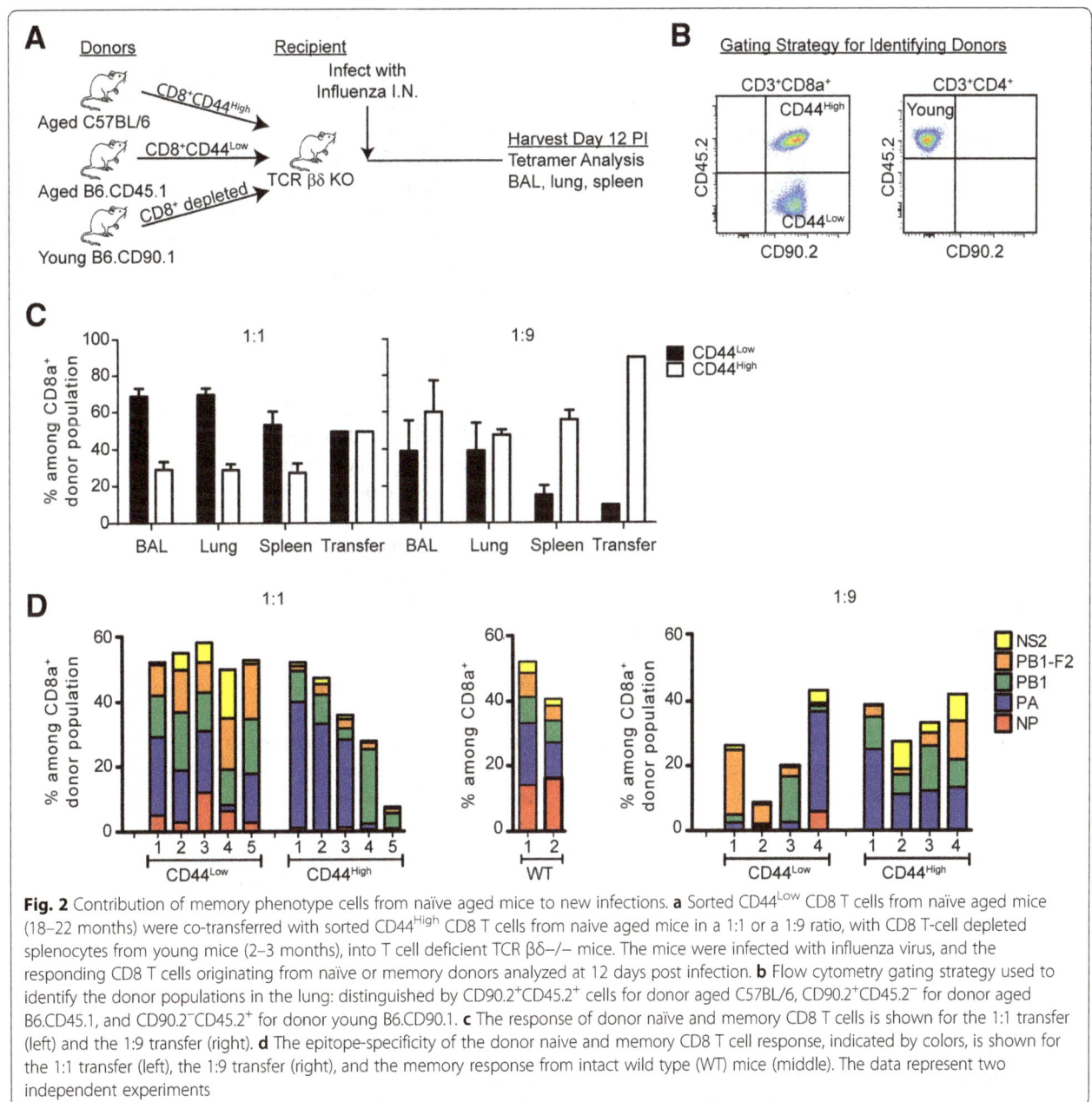

Fig. 2 Contribution of memory phenotype cells from naïve aged mice to new infections. a Sorted CD44^{Low} CD8 T cells from naïve aged mice (18–22 months) were co-transferred with sorted CD44^{High} CD8 T cells from naive aged mice in a 1:1 or a 1:9 ratio, with CD8 T-cell depleted splenocytes from young mice (2–3 months), into T cell deficient TCR βδ–/– mice. The mice were infected with influenza virus, and the responding CD8 T cells originating from naïve or memory donors analyzed at 12 days post infection. b Flow cytometry gating strategy used to identify the donor populations in the lung: distinguished by CD90.2$^+$CD45.2$^+$ cells for donor aged C57BL/6, CD90.2$^+$CD45.2$^-$ for donor aged B6.CD45.1, and CD90.2$^-$CD45.2$^+$ for donor young B6.CD90.1. c The response of donor naïve and memory CD8 T cells is shown for the 1:1 transfer (left) and the 1:9 transfer (right). d The epitope-specificity of the donor naive and memory CD8 T cell response, indicated by colors, is shown for the 1:1 transfer (left), the 1:9 transfer (right), and the memory response from intact wild type (WT) mice (middle). The data represent two independent experiments

diverse, and consisted of responses to all 5 epitopes tested, reflective of the repertoire of wild type mice. In contrast, the repertoire of the responding memory cells in both the 1:1 and the 1:9 transfer was skewed from the normal response of naïve CD8 T cells, and varied greatly in individual mice. Together, these data support the hypothesis that cross-reactive memory CD8 T cells, not generated in response to influenza virus infection, make a major contribution to the response to a newly-encountered antigen in aged mice, with skewed repertoire diversity.

Distribution of peripheral memory CD8 T cells in influenza memory mice infected when young or aged

The previous data supported our hypothesis that in aged mice the naïve CD8 T cell repertoire may become so constrained that responses to newly-encountered pathogens are mediated primarily by fortuitously cross reactive memory CD8 T cells, previously generated in response to unrelated antigens. The composition of the peripheral CD8 T cells in the spleen and lung of young mice is predominately of a naïve phenotype (CD44^{Low}), whereas the composition in aged mice is predominantly a memory phenotype (CD44^{High}), consistent with published data [42] (Fig. 3). Furthermore, memory phenotype cells in young mice were predominantly CM whereas aged mice had a large percentage of EM in addition to CM. Further analysis of the phenotype of the CM using the phenotypic markers CD62L and CD49d showed that cells with a virtual memory (VM) phenotype dominated the CM population in both young and aged mice. We termed the memory cells without a VM phenotype (CD49d^{High}), true memory (TM) cells. The low number of TM in aged mice raised the possibility that memory T cells of a VM rather than a TM phenotype responded to de novo influenza infection. Thus we next investigated whether the adoptively-transferred CD8 memory T cells responding to a primary influenza infection in aged mice originated from VM or TM cells.

VM dominate the response of memory CD8 T cells from aged naïve mice to primary influenza virus infection

To determine if the memory CD8 T cells that were responding during influenza infection of aged mice were of the TM or VM phenotype, the two populations were sorted from aged naïve B6 and congenic (B6.CD45.1) mice based on CD49d expression. Cells were then adoptively transferred into T cell-deficient (TCR βδ$^{-/-}$) mice, along with CD8-depleted T cells from young congenic mice (B6.CD90.1), and infected with influenza virus, as shown (Fig. 4a). We then followed the response to PA$_{224}$/D^b since our previous findings demonstrated the low and variable nature of the NP$_{366}$/D^b response in aged mice (Figs. 1b and 2d). As shown in Fig. 4c, the influenza antigen-specific T cell response to the PA$_{224}$/D^b epitope was dominated by VM cells, with only a very small

component arising from the adoptively transferred TM cells. Further examination of the antigen-specific T cell repertoire to the five major influenza epitopes in C57BL/6 mice reinforced the conclusion that the influenza-specific response of aged mice predominantly derives from VM cells (Fig. 4e). We also examined the phenotype of the antigen-specific T cells that developed in response to the influenza infection and found that all of the cells had up-regulated CD49d, switching to a TM phenotype (Fig. 4d). Taken together, the data show that the response of memory CD8 T cells from influenza-naïve aged mice to a new influenza infection is predominantly mediated by VM cells and these VM cells then convert to a TM phenotype, consistent with previous observations [48].

VM cells from aged mice generate functional effector cells

In order to determine whether influenza virus reactive VM CD8 T cells were functional, we analyzed granzyme responses (Fig. 5a). Granzyme staining from representative individual mice is shown in Fig. 5b. The plotted data from two independent experiments (Fig. 5c) show the VM cells from aged, influenza-naïve mice developed a granzyme response at least as strong as that developed by the naïve T cells from young mice at day 6. By day 9 the response of both populations had waned.

The delay in viral clearance of influenza infection in aged mice has been well established [49]. However, our observations that naïve CD8 T cells from young mice and VM CD8 T cells from aged mice generate comparable granzyme responses prompted us to examine viral clearance (Fig. 6a). Therefore, we compared viral clearance mediated by young CD8 T cells (mostly naïve) and aged CD8 T cells (mostly VM). Unexpectedly, the kinetics of viral clearance in TCR βδ $-/-$ mice into which young or aged CD8 T cells had been transferred was comparable. In order to rule out the possible participation of cytotoxic young CD4 T cells [50, 51], we eliminated young CD4 T cells from the co-transfer. The data (Fig. 6b) showed that the kinetics of viral clearance remained comparable between transferred CD8 T cells from young mice, which have mostly naïve CD8 T cells and aged mice, which have mostly VM CD8 T cells. TCR βδ$-/-$ mice that received no transferred T cells (Fig. 6c) failed to clear virus, indicating that the viral clearance we are detecting in panel B is mediated by the transferred T cells.

Together, our data show that VM effectively produce granzyme and mediate viral clearance. These data are consistent with previous reports that VM protect against infectious challenge and mediate rapid effector function [48, 52, 53], although it is possible that there are kinetic differences compared with TM, which have not been examined (in isolation) in this study.

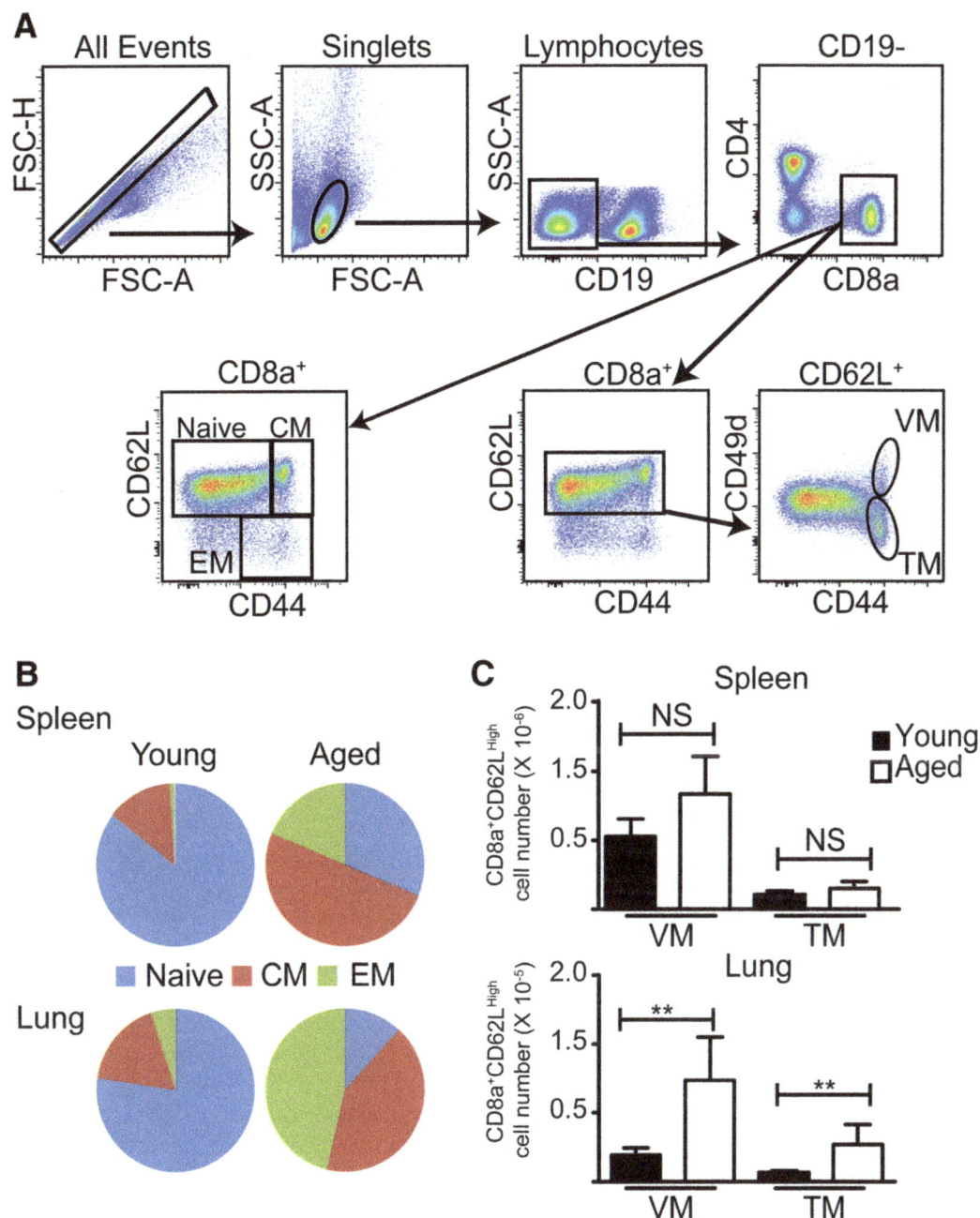

Fig. 3 Distribution of peripheral CD8 T cells in naïve young and aged mice. **a** Representative flow cytometry staining from spleen illustrating the gating strategy for identifying CD8 subsets in B and C. **b** The distribution of naïve (CD62L^{High}/CD44L^{Low}), CM (CD62L^{High}/CD44^{High}) and EM (CD62L^{Low}/CD44^{High}) in the spleen and lung of young (2–3 months) and aged (18–22 months) SPF mice. **c** The number of VM (CD49d^{Low}) and TM (CD49d^{High}) among the CM population in the spleen and lung of young and aged mice. Bars represent the mean ± SD. The data are from a single experiment, $n = 5$ mice/group, and are consistent with published data [42]. Data were analyzed by unpaired, two-tailed T test (**$p < 0.01$)

Discussion

It is well-established that there is a dramatic reduction in the number of naïve CD8 T cells and a corresponding increase in the number of memory phenotype CD8 T cells in the periphery of aged mice. Because of the decline in numbers (and, consequently, repertoire diversity) of naïve cells, we hypothesized that the response of aged mice to new infections would be dominated by cross-reactive memory cells previously generated in response to other antigens during the lifespan, rather than from the pool of naïve cells [6, 54]. Using an adoptive transfer system, we have shown that, indeed, memory CD8 T cells from aged, influenza-naïve mice are capable of responding to influenza virus and developing into effector T cells that could

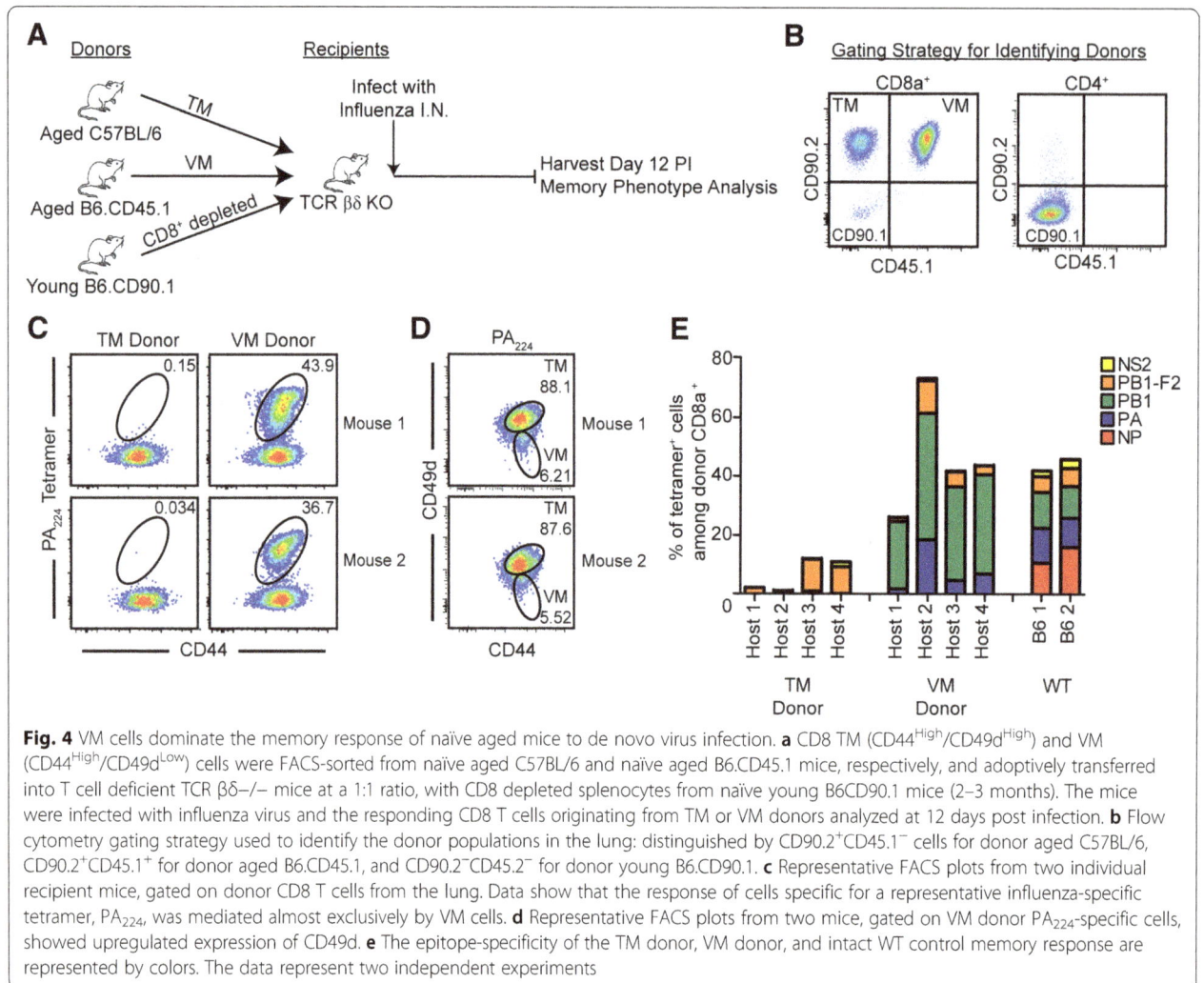

Fig. 4 VM cells dominate the memory response of naïve aged mice to de novo virus infection. **a** CD8 TM (CD44^{High}/CD49d^{High}) and VM (CD44^{High}/CD49d^{Low}) cells were FACS-sorted from naïve aged C57BL/6 and naïve aged B6.CD45.1 mice, respectively, and adoptively transferred into T cell deficient TCR βδ–/– mice at a 1:1 ratio, with CD8 depleted splenocytes from naïve young B6CD90.1 mice (2–3 months). The mice were infected with influenza virus and the responding CD8 T cells originating from TM or VM donors analyzed at 12 days post infection. **b** Flow cytometry gating strategy used to identify the donor populations in the lung: distinguished by CD90.2$^+$CD45.1$^-$ cells for donor aged C57BL/6, CD90.2$^+$CD45.1$^+$ for donor aged B6.CD45.1, and CD90.2$^-$CD45.2$^-$ for donor young B6.CD90.1. **c** Representative FACS plots from two individual recipient mice, gated on donor CD8 T cells from the lung. Data show that the response of cells specific for a representative influenza-specific tetramer, PA$_{224}$, was mediated almost exclusively by VM cells. **d** Representative FACS plots from two mice, gated on VM donor PA$_{224}$-specific cells, showed upregulated expression of CD49d. **e** The epitope-specificity of the TM donor, VM donor, and intact WT control memory response are represented by colors. The data represent two independent experiments

migrate to the sites of infection. Our dual adoptive transfer experiments showed that when naïve and memory CD8 T cells were co-transferred at a ratio consistent with that found in aged mice (1:9), the memory T cells dominated the response. Yet the ability of adoptively transferred aged CD8 T cells to respond was outcompeted by the naïve CD8 T cells when transferred at the 1:1 ratio. Furthermore, the epitope specificity of the memory T cell response was substantially constricted compared with naïve T cells, and heterogeneous in individual mice, particularly with regard to the normally immunodominant epitope, NP (Fig. 1b). These data are consistent with previous studies by us [7] and others [9], showing reduced repertoire diversity following primary infection of intact aged mice.

Thus, our data support the hypothesis that the response to new antigens in aged mice is dominated by cross-reactive memory CD8 T cells. However, phenotypic analysis revealed that the memory cells were not "true" memory cells (TM), as would have been generated to previous infections. Instead, the memory cells had characteristics of VM, which are generated in the absence of antigen [38, 53, 55, 56]. Importantly, the cells were found to be functional in terms of granzyme production and cleared virus upon influenza infection after adoptive transfer into young, T cell-deficient mice.

VM cells in mice appear in the periphery soon after birth in the absence of antigen [38, 48, 56–58], and accumulate with age in naïve specific pathogen free (spf) mice [2, 41, 42, 59]. While the factors influencing the generation of VM are not completely understood, it has been hypothesized that these cells arise via different mechanisms in young and aged mice. For example, secondary TCRα rearrangements have been shown to be necessary for the age-related dominance of VM, indicating a requirement for TCR ligation in the generation of VM in aged mice, which was not a requirement in young mice [59]. Clearly, the mechanisms involved in VM cell generation, as well as the maintenance of these cells, need to be studied in both young and aged mice.

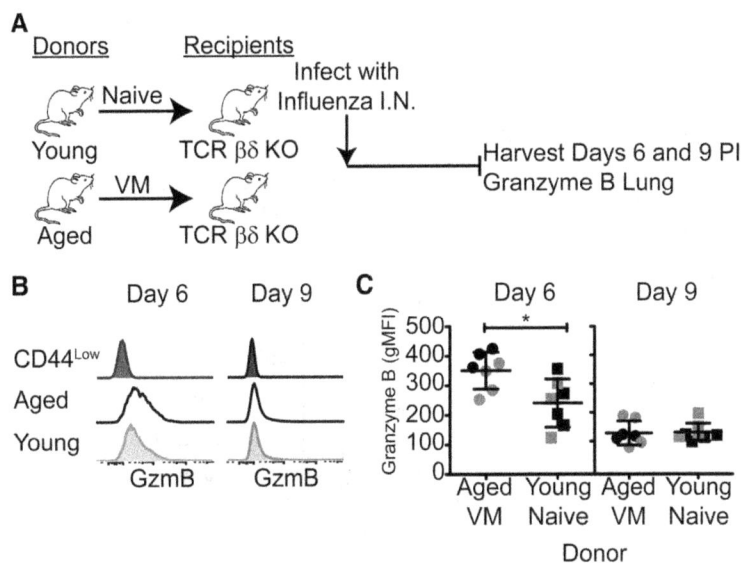

Fig. 5 VM cells from aged mice express Granzyme B following response to influenza infection. **a** Pooled CD8 VM cells (CD44^{High}/CD62L^{High}/CD49d^{Low}) from aged C57BL/6 donors and pooled CD8 naïve cells (CD44^{Low}/CD62L^{High}) from young C57BL/6 donors were FACS-sorted and adoptively transferred into individual T cell deficient TCR βδ−/− mice, infected with influenza, and assessed for Granzyme B expression at days 6 and 9 post infection. **b** Representative histograms gated on the donor CD8 T cell population show Granzyme B expression in the lung at the indicated time points after infection. **c** Summary graphs show plots of of Granzyme B expression (gMFI) in lung donor CD8 T cell populations from individual recipient mice at the indicated times after infection. Data from two independent experiments, pooled for statistical analysis, are represented in separate shades. Bars represent the mean ± SD. Data were analyzed by unpaired, two-tailed T test (p < 0.05)

It has been shown that VM proliferate more robustly than naïve CD8 T cells after antigen stimulation of young mice [38, 48]. However, we observed that aged memory cells were outcompeted by aged naïve CD8 T cells after influenza infection when transferred 1:1. This is consistent with the observation that VM in aged mice exhibit impaired TCR-mediated proliferation [59]. It has also been suggested that the antigen diversity of VM and naïve T cells is similar, because tetramer positive cells were identified in unprimed (young) animals to all epitopes tested [38]. However, this was not observed in our studies, as we saw a greater degree of epitope diversity in the response of naïve compared to VM CD8 T cells following influenza infection of aged mice (Fig. 2d).

Since our results demonstrated that the vast majority of the responding CD8 T cells that develop in the aged mice in response to influenza infection were from the population of VM cells, it was important to determine if these cells were capable of effector function. It has been shown that VM produce IFNγ, both in response to cognate antigen as well as cytokine-mediated, antigen independent stimulation [38, 39, 48]. In addition, VM have been shown to express granzyme, and can mediate antigen-independent bystander killing [39, 53]. Consistent with these published data, our results show that VM cells from aged mice have the capacity to become granzyme-secreting effectors and clear virus with kinetics comparable to CD8 T cells from young, influenza-naïve mice. Interestingly,

it has been shown that VM preferentially differentiate into CM after stimulation, whereas TM cells tend to become EM upon secondary challenge [48], suggesting that the response of VM to influenza infection may actually contribute to strong maintenance of memory. This intriguing idea was not directly examined in the current study.

A key question in the field of aging immunity is the relevance of the aged mouse model to elderly humans. Whereas naïve CD8 T cell repertoire diversity in the mouse declines to the extent that the ability to respond to new infections is impaired [3–6, 13, 22, 23] and "holes" in the repertoire can develop [7], it has been shown that there is only a modest (3–5-fold) reduction in CD8 T cell repertoire diversity with age in humans [60, 61]. Thus, partly because of the increased total number of T cells in the human compared to mouse (3 × 10^{11} compared to 1–2 × 10^8) [62–64], the CD8 T cell repertoire in human remains reasonably diverse and unlikely to develop holes [65], as we have shown in the mouse [7]. However, in very old individuals, clonal expansions and loss of the proliferative capacity of T cells result in more dramatic reduction of the human T cell repertoire [18, 63, 66, 67], making the results in aged mice relevant.

Another important question is whether VM are found in humans and whether they increase with age, as has been shown for the mouse. Importantly, although the phenotypic markers differ from VM in mouse, a

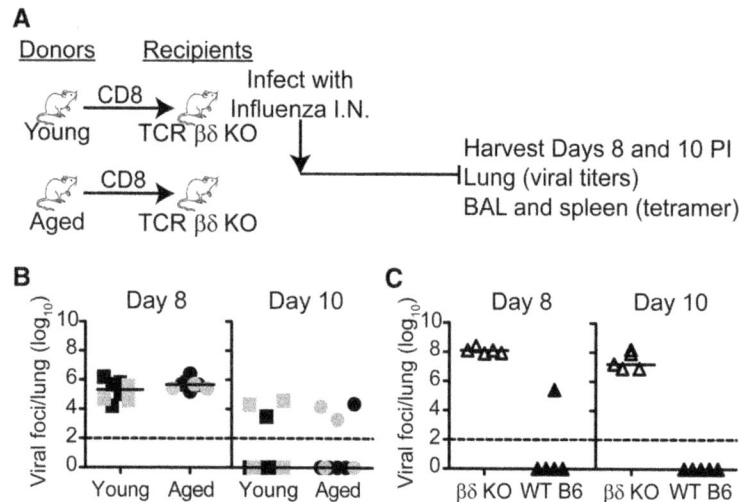

Fig. 6 Transferred CD8 cells from naïve aged and young mice clear virus with similar kinetics. **a** CD8 T cells from naive aged or young mice were enriched from splenocytes using negative selection, adoptively transferred into individual T cell deficient βδ−/− mice, infected with influenza virus, and the lungs were harvested at days 8 and 10 post-infection to determine viral titers. **b** Summary graphs of the viral foci/lung on days 8 and 10 post infection. Data from two independent experiments, pooled for statistical analysis, are represented in separate shades. Bars represent the median. Viral titers on day 8 or on day 10 in the two groups did not differ significantly ($p > 0.05$). Data were analyzed by Mann-Whitney Test. **c** Graph of the viral foci/lung on days 8 and 10 post infection for control individual WT C57BL/6 mice and individual T cell deficient βδ−/− mice that did not receive adoptively transferred CD8 T cells

population of CD8 T cells that functionally resembles VM has been identified in human, and these cells have been shown to increase with age in splenocytes and liver in human [39, 53]. For example, the data showed an increase in human VM cells in the spleen from ~ 5% at age 30 to ~ 20% at age 65 [53]. The studies reported here show VM cells play a major role in the response of aged mice to new infections, whereas the impact of human VM cells on responsiveness of the elderly to new infections is unknown. To add to the complexity of peripheral memory CD8 T cells in aging, a novel population of memory cells with a naïve phenotype has recently been shown to accumulate with age in humans [68]. It remains to be determined if a similar population is found in aged mice.

In our studies, the CD8 memory T cell population in aged SPF mice was dominated by VM cells. We hypothesized that aged mice that have experienced infections during their lifespan comparable to humans would have a higher ratio of TM to VM. It has been argued that VM are not an artifact of spf housing of mice because VM are generated and persist after bystander activation during deliberate, unrelated infections [56] However, a single infection in the mouse is not comparable to a lifetime of infections, including persistent infections, in human. Newly-developed "dirty" mouse models will allow testing the possibility that spf housing explains the large population of VM cells [69–72]. It has not yet been determined whether VM dominate the peripheral

repertoire of CD8 T cells in antigen-experienced (dirty), aged mice.

The knowledge that T cell immunity is long-lived has raised the suggestion that aggressive immunization in youth and middle age would prevent the decline in repertoire and function of CD8 T cells associated with aging, and provide an approach to enhancing vaccination efficacy for the elderly. In support of this, it has been shown that priming of mice at an early age to influenza virus results in preservation of numbers, repertoire and function of virus-specific memory CD8 T cells [9, 73]. This is in stark contrast to the reduced repertoire diversity and impaired response of CD8 T cells that are observed following primary infection of aged mice [7, 9, 41]. Despite the apparent ability of VM cells to clear virus in the absence of specific immunization, it should be remembered that the response of TM out-competes the response of VM when directly compared [52, 55]. Thus, specifically increasing the population of TM by vaccination will likely reduce the impact of VM in aged, specific pathogen free mice to influenza virus infection, supporting the concept of vaccinations early in life. In light of the observation that VM differentiate into long-lived CM phenotype cells after priming [48], whereas TM develop preferentially into short-lived EM, it will be important in future studies to determine the contribution of VM and TM in response to infection in young mice and the contribution of each cell type to long-term maintenance of memory.

Conclusions

In conclusion, the declining response of the elderly to new infections and vaccines is well-established and provides a compelling rationale for dissecting the impact of age-associated changes in the CD8 T cell repertoire and functional immune response to new infections, using the mouse model. Although the mouse model is robust, it is important to keep in mind differences between humans and mice and, where possible, validate findings in the mice with experiments in humans.

In the current studies, we have tested the hypothesis that in the face of declining numbers and repertoire diversity of naïve CD8 T cells in aged mice, responses are dominated by fortuitously cross-reactive memory cells. Adoptive transfer studies confirmed that memory CD8 T cells from influenza-naïve aged mice can respond to de novo infection with influenza virus in influenza-naïve aged mice with a highly constricted T cell receptor repertoire for the well characterized epitopes in C57BL/6 mice. Unexpectedly, the response was mediated by CD8 T cells with a virtual memory phenotype, rather than by true memory CD8 T cells previously generated in response to unrelated antigens. The VM CD8 T cells that dominated the repertoire in aged mice became functional granzyme B-producing effector cells and were able to clear influenza virus with a comparable kinetics to cells from young naïve mice. These data confirm the complexity of aging effects on the peripheral CD8 T cell repertoire.

Methods

Mice and viral infections

Female C57BL/6, B6.SJL-Ptprca Pepcb/BoyJ (B6.CD45.1), B6.PL-Thy1a/Cy (B6.CD90.1) and B6.129P2-Tcrb$^{\text{tm1Mom}}$ Tcrd$^{\text{tm1Mom}}$/J (TCRβδ$^{-/-}$) were obtained from the Trudeau Institute animal facility or purchased from Jackson Laboratory and maintained under specific pathogen-free conditions. Often, but not always, impaired immune function has been attributed to the presence of large TCEs in the CD8 population [4, 7]. To avoid this complicating factor, peripheral blood lymphocytes of all aged mice were pre-screened for major CD8 T cell Vβ expansions, and those that exhibited TCR Vβ8, Vβ7 or Vβ8.3 staining ± 4 SD over that observed with young C57BL/6 mice were omitted from the study. Mice were anesthetized with 2,2,2,-tribromoethanol and infected intranasally (i.n.) with 3000 EID$_{50}$ A/HK-× 31 (× 31, H3N2). All experiments were approved by the Institutional Animal Care and Use Committee of the Trudeau Insitute.

Lymphocyte isolation and flow cytometry

Lung tissue was prepared by coarsely chopping the tissue followed by incubation in a 0.5 mg/mL solution of collagenase D (Roche) and DNase (Sigma Aldrich) for 30–45 min at 37 °C. Lymphocytes were enriched from digested lung tissue by differential centrifugation, using a gradient of 40/80% Percoll (GE Healthcare). Single-cell suspensions were prepared from lymph nodes and spleens by dispersing the tissues through a 70 μm cell mesh. Single-cell suspensions were incubated with Fc-block (anti-CD16/32) for 15 min on ice followed by staining with MHC class I tetramer reagents for one hour at room temperature. Tetramer-labeled cells were then washed and stained with fluorochrome-conjugated antibodies against CD4, CD8α, CD19, CD90.2 (BD); CD44, CD45.1, CD45.2, CD62L (BioLegend); CD44 and CD49d (eBioscience) for 30 min on ice. MHC class I peptide tetramers specific for influenza virus NP$_{366}$/D^{b}, PA$_{224}$/D^{b}, PB1$_{703}$/K^{b}, PB1-F2$_{62}$/D^{b}, and NS2$_{114}$/K^{b} were generated by the Trudeau Institute Molecular Biology Core Facility. For granzyme B staining, cells were fixed and permeabilized using the Cytofix/Cytoperm kit (BD) after tetramer and surface marker staining. Cells were stained with anti–granzyme B (or isotype control) antibody conjugated to PE (Invitrogen). Stained samples were run on a FACS Canto II or LSRII flow cytometer (BD Biosciences) and data were analyzed with FloJo software (TreeStar).

Isolation of CD8 T cell subpopulations

Spleen and superficial lymph nodes were harvested from young (2–3 months) or aged (18–22 months) mice, processed into single-cell suspensions as described above, and further enriched by negative selection for CD8 cells using the BD Mouse CD8 T Lymphocyte Enrichment Kit. Sorting was performed on a BD Influx cell sorter with BD FACS Sortware software. Combinations of CD45 and CD90 alleles were chosen to allow discrimination of co-transferred populations, as shown in figures, where applicable.

In studies described in Figs. 1, 2 and 4, sorted cell populations were transferred, along with CD8-depleted splenocytes from young (2–3 month) B6.CD90.1 donors, into young TCR-deficient hosts (TCRβδ$^{-/-}$) via intravenous injection. For the studies described in Fig. 1, CD8 T cells were enriched from pooled spleen and lymph nodes from individual naive aged (18–22 months) mice and sorted to isolate the CD44^{High} CD8 T cells. Total sorted cells, along with CD8 depleted splenocytes from young (2–3 month) B6.CD90.1 donors, were transferred into individual young TCRβδ$^{-/-}$ hosts via intravenous injection. Recipient mice were infected i.n. with X-31 influenza virus (H3N2, 3000 EID$_{50}$/mouse) 1 day after transfer. BAL, lung and spleen were harvested for analyses at day 12 following infection. Responding donor CD8 T cells were identified and enumerated through the use of antibody staining and MHC class I tetramers.

For studies described in Fig. 2, CD8 T cells were enriched from pooled spleen and lymph nodes from naïve aged (18–22 months) B6.CD45.1 or C57BL/6 mice and sorted to isolate the $CD44^{High}$ and $CD44^{Low}$ CD8 T cells. After sorting, the cells were transferred at either a 1:1 or 1:9 ratio of $CD44^{Low}$:$CD44^{High}$, along with CD8-depleted splenoctyes from young (2–3 month) B6.CD90.1 donors, into young $TCR\beta\delta^{-/-}$ hosts. Recipient mice were infected i.n. with X-31 influenza virus (H3N2, 3000 EID_{50}/mouse) 1 day after transfer. BAL, lung and spleen were harvested for analyses at day 12 following infection. Responding donor CD8 T cells were identified and enumerated through the use of antibody staining and MHC class I tetramers.

For studies described in Fig. 4, CD8 T cells were enriched from pooled spleen and lymph nodes from naïve aged (18–22 months) B6.CD45.1 or B6.CD45.2 mice and sorted to isolate the TM ($CD62L^{High}CD44^{High}CD49d^{High}$) and the VM ($CD62L^{High}CD44^{High}CD49d^{Low}$) CD8 T cells. The sorted cells were adoptively transferred into young $TCR\beta\delta^{-/-}$ hosts at a 1:1 ratio. Recipient mice were infected i.n. with X-31 influenza virus (H3N2, 3000 EID_{50}/mouse) 1 day after transfer. BAL, lung and spleen were harvested for analyses at day 12 following infection. Responding donor CD8 T cells were identified and enumerated through the use of antibody staining and MHC class I tetramers.

For studies described in Fig. 5, CD8 T cells were enriched from pooled spleen and lymph nodes from naïve young (2–3 months) or naïve aged (18–22 months) mice and sorted to isolate the $CD44^{Low}$ CD8 T cells or the $CD62L^{High}CD44^{High}CD49d^{Low}$ CD8 T cells, respectively. Sorted cells from young or aged mice were transferred into young $TCR\beta\delta^{-/-}$ hosts. Recipient mice were infected i.n. with X-31 influenza virus (H3N2, 3000 EID_{50}/mouse) 1 day after transfer. BAL, lung and spleen were harvested for analyses at days 6 and 9 following infection. Responding donor CD8 T cells were identified and enumerated through the use of antibody staining and MHC class I tetramers, and evaluated for Granzyme B expression.

For studies described in Fig. 6, spleen and superficial lymph nodes were harvested from naïve young (2–3 months) or aged (18–22 months) mice, pooled, and enriched by negative selection for $CD8^{+}$ cells using the BD Mouse CD8 T Lymphocyte Enrichment Kit. 2.5×10^6 enriched CD8 T cells from either young or aged mice were transferred into young $TCR\beta\delta^{-/-}$ hosts. Recipient mice were infected i.n. with X-31 influenza virus (H3N2, 3000 EID_{50}/mouse) 1 day after transfer. Lungs were harvested from recipient mice at days 8 and 10 and processed for viral titers. In a separate control experiment, young $TCR\beta\delta^{-/-}$ with no T cell transfer and young C57BL/6 mice were infected i.n. with X-31 influenza virus (H3N2, 3000 EID_{50}/mouse). Lungs were harvested at days 8 and 10 and processed for viral titers.

Measurement of viral load

Whole lung tissue was harvested in PBS at the indicated times, homogenized, and stored at $-70\,°C$. Virus titers were measured with a standard plaque assay by infecting MDCK cell monolayers with serial 5-fold dilutions of lung suspension in duplicate. Eighteen to twenty-four hours after infection, monolayers were washed and fixed with 80% acetone in water. Infected cell clusters were detected with a biotin-labeled mouse anti-influenza A monoclonal antibody (Chemicon), followed by staining with streptavidin-AP, and visualized with Sigma Fast BCIP/NBT substrate (Sigma). The number of viral-foci units (VFUs) was counted, and the data were shown as the VFU/lung.

Statistical analysis

Statistical analysis was performed with GraphPad Prism 5 software (GraphPad, San Diego, CA). Differences were considered significant at p value < 0.05.

Abbreviations

BAL: Bronchoalveolar lavage; CM: Central memory; EM: Effector memory; NP: Nucleoprotein; TM: "True" memory; T_{RM}: Resident memory; VM: Virtual memory

Acknowledgements

We thank Drs. David Woodland and Laura Haynes for helpful discussion and reviewing the manuscript, Dr. Larry Johnson for help with statistical analysis and Drs. Suzy Swain and Janet McElhaney for comments and discussion. We thank the Molecular Biology Core at Trudeau Institute for providing the MHC class I tetramers and the Animal Care facility at Trudeau Institute for breeding and maintaining the aged mice.

Funding

This work was supported by the National Institutes of Health grants P01 AG021600, project 4 (M.A.B), R01 AG039485 (M.A.B) and funds from the Trudeau Institute.

Authors' contributions

MAB designed experiments, performed data interpretation, and wrote the manuscript. KLG designed and performed experiments, performed data analysis and assisted with manuscript preparation. TC performed experiments and assisted with data analysis. WWR designed experiments, assisted with data interpretation and assisted with manuscript preparation. All authors read and approved the final manuscript.

Ethics approval

Animal housing and procedures were approved by the Animal Care and Use Committee of Trudeau Institute.

Competing interests

The authors declare that they have no competing interests.

References

1. Yewdell JW, Haeryfar SM. Understanding presentation of viral antigens to CD8 (+) T cells in vivo: the key to rational vaccine design *. Annu Rev Immunol. 2005;23:651–82.

2. Rudd BD, Venturi V, Li G, Samadder P, Ertelt JM, Way SS, et al. Nonrandom attrition of the naive CD8+ T-cell pool with aging governed by T-cell receptor:pMHC interactions. Proc Natl Acad Sci U S A. 2011;108:13694–9.

3. Messaoudi I, Guevara Patino JA, Dyall R, LeMaoult J, Nikolich-Zugich J. Direct link between MHC polymorphism, T cell avidity, and diversity in immune defense. Science. 2002;298:1797–800.

4. Messaoudi I, Lemaoult J, Guevara-Patino JA, Metzner BMNikolich-Zugich J. Age-related CD8 T cell clonal expansions constrict CD8 T cell repertoire and have the potential to impair immune defense. J Exp Med. 2004; 200:1347–58.

5. Nikolich-Zugich J, Slifka MK, Messaoudi I. The many important facets of T-cell repertoire diversity. Nat Rev Immunol. 2004;4:123–32.

6. Woodland DL, Blackman MA. Immunity and age: living in the past? Trends Immunol. 2006;27:303–7.

7. Yager EJ, Ahmed M, Lanzer K, Randall TD, Woodland DL, Blackman MA. Age-associated decline in T cell repertoire diversity leads to holes in the repertoire and impaired immunity to influenza virus. J Exp Med. 2008;205:711–23.

8. Ahmed M, Lanzer KG, Yager EJ, Adams PS, Johnson LL, Blackman MA. Clonal expansions and loss of receptor diversity in the naive CD8 T cell repertoire of aged mice. J Immunol. 2009;182:784–92.

9. Valkenburg SA, Venturi V, Dang TH, Bird NL, Doherty PC, Turner SJ, et al. Early priming minimizes the age-related immune compromise of CD8(+) T cell diversity and function. PLoS Pathog. 2012;8:e1002544.

10. Johnson PL, Goronzy JJ, Antia R. A population biological approach to understanding the maintenance and loss of the T-cell repertoire during aging. Immunology. 2014;142:167–75.

11. Gil A, Yassai MB, Naumov YN, Selin LK. Narrowing of human influenza a virus-specific T cell receptor alpha and beta repertoires with increasing age. J Virol. 2015;89:4102–16.

12. Yoshida K, Cologne JB, Cordova K, Misumi M, Yamaoka M, Kyoizumi S, et al. Aging-related changes in human T-cell repertoire over 20 years delineated by deep sequencing of peripheral T-cell receptors. Exp Gerontol. 2017;96: 29–37.

13. Smithey MJ, Li G, Venturi V, Davenport MP, Nikolich-Zugich J. Lifelong persistent viral infection alters the naive T cell pool, impairing CD8 T cell immunity in late life. J Immunol. 2012;189:5356–66.

14. Britanova OV, Putintseva EV, Shugay M, Merzlyak EM, Turchaninova MA, Staroverov DB, et al. Age-related decrease in TCR repertoire diversity measured with deep and normalized sequence profiling. J Immunol. 2014;192:2689–98.

15. Lee JB, Oelke M, Ramachandra L, Canaday DH, Schneck JP. Decline of influenza-specific CD8+ T cell repertoire in healthy geriatric donors. Immun Ageing. 2011;8:6.

16. Sempowski GD, Gooding ME, Liao HX, Le PT, Haynes BF. T cell receptor excision circle assessment of thymopoiesis in aging mice. Mol Immunol. 2002;38:841–8.

17. Effros RB, Cai Z, Linton PJ. CD8 T cells and aging. Crit Rev Immunol. 2003;23:45–64.

18. Naylor K, Li G, Vallejo AN, Lee WW, Koetz K, Bryl E, et al. The influence of age on T cell generation and TCR diversity. J Immunol. 2005;174:7446–52.

19. Lerner A, Yamada T, Miller RA. Pgp-1hi T lymphocytes accumulate with age in mice and respond poorly to concanavalin a. Eur J Immunol. 1989;19:977–82.

20. Callahan JE, Kappler JW, Marrack P. Unexpected expansions of CD8-bearing cells in old mice. J Immunol. 1993;151:6657–69.

21. Posnett DN, Sinha R, Kabak S, Russo C. Clonal populations of T cells in normal elderly humans: the T cell equivalent to "benign monoclonal gammapathy". J Exp Med. 1994;179:609–18.

22. Brien JD, Uhrlaub JL, Hirsch A, Wiley CA, Nikolich-Zugich J. Key role of T cell defects in age-related vulnerability to West Nile virus. J Exp Med. 2009;206: 2735–45.

23. Cicin-Sain L, Smyk-Pearson S, Currier N, Byrd L, Koudelka C, Robinson R, et al. Loss of naive T cells and repertoire constriction predict poor response to vaccination in old primates. J Immunol. 2010;184:6739–45.

24. Brehm MA, Pinto AK, Daniels KA, Schneck JP, Welsh RM, Selin LK. T cell immunodominance and maintenance of memory regulated by unexpectedly cross-reactive pathogens. Nat Immunol. 2002;3:627–34.

25. Shimojo N, Cowan EP, Engelhard VH, Maloy WL, Coligan JE, Biddison WE. A single amino acid substitution in HLA-A2 can alter the selection of the cytotoxic T lymphocyte repertoire that responds to influenza virus matrix peptide 55-73. J Immunol. 1989;143:558–64.

26. Selin LK, Cornberg M, Brehm MA, Kim SK, Calcagno C, Ghersi D, et al. CD8 memory T cells: cross-reactivity and heterologous immunity. Semin Immunol. 2004;16:335–47.

27. Selin LK, Welsh RM. Plasticity of T cell memory responses to viruses. Immunity. 2004;20:5–16.

28. Welsh RM, Selin LK, Szomolanyi-Tsuda E. Immunological memory to viral infections. Annu Rev Immunol. 2004;22:711–43.

29. Kim SK, Cornberg M, Wang XZ, Chen HD, Selin LK, Welsh RM. Private specificities of CD8 T cell responses control patterns of heterologous immunity. J Exp Med. 2005;201:523–33.

30. Welsh RM, Che JW, Brehm MA, Selin LK. Heterologous immunity between viruses. Immunol Rev. 2010;235:244–66.

31. Che JW, Selin LK, Welsh RM. Evaluation of non-reciprocal heterologous immunity between unrelated viruses. Virol. 2015;482:89–97.

32. Su LF, Kidd BA, Han A, Kotzin JJ, Davis MM. Virus-specific CD4 (+) memory-phenotype T cells are abundant in unexposed adults. Immunity. 2013;38:373–83.

33. Mason D. A very high level of crossreactivity is an essential feature of the T-cell receptor. Immunol Today. 1998;19:395–404.

34. Sallusto F, Lenig D, Forster R, Lipp M, Lanzavecchia A. Two subsets of memory T lymphocytes with distinct homing potentials and effector functions. Nature. 1999;401:708–12.

35. Masopust D, Vezys V, Marzo AL, Lefrancois L. Preferential localization of effector memory cells in nonlymphoid tissue. Science. 2001;291:2413–7.

36. Sallusto F, Geginat J, Lanzavecchia A. Central memory and effector memory T cell subsets: function, generation, and maintenance. Annu Rev Immunol. 2004;22:745–63.

37. Gerlach C, Loughhead SM, von Andrian UH. Figuring fact from fiction: unbiased polling of memory T cells. Cell. 2015;161:702–4.

38. Haluszczak C, Akue AD, Hamilton SE, Johnson LD, Pujanauski L, Teodorovic L, et al. The antigen-specific CD8+ T cell repertoire in unimmunized mice includes memory phenotype cells bearing markers of homeostatic expansion. J Exp Med. 2009;206:435–48.

39. White JT, Cross EW, Kedl RM. Antigen-inexperienced memory CD8+ T cells: where they come from and why we need them. Nat Rev Immunol. 2017; 17(6):391.

40. Lee YJ, Jameson SC, Hogquist KA. Alternative memory in the CD8 T cell lineage. Trends Immunol. 2011;32:50–6.

41. Decman V, Laidlaw BJ, Doering TA, Leng J, Ertl HC, Goldstein DR, et al. Defective CD8 T cell responses in aged mice are due to quantitative and qualitative changes in virus-specific precursors. J Immunol. 2012; 188:1933–41.

42. Chiu BC, Martin BE, Stolberg VR, Chensue SW. Cutting edge: central memory CD8 T cells in aged mice are virtual memory cells. J Immunol. 2013;191:5793–6.

43. Belz GT, Xie W, Altman JD, Doherty PC. A previously unrecognized H-2D (b)-restricted peptide prominent in the primary influenza a virus-specific CD8 (+) T-cell response is much less apparent following secondary challenge. J Virol. 2000;74:3486–93.

44. Crowe SR, Turner SJ, Miller SC, Roberts AD, Rappolo RA, Doherty PC, et al. Differential antigen presentation regulates the changing patterns of CD8+ T cell immunodominance in primary and secondary influenza virus infections. J Exp Med. 2003;198:399–410.

45. Ballesteros-Tato A, Leon B, Lee BO, Lund FE, Randall TD. Epitope-specific regulation of memory programming by differential duration of antigen presentation to influenza-specific CD8 (+) T cells. Immunity. 2014;41:127–40.

46. LeMaoult J, Messaoudi I, Manavalan JS, Potvin H, Nikolich-Zugich D, Dyall R, et al. Age-related dysregulation in CD8 T cell homeostasis: kinetics of a diversity loss. J Immunol. 2000;165:2367–73.

47. Kohlmeier JE, Connor LM, Roberts AD, Cookenham T, Martin K, Woodland DL. Nonmalignant clonal expansions of memory CD8+ T cells that arise with age vary in their capacity to mount recall responses to infection. J Immunol. 2010;185:3456–62.

48. Lee JY, Hamilton SE, Akue AD, Hogquist KA, Jameson SC. Virtual memory CD8 T cells display unique functional properties. Proc Natl Acad Sci U S A. 2013;110:13498–503.

49. Toapanta FR, Ross TM. Impaired immune responses in the lungs of aged mice following influenza infection. Respir Res. 2009;10:112.

50. Brown DM, Roman E, Swain SL. CD4 T cell responses to influenza infection. Semin Immunol. 2004;16:171–7.

51. Brown DM, Dilzer AM, Meents DL, Swain SL. CD4 T cell-mediated protection from lethal influenza: perforin and antibody-mediated mechanisms give a one-two punch. J Immunol. 2006;177:2888–98.

52. Hamilton SE, Wolkers MC, Schoenberger SP, Jameson SC. The generation of protective memory-like CD8+ T cells during homeostatic proliferation requires CD4+ T cells. Nat Immunol. 2006;7:475–81.

53. White JT, Cross EW, Burchill MA, Danhorn T, McCarter MD, Rosen HR, et al. Virtual memory T cells develop and mediate bystander protective immunity in an IL-15-dependent manner. Nat Commun. 2016;7:11291.

54. Blackman MA, Woodland DL. The narrowing of the CD8 T cell repertoire in old age. Curr Opin Immunol. 2011;23:537–42.

55. Cheung KP, Yang E, Goldrath AW. Memory-like CD8+ T cells generated during homeostatic proliferation defer to antigen-experienced memory cells. J Immunol. 2009;183:3364–72.

56. Akue AD, Lee JY, Jameson SC. Derivation and maintenance of virtual memory CD8 T cells. J Immunol. 2012;188:2516–23.

57. Goldrath AW. Maintaining the status quo: T-cell homeostasis. Microbes Infect. 2002;4:539–45.

58. Jameson SC, Lee YJ, Hogquist KA. Innate memory T cells. Adv Immunol. 2015;126:173–213.

59. Renkema KR, Li G, Wu A, Smithey MJ, Nikolich-Zugich J. Two separate defects affecting true naive or virtual memory T cell precursors combine to reduce naive T cell responses with aging. J Immunol. 2014;192:151–9.

60. Kim C, Fang F, Weyand CM, Goronzy JJ. The life cycle of a T cell after vaccination - where does immune ageing strike? Clin Exp Immunol. 2017;187:71–81.

61. Qi Q, Liu Y, Cheng Y, Glanville J, Zhang D, Lee JY, et al. Diversity and clonal selection in the human T-cell repertoire. Proc Natl Acad Sci U S A. 2014;111: 13139–44.

62. Arstila TP, Casrouge A, Baron V, Even J, Kanellopoulos J, Kourilsky P. A direct estimate of the human alphabeta T cell receptor diversity. Science. 1999; 286:958–61.

63. Goronzy JJ, Weyand CM. T cell development and receptor diversity during aging. Curr Opin Immunol. 2005;17:468–75.

64. Casrouge A, Beaudoing E, Dalle S, Pannetier C, Kanellopoulos J, Kourilsky P. Size estimate of the alpha beta TCR repertoire of naive mouse splenocytes. J Immunol. 2000;164:5782–7.

65. Goronzy JJ, Qi Q, Olshen RA, Weyand CM. High-throughput sequencing insights into T-cell receptor repertoire diversity in aging. Genome Med. 2015;7:117.

66. Hadrup SR, Strindhall J, Kollgaard T, Seremet T, Johansson B, Pawelec G, et al. Longitudinal studies of clonally expanded CD8 T cells reveal a repertoire shrinkage predicting mortality and an increased number of dysfunctional cytomegalovirus-specific T cells in the very elderly. J Immunol. 2006;176:2645–53.

67. Schwanninger A, Weinberger B, Weiskopf D, Herndler-Brandstetter D, Reitinger S, Gassner C, et al. Age-related appearance of a CMV-specific high-avidity CD8+ T cell clonotype which does not occur in young adults. Immun Ageing. 2008;5:14.

68. Pulko V, Davies JS, Martinez C, Lanteri MC, Busch MP, Diamond MS, et al. Human memory T cells with a naive phenotype accumulate with aging and respond to persistent viruses. Nat Immunol. 2016;17(8):966.

69. Reese TA, Bi K, Kambal A, Filali-Mouhim A, Beura LK, Burger MC, et al. Sequential infection with common pathogens promotes human-like immune gene expression and altered vaccine response. Cell Host Microbe. 2016;19:713–9.

70. Beura LK, Hamilton SE, Bi K, Schenkel JM, Odumade OA, Casey KA, et al. Normalizing the environment recapitulates adult human immune traits in laboratory mice. Nature. 2016;532:512–6.

71. Abolins S, King EC, Lazarou L, Weldon L, Hughes L, Drescher P, et al. The comparative immunology of wild and laboratory mice, *Mus muscdomesticus*. Nat Commun. 2017;8:14811.

72. Rosshart SP, Vassallo BG, Angeletti D, Hutchinson DS, Morgan AP, Takeda K, et al. Wild mouse gut microbiota promotes host fitness and improves disease resistance. Cell. 2017;171(5):1015–28.

73. Kedzierska K, Valkenburg SA, Doherty PC, Davenport MP, Venturi V. Use it or lose it: establishment and persistence of T cell memory. Front Immunol. 2012;3:357.

Porphyromonas gingivalis, a periodontitis causing bacterium, induces memory impairment and age-dependent neuroinflammation in mice

Ye Ding[1], Jingyi Ren[1], Hongqiang Yu[1], Weixian Yu[2*] and Yanmin Zhou[1*]

Abstract

Background: A possible relationship between periodontitis and Alzheimer's disease (AD) has been reported. However, there is limited information on the association between the *Porphyromonas gingivalis* (*P. gingivalis*) periodontal infection and the pathological features of AD. The hypothesis that *P. gingivalis* periodontal infection may cause cognitive impairment via age-dependent neuroinflammation was tested.

Results: Thirty 4-week-old (young) female C57BL/6 J mice were randomly divided into two groups, the control group and the experimental group. Thirty 12-month-old (middle-aged) were grouped as above. The mouth of the mice in the experimental group was infected with *P. gingivalis*. Morris water maze(MWM) was performed to assess the learning and memory ability of mice after 6 weeks. Moreover, the expression levels of the pro-inflammatory cytokines TNF-α, IL-6, and IL-1β in the mice brain tissues were determined by Quantitative real-time polymerase chain reaction (qRT-PCR), Enzyme Linked Immunosorbent Assay(ELISA) and immunohistochemistry. Our results showed that the learning and memory abilities of the middle-aged *P. gingivalis* infected mice were impaired. Moreover, the expression levels of the pro-inflammatory cytokines TNF-α, IL-6, and IL-1β in the brain tissues of the middle-aged *P. gingivalis* infected mice were increased.

Conclusions: These results suggest that *P. gingivalis* periodontal infection may cause cognitive impairment via the release of the pro-inflammatory cytokines TNF-α, IL-6, and IL-1β in the brain tissues of middle-aged mice.

Keywords: Porphyromonas gingivalis (*P. gingivalis*), Periodontitis, Cognition, Neuroinflammation, Alzheimer's disease(AD)

Background

Periodontium is composed of gingiva, periodontal ligament, alveolar bone and cementum. Infection of the periodontium, known as periodontitis, is a chronic peripheral inflammatory disease, initiated by microbes residing in the oral cavity. It is commonly caused by specific bacteria, such as *P. gingivalis*, a Gram-negative bacterium, which is a key periodontal pathogen. *P. gingivalis* and its toxic components, including fimbria, gingipains, and lipopolysaccharide (LPS), are closely related to periodontitis. Clinically, chronic periodontitis is characterized by the presence of gingival erythema, edema, periodontal pockets, and destruction of the tissue supporting the teeth [1–3]. Periodontal microorganisms and their products may enter into the circulation leading to bacteremia and systemic dissemination of bacterial products [4]. Moreover, periodontitis can induce systemic effects by promoting the expression of inflammatory mediators such as pro-inflammatory cytokines. Thus, periodontitis has been confirmed to be associated with systemic diseases including cardiovascular disease, diabetes, atherosclerotic, and respiratory diseases [5].

* Correspondence: ywx461@163.com; zhouym62@126.com
[2]Key laboratory of Mechanism of Tooth Development and Jaw Bone Remodeling and Regeneration in Jilin Province, Qinghua Road 1500, Chaoyang District, Changchun 130021, China
[1]Department of Implantology, School and Hospital of Stomatology, Jilin University, Qinghua Road 1500, Chaoyang District, Changchun 130021, China

In recent years, AD, well known as a progressive neurodegenerative disease, has been recognized as the leading cause of cognitive and behavioral damage [6]. It has been increasingly claimed that peripheral infections could activate already primed microglial cells within the central nervous system (CNS) which promotes the development of neurodegeneration in AD [7]. The mechanism by which peripheral pro-inflammatory molecules might increase the brain's molecular inflammatory pool involves at least two pathways, the systemic circulation and/or the neural pathways. Once in the brain, pro-inflammatory molecules might directly elevate the expression levels of the pro-inflammatory cytokine pool locally, or indirectly activate glial cells by regulating the secretion of additional pro-inflammatory cytokines. Therefore, Kamer et al. first proposed that the pool of the inflammatory molecules in the brain could be enhanced by periodontitis, which is characterized by elevated inflammatory levels, and consequently promoting the development of AD [5]. Recently, there are increasing studies supporting this hypothesis. A close relationship between immunological mediators, such as TNF-α and antibodies against periodontal pathogens, and AD, has been reported. Furthermore, these mediators can be used as AD diagnostic factors [8]. In addition, a report stated that poor dentition is associated with cognitive impairment [9]. A positive correlation between cognitive decline in AD patients and both acute and chronic inflammation was revealed by a human trial [10]. Moreover, a study conducted by Sophie et al. reported that LPS from periodontal pathogens could gain access to the brain tissue of AD patients during life, demonstrating the vital role of inflammatory factors in the pathology of AD [11]. Therefore, these reports suggest a possible connection between periodontitis and AD. However, most of the previous studies have not demonstrated a clear causative relationship between periodontitis and cognitive impairment. The experimental model used in this study was more representative of periodontitis infection as it utilizes the entire *P. gingivalis* in order to take into consideration all the bacteria components and secreted compounds which might be contributing to the development of periodontitis and might also affect cognitive memory. Therefore, in this study we test our hypothesis that periodontitis may cause cognitive impairment via age-dependent neuroinflammation in the *P. gingivalis* infection animal model.

Methods
Animal model
All animal experiments protocols were approved by the Animal Ethics Committee of Jilin University Medical Centre (Jilin, China). Thirty 4-week-old (young) and thirty 12-month-old (middle-aged) female C57BL/6 J mice (Animal Experiment Center of Jilin University) were respectively maintained with autoclaved food, water and bedding. Fifteen young and fifteen middle-aged mice were allocated to the *P. gingivalis* infection group. The remaining mice composed the control group. Mice were treated prior to infection with kanamycin (1 mg/ml water) for 7 days to suppress resident flora growth. Mice were infected with live *P. gingivalis* ATCC33277 by oral gavage using feeding needles. The periodontitis group received 0.1 ml of *P. gingivalis* (10^9 CFU/ml) in 2% carboxymethyl cellulose (CMC), once every 48 h, and this process repeated for the following 6 weeks. The control group received 0.1 ml of phosphate buffer saline (PBS) in 2% CMC. Mice were sacrificed 6 weeks after the first infection.

Behavioral evaluation
MWM tests were carried out as described by M.K. et al. with few modifications [12]. MWM is used in behavioral neuroscience to study spatial learning and memory [13]. The water pool was 1.2 m in diameter and 50 cm deep. The pool was filled with nontoxic white paint opaque water. The temperature was held constant at 23 ± 1 °C. The pool was separated into four equal quadrants. A platform (10 cm^2) laid 1 cm below the level of the surface of the water, in the center of one of these four quadrants, was considered the target quadrant. During the training days, the location of the platform remained the same. The mice were given four tests a day for four days. During the successive four days, mice were allowed to flee to hidden platforms. In the fourth trial, each experiment used a different starting point. If the mouse couldn't find the hidden platform in 60 s, it was gently guided to the platform, and allowed to stay there for 20 s. The time taken to reach the platform (escape latency) was recorded. On the fifth day, the platform was removed from the pool. During the probe test, the mice were freed into the pool for 120 s. The amount of times the mice crossed the area where the platform had been placed were calculated by a visual tracing system (XR-XM101, Chengdu Techman Software Co. LTD).

Immunohistochemistry
The immunohistochemical staining was performed as described by Li et al. with slight modifications [14]. Mice were sacrificed under deep anesthesia and the brains were removed. After fixing in 4% paraformaldehyde overnight at 4 °C, the brains were embedded in paraffin and then cut coronally at a thickness of 5 μm. The sections for staining were deparaffinized and washed. Following, they were heated in 0.01 M sodium citrate buffer (pH 6.0) for antigen retrieval. Endogenous peroxide activity was quenched with 3% hydrogen peroxide. Sections were incubated with primary antibodies against

TNF-α (Abcam, ab6671, 1:100), IL-6 (Bioss, bs-0379R, 1:100), IL-1β (Bioss, bs-0812R, 1:100) for 1 h at 37 °C, followed by Polymer Helper and anti-rabbit IgG polymer (ZSGB-BIO, PV-9001). Finally, color was developed with 3,3-diaminobenzidine DAB (ZSGB-BIO, ZLI-9018), and then it was counterstained with hematoxylin. Images were captured using the Olympus cellSens Dimension–Experimental systems in combination with light microscopy (Olympus BX 51, Japan).

qRT-PCR analysis

The total RNA was extracted with Trizol reagent (Invitrogen), according to the manufacturer's instructions. A total of 1000 ng of extracted RNA was reverse transcribed to cDNA using the PrimeScript RT reagent Kit with gDNA Eraser (TaKaRa DRRO47A). 25 ng of cDNA was used to perform qRT-PCR on the QPCR Mx3005P system (Agilent Technologies Stratagene) in a final volume of 25 µl using the SYBR Premix Ex Taq II (TaKaRa RR420Q). The data were evaluated using the MxPro-Mx3005P QPCR software program. For data normalization, mouse β-actin was used to control for the cDNA input, and the relative units were calculated by a comparative Ct method. All experiments were repeated three times.

The primer sequences used for qRT-PCR are as follows:

IL-1β: 5′- TCCAGGATGAGGACATGAGCAC-3' and 5'-GAACGTCACACACCAGCAGGTTA-3′;

IL-6: 5'-CCACTTCACAAGTCGGAGGCTTA-3' and 5'-CCAGTTTGGTAGCATCCATCATTTC-3';

TNF-α:5'-ACTCCAGGCGGTGCCTATGT-3' and 5'- G TGAGGGTCTGGGCCATAGAA-3';

β-actin:5'-CATCCGTAAAGACCTCTAGCCAAC-3' and 5'-ATGGAGCCACCGATCCACA-3'.

ELISA

The ELISA was carried out as described by Xu Wu et al. with few modifications [15]. The mice were sacrificed by decollation. The brain tissues were quickly removed and the cerebral cortex was carefully isolated with microscopic forceps. The isolated tissues were homogenized in PBS (pH 7.4) and then centrifuged. The supernatant was recovered and used as the test sample. The levels of TNF-α, IL-6, and IL-1β were determined by the ELISA kit (Lengton Bioscience Company), following the manufacturer's instructions. The monoclonal antibodies specific for mouse TNF-a, IL-6, and IL-1β were aliquoted in 96-well plates. The wells were incubated for 30 min at room temperature and then the test samples were added. The biotin-labelled antibodies against the mouse TNF-a, IL-6, IL-1β and the streptavidin-HRP were added successively. After color development, the absorbance of each well was recorder at 450 nm.

Statistical analysis

All the data are presented as mean ± SEM from at least three independent experiments. Morris water maze was analyzed with repeated measurements ANOVA. Comparisons between the periodontitis and the control group were evaluated by the Student's t-test. All statistical analyses were performed using the SPSS Statistics software (17.0). Differences with $P < 0.05$ were considered statistically significant.

Results

MWM spatial learning and memory tests in young and middle-aged mice

During the training days, escape latency was analyzed with repeated measurements ANOVA. The escape latency of middle-aged P. gingivalis infected mice was not significantly reduced during the 4 successive days. In contrast, escape latency of the middle-aged mice control group was gradually reduced, especially on day 4 compared to day 1. Both young P. gingivalis infected and control mice progressively decreased the time of finding the platform, with the difference being more obvious on day 4 when compared to day 1. There was no significant effect in the escape latency between the young P. gingivalis infected and the control mice on day 1. However, the escape latency of the middle-aged P. gingivalis infected mice was statistically different from the control group on day 2, day 3 and day 4 (Fig. 1a). During the probe test, no significant variations in the number of crossing times were observed between the young P. gingivalis infected and the control mice. As for the middle-aged mice, the P. gingivalis infected mice crossed the area where the platform had been located more times than the control group (Fig. 1b). These results clearly indicate that P. gingivalis infection can impair the spatial learning and memory abilities of the middle-aged mice. However, P. gingivalis infection did not significantly affect the cognitive competence of young mice.

mRNA expression of TNF-α, IL-6, and IL-1β in brain tissues

It has been revealed that periodontal-induced pro-inflammatory mediators, microorganisms, and products of bacteria can reach the brain through systemic circulation and/or neural pathways and increase the brain cytokine levels [16]. In order to investigate whether P. gingivalis periodontal infection could induce inflammatory responses and cause the release of pro-inflammatory cytokines in young and middle-aged mice, we examined the mRNA expression of TNF-α in the brains of mice. We were able to show that the mean mRNA expression levels of TNF-α in the brain tissues of the middle-aged P. gingivalis infected mice was increased, in comparison to the control group. However, no significant effect in the mRNA levels of TNF-α in the young mice group was observed

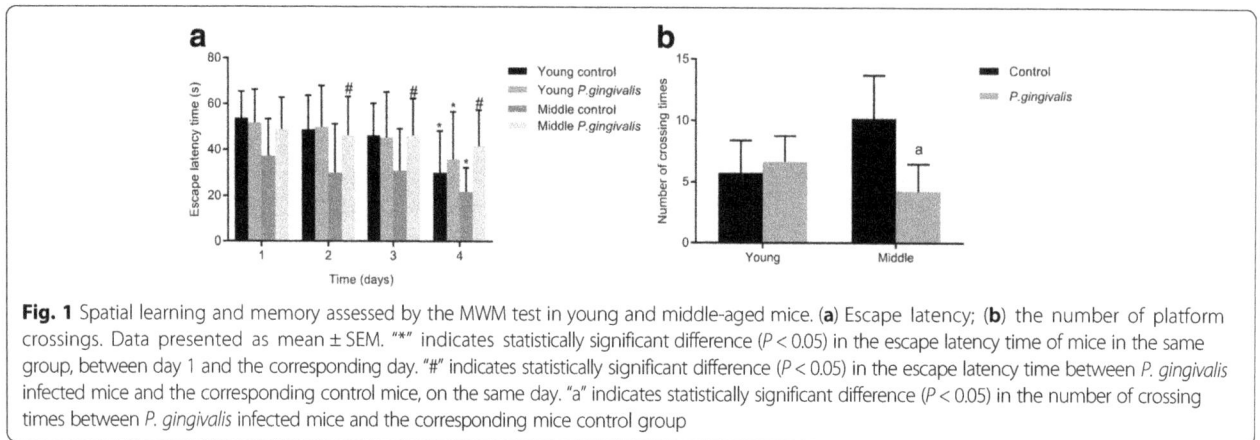

Fig. 1 Spatial learning and memory assessed by the MWM test in young and middle-aged mice. (**a**) Escape latency; (**b**) the number of platform crossings. Data presented as mean ± SEM. "*" indicates statistically significant difference ($P < 0.05$) in the escape latency time of mice in the same group, between day 1 and the corresponding day. "#" indicates statistically significant difference ($P < 0.05$) in the escape latency time between *P. gingivalis* infected mice and the corresponding control mice, on the same day. "a" indicates statistically significant difference ($P < 0.05$) in the number of crossing times between *P. gingivalis* infected mice and the corresponding mice control group

(Fig. 2a). Similarly, assessment of other pro-inflammatory cytokines revealed that IL-6 and IL-1β mRNA levels increased only in middle-aged *P. gingivalis* infected mice, but not in young mice (Fig. 2b, c).

Protein levels of TNF-α, IL-6, and IL-1β in brain tissues

We next determined the protein content of TNF-α, IL-6, and IL-1β in the brain tissues. The levels of all of the three pro-inflammatory cytokines were significantly higher in middle-aged *P. gingivalis* infected mice than in control mice. In contrast, the concentration of TNF-α, IL-6, and IL-1β did not differ within the young mice groups (Fig. 3a-c). These findings were also supported by immunohistochemistry analyses. As show in Fig. 3g, the brains of the middle-aged *P. gingivalis* infected mice showed an increased expression of TNF-α compared to the brain tissues from the control group. There was little TNF-α immunoreactivity found in both young *P. gingivalis* infected and control mice group (Fig. 3d, e). Similar to the TNF-α results, IL-6 and IL-1β expression in the *P. gingivalis* infected mice was higher than in the control group of the middle-aged mice. However, IL-6, IL-1β were expressed at low levels, particularly in young mice. These results suggest that *P. gingivalis* infection may promote neuroinflammation by increasing the expression of the

pro-inflammatory cytokines TNF-α, IL-6, and IL-1β in the brain tissues of middle-aged mice. Summary tables for statistical analysis are presented in Additional file 1.

Discussion

The major result of the current study is that *P. gingivalis* infection may cause memory impairment through induced age-dependent neuroinflammatory responses via modulation of pro-inflammatory cytokines release in the middle-aged mice.

Periodontitis is a chronic inflammatory disease, which could induce systemic host responses. Numerous reports have shown that periodontitis could raise the serum pro-inflammatory state, characterized by increased levels of C Reactive Protein (CRP) and pro-inflammatory cytokines (e.g. TNF-α), and decreased levels of anti-inflammatory markers (e.g. IL-10) [17]. Several studies have reported that peripheral inflammation could activate microglia cells and promote the generation of pro-inflammatory cytokines, including IL-1β, IL-6 and TNF-α, in the brain, resulting in neuroinflammation [18]. Neuroinflammation, including activation of microglia cells, participation of astrocytes, and involvement of neurons, has been suggested to contribute to the development of neurodegenerative diseases such as AD,

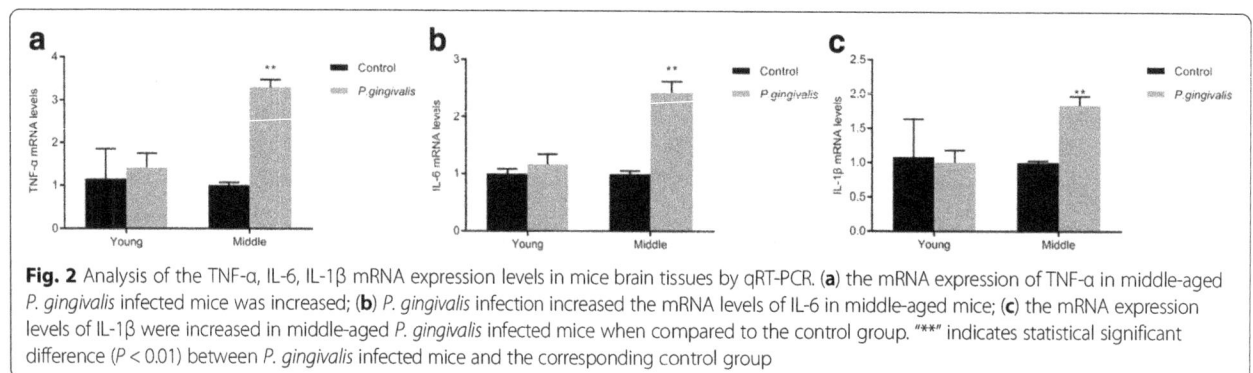

Fig. 2 Analysis of the TNF-α, IL-6, IL-1β mRNA expression levels in mice brain tissues by qRT-PCR. (**a**) the mRNA expression of TNF-α in middle-aged *P. gingivalis* infected mice was increased; (**b**) *P. gingivalis* infection increased the mRNA levels of IL-6 in middle-aged mice; (**c**) the mRNA expression levels of IL-1β were increased in middle-aged *P. gingivalis* infected mice when compared to the control group. "**" indicates statistical significant difference ($P < 0.01$) between *P. gingivalis* infected mice and the corresponding control group

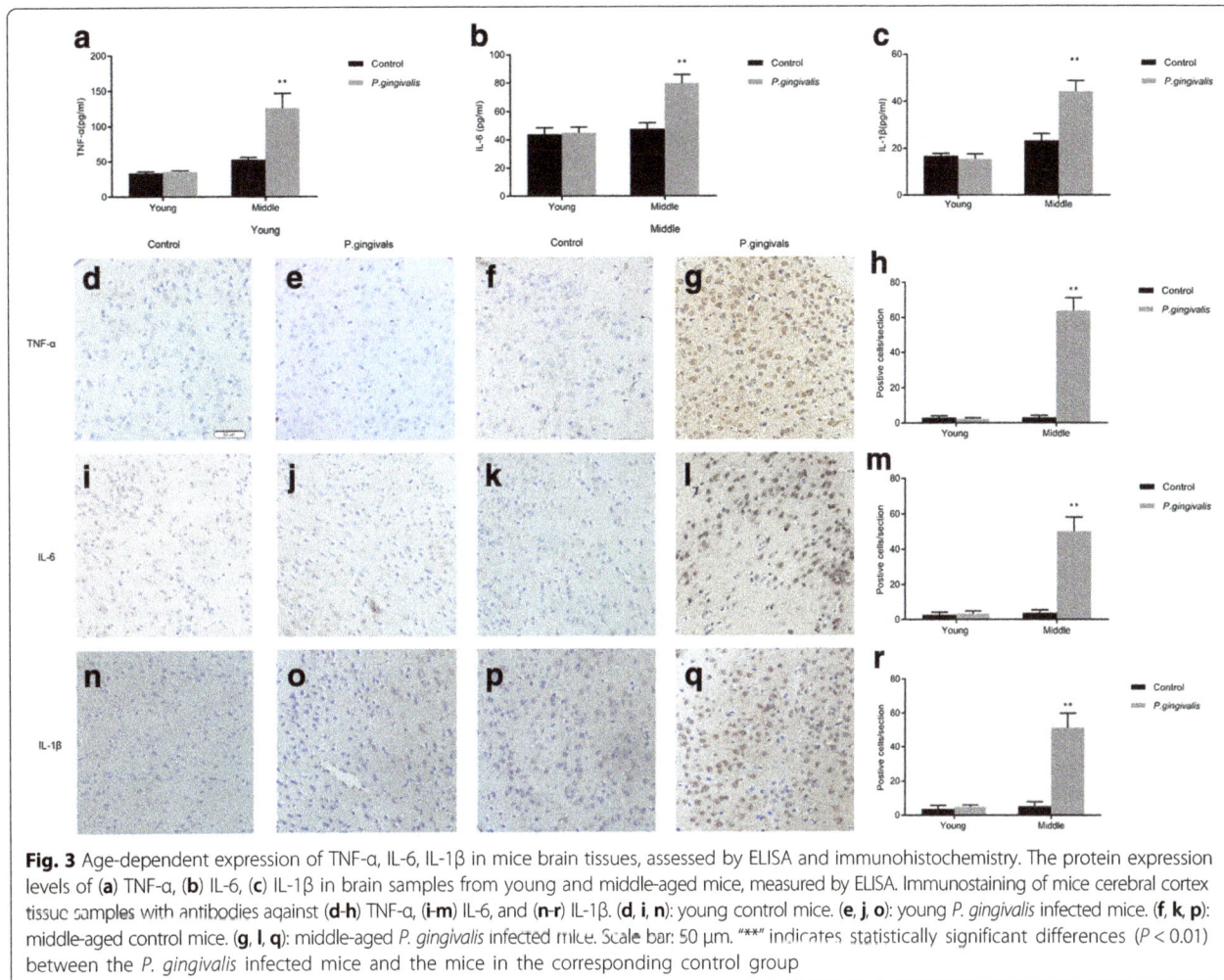

Fig. 3 Age-dependent expression of TNF-α, IL-6, IL-1β in mice brain tissues, assessed by ELISA and immunohistochemistry. The protein expression levels of (**a**) TNF-α, (**b**) IL-6, (**c**) IL-1β in brain samples from young and middle-aged mice, measured by ELISA. Immunostaining of mice cerebral cortex tissue samples with antibodies against (**d-h**) TNF-α, (**i-m**) IL-6, and (**n-r**) IL-1β. (**d**, **i**, **n**): young control mice. (**e**, **j**, **o**): young *P. gingivalis* infected mice. (**f**, **k**, **p**): middle-aged control mice. (**g**, **l**, **q**): middle-aged *P. gingivalis* infected mice. Scale bar: 50 μm. "**" indicates statistically significant differences (*P* < 0.01) between the *P. gingivalis* infected mice and the mice in the corresponding control group

Parkinson's disease, amyotrophic lateral sclerosis, and multiple sclerosis [14, 15, 19, 20]. Therefore, many studies focus on the correlation between periodontitis and AD. In addition, several reports support the hypothesis that periodontal inflammation can affect cognition. Kamer et al. found that older Danish adults with periodontitis or severe tooth loss exhibit impaired cognition in comparison to healthy subjects [4]. Animal studies have also provided evidence on the impact of tooth loss on neuroinflammation and cognition. Female transgenic mice after tooth extraction were significantly impaired in learning and memory abilities which confirmed that neuronal cell loss in the hippocampus could be triggered by tooth loss causing memory impairment [21]. Although tooth loss can occur for several reasons, periodontitis is one of the major causative factors [22]. Additionally, *P. gingivalis* has been shown to secrete other components associated with periodontitis, which might also affect cognitive function [23]. These results indicate that periodontitis may impair cognition. However, there is limited information on the association

between *P. gingivalis* infection and cognition. In the present study, we have observed that *P. gingivalis* infection elevated the expression levels of the pro-inflammatory cytokines TNF- α, IL-6, and IL-1β in the brains of middle-aged mice. It was also noted that middle-aged *P. gingivalis* infected mice displayed impaired learning and memory abilities. These findings provided further evidence for supporting the association between *P. gingivalis* periodontal infection and cognitive impairment.

In order to assess the learning and memory abilities of mice, behavioral tests are required. The MWM test was used to assess learning and memory [24]. It is a maze where the animals must search for a hidden platform which is submerged under the water surface and placed in a fixed location [25]. Our setup is free from motivational stimuli, like deprived food and water, electrical stimuli, and buzzer sounds, which are likely to impact the normal process of memory. Thus, this task is more precise than active/passive avoidance tasks as it eliminates factors which may interfere with the learning and memory like visual acuity and motor function [12, 26]. In general, the MWM is an effective and accurate test for assessing learning and memory abilities. The escape latency data could be interpreted as spatial learning. During the training days, mice spent less time finding the platform, indicating that they have learned and memorized the location of the platform [26]. The number of times of crossing the platform is regarded as the evaluation outcome of the memory assessment of the mice, and a reduction of the crossing times through the platform indicates memory impairment. In our present study, the results showed that the escape latency and the crossing times were statistically significant different between middle-aged mice with *P. gingivalis* periodontal infection and control mice. Therefore, it is possible that *P. gingivalis* periodontal infection promotes age-dependent neuroinflammatory responses though pro-inflammatory cytokines release.

It has been demonstrated that inflammation induces alterations in neurovascular functions, resulting in an increase in the blood–brain barrier permeability, reduction of nutrient supplements, and aggregation of toxins. Elevated levels of pro-inflammatory mediators in the blood, such as IL-β and TNF-α, can lead to their direct or indirect transport to the brain, which might accelerate the development of brain impairment [27]. During the process of neuroinflammation, pro-inflammatory cytokines (TNF-α, IL-6, IL-1β, and others) are essential neuroinflammation mediating signaling molecules [28]. TNF-α has been reported to play a pivotal role in the development and functions of the CNS, including neuron compliance, cognition, and behavior [29]. In the brain, trauma, infection, or the presence of endogenic abnormal protein aggregates, such as amyloid-β (Aβ) peptides in AD, can activate the secretion of TNF-α, primarily produced by glial cells. In addition, TNF-α has been proven to activate immune/glial cells leading to the augment of amyloid-β precursor protein and Aβ deposits in vitro [20]. One study demonstrated that a single intraperitoneal LPS injection in mice caused peripheral TNF-α expression, both at the mRNA and the protein levels, in the brain [30]. As a key molecule, IL-1β is capable of triggering the production of various inflammatory mediators via activating microglia cells. Thus, there is a close correlation between IL-1β levels and neuroinflammation in AD [31]. Some reports have deduced that afferent neurons can respond directly to peripheral cytokines, like IL-1, for vagal sensory nerve activation. IL-1β has been proven to promote the transformation of Aβ from its non-fibrillar form to insoluble Aβ fibers, leading to increase in plaque formation [32]. Concerning IL-6, its up-regulation in the brain of transgenic mice has been shown to be associated with severe neurological dysfunction. Another study using radial arm maze test to examine the spatial learning of mice showed that IL-6

deficient mice exhibit better and faster acquisition of learning and memory abilities [14].

Our approach to study the association between periodontitis and cognition differed from previous studies, as we have used the *P. gingivalis* periodontal infection animal model. We have assessed the effect of the entire *P. gingivalis* on healthy mice, rather than assessing the individual components of *P. gingivalis*. In addition, we directly measured the mRNA and protein levels of TNF-α, IL-1β, and IL-6, in the brains of mice by qRT-PCR and ELISA. We found that the expression of these cytokines showed differences between young and middle-aged mice. Therefore, the effects of aging on neuroinflammation need to be considered. Most studies have used middle-aged or older mice for research purposes. In our study we chose both young and middle-aged mice and found that, unlike the middle-aged animals, the young mice with *P. gingivalis* periodontal infection neither displayed impaired cognition nor over-expressed pro-inflammatory factors. These differences between the young and middle-aged mice might be attributed to chronic inflammation due to aging, which exerts additional stress to the brain nerve cells of older mice and makes them more vulnerable to infection [33]. Moreover, aging-related alterations, like decreased density and plasticity of synapses, and the amount of the pathological neurofibrillary tangle formation required to cause dementia, increase with age [34, 35]. Additionally, during systemic inflammation, the functions of the blood-cerebrospinal fluid barrier (BCSFB) were significantly affected by the differential responses of glial cells to age-dependent cytokines [36]. Recent reports showed that chronic systemic inflammatory processes promoted the transformation of microglia and astrocytes into anti-inflammatory cell types in young rats, while a pro-inflammatory cell phenotype was detected in middle-aged rats [37]. Furthermore, aging is the major risk factor of AD and is correlated with elevated glial responsiveness, which might increase the brain's susceptibility to injury and disease [21, 38]. One study supports this view by showing that the age-associated progression of the AD-like phenotype in WT mice could be initiated by chronic inflammatory conditions with enhanced accumulations of APP [39].

The present study has some limitations. First, although over-activation of microglia has been reported to be a hallmark of neuroinflammation [40], we did not investigate the activation of microglia in our study. However, the objective of this paper was to determine whether *P. gingivalis* periodontal infection can promote cognitive impairment via inducing neuroinflammation, which was assessed by measuring the levels of the main pro-inflammatory cytokines. Second, the brain inflammation induced by *P. gingivalis* periodontal infection may be mediated via the systemic circulation and/or direct neural pathways. In this study we did not access which mediating pathway is involved, which needs to be considered in the future. In addition, although TNF-α, IL-6, and IL-1β are the most reported molecules to be implicated in neuroinflammation, they cannot represent the whole range of inflammatory cytokines. Therefore, other inflammatory cytokines associated with neuroinflammation remain to be considered.

Conclusion

We have shown that *P. gingivalis* periodontal infection may induce an age-dependent brain inflammation, which increases the TNF- α, IL-6, and IL-1 β levels in middle-aged mice. Moreover, the middle-aged *P. gingivalis* infected mice displayed impaired cognition. Although we have not demonstrated that periodontitis is a risk factor for AD, these findings showed that *P. gingivalis* periodontal infection can cause memory impairment, which suggests that periodontitis might have a similar effect on the development of AD.

Abbreviations
AD: Alzheimer's disease; Aβ: Amyloid-β; BCSFB: Blood-cerebrospinal fluid barrier; CMC: Carboxymethyl cellulose; CNS: Central nervous system; CPR: C Reactive Protein; LPS: Lipopolysaccharide; MWM: Morris water maze; *P. gingivalis*: *Porphyromonas gingivalis*; PBS: Phosphate buffer saline

Acknowledgements
Not applicable.

Funding
This work was supported partly by The National Natural Science Foundation of China to Yanmin Zhou (81570983).

Authors' contributions
YZ and WY conceived the original idea. YD and JR performed the experiments and drafted the manuscript. YQ acquired all data. All authors read and approved the final manuscript.

Ethics approval
The present study was performed in accordance with the guidelines of the National Institutes of Health Guide for the Care and Use of Laboratory Animals (NIH Pub. No. 85–23, revised 1996) and was approved by Animal Care and Use Committee of the Jilin University Medical Centre (Jilin, China).

Competing interests
The authors declare that they have no competing interests.

References

1. Kamer AR, Fortea JO, Videla S, Mayoral A, Janal M, Carmona-Iragui M, et al. Periodontal disease's contribution to Alzheimer's disease progression in down syndrome. Alzheimers Dement. 2016;2:49–57.
2. Hajishengallis G. Periodontitis: from microbial immune subversion to systemic inflammation. Nat Rev Immunol. 2015;15:30–44.
3. Ke X, Lei L, Li H, Li H, Yan F. Manipulation of necroptosis by Porphyromonas gingivalis in periodontitis development. Mol Immunol. 2016;77:8–13.
4. Kamer AR, Morse DE, Holm-Pedersen P, Mortensen EL, Avlund K. Periodontal inflammation in relation to cognitive function in an older adult Danish population. J Alzheimers Dis. 2012;28:613–24.
5. Kamer AR, Craig RG, Dasanayake AP, Brys M, Glodzik-Sobanska L, de Leon MJ. Inflammation and Alzheimer's disease: possible role of periodontal diseases. Alzheimers Dement. 2008;4:242–50.
6. Hill JM, Clement C, Pogue AI, Bhattacharjee S, Zhao Y, Lukiw WJ. Pathogenic microbes, the microbiome, and Alzheimer's disease (AD). Front Aging Neurosci. 2014;6:127.
7. Holmbs C, Coterell D. Role of infection in the pathogenesis of Alzheimer's disease: implications for treatment. CNS Drugs. 2009;23:993–1002.
8. Kamer AR, Craig RG, Pirraglia E, Dasanayake AP, Norman RG, Boylan RJ, et al. TNF-alpha and antibodies to periodontal bacteria discriminate between Alzheimer's disease patients and normal subjects. J Neuroimmunol. 2009; 216:92–7.
9. Stewart R, Hirani V. Dental health and cognitive impairment in an English national survey population. J Am Geriatr Soc. 2007;55:1410–4.
10. Krstic D, Knuesel I. Deciphering the mechanism underlying late-onset Alzheimer disease. Nat Rev Neurol. 2013;9:25–34.
11. Poole S, Singhrao SK, Kesavalu L, Curtis MA, Crean S. Determining the presence of periodontopathic virulence factors in short-term postmortem Alzheimer's disease brain tissue. J Alzheimers Dis. 2013;36:665–77.
12. Saraf MK, Prabhakar S, Anand A. Bacopa monniera alleviates N(omega)-nitro-L-arginine arginine-induced but not MK-801-induced amnesia: a mouse Morris watermaze study. Neuroscience. 2009;160:149–55.
13. Hooge RD, Deyn PPD. Applications of the Morris water maze in the study of learning and memory. Brain Res Rev. 2001;36:60–90.
14. Li Y, Shen R, Wen G, Ding R, Du A, Zhou J, et al. Effects of ketamine on levels of inflammatory cytokines IL-6, IL-1beta, and TNF-alpha in the hippocampus of mice following acute or chronic administration. Front Pharmacol. 2017;8:139.
15. Wu X, Lu Y, Dong Y, Zhang G, Zhang Y, Xu Z, et al. The inhalation anesthetic isoflurane increases levels of proinflammatory TNF-α, IL-6, and IL-1β. Neurobiol Aging. 2012;33:1364–78.
16. Kamer AR, Pirraglia E, Tsui W, Rusinek H, Vallabhajosula S, Mosconi L, et al. Periodontal disease associates with higher brain amyloid load in normal elderly. Neurobiol Aging. 2015;36:627–33.
17. Ide M, Harris M, Stevens A, Sussams R, Hopkins V, Culliford D, et al. Periodontitis and cognitive decline in Alzheimer's disease. PLoS One. 2016;11:e0151081.
18. Ho YH, Lin YT, CW W, Chao YM, Chang AY, Chan JY. Peripheral inflammation increases seizure susceptibility via the induction of neuroinflammation and oxidative stress in the hippocampus. J Biomed Sci. 2015;22:46.
19. Fan K, Wu X, Fan B, Li N, Lin Y, Yao Y, et al. Up-regulation of microglial cathepsin C expression and activity in lipopolysaccharide-induced neuroinflammation. J Neuroinflammation. 2012;9:1–13.
20. Tweedie D, Ferguson RA, Fishman K, Frankola KA, Van Praag H, Holloway HW, et al. Tumor necrosis factor-alpha synthesis inhibitor 3,6′-dithiothalidomide attenuates markers of inflammation, Alzheimer pathology and behavioral deficits in animal models of neuroinflammation and Alzheimer's disease. J Neuroinflammation. 2012;9:106.
21. Oue H, Miyamoto Y, Okada S, Koretake K, Jung CG, Michikawa M, et al. Tooth loss induces memory impairment and neuronal cell loss in APP transgenic mice. Behav Brain Res. 2013;252:318–25.
22. Shaik M, Ahmad S, Gan S, Abuzenadah A, Ahmad E, Tabrez S, et al. How do periodontal infections affect the onset and progression of Alzheimer's disease? CNS Neurol Disord Drug Targets. 2014;13:460–6.
23. Singhrao SK, Harding A, Poole S, Kesavalu L, Crean S. Porphyromonas gingivalis periodontal infection and its putative links with Alzheimer's disease. Mediat Inflamm. 2015;2015:137357.
24. Morris R. Developments of a water-maze procedure for studying spatial learning in the rat. J Neurosci Methods. 1984;11:47–60.
25. Vorhees CV, Williams MT. Morris water maze: procedures for assessing spatial and related forms of learning and memory. Nat Protoc. 2006;1:848–58.
26. Barnhart CD, Yang D, Lein PD. Using the Morris water maze to assess spatial learning and memory in weanling mice. PLoS One. 2015;10:e0124521.

27. Xia MX, Ding X, Qi J, Gu J, Hu G, Sun XL. Inhaled budesonide protects against chronic asthma-induced neuroinflammation in mouse brain. J Neuroimmunol. 2014;273:53–7.

28. Lee YJ, Choi DY, Yun YP, Han SB, Oh KW, Hong JT. Epigallocatechin-3-gallate prevents systemic inflammation-induced memory deficiency and amyloidogenesis via its anti-neuroinflammatory properties. J Nutr Biochem. 2013;24:298–310.

29. Garay PA, Mcallister AK. Novel roles for immune molecules in neural development: implications for neurodevelopmental disorders. Frontiers in Synaptic Neuroscience. 2010;2:136.

30. Qin L, Wu X, Block ML, Liu Y, Breese GR, Hong JS, et al. Systemic LPS causes chronic neuroinflammation and progressive neurodegeneration. Glia. 2007; 55:453–62.

31. Wu Z, Nakanishi H. Connection between periodontitis and Alzheimer's disease: possible roles of microglia and leptomeningeal cells. J Pharmacol Sci. 2014;126:8–13.

32. Gaur S, Agnihotri R. Alzheimer's disease and chronic periodontitis: is there an association? Geriatr Gerontol Int. 2015;15:391–404.

33. Herrup K. Reimagining Alzheimer's disease–an age-based hypothesis. J Neurosci. 2010;30:16755–62.

34. Ganguli M, Rodriguez E. Age, Alzheimer's disease, and the big picture. Int Psychogeriatr. 2011;23:1531–4.

35. Dolan D, Troncoso J, Resnick SM, Crain BJ, Zonderman AB, O'Brien RJ. Age, Alzheimer's disease and dementia in the Baltimore longitudinal study of ageing. Brain. 2010;133:2225–31.

36. Wu Z, Tokuda Y, Zhang XW. Nakanishi. Age-dependent responses of glial cells and leptomeninges during systemic inflammation. Neurobiol Dis. 2008; 32:543–51.

37. Liu X, Wu Z, Hayashi Y, Nakanishi H. Age-dependent neuroinflammatory responses and deficits in long-term potentiation in the hippocampus during systemic inflammation. Neuroscience. 2012;216:133–42.

38. Kyrkanides S, O'Banion MK, Whiteley PE, Daeschner JC, Olschowka JA. Enhanced glial activation and expression of specific CNS inflammation-related molecules in aged versus young rats following cortical stab injury. J Neuroimmunol. 2001;119:269–77.

39. Krstic D, Madhusudan A, Doehner J, Vogel P, Notter T, Imhof C, et al. Systemic immune challenges trigger and drive Alzheimer-like neuropathology in mice. J Neuroinflammation. 2012;9:151.

40. Liu Z, Chen Y, Qiao Q, Sun Y, Liu Q, Ren B, et al. Sesamol supplementation prevents systemic inflammation-induced memory impairment and amyloidogenesis via inhibition of nuclear factor kappaB. Mol Nutr Food Res. 2016; https://doi.org/10.1002/mnfr.201600734.

Effects of a new nutraceutical combination on cognitive function in hypertensive patients

Giuseppe Giugliano[1], Alessia Salemme[2], Sara De Longis[3], Marialuisa Perrotta[4], Valentina D'Angelosante[4], Alessandro Landolfi[4], Raffaele Izzo[3*] (iD) and Valentina Trimarco[5]

Abstract

Background: Chronic increased arterial blood pressure has been associated with executive dysfunction, slowing of attention and mental processing speed, and later with memory deficits. Due to the absence of a concrete therapeutic approach to this pathophysiological process, in the last decades there has been an increasing interest in the use of nutraceuticals, especially those with antioxidant properties, which own strong neuroprotective potential, that may help to improve cognitive function and to delay the onset of dementia.

Results: We evaluated the effects of the treatment with a new nutraceutical preparation containing different molecules with potent antioxidant properties (AkP05, IzzeK®) and placebo on a cohort of thirty-six hypertensive patients. At baseline, neuropsychological evaluation, arterial stiffness and biochemical parameters of the subjects were comparable. After 6 months of treatment, there was a significant reduction of the augmentation index in the AkP05-treated group. Moreover, the measurement of cognitive function, evaluated with MoCA test and Word Match Testing, showed a significant improvement in patients receiving the active treatment. In addition, the group treated with nutraceutical reached a better Stroop test score, while subjects that received placebo did not showed any improvement. Finally, a positive relationship between SBP variation and the psychometric assessment with the EQ-VAS scale was observed only in the active treatment group.

Conclusions: In this study, we demonstrated that the therapy with a new nutraceutical preparation is able to significantly increase the scores of important neuropsychological tests in hypertensive patients already on satisfactory blood pressure control. Although future studies are needed to better characterize the molecular mechanisms involved, these results candidate the new nutraceutical combination as a possible therapeutic strategy to support the cerebrovascular functions and delay the onset of dementia in hypertensive patients.

Keywords: Nutraceutical, Neuropsychological evaluation, Arterial stiffness

Background

One of the most common neurological disorders in the elderly is represented by a progressive and unremitting deterioration of cognitive functions, a condition globally referred to as dementia [1, 2]. In consideration of the lack of effective treatments and the demographic conditions shifting the population toward older adults, the incidence of dementia is predicted to exponentially increase in the future. Basically, for the vast majority of cases, cognitive impairment can be ascribed to two main causes: Alzheimer's Disease (AD) and cerebrovascular diseases. Although it has been generally thought that AD represents those cases of dementia related to genetic alterations that leads to an increased production of the Aβ (amyloid β-peptide) and accumulation of plaques, we are now aware that a clear-cut distinction of AD and cerebrovascular diseases is not always found in the clinical practice, having patients a mixture of both pathologies [3]. On this notice, experimental models have shown that, even when no evident increase of Aβ production does exist, alterations of

* Correspondence: raffaele.izzo@unina.it
[3]Hypertension Research Center; Department of Translational Medical Sciences, Federico II University, via Pansini 5, 80131 Naples, Italy
Full list of author information is available at the end of the article

cerebrovascular homeostasis can determine a failure in the mechanisms responsible for the clearance of Aβ from the brain [4–6]. Thus, the definition of vascular cognitive impairment (VCI) predicts to recapitulate a wide range of cognitive deficits caused by vascular factors, and contributing to the development of later dementia, a condition where cognitive decline is irreversible and impairs even day-to-day functioning [7]. It is generally accepted that, whichever the primary cause, the outcome toward dementia and/or AD is a stage where no strategy is available to improve or at least counteracts the symptomatic manifestations of the disease.

Hypertension, a highly prevalent disease, representing nowadays one of the most impacting cause of disease burden and disability, is the major risk factor for cerebrovascular diseases [1]. Chronic increased arterial blood pressure has been associated with executive dysfunction, slowing of attention and mental processing speed, and later with memory deficits. Similarly, experimental models of hypertension allowed to unravel several pathophysiological mechanisms involved in this deleterious association [4, 8–10]. In addition, the intertwining of cerebrovascular diseases and AD can be also inferred from the neuropathological hallmarks of the two conditions, showing amyloid plaques and neurofibrillary tangles but also microvascular and ischemic lesions.

Taken together the neuropathological traits of brains affected by dementia have suggested over years the existence of an oxidative and inflammatory burden, deriving from the molecular lesions identified. Recent evidence suggests that immune and inflammatory processes significantly contribute to the progression of pathological hallmarks [11–15]. On a similar notice, inflammation and immune activation are clearly recognized as crucial aspects of hypertension and related target organ damage [16, 17].

The idea to counteract the inflammatory burden in early stages of cognitive deterioration and in those predisposing conditions, like hypertension and vascular risk factors, where pro-inflammatory and oxidative mechanisms have a considerable impact as well, raised an expanding area of research aimed at testing the potential beneficial effects of therapeutic strategies enhancing the global anti-oxidant and anti-inflammatory power. On this notice, several evidence in animal models support the use of combined nutraceutical supplementations in the prevention of cognitive decline [18–21]. At this regard different molecules with potent antioxidant properties, including Gingko biloba, extract of Bacopa monniera, Phosphatidylserine, a phospholipid component of the neuronal membrane, Green tea polyphenols and Epigallocathechin, although with mixed results, have shown to have positive effects on cognitive function also in humans [22–36].

According to these promising results, the present study was planned to asses in a double blind, parallel group versus placebo, the effects of a chronic treatment with a novel nutraceutical combination containing dry extract of Gingko biloba, Bacopa monniera, Green tea, phosphatidylserine and catechins on blood pressure, metabolic profile, arterial stiffness and cognitive function in hypertensive patients with a satisfactory blood pressure control obtained by an adequate antihypertensive therapy.

Methods
Study design
The study was conducted in accordance with the guidelines of the declaration of Helsinki and was approved by the Ethic Committee of the IRCCS Neuromed, Pozzilli (Isernia), Italy, which designed and registered the study protocol (ClinicalTrials.gov ID: NCT02572219). Written informed consent was obtained from each subject.

This was a randomized, double blind, placebo-controlled study with a 6-months follow-up, during which patients were randomized to receive placebo or active treatment of a nutraceutical preparation (AkP05, IzzeK®) containing: dry plant extract of *Bacopa monnieri* 300 mg + dry extract of *Ginkgo biloba* leaves 50 mg + Phosphatidylserine 25 mg + dry extract of green tea leaves 40 mg + Catechin 20 mg. Akademy Pharma produced the nutraceutical preparation. The company also produced the placebo, similar in appearance and organoleptic properties to the nutraceutical preparation.

Thirty-six patients were enrolled in the study between January 2017 and March 2017. Subjects of both sexes aged between 40 and 70 with diagnosis of essential hypertension were screened for assessment of the following exclusion criteria. Exclusion criteria were any of the following: previous cardiac or cerebrovascular event; heart failure; diabetes mellitus; history of atrial fibrillation or other severe arrhythmias; chronic kidney disease (defined as serum creatinine levels >1.4 mg/dL); pre-existing psychiatric disorders; neurodegenerative diseases such as multiple sclerosis, amyotrophic lateral sclerosis, Parkinson's disease, early onset/genetic Alzheimer's disease, neuromuscular pathologies, epilepsy; diagnosis of dementia. In addition, patients requiring any pharmacological treatment beyond antihypertensive drugs or with intolerance to nutraceutical compounds, pregnant women and women planning to conceive were also excluded from the study. Only hypertensive patients on pharmacological therapy and with a satisfactory and stable blood pressure control were enrolled, in order to rule out the possibility of an interference of potential additional antihypertensive drugs on cognitive function.

Eighteen were assigned to the nutraceutical treatment group and 18 to the placebo group, according to a computer based randomization double-blinded scheme.

Procedures

Clinical history, risk factors and current pharmacological therapies were assessed at the baseline evaluation. Smokers included current and former smokers. Hypertension was diagnosed if systolic arterial pressure exceeded 140 mmHg and/or diastolic arterial pressure exceeded 90 mmHg, or if the patient was in antihypertensive drugs. Systolic and diastolic BP were measured by standard sphygmomanometer after 5 min in the supine position, according to the guidelines of the European Society of Hypertension/ European Society of Cardiology [37].

All patients suitable for enrollment underwent 2 pre-randomization visits: at baseline and after 2 weeks of run-in period in order to assess the stable and satisfactory blood pressure control. At the end of the run-in period, all randomized patients underwent the following evaluations:

- *Neuropsychological evaluation:* a battery of neuropsychological tests was administered to profile specific aspects of cognitive domains such as associative memory, visual-spatial memory, working memory, attentive skills, and reasoning skills. Cognitive assessment was administered by a well-trained psychologist (A.S.). The specific tests used were: the Montreal Cognitive Assessment (MoCA); Word pairing learning test; Stroop test; Visual analogue scale (EQ-VAS). The execution of all the neuropsychological tests was completed always in the same order.
- *Evaluation of arterial stiffness* was obtained by measuring the augmentation index (AI) with the SphygmoCor pulse wave analysis system (AtCor Medical Pty. Ltd., Sydney, Australia).
- *Peripheral blood sampling* for assessment of glucose and lipid profile.

Neuropsychological tests

Montreal cognitive assessment (MoCA)

This test was designed as a tool for screening of mild cognitive deterioration and has been validated as a gold standard evaluation in vascular-related dementias [38]. The specific cognitive subdomains assessed are the following: attention, executive functions, memory, language, visuo-spatial abilities. The MoCA administration time is 10 min. The maximum possible score is 30 points; a score equal to or greater than 26 is considered normal.

Word match testing

The standard procedure requires reading a list of 10 pairs of words in the fixed order at the rate of a pair every 2 s. Next, in a different order from the first reading, the first member of each pair is read, and the subject is asked to recall the second. This procedure is repeated for 3 times. 5 pairs of words' associations are usually easier (i.e. back and forth), while the other 5 are difficult (i.e. explosion-stamp). The test evaluates the associative memory in simple voluntary learning conditions.

Stroop test

This is a good example of the interference effect on highly automated tasks such as reading. The subject is asked to read the words in the first test, to name the colors in the second and third tests. It is necessary to mark both the mistakes made by the subject, but also the time spent in each trial. Results of the test are provided as two scores: 1) number of errors (Stroop E); and 2) number corrected for time and referred to as interference time (Stroop T).

Visual analogue scale (EQ-VAS)

Visual analogue scale is the second part of the EQ-5D test, in which the subject is asked to mark health status on the day of the interview on a 20 cm vertical scale with end points of 0 and 100. There are notes at the both ends of the scale that the bottom rate (0) corresponds to "the worst health you can imagine", and the highest rate (100) corresponds to "the best health you can imagine".

Participants were allowed to take a 5 min break if necessary to minimize tiredness and maintain motivation. The average duration of the whole neuropsychological evaluation was about of 30 min. For the first 3 tests, the scores obtained were corrected for age and level of education, following correction matrices developed according to validation rules for the Italian population [39]. Adjusted scores were then converted to a five-point interval scale, from 0 to 4 equivalent scores (ES) [39]. The five-point interval scale was divided as follows: 0 = below average scores; 1 = low average scores; 2 = average scores; 3 = high average scores; 4 = above average scores [39].

Arterial stiffness

AI, a validated index of arterial stiffness, was measured by applanation tonometry. To record the central pressure waveform, the indirect method of arterial tonometry was used. Briefly, pressure waveform was recorded at the left radial artery and, using the generalized transfer function, it was converted into a calculated central pressure waveform [40]. All measurements were performed with the SphygmoCor device and designated software (AtCor Medical Pty. Ltd., Sydney, Australia). SphygmoCor uses a high fidelity Millar strain-gauge transducer (Millar Instruments, Houston, TX) allowing for measurement of the first systolic peak (P1), the second systolic peak (P2), and the central pulse pressure (PP) from the calculated aortic waveform. AIx was then calculated as: AI (%) = (P2-P1)PP*100. All patients were maintained without smoking, alcohol or caffeine, starting from the night before the evaluation. All measurements were performed with the patient in supine position in a quiet temperature-controlled laboratory (26 ± 1 °C).

Endpoints

The primary endpoint was the effect of the two treatments (placebo vs active compound) on the score obtained at the Montreal Cognitive Assessment (MoCA) test. Secondary endpoints were the effects on other neuropsychological tests, arterial stiffness, as evaluated by SphygmoCor technology, and metabolic parameters.

Statistical analysis

Based on preliminary data and previous studies assessing the impact of hypertension on cognitive functions, we hypothesized that 50% of patients treated with the nutraceutical preparation would experience an increase of at least one equivalent score (ES) of MoCA test (primary endpoint) with respect to 10% of subjects assuming placebo.

On this assumption, a sample size of 17 subjects in each group would have provided a power of 80% with a two-tailed α-error of 5%. In addition, expecting a dropout rate of about 5%, due to the documented good tolerability of nutraceutical therapies, the total number of patients enrolled was of 36 (18 in each group). Data were analyzed using SPSS (version 22.0; SPSS, Chicago, Illinois, USA) and expressed as number and percentages or means $\pm$ SD. Differences between the two groups at baseline were evaluated by independent sample t-test or chi-square test, as appropriate. A general linear model (GLM) for repeated measures with correction for treatment was performed to evaluate the treatment effect in both groups. Pearson correlation coefficients were used to assess correlations between changes in clinical variables and changes in neuropsychological tests. For all tests, a p value <0.05 was considered statistically significant.

Results

All the 36 patients enrolled completed the entire protocol of the study. Patients included in the study were predominantly males (75%) with a mean age of 58.1 ± 7.2 years, mean body mass index of 26.9 ± 3.0, mean SBP of 134.4 ± 15.1, and mean DBP of 85.0 ± 10.7 mmHg. At baseline, the patients of the two arms were comparable for all clinical and metabolic characteristics, arterial stiffness, and neuropsychological evaluation (Table 1). Also antihypertensive treatments were not different between the two study arms (Table 1).

After 6 months, patients were subjected to the assessment of the same clinical and biochemical variables, as well as the cognitive profile. All the variables resulted unchanged in both placebo and active treatment groups, with respect to the baseline condition (Table 2), with the exception of AI which was significantly reduced in

Table 1 Baseline characteristics according to the treatment protocol group

	Placebo ($n = 18$)	Active treatment ($n = 18$)	p
Age (yrs)	57.9 ± 6.7	58.2 ± 8.0	0.910
Males	14 (77.8)	13 (72.2)	0.700
Height (cm)	170.0 ± 9.2	170.2 ± 8.6	0.955
Weight (kg)	75.9 ± 11.0	80.2 ± 15.7	0.351
Body Mass Index (kg/m^2)	26.3 ± 3.1	27.7 ± 2.8	0.161
SBP (mmHg)	133.3 ± 16.9	135.6 ± 13.5	0.666
DBP (mmHg)	84.1 ± 12.3	85.8 ± 9.1	0.636
Heart rate (bpm)	68.8 ± 6.8	66.4 ± 7.9	0.350
Total cholesterol (mg/dl)	198.2 ± 23.7	201.9 ± 27.5	0.667
HDL cholesterol (mg/dl)	47.6 ± 7.9	51.3 ± 7.2	0.144
LDL cholesterol (mg/dl)	129.2 ± 26.1	126.7 ± 30.4	0.789
Triglycerides (mg/dl)	107.1 ± 34.8	119.5 ± 27.9	0.245
Uric acid (mg/dl)	5.8 ± 1.1	5.4 ± 0.8	0.175
Serum creatinine (mg/dl)	0.94 ± 0.14	0.99 ± 0.20	0.402
Glycaemia (mg/dl)	95.7 ± 11.2	93.1 ± 7.5	0.407
MoCA test ES	1.94 ± 0.94	1.89 ± 1.08	0.870
Word Match Testing ES	2.00 ± 0.97	2.50 ± 1.20	0.178
Stroop test E ES	2.22 ± 0.88	1.67 ± 1.65	0.215
Stroop test T ES	2.67 ± 0.91	2.28 ± 1.67	0.392
EQ-VAS	65.3 ± 12.8	68.1 ± 12.8	0.520
Augmentation Index (%)	14.19 ± 10.00	18.59 ± 18.21	0.400
Antihypertensive therapy			
ACE-inhibitors	2 (11.1)	2 (11.1)	1.000
ATII receptor blockers	13 (72.2)	14 (77.8)	0.700
Beta-blockers	4 (22.2)	5 (27.8)	0.700
Calcium channel antagonists	7 (38.9)	6 (33.6)	0.729
Diuretics	9 (50.0)	9 (50.0)	1.000

Values are numbers (percentage) or means $\pm$ standard deviation
SBP = systolic blood pressure; DBP = diastolic blood pressure; HDL = high-density lipoprotein; LDL = low-density lipoprotein; MoCa = Montreal Cognitive Assessment; ES = equivalent score; EQ-VAS = EQ-5D test visual analogue scale

patients receiving the active nutraceutical compound (Table 2 and Fig. 1). When tested for the cognitive functions, the hypertensive patients in the active treatment group performed significantly better test than the placebo group, as compared to the baseline condition (Table 3 and Fig. 2). In particular, there was a significant improvement in the performance obtained at the MoCA test and Word Match Testing (Table 3 and Fig. 2) for patients receiving the nutraceutical active compound. With a trend toward significance, the same group of hypertensive patients executed the Stroop test with improved scores, whereas no variation was observed for patients receiving the placebo. The psychometric assessment with the EQ-VAS scale revealed a significant amelioration in the active treatment group (Table 3 and Fig. 3) but

Table 2 Characteristics of patients at baseline and after 6 months of treatment

	Baseline	6-months	Treatment effect[a]
SBP (mmHg)			
Control group	133.3 ± 16.9	133.1 ± 15.7	0.132
Active treatment group	135.6 ± 13.5	130.6 ± 11.4	
DBP (mmHg)			
Control group	84.1 ± 12.3	83.1 ± 8.8	0.402
Active treatment group	85.8 ± 9.1	81.5 ± 8.5	
Heart rate (bpm)			
Control group	68.8 ± 6.8	68.2 ± 5.3	0.209
Active treatment group	66.4 ± 7.9	68.3 ± 8.3	
Total cholesterol (mg/dl)			
Control group	198.2 ± 23.7	210.8 ± 21.7	0.132
Active treatment group	201.9 ± 27.5	204.4 ± 23.6	
HDL cholesterol (mg/dl)			
Control group	47.6 ± 7.9	51.3 ± 11.9	0.740
Active treatment group	51.3 ± 7.2	54.3 ± 7.7	
LDL cholesterol (mg/dl)			
Control group	129.2 ± 26.1	138.9 ± 22.4	0.179
Active treatment group	126.7 ± 30.4	126.9 ± 25.0	
Triglycerides (mg/dl)			
Control group	107.1 ± 34.8	103.1 ± 35.0	0.946
Active treatment group	119.5 ± 27.9	115.9 ± 24.3	
Glycaemia (mg/dl)			
Control group	95.7 ± 11.2	96.6 ± 13.3	0.746
Active treatment group	93.1 ± 7.5	93.0 ± 8.0	
Augmentation Index (%)			
Control group	14.19 ± 10.00	14.69 ± 11.79	0.028
Active treatment group	18.59 ± 18.21	12.24 ± 12.30	

Values are means ± standard deviation
SBP = systolic blood pressure; DBP = diastolic blood pressure; HDL = high-density lipoprotein; LDL = low-density lipoprotein
[a] = active treatment versus placebo, GLM analysis

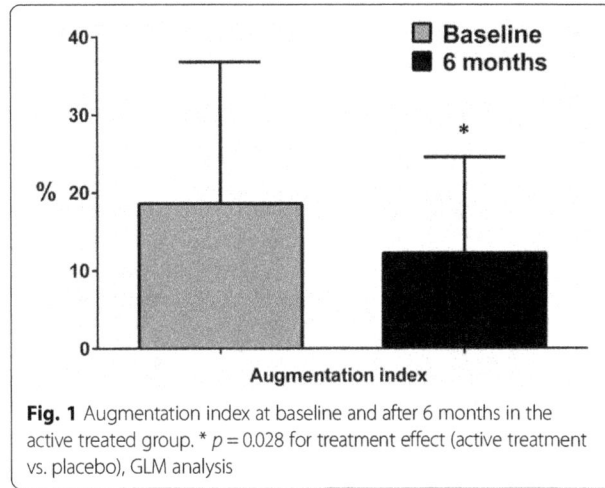

Fig. 1 Augmentation index at baseline and after 6 months in the active treated group. * $p = 0.028$ for treatment effect (active treatment vs. placebo), GLM analysis

containing dry plant extracts of *Bacopa monnieri*, *Ginkgo biloba* and Green tea, plus Phosphatidylserine and Catechins, significantly improved the cognitive performance at MoCA test, Word Match Testing, Stroop test, and EQ-VAS, in a population of hypertensive patients on satisfactory blood pressure control. In contrast, the hypertensive patients treated with the placebo composition, had no significant modification in the scores obtained at the various cognitive tests. Thus, the improvement observed in patients treated with the active nutraceutical preparation could be ascribed to positive effects

Table 3 Characteristics of patients at baseline and after 6 months of treatment

	Baseline	6-months	Treatment effect[a]
MoCA test ES			
Control group	1.94 ± 0.94	1.83 ± 0.79	<0.001
Active treatment group	1.89 ± 1.08	2.89 ± 1.08	
Word Match Testing ES			
Control group	2.00 ± 0.97	1.72 ± 0.89	0.023
Active treatment group	2.50 ± 1.20	2.94 ± 1.21	
Stroop test E ES			
Control group	2.22 ± 0.88	1.94 ± 1.11	0.050
Active treatment group	1.67 ± 1.65	2.00 ± 1.41	
Stroop test T ES			
Control group	2.67 ± 0.91	2.22 ± 1.11	0.124
Active treatment group	2.28 ± 1.67	2.61 ± 1.42	
EQ-VAS			
Control group	65.3 ± 12.8	63.6 ± 12.3	<0.001
Active treatment group	68.1 ± 12.8	80.6 ± 12.0	

Values are means ± standard deviation
MoCa = Montreal Cognitive Assessment; ES = equivalent score; EQ-VAS = EQ-5D test visual analogue scale
[a] = active treatment versus placebo, GLM analysis

not in the control group receiving placebo (Table 3 and Fig. 3).

When we analyzed the potential correlations between changes of clinical and biochemical parameters with changes in neuropsychological scores obtained in the active treatment group, a positive relationship between SBP variation (from baseline to 6 months values) and EQ-VAS change was observed ($r = 0.554$, $p = 0.017$, Fig. 4).

Discussion

The present randomized, double blind, placebo-controlled study demonstrated that a 6-month treatment with the novel nutraceutical preparation (AkP05, IzzeK®),

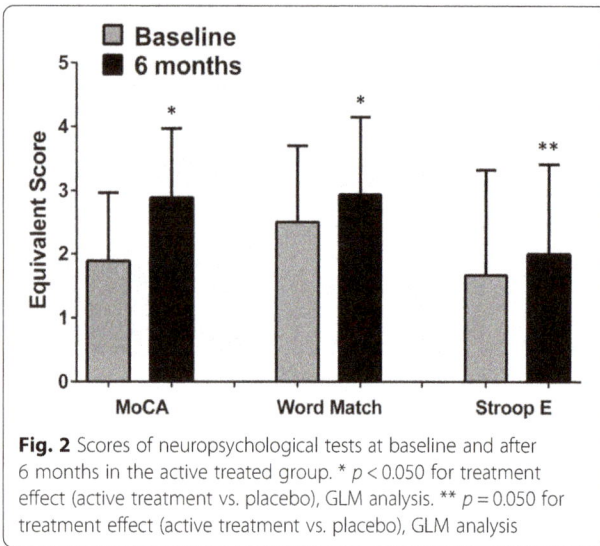

Fig. 2 Scores of neuropsychological tests at baseline and after 6 months in the active treated group. * $p < 0.050$ for treatment effect (active treatment vs. placebo), GLM analysis. ** $p = 0.050$ for treatment effect (active treatment vs. placebo), GLM analysis

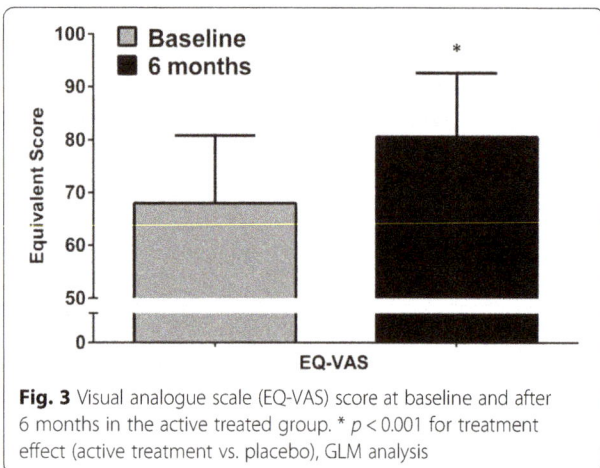

Fig. 4 Correlation between change in systolic blood pressure and change in visual analogue scale (EQ-VAS) after 6 months of treatment in the active treated group

on cognitive performance, ruling out the possibility of a placebo effect or potential habituation effects in performing the tests. In addition, hypertensive patients on active nutraceutical treatment displayed a significant improvement of arterial stiffness, as assessed by AI.

In this study, cognitive function was assessed accordingly to the most common measures used in general studies testing the impact of hypertension on cerebrovascular homeostasis. Basically, we tested how the nutraceutical compound under examination affected the most typically impaired cognitive domains of memory, executive function, and processing speed. The results obtained at the MoCA test after 6-months of treatment (active compound vs placebo), showed a significant improvement in the group of hypertensive patients receiving the nutraceutical preparation and no variation in the placebo group. Taking into consideration the fact that the battery of MoCA tests comprises a series of assessments capable to discriminate among different cognitive domains (memory and attention, visuospatial and executive functions, and

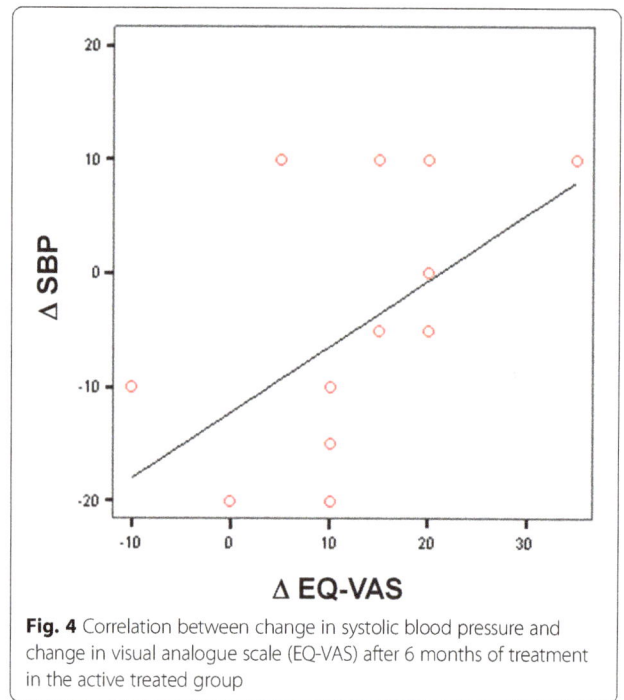

Fig. 3 Visual analogue scale (EQ-VAS) score at baseline and after 6 months in the active treated group. * $p < 0.001$ for treatment effect (active treatment vs. placebo), GLM analysis

language), we also evaluated more specific subdomains of cognition. Word-matching test highlighted a similar significant trend of improved learning abilities of the memory domain in patients receiving the active nutraceutical compound as compared to the placebo. The better performance in executive functions and processing speed was also confirmed when patients were subjected to the Stroop test, which showed enhanced functions in patients on active nutraceutical preparation. Lastly, the significantly increased score obtained in the VAS scale, indicative of patients' awareness on their health status, was also suggestive that the benefit obtained with the 6-months treatment with the active nutraceutical compound was positively perceived by patients themselves.

Although several mechanisms may be involved in the improved overall cognitive function displayed by hypertensive patients treated with the nutraceutical compound, it could be envisaged that the concomitant reduction in arterial stiffness may be causally related. In fact, at the clinical level, indexes of aortic and large-artery stiffening are considered valuable predictors of cerebrovascular events and VCI [41, 42]. In this study, we observed that a 6-months treatment with the active nutraceutical compound induced a significant reduction in the AI, a parameter correlated with arterial stiffness. No significant variation of the AI was found in the group of patients receiving the placebo for 6 months. Although we failed to detect significant correlations between the changes in AI and any of the measured cognitive parameters, we could speculate that the improvement in arterial stiffness positively influenced cerebral circulation, eventually enhancing cognitive functions.

Chronic hypertension is also accompanied with hypertrophic remodeling of cerebral arteries and arterioles, a phenomenon well described in experimental models of hypertension and supported by evidence in patients. A critical aspect regarding cerebral circulation at the level of smaller arterioles consists in the disruption of the Blood-Brain Barrier (BBB), often leading to a potent inflammatory reaction, typically associated with the production of reactive oxygen species. A trait that can be commonly found in all the phenomena described above (hypertension, arterial stiffness, VCI and arterial stiffness) is the presence of a chronic low-grade inflammation, a process thought to contribute to pathogenesis of several diseases [14, 15]. Several experimental evidence suggests that the use of nutraceutical compounds can be effective in hampering cognitive decline in experimental models [18–21]. Thus, the possibility that hypertension could influence onset/progression of late-life dementia/sporadic AD by promoting neuroinflammatory processes through an increase in oxidative stress [43–46], accounts for the use of nutritional supplements with antioxidant action to counteract the development of cognitive decline in hypertensive patients. The nutraceutical preparation tested in the present study contains different molecules with potent antioxidant properties which, although with mixed results, have shown to have positive effects on cognitive function also in humans [22–32, 34], thus supporting the hypothesis that the improvement in cognitive function observed in our study is mediated by a reduction of the oxidative stress.

Conclusions

The potential to counteract cognitive decline in hypertensive patients is of utmost importance. Although some studies [47–50] have shown little benefit from using antioxidant or anti-hypertensive drugs, they are often generally not well accepted as long-term preventive tools by the general population. By contrast, the use of dietary supplements and nutraceutical preparations is becoming more common and widespread, since they are often seen as a useful tool, associated with a healthy lifestyle, to deal with health problems that inevitably arise over time, in the presence of predisposing risk factors.

In this study, we demonstrated that the therapy with a novel nutraceutical preparation (AkP05, IzzeK®) containing *Bacopa monnieri*, *Ginkgo biloba*, Phosphatidylserine, Green tea and Catechins is able to significantly increase the scores of important neuropsychological tests such as the MoCA battery of tests, the Word Match Testing and Stroop test. The positive variation in the EQ-VAS was also suggestive that patients increased their perception of a better health status. The fact that an enhancement of performance in specific cognitive domain was obtained in patients already on satisfactory control of blood pressure

levels, could reflect that the effect was exerted at the level of target organ damage, probably supporting cerebrovascular function by reducing oxidative stress at the level of brain microcirculation. Future pharmacological and pathophysiological studies are needed to better clarify the mechanisms underlying this effect.

Abbreviations

AD: Alzheimer's Disease; AI: augmentation index; Aβ: amyloid β-peptide; BBB: Blood-Brain Barrier; BP: blood pressure ; DBP: diastolic blood pressure; ES: equivalent score; GLM: general linear model; MoCA: Montreal Cognitive Assessment; P1: first systolic peak; PP: pulse pressure; SBP: systolic blood pressure; VAS: Visual analogue scale; VCI: vascular cognitive impairment

Acknowledgements

The authors wish to thank nurses Maria Abbate, Valeria Celestino, Maria Rosaria Cipro and Marco Colonna and their coordinator Anna Vitiello for their invaluable support in the management of patients.

Funding

The present research received no funding.

Authors' contributions

GG, AS, SDL, MLP, VDA, conceived and drafted the paper; AL, RI, VT made critical revisions to the draft. All authors read and approved the final manuscript.

Competing interests

The authors declare that they have no competing interests.

Author details

[1]Hypertension Research Center; Department of Advanced Biomedical Sciences, Federico II University, Naples, Italy. [2]Federico II University, Naples, Italy. [3]Hypertension Research Center; Department of Translational Medical Sciences, Federico II University, via Pansini 5, 80131 Naples, Italy. [4]Department of Angiocardioneurology and Translational Medicine, IRCCS Neuromed, Pozzilli, Isernia, Italy. [5]Hypertension Research Center; Department of Neurosciences, Federico II University, Naples, Italy.

References

1. Iadecola C, Yaffe K, Biller J, Bratzke LC, Faraci FM, Gorelick PB, Gulati M, Kamel H, Knopman DS, Launer LJ, et al. Impact of hypertension on cognitive function: a scientific statement from the American Heart Association. Hypertension. 2016;68(6):e67–94.
2. Prince M, Bryce R, Albanese E, Wimo A, Ribeiro W, Ferri CP. The global prevalence of dementia: a systematic review and metaanalysis. Alzheimers Dement. 2013;9(1):63–75. e62
3. Fotuhi M, Hachinski V, Whitehouse PJ. Changing perspectives regarding late-life dementia. Nat Rev Neurol. 2009;5(12):649–58.
4. Carnevale D, Mascio G, D'Andrea I, Fardella V, Bell RD, Branchi I, Pallante F, Zlokovic B, Yan SS, Lembo G. Hypertension induces brain beta-amyloid accumulation, cognitive impairment, and memory deterioration through

activation of receptor for advanced glycation end products in brain vasculature. Hypertension. 2012;60(1):188–97.

5. Zlokovic BV. The blood-brain barrier in health and chronic neurodegenerative disorders. Neuron. 2008;57(2):178–201.

6. Deane R, Du Yan S, Submamaryan RK, LaRue B, Jovanovic S, Hogg E, Welch D, Manness L, Lin C, Yu J, et al. RAGE mediates amyloid-beta peptide transport across the blood-brain barrier and accumulation in brain. Nat Med. 2003;9(7):907–13.

7. Gorelick PB, Scuteri A, Black SE, Decarli C, Greenberg SM, Iadecola C, Launer LJ, Laurent S, Lopez OL, Nyenhuis D, et al. Vascular contributions to cognitive impairment and dementia: a statement for healthcare professionals from the american heart association/american stroke association. Stroke. 2011;42(9):2672–713.

8. Carnevale D, Mascio G, Ajmone-Cat MA, D'Andrea I, Cifelli G, Madonna M, Cocozza G, Frati A, Carullo P, Carnevale L, et al. Role of neuroinflammation in hypertension-induced brain amyloid pathology. Neurobiol Aging. 2012; 33(1):205;e219–29.

9. Gentile MT, Poulet R, Di Pardo A, Cifelli G, Maffei A, Vecchione C, Passarelli F, Landolfi A, Carullo P, Lembo G. Beta-amyloid deposition in brain is enhanced in mouse models of arterial hypertension. Neurobiol Aging. 2009;30(2):222–8.

10. Faraco G, Park L, Zhou P, Luo W, Paul SM, Anrather J, Iadecola C. Hypertension enhances Abeta-induced neurovascular dysfunction, promotes beta-secretase activity, and leads to amyloidogenic processing of APP. J Cereb Blood Flow Metab. 2016;36(1):241–52.

11. Spangenberg EE, Green KN. Inflammation in Alzheimer's disease: lessons learned from microglia-depletion models. Brain Behav Immun. 2017;61:1–11.

12. Faraco G, Sugiyama Y, Lane D, Garcia-Bonilla L, Chang H, Santisteban MM, Racchumi G, Murphy M, Van Rooijen N, Anrather J, et al. Perivascular macrophages mediate the neurovascular and cognitive dysfunction associated with hypertension. J Clin Invest. 2016;126(12):4674–89.

13. Park L, Uekawa K, Garcia-Bonilla L, Koizumi K, Murphy M, Pistik R, Younkin L, Younkin S, Zhou P, Carlson G, et al. Brain perivascular macrophages initiate the neurovascular dysfunction of Alzheimer Abeta peptides. Circ Res. 2017;121(3):258–69.

14. Minghetti L. Role of inflammation in neurodegenerative diseases. Curr Opin Neurol. 2005;18(3):315–21.

15. Wyss-Coray T. Inflammation in Alzheimer disease: driving force, bystander or beneficial response? Nat Med. 2006;12(9):1005–15.

16. Li JJ, Chen JL. Inflammation may be a bridge connecting hypertension and atherosclerosis. Med Hypotheses. 2005;64(5):925–9.

17. Marvar PJ, Lob H, Vinh A, Zarreen F, Harrison DG. The central nervous system and inflammation in hypertension. Curr Opin Pharmacol. 2011;11(2):156–61.

18. Koh SH, Lee SM, Kim HY, Lee KY, Lee YJ, Kim HT, Kim J, Kim MH, Hwang MS, Song C, et al. The effect of epigallocatechin gallate on suppressing disease progression of ALS model mice. Neurosci Lett. 2006;395(2):103–7.

19. Rezai-Zadeh K, Arendash GW, Hou H, Fernandez F, Jensen M, Runfeldt M, Shytle RD, Tan J. Green tea epigallocatechin-3-gallate (EGCG) reduces beta-amyloid mediated cognitive impairment and modulates tau pathology in Alzheimer transgenic mice. Brain Res. 2008;1214:177–87.

20. Lee YK, Yuk DY, Lee JW, Lee SY, Ha TY, Oh KW, Yun YP, Hong JT. Epigallocatechin-3-gallate prevents lipopolysaccharide-induced elevation of beta-amyloid generation and memory deficiency. Brain Res. 2009;1250:164–74.

21. Araujo JA, Landsberg GM, Milgram NW, Miolo A. Improvement of short-term memory performance in aged beagles by a nutraceutical supplement containing phosphatidylserine, Ginkgo Biloba, vitamin E, and pyridoxine. Can Vet J. 2008;49(4):379–85.

22. Stough C, Lloyd J, Clarke J, Downey LA, Hutchison CW, Rodgers T, Nathan PJ. The chronic effects of an extract of Bacopa monniera (Brahmi) on cognitive function in healthy human subjects. Psychopharmacology. 2001;156(4):481–4.

23. Roodenrys S, Booth D, Bulzomi S, Phipps A, Micallef C, Smoker J. Chronic effects of Brahmi (Bacopa Monnieri) on human memory. Neuropsychopharmacology. 2002;27(2):279–81.

24. Calabrese C, Gregory WL, Leo M, Kraemer D, Bone K, Oken B. Effects of a standardized Bacopa Monnieri extract on cognitive performance, anxiety, and depression in the elderly: a randomized, double-blind, placebo-controlled trial. J Altern Complement Med. 2008;14(6):707–13.

25. Morgan A, Stevens J. Does Bacopa Monnieri improve memory performance in older persons? Results of a randomized, placebo-controlled, double-blind trial. J Altern Complement Med. 2010;16(7):753–9.

26. Stough C, Clarke J, Lloyd J, Nathan PJ. Neuropsychological changes after 30-day Ginkgo Biloba administration in healthy participants. Int J Neuropsychopharmacol. 2001;4(2):131–4.

27. Schneider LS, DeKosky ST, Farlow MR, Tariot PN, Hoerr R, Kieser M. A randomized, double-blind, placebo-controlled trial of two doses of Ginkgo Biloba extract in dementia of the Alzheimer's type. Curr Alzheimer Res. 2005;2(5):541–51.

28. Woelk H, Arnoldt KH, Kieser M, Hoerr R. Ginkgo Biloba special extract EGb 761 in generalized anxiety disorder and adjustment disorder with anxious mood: a randomized, double-blind, placebo-controlled trial. J Psychiatr Res. 2007;41(6):472–80.

29. Cenacchi T, Bertoldin T, Farina C, Fiori MG, Crepaldi G. Cognitive decline in the elderly: a double-blind, placebo-controlled multicenter study on efficacy of phosphatidylserine administration. Aging (Milano). 1993;5(2):123–33.

30. Kesse-Guyot E, Fezeu L, Andreeva VA, Touvier M, Scalbert A, Hercberg S, Galan P. Total and specific polyphenol intakes in midlife are associated with cognitive function measured 13 years later. J Nutr. 2012;142(1):76–83.

31. Mohamed S, Lee Ming T, Jaffri JM. Cognitive enhancement and neuroprotection by catechin-rich oil palm leaf extract supplement. J Sci Food Agric. 2013;93(4):819–27.

32. Snitz BE, O'Meara ES, Carlson MC, Arnold AM, Ives DG, Rapp SR, Saxton J, Lopez OL, Dunn LO, Sink KM, et al. Ginkgo Biloba for preventing cognitive decline in older adults: a randomized trial. JAMA. 2009; 302(24):2663–70.

33. Nurk E, Refsum H, Drevon CA, Tell GS, Nygaard HA, Engedal K, Smith AD. Intake of flavonoid-rich wine, tea, and chocolate by elderly men and women is associated with better cognitive test performance. J Nutr. 2009;139(1):120–7.

34. Kuriyama S, Hozawa A, Ohmori K, Shimazu T, Matsui T, Ebihara S, Awata S, Nagatomi R, Arai H, Tsuji I. Green tea consumption and cognitive function: a cross-sectional study from the Tsurugaya project 1. Am J Clin Nutr. 2006;83(2):355–61.

35. Letenneur L, Proust-Lima C, Le Gouge A, Dartigues JF, Barberger-Gateau P. Flavonoid intake and cognitive decline over a 10-year period. Am J Epidemiol. 2007;165(12):1364–71.

36. Mastroiacovo D, Kwik-Uribe C, Grassi D, Necozione S, Raffaele A, Pistacchio L, Righetti R, Bocale R, Lechiara MC, Marini C, et al. Cocoa flavanol consumption improves cognitive function, blood pressure control, and metabolic profile in elderly subjects: the Cocoa, cognition, and aging (CoCoA) study–a randomized controlled trial. Am J Clin Nutr. 2015;101(3):538–48.

37. Mancia G, Fagard R, Narkiewicz K, Redon J, Zanchetti A, Bohm M, Christiaens T, Cifkova R, De Backer G, Dominiczak A, et al. 2013 ESH/ESC guidelines for the Management of Arterial Hypertension: the task force for the management of arterial hypertension of the European Society of Hypertension (ESH) and of the European Society of Cardiology (ESC). Eur Heart J. 2013;34(28):2159–219.

38. Popovic IM, Seric V, Demarin V. Mild cognitive impairment in symptomatic and asymptomatic cerebrovascular disease. J Neurol Sci. 2007;257(1–2):185–93.

39. Spinnler HTG. Standardizzazione e taratura italiana di test neuropsicologici. Ital J Neurol Sci. 1987;6:8–120.

40. Chen CH, Nevo E, Fetics B, Pak PH, Yin FC, Maughan WL, Kass DA. Estimation of central aortic pressure waveform by mathematical transformation of radial tonometry pressure. Validation of generalized transfer function. Circulation. 1997;95(7):1827–36.

41. Matsumoto A, Satoh M, Kikuya M, Ohkubo T, Hirano M, Inoue R, Hashimoto T, Hara A, Hirose T, Obara T, et al. Day-to-day variability in home blood pressure is associated with cognitive decline: the Ohasama study. Hypertension. 2014;63(6):1333–8.

42. Bohm M, Schumacher H, Leong D, Mancia G, Unger T, Schmieder R, Custodis F, Diener HC, Laufs U, Lonn E, et al. Systolic blood pressure variation and mean heart rate is associated with cognitive dysfunction in patients with high cardiovascular risk. Hypertension. 2015;65(3):651–61.

43. Minuz P, Patrignani P, Gaino S, Degan M, Menapace L, Tommasoli R, Seta F, Capone ML, Tacconelli S, Palatresi S, et al. Increased oxidative stress and platelet activation in patients with hypertension and renovascular disease. Circulation. 2002;106(22):2800–5.

44. Morris MC, Evans DA, Tangney CC, Bienias JL, Wilson RS. Associations of vegetable and fruit consumption with age-related cognitive change. Neurology. 2006;67(8):1370–6.

45. Craft S, Foster TC, Landfield PW, Maier SF, Resnick SM, Yaffe K, Session III. Mechanisms of age-related cognitive change and targets for intervention: inflammatory, oxidative, and metabolic processes. J Gerontol A Biol Sci Med Sci. 2012;67(7):754–9.

46. Poulet R, Gentile MT, Vecchione C, Distaso M, Aretini A, Fratta L, Russo G, Echart C, Maffei A, De Simoni MG, et al. Acute hypertension induces oxidative stress in brain tissues. J Cereb Blood Flow Metab. 2006;26(2):253–62.

47. Saxby BK, Harrington F, Wesnes KA, McKeith IG, Ford GA. Candesartan and cognitive decline in older patients with hypertension: a substudy of the SCOPE trial. Neurology. 2008;70(19 Pt 2):1858–66.

48. Hanon O, Berrou JP, Negre-Pages L, Goch JH, Nadhazi Z, Petrella R, Sedefdjian A, Sevenier F, Shlyakhto EV, Pathak A. Effects of hypertension therapy based on eprosartan on systolic arterial blood pressure and cognitive function: primary results of the observational study on cognitive function and systolic blood pressure reduction open-label study. J Hypertens. 2008;26(8):1642–50.

49. Anderson C, Teo K, Gao P, Arima H, Dans A, Unger T, Commerford P, Dyal L, Schumacher H, Pogue J, et al. Renin-angiotensin system blockade and cognitive function in patients at high risk of cardiovascular disease: analysis of data from the ONTARGET and TRANSCEND studies. Lancet Neurol. 2011;10(1):43–53.

50. Katada E, Uematsu N, Takuma Y, Matsukawa N. Comparison of effects of valsartan and amlodipine on cognitive functions and auditory p300 event-related potentials in elderly hypertensive patients. Clin Neuropharmacol. 2014;37(5):129–32.

Anti-cytomegalovirus IgG antibody titer is positively associated with advanced T cell differentiation and coronary artery disease in end-stage renal disease

Feng-Jung Yang[1,2], Kai-Hsiang Shu[3,4], Hung-Yuan Chen[3], I-Yu Chen[3], Fang-Yun Lay[3,4], Yi-Fang Chuang[5], Chien-Sheng Wu[3], Wan-Chuan Tsai[3], Yu-Sen Peng[3], Shih-Ping Hsu[3], Chih-Kang Chiang[6], George Wang[7] and Yen-Ling Chiu[1,3,8*]

Abstract

Background: Accumulating evidence indicates that persistent human cytomegalovirus (HCMV) infection is associated with several health-related adverse outcomes including atherosclerosis and premature mortality in individuals with normal renal function. Patients with end-stage renal disease (ESRD) exhibit impaired immune function and thus may face higher risk of HCMV-related adverse outcomes. Whether the level of anti-HCMV immune response may be associated with the prognosis of hemodialysis patients is unknown.

Results: Among 412 of the immunity in ESRD study (iESRD study) participants, 408 were HCMV seropositive and were analyzed. Compared to 57 healthy individuals, ESRD patients had higher levels of anti-HCMV IgG. In a multivariate-adjusted logistic regression model, the log level of anti-HCMV IgG was independently associated with prevalent coronary artery disease (OR = 1.93, 95% CI = 1.2~ 3.2, p = 0.01) after adjusting for age, sex, hemoglobin, diabetes, calcium phosphate product and high sensitivity C-reactive protein. Levels of anti-HCMV IgG also positively correlated with both the percentage and absolute number of terminally differentiated CD8+ and CD4+ CD45RA+ CCR7- T_{EMRA} cells, indicating that immunosenescence may participate in the development of coronary artery disease.

Conclusion: This is the first study showing that the magnitude of anti-HCMV humoral immune response positively correlates with T cell immunosenescence and coronary artery disease in ESRD patients. The impact of persistent HCMV infection should be further investigated in this special patient population.

Keywords: Cytomegalovirus, End-stage renal disease, Cardiovascular disease, Immunosenescence, Immunology

Background

Human cytomegalovirus (HCMV), a member of the β-herpesvirus family, contains a double-stranded DNA genome and persists in certain host cells indefinitely after primary infection [1]. Worldwide HCMV seroprevalence among women of reproductive age is about 45–100% [2]. Overall seroprevalence rate increases with age [3], reaching above 60% among people older than 50 and is considerably higher in Asian countries [4, 5]. Importantly, in addition to causing opportunistic infections, congenital infections, and mononucleosis, HCMV infection also possess long-term threats to immunocompetent individuals. Mounting evidence strongly suggests the implication of persistent HCMV infection in autoimmunity, cancer, poor response toward vaccination, cardiovascular disease and mortality [6–8].

Large-scale epidemiological studies and meta-analysis have suggested an association between HCMV seropositivity and cardiovascular disease [9, 10]. Earlier observations noted that HCMV seropositivity is associated with restenosis after coronary atherectomy [11]. HCMV can

* Correspondence: yenlingchiu@ntu.edu.tw
[1]Graduate Institute of Clinical Medicine, College of Medicine, National Taiwan University, Taipei, Taiwan
[3]Department of Internal Medicine, Far Eastern Memorial Hospital, New Taipei City, Taiwan
Full list of author information is available at the end of the article

infect endothelial cells, which explains why its viral DNA is often found at sites of arterial disease [12]. HCMV could also contribute to cardiovascular disease via indirect mechanisms such as inducing systemic inflammation, cytokine release [13], and an increase in blood pressure [14]. Several studies based on HCMV-specific IgG titers also showed that higher IgG titers against HCMV, but not antibodies against herpes simplex virus 1, are significantly associated with incident coronary artery events [15, 16]. Since HCMV IgG increases in individuals with virus shedding [17] and its level positively correlates with HCMV-specific IgM [18], an increase of HCMV IgG during latency might indicate frequent or recent virus reactivation.

Of note, HCMV infection also leads to an imbalance of the T cell homeostasis, causing significant loss of naïve CD8+ T cells, accumulation of terminally differentiated memory CD4+ and CD8+ cells – premature aging of T cells, also known as "immunosenescence" [19, 20]. This perturbation of immune system not only causes impaired vaccine response [21], but also poor survival [22]. These terminally differentiated memory T cells might be preferentially recruited to vascular endothelium via upregulation of CX3CR1 and participate in the process of atherosclerosis [23, 24].

Cardiovascular mortality is the most important cause of death in ESRD (end stage renal disease) patients worldwide [25, 26]. ESRD patients exhibit a striking 20–400 fold higher risk of cardiovascular death compared to age-matched healthy individuals. However, traditional cardiovascular disease risk factors only explain a relatively small proportion of such high cardiovascular disease burden [27]. Similar to healthy individuals, CMV seropositivity is related to the amount of terminally differentiated T cells in patients with ESRD [28, 29]. To our knowledge, no study has attempted to study the relationship between the titer of HCMV-specific IgG with either immunosenescence or atherosclerotic heart disease in ESRD. We thus established the "immunity in ESRD" (iESRD) study, which is an ongoing longitudinal study aiming to investigate the impacts of immunological mechanisms on cardiovascular outcome in ESRD patients. The current study reports the association between HCMV IgG titer with immunosenescence and cardiovascular co-morbidities based on the baseline data from this cohort study.

Methods

Participants

The immunity in ESRD (iESRD) study is a cohort study investigating the effect of immunological factors on outcomes of hemodialysis patients. Patients and healthy controls were recruited from Far Eastern Memorial Hospital and National Taiwan University Hospital Yun Lin Branch. Far Eastern Memorial Hospital is located in

New Taipei City in northern Taiwan and National Taiwan University Yun Lin Branch is located in southern Taiwan. A total of 432 patients signed informed consent to join the study and were screened for eligibility. Those with recent hospitalization within three months, active or chronic infection requiring antibiotics, incomplete blood test results or poor blood samples quality were excluded, resulting in 412 patients enrolled in the iESRD study (198 from Far Eastern Memorial Hospital and 214 from National Taiwan University Hospital). Among these patients, 408 were CMV seropositive and were analyzed in the current study. Most patients (99.5%) received hemodialysis at least 4 h per session, thrice a week; only two patients underwent twice a week hemodialysis. All patients were treated by their primary care nephrologists according to the Kidney Disease Outcomes Quality Initiative (KDOQI) guidelines.

Data collections and laboratory exams

Blood samples were collected before the start of hemodialysis sessions in the middle of week. In addition to hematological and biochemical tests, peripheral blood mononuclear cells (PBMC) were sampled. Intact-parathyroid hormone (i-PTH) immunoradiometric assay (Cisbio) and high sensitive C-reactive protein (hs-CRP) nephelometry (Siemens) were also tested. By history taking and detailed chart reviews, baseline co-morbidities and clinical laboratory data were recorded. HCMV-specific IgG titer was measured by ELISA (Roche Elecsys assay) at Far Eastern Memorial Hospital. Plasma level of inflammatory cytokines were measured using the human IL-6 Quantikine HS ELISA kit and human TNFα Quantikine ELISA Kit from R&D systems.

Immunophenotyping and multicolor flow cytometry

After blood collection, peripheral blood mononuclear cells (PBMCs) were immediately isolated by Ficoll-Paque PLUS gradient centrifugation following the manufacturer's protocol (GE Healthcare). For flow cytometry analysis, briefly, singlets were collected by forward scatter area and height. CD3-AF700 (clone UCHT1, BioLegend) was used to identify CD3+ T cells from the lymphocytes gated by forward and side scatter properties. CD4+ and CD8+ T cells were determined by CD4-PerCP-Cy5.5 and CD8-APC-Cy7 (clone OKT4 and SK1, BioLegend) respectively, and the T cell differentiation states were determined by CCR7-APC, CD45RA-Alexa488 (clone G043H7 and HI100, BioLegend) and CD28-PE-Cy7 (clone 28.2, eBioscience).

Monocyte staining was performed according to previous studies performed by Zawada et al., which indicated that a pan-monocyte marker such as CD86 is necessary to correctly enumerate monocyte subsets [30]. After gating on the forward scatter/side scatter, monocytes were determined by expression of CD86-PE (clone IT2.2, eBioscience), and were further classified as classical (CD14 ++CD16-), intermediate (CD14++CD16+), and non-classical (CD14 + CD16++) by CD14-FITC and CD16-APC (clone M5E2, Biolegend and clone 3G8, eBioscience). In general, the percentage calculated for a specific immune cell subset refers to the percentage of a specific cell subset among the mother population on flow cytometry.

Cardiovascular co-morbidities

Medical comorbidity status of all patients were determined by careful review of medical history and radiological reports. The documented coronary artery disease (CAD) was defined as either 1) > 50% stenosis of at least one coronary artery on coronary angiography or 2) documented perfusion defect(s) on stressed cardiac nuclear scan. Cardiovascular disease (CVD) was defined as having documented CHF, CAD, stroke and/or peripheral arterial disease (PAOD). Congestive heart failure (CHF) was diagnosed clinically as a syndrome in which patients have symptoms and signs resulting from an abnormal cardiac structure or function by cardiologists.

Statistical analyses

Patient characteristics were described as mean ± standard deviation for continuous variables and frequency for categorical variables. These variables were analyzed by ANOVA and Chi-square test, respectively. Pearson correlation was applied to evaluate the correlation of log-transformed HCMV-specific IgG with immune cell subsets frequencies and absolute cell numbers.

Binary and ordered logistic regression models were used to calculate the predictive value of HCMV IgG level on cardiovascular co-morbidities. Univariate logistic regression was performed to calculate the p for trend value for determining the relationship between HCMV IgG quintiles and individual medical co-morbidity. Multivariable-adjusted logistic regression models, including age, gender, diabetes mellitus, albumin, hemoglobin, calcium phosphate product and high sensitivity-CRP were used to investigate the association between HCMV IgG level and co-morbidities. All statistical tests were two-tailed, and a p value of less than 0.05 was considered be significant. The statistical analyses were performed with SPSS Version 25 (IBM) and STATA version 14.2 (StataCorp).

Results

HCMV IgG levels in ESRD patients are elevated compared to control individuals

First, we compared HCMV IgG levels between 408 CMV seropositive ESRD patients from the iESRD cohort and 57 CMV seropositive healthy individuals. The age of ESRD patients and healthy individuals were not statistically different (mean ± SD, ESRD: 62.0 ± 11.9; Healthy: 58.9 ± 6.8). Despite general belief of a more immunosuppressed state, ESRD patients exhibit significantly higher levels of HCMV IgG compared to healthy individuals (Fig. 1a, medium = 391.9 U/mL, IQR 181.5 ~ 818.5 versus medium = 305.8 U/mL, IQR 132.1 ~ 624.1). We further stratified HCMV IgG levels into quintiles and investigated the differences in demographic, clinical and laboratory data among groups. As Table 1 shows, patients in the highest HCMV IgG quintile tend to be older, have lower levels of hemoglobin, creatinine, phosphate and normalized protein catabolic rate, although most of these differences were not statistically significant.

Elevated HCMV IgG levels is not associated with systemic inflammation in ESRD

Since premature aging and systemic inflammation are important features of ESRD patients [31], we tested the associations between HCMV-specific IgG level with chronological age and circulatory inflammatory markers. We found a significant association between age and log-transformed HCMV IgG level (R = 0.15, p value = 0.003). Nevertheless, there was no relationship between HCMV IgG level and systemic inflammation, as measured by high-sensitivity C-reactive protein levels, TNFα levels and IL-6 (by Pearson correlation, all p value > 0.05). It has been suggested that elevated HCMV IgG level in asymptomatic individuals reflects virus reactivation and shedding [17]. As a result, augmented humoral response toward CMV in ESRD patients may be a unique immunological phenomenon that reflects aging and subclinical viral reactivation but not simply a status of non-specific systemic inflammation.

Higher CMV-IgG level is associated with advanced T cell differentiation but not monocyte subset distribution in ESRD

Previous studies indicated that certain T cell and monocyte subsets [32–34] are associated with cardiovascular disease and/or atherosclerosis. Although it is known that CMV infection profoundly affects the adaptive human immune system [35, 36], much less is known about the effect of CMV infection on monocytes. We performed peripheral blood T cell and monocyte immunophenotyping in all the 408 CMV seropositive iESRD participants and tested the relationship between log-transformed HCMV-specific IgG level with distinct immune subsets, in either relative (percentage of mother population) or absolute (absolute cell number per μl of blood) terms. The representative multicolor flow cytometry staining is shown in Fig. 1b. Human T cells were separated into the CCR7+ CD45RA+ T_{NAIVE} subset, the CCR7+ CD45RA- T_{CM} subset, the CCR7-CD45RA-T_{EM} subset and the CCR7-CD45RAT_{EMRA} subset and the T_{EM} and T_{EMRA} subsets are known to increase in HCMV-infected individuals. As shown in Table 2, stronger humoral response

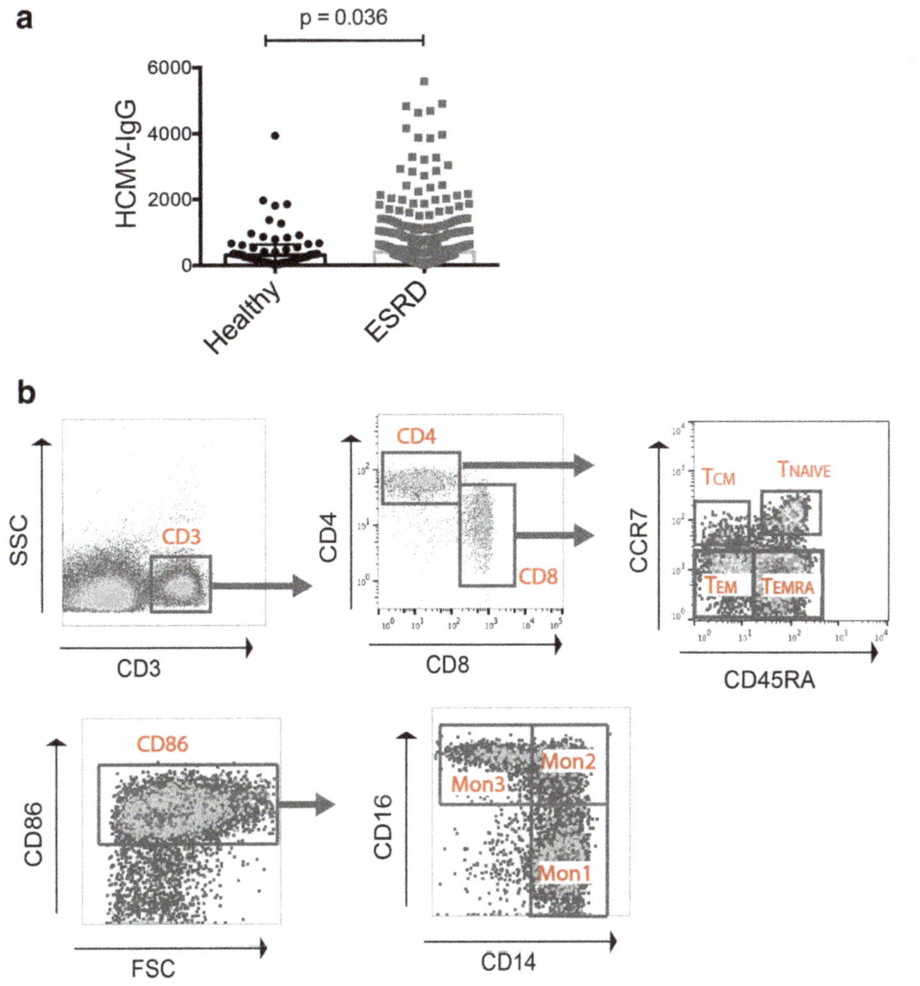

Fig. 1 a Levels of HCMV-specific IgG (U/mL) were compared between healthy individuals and ESRD patients. The lines indicate medium and interquartile range. Statistical calculation of p value was performed using Mann-Whitney *U* non-parametric test. **b** Representative multicolor flow cytometry staining of T cell subsets (above) and monocyte subsets (below). T$_{NAIVE}$, naïve T cells; T$_{CM}$, central memory T cells; T$_{EM}$, effector memory T cells; T$_{EMRA}$, effector memory T cells with RA expression. Mon1, classical monocytes; Mon2, intermediate monocytes; Mon3, non-classical monocytes

against HCMV is associated with significant disturbance in the adaptive T cell homeostasis in ESRD. Patients with higher titer of HCMV-specific IgG exhibit lower percentages of CD4+ and CD8+ T cells but higher percentages of CD4 + CD28null and CD8+ terminally differentiated T$_{EMRA}$ cells. Similar trends were observed when absolute cell number of each T cell subsets was analyzed and were also present in healthy controls (Additional file 1: Table S1). Higher titer of HCMV-specific IgG was associated with increased numbers of advanced differentiated CD4+ T cells. In contrast, HCMV-specific IgG level did not correlate with any specific monocyte subset changes. Previous studies in the literature only have compared T cell differentiation between HCMV seropositive and seronegative individuals. To our knowledge, this is the first description that the magnitude of humoral response against HCMV positively correlates with level of advanced

terminal differentiation of both CD4+ and CD8+ T cells in ESRD patients. Overall, these results support the hypothesis that less-well controlled HCMV infection in ESRD patients drives the host adaptive immune system toward advanced terminal differentiation.

Cardiovascular co-morbidities stratified by HCMV IgG levels
As reviewed in the introduction, previous studies performed on non-renal failure individuals have implicated HCMV infection in atherosclerotic vascular disease [37, 38]. As shown above, HCMV IgG level positively associates with the accumulation of terminally differentiated immunosenescent T cells. These cells have high atherogenic potentials, characterized by high CX3CR1 expression (thus allowing binding to injured endothelium) and capability of inducing endothelium damage [23, 24], eventually leading to atherosclerotic vascular diseases. These effector cells are

Table 1 Baseline demographic, clinical and laboratory measurements stratified by HCMV-specific IgG titer

	1 st Quintile ($n = 73$)	2nd Quintile ($n = 75$)	3rd Quintile ($n = 80$)	4th Quintile ($n = 87$)	5th Quintile ($n = 93$)	p value
HCMV-IgG (U/ml)	76.9(35.4)	214.1(50.9)	367.6(48.5)	618.4(129)	1813(1079)	< 0.001*
Age (yr)	59.3(11.4)	62.9(13.4)	61.2(11.5)	62.4(12.0)	63.8(11.0)	0.16
Male (%)	56	49	51	52	46	0.79
Diabetes (%)	55	31	30	46	41	0.07
Dialysis vintage (yr)	4.7(3.5)	6.6(4.9)	6.1(4.7)	6.4(4.8)	6.7(6.2)	0.11
Albumin (g/dl)	4.1(0.33)	4.0(0.40)	4.1(0.30)	4.0(0.48)	4.0(0.42)	0.09
WBC (K/ul)	6.4(2.0)	6.2(2.0)	6.3(1.7)	6.6(2.2)	6.5(2.2)	0.75
Hemoglobin (g/dl)	11.1(1.3)	10.7(1.3)	11.3(1.1)	10.8(1.6)	10.6(1.4)	0.01*
BUN (mg/dl)	81.1(20.3)	79.5(20.3)	78.9(20.8)	79.5(20.6)	76.8(18.1)	0.72
Creatinine (mg/dl)	11.7(2.3)	11.1(2.7)	11.9(2.4)	10.7(2.4)	10.6(2.3)	0.001*
T-Cholesterol (mg/dl)	145(38.1)	151(34.0)	159(36.1)	154(42.6)	148(33.7)	0.15
Triglyceride (mg/dl)	148(93.9)	139(92.1)	146(100.3)	160(94.0)	143(92.1)	0.71
intact-PTH (pg/ml)	344(37.1)	405(46.9)	307(38.3)	308(37.8)	443(58.1)	0.12
Calcium (mg/dl)	9.2(0.7)	9.4(0.9)	9.4(0.7)	9.3(0.8)	9.4(0.8)	0.87
Phosphate (mg/dl)	5.2(1.5)	5.2(1.5)	5.1(1.2)	4.7(1.4)	4.6(1.3)	0.005*
Kt/V (Gotch)	1.35(0.2)	1.41(0.2)	1.40(0.2)	1.38(0.2)	1.39(0.2)	0.48
nPCR (g/Kg)	1.15(0.3)	1.23(0.4)	1.23(0.3)	1.21(0.3)	1.11(0.7)	0.40

Demographic and clinic data were compared between groups of CMV-IgG quintiles in 408 ESRD patients. Quintile cut-offs were derived from HCMV-IgG levels of healthy controls. Values were expressed as mean (SD)
nPCR normalized protein catabolic rate
*p value < 0.05

Table 2 Correlations between HCMV-specific IgG titer with levels of immune cells among ESRD patients

	Cell frequency		Absolute cell number	
	R	p value	R	p value
CD4+ T cells				
Naïve T cells	−0.33	NS	−0.05	NS
Stem Memory T cells	−0.03	NS	−0.12	NS
Central Memory T cells	−0.12	0.013*	−0.13	0.007*
Effector Memory T cells	0.14	0.006*	0.06	NS
Terminally Differentiated T cells	0.11	0.035*	0.010	0.003*
CD28 null cells	0.15	0.002*	0.12	0.02*
CD8+ T cells				
Naïve T cells	−0.15	0.003*	−0.18	< 0.001*
Stem Memory T cells	0.006	NS	−0.16	0.002*
Central Memory T cells	−0.10	0.039*	−0.15	0.003*
Effector Memory T cells	−0.03	NS	−0.03	NS
Terminally Differentiated T cells	0.20	< 0.001*	0.09	0.07
Monocytes				
Classical Monocytes	0.02	NS	0.04	NS
Intermediate Monocytes	0.01	NS	0.04	NS
Non-Classical Monocytes	−0.03	NS	−0.006	NS

Pearson correlation was applied to investigate the relationship between log transformed HCMV-specific IgG titer and immune cell levels, including percentages as well as absolute cell counts of naïve (T_{NAIVE}), stem cell memory (T_{SCM}), central memory (T_{CM}), effector memory (T_{EM}), terminally differentiated (T_{EMRA}) subsets and three monocyte subsets (classical monocytes, intermediate monocytes, non-classical monocytes)
NS non-significant, *P* value > 0.1
*p value < 0.05

likely to be HCMV-specific, and we previously have shown that HCMV-specific cells are of high degree of cytokine production as well as cytotoxic functions [39]. We thus compared the percentage of patients with various cardiovascular complications among patients belonging to different HCMV IgG quintiles. As shown in Fig. 2, patients within the highest IgG quintile had the highest prevalence of congestive heart failure (CHF), coronary artery disease (CAD), and history of old myocardial infarction. However, the prevalence of stroke (including both ischemic and hemorrhagic stroke) was not associated with higher of HCMV IgG levels (data not shown). When the relationship between HCMV IgG quintile and individual comorbidity were analyzed in regression models, higher IgG quintile was significantly associated with CAD (odds ratio = 1.25, p for trend = 0.006), CHF (odds ratio = 1.22, p for trend = 0.036), and history of MI (odds ratio = 1.48, p for trend = 0.014), but not with stroke (odds ratio = 0.84, p for trend = 0.19) and CVD (odds ratio = 1.13, p for trend = 0.32).

HCMV IgG level independently associates with prevalent CAD

We next tested the independent association of HCMV-specific IgG level with CAD and CVD. Besides CAD, other individual co-morbidities were not tested because the percentages of patient with those co-morbidities were much lower. As shown in Table 3, higher HCMV-specific IgG quintile independently associated with prevalent CAD in both regression models, after adjusting for age, gender and other traditional and non-traditional cardiovascular risk factors. Nevertheless, the independent association between CVD and CMV IgG was not statistically significant. Similarly results were found when log-transformed IgG level was used in the regression model instead of HCMV IgG quintile (Additional file 1: Table S2).

Discussion

In the general population, HCMV infection is related to many adverse clinical conditions; atherosclerotic vascular complications are by far one of the best studied [37,

40]. In this study, we successfully demonstrated the association between higher anti-HCMV IgG titer in ESRD patients and higher risk for CAD, and suggested a potential mechanistic link between subclinical HCMV reactivation, aggravated T cell effector differentiation and coronary artery disease in this patient population. Our results indicate that it is necessary to continue investigating the long-term impact of immune response against HCMV in ESRD in longitudinal studies.

ESRD patients are characterized by a marked status of chronic systemic inflammation [41]. Interestingly, although HCMV IgG titer does not correlate with systemic inflammation in our study, previous studies indicate persistent HCMV infection has stronger impact in individuals with chronic inflammation. In a study involving 989 non-renal patients with CAD [42], HCMV seropositivity was independently associated with a 3.2-fold increase in risk of future cardiac death only in patients with high IL-6 levels, whereas in individuals without IL-6 elevation, HCMV had no effect on cardiac mortality. Another study showed that HCMV seropositivity in combination with elevated hsCRP is a strong, independent predictor of future cardiac death [38]. Because chronic inflammation is a pertinent feature of renal failure patients, ESRD patients might be prone to suffer from HCMV-associated adverse effects on cardiovascular complications.

Our study also found that HCMV-specific IgG level positively correlated with advanced T cell differentiation. Cantisan et al. had found that the loss of CD27 and CD28 on HCMV-specific T cells post solid organ transplantation correlated with HCMV replication and this process was age-dependent [43]. Advanced T cell differentiation has been found in ESRD seropositive for HCMV [44], and ESRD patients also demonstrate a shift in their T cell receptor Vβ chain repertoire [45], which is correlated with age. It remains unknown if level of HCMV-specific IgG correlates with Vβ diversity in ESRD patients.

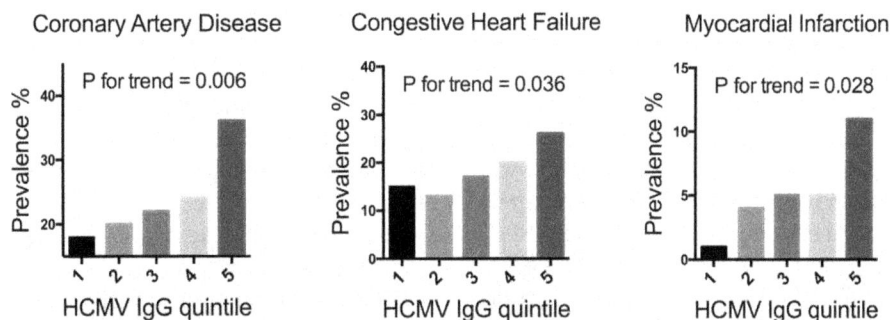

Fig. 2 Percentage of patients with each specified co-morbidity among each HCMV-IgG quintile group is shown. Univariate regression analysis was performed to investigate the associations between IgG quintile and prevalence of individual co-morbidity

Table 3 Association between HCMV-specific IgG quintile and coronary artery disease or cardiovascular disease

Variables in model (independent variable: CAD)	OR (95% CI)	P value
Model 1		
Age	1.03(1.01–1.05)	0.01*
Gender (Male)	1.43(0.90–2.29)	0.14
Diabetes	2.90(1.82–4.64)	< 0.001*
HCMV-specific IgG quintile	1.25(1.06–1.48)	0.007*
Model 2		
Age	1.04(1.01–1.06)	0.003*
Gender (Male)	1.39(0.86–2.25)	0.18
Diabetes	2.87(1.77–4.64)	< 0.001*
Albumin (g/dL)	1.44(0.67–3.12)	0.35
Hemoglobin (g/dL)	1.17(0.97–1.43)	0.10
Ca × P product (mg^2/dL^2)	1.01 (1.0–1.03)	0.27
hs-CRP (mg/dL)	1.37(1.12–1.67)	0.002*
HCMV-specific IgG quintile	1.27(1.07–1.51)	0.007*
Variables in model (independent variable: CVD)	OR (95% CI)	P value
Model 1		
Age	1.04(1.02–1.06)	< 0.001*
Gender (Male)	1.36(0.88–2.11)	0.17
Diabetes	2.88(1.86–4.48)	< 0.001*
HCMV-specific IgG quintile	1.13(0.97–1.32)	0.13
Model 2		
Age	1.03(1.02–1.06)	< 0.001*
Gender (Male)	1.32(0.84–2.08)	0.22
Diabetes	2.84(1.80–4.44)	< 0.001*
Albumin (g/dL)	1.07(0.52–2.16)	0.87
Hemoglobin (g/dL)	1.20(1.00–1.44)	0.048*
Ca × P product (mg^2/dL^2)	1.01 (0.99–1.03)	0.32
hs-CRP (mg/dL)	1.32(1.08–1.60)	0.005*
HCMV-specific IgG quintile	1.13(0.96–1.33)	0.13

Multivariable-adjusted logistic regression models, including age, gender, diabetes mellitus, albumin, hemoglobin, calcium phosphate product and high sensitivity-CRP were used to investigate the independent association between HCMV IgG quintile and co-morbidities. *: p value < 0.05

Only few cohort studies have investigated the role of HCMV-specific IgG in cardiovascular mortality in the general population. In the population-based Atherosclerosis Risk in Community (ARIC) study, people with the highest level of anti-HCMV IgG exhibited a 1.76-fold higher risk for coronary artery disease during a five-year follow-up when compared to the lowest level group [16]. People with diabetes are also affected by HCMV infection, with a relative risk of 9.2. In another population-based study (EPIC-Norfolk), individuals with the highest level of anti-HCMV IgG also had a 1.22-fold higher risk for ischemic heart disease when compared to seronegative individuals [15]. Our current study in ESRD patients indicates elevated HCMV IgG titer is related to coronary artery disease and history of myocardial infarction, but we did not find significant association between IgG titer and stroke. Interestingly, while CMV viral DNA is frequently found in coronary artery atherosclerotic plaques, some studies had reported the lack of CMV DNA in carotid artery plaques [46].

The exact mechanisms by which persistent HCMV infection results in higher cardiovascular mortality remain elusive [47], but the accumulation of terminally differentiated T cells could be a plausible mechanism. Our recent studies showed anti-HCMV IgG level positively correlates with the total size of virus-specific T cell pool [39] and inversely correlated with T cell receptor diversity [48] in individuals without renal disease. A recent report further showed that HCMV-specific senescent T cells are associated with arterial stiffness [49]. After adherence to activated vascular endothelium via CXCR3, these cyto-toxic T cells further participate in atherogenesis by directly causing endothelial damage [24] and they also secrete high level of TNFα [39], the critical cytokine to activate macro-phages. Intermediate monocytes (CD14++CD16+) are known to participate in atherosclerosis [50] but we discovered that HCMV-specific IgG did not affect the level of intermediate monocyte, indicating a different mechanism for monocyte activation in ESRD patients. Since our study did not measure the extent of atherosclerosis or arteriosclerosis, we could not analyze the impact of immune response on these pathological parameters separately. Animal studies of MCMV infection in renal failure mice will help to provide more detailed information.

There are additional limitations with this study. First, because the study is built on cross-sectional data only, we could not yet establish the causal relationship between levels of anti-HCMV IgG and cardiovascular complications. In addition, it remains technically difficult to detect subclinical HCMV reactivation, as attempts to analyze serum viral load turned out negative for all of our patients (data not shown). As a result, the mechanism for variable HCMV-specific IgG titers in ESRD patients is still unknown. Finally, it remains unknown if HCMV-specific IgG level is dynamic or stable in ESRD patients and follow-up data from our ongoing iESRD cohort will provide insight into this question.

In conclusion, our current study is the first to demonstrate that anti-HCMV IgG titer is elevated in ESRD patients with persistent HCMV infection and associates with prevalent coronary artery disease. The effect is significant and independent of traditional or non-traditional cardiovascular risk factors, including inflammation. Level of HCMV IgG also positively correlates with T cell terminal differentiation, which could serve as the mediator for this association. This implies a pathogenic role of HCMV reactivation in ESRD patients, and further studies are warranted to continue investigating the long-term effects of persistent HCMV infection in this susceptible population.

Conclusions

Our study indicates that anti-HCMV specific IgG is elevated in ESRD patients, who are at high risk of CAD. The elevation of HCMV-specific IgG positively correlates with advanced T cell differentiation but does not with monocyte subset homeostasis. In ESRD patients, HCMV-specific IgG level is independently associated with prevalent of CAD. The impact of persistent HCMV infection on CAD should be further investigated in this patient population.

Abbreviations
CAD: Coronary artery disease; CHF: Congestive heart failure; CVD: Cardiovascular disease; ESRD: End-stage renal disease; HCMV: Human cytomegalovirus

Acknowledgements
The authors thank Ms. Priscilla Tsai for her expertise and assistance with multicolor flow cytometry.

Funding
This work was supported by Far Eastern Memorial Hospital grant FEMH-2015-C-007, FEMH-NTUH joint grant-104-FTN-17, Ministry of Science and Technology grant 104–2314-B-418-017, and National Taiwan University Hospital Yunlin Branch grant NTUHYL105.X010, NTUHYL106.X009.

Authors' contributions
FJY, KHS and YLC designed the study; FJY, HYC, WCT, YSP, SPH and YLC recruited study participants; IYC, FYL and KHS performed the experiments and multicolor flow cytometry; YFC and FJY performed statistical analyses; FJY, KHS and YLC wrote the manuscript; CSW and GW provided expert opinions for study design, execution and edited the manuscript; all authors participated in discussion, interpretation and final preparation of the manuscript. All authors read and approved the final manuscript.

Competing interests
Non-declared. The authors declare that the research was conducted in the absence of any commercial or financial relationships that serves as a potential conflict of interest. The results presented in this paper have not been published previously in whole or part, except in abstract format.

Author details
[1]Graduate Institute of Clinical Medicine, College of Medicine, National Taiwan University, Taipei, Taiwan. [2]Department of Internal Medicine, National Taiwan University Hospital Yun Lin Branch, Douliu, Taiwan. [3]Department of Internal Medicine, Far Eastern Memorial Hospital, New Taipei City, Taiwan. [4]Graduate Institute of Immunology, College of Medicine, National Taiwan University, Taipei, Taiwan. [5]Institute of Public Health, School of Medicine, National Yang Ming University, Taipei, Taiwan. [6]Department of Medicine, National Taiwan University Hospital, Taipei, Taiwan. [7]Biology of Healthy Aging Program, Division of Geriatric Medicine and Gerontology, Johns Hopkins University School of Medicine, Baltimore, MD, USA. [8]Graduate Program in Biomedical Informatics, Yuan Ze University, Taoyuan City, Taiwan.

References
1. Dolan A, Cunningham C, Hector RD, Hassan-Walker AF, Lee L, Addison C, Dargan DJ, McGeoch DJ, Gatherer D, Emery VC, et al. Genetic content of wild-type human cytomegalovirus. J Gen Virol. 2004;85:1301–12.
2. Cannon MJ, Schmid DS, Hyde TB. Review of cytomegalovirus seroprevalence and demographic characteristics associated with infection. Rev Med Virol. 2010;20:202–13.
3. Staras SA, Dollard SC, Radford KW, Flanders WD, Pass RF, Cannon MJ. Seroprevalence of cytomegalovirus infection in the United States, 1988-1994. Clin Infect Dis. 2006;43:1143–51.
4. Taniguchi K, Watanabe N, Sato A, Jwa SC, Suzuki T, Yamanobe Y, Sago H, Kozuka K. Changes in cytomegalovirus seroprevalence in pregnant Japanese women-a 10-year single center study. J Clin Virol. 2014;59:192–4.
5. Chen HY, Chiang CK, Wang HH, Hung KY, Lee YJ, Peng YS, Wu KD, Tsai TJ. Cognitive-behavioral therapy for sleep disturbance in patients undergoing peritoneal Dialysis: a pilot randomized controlled trial. Am J Kidney Dis. 2008;52(2):314–23.
6. Spyridopoulos I, Martin-Ruiz C, Hilkens C, Yadegarfar ME, Isaacs J, Jagger C, Kirkwood T, von Zglinicki T. CMV seropositivity and T-cell senescence predict increased cardiovascular mortality in octogenarians: results from the Newcastle 85+ study. Aging Cell. 2015;15(2):389–92.

7. Wang GC, Kao WH, Murakami P, Xue QL, Chiou RB, Detrick B, McDyer JF, Semba RD, Casolaro V, Walston JD, Fried LP. Cytomegalovirus infection and the risk of mortality and frailty in older women: a prospective observational cohort study. Am J Epidemiol. 2010;171:1144–52.

8. Aiello AE, Chiu YL, Frasca D. How does cytomegalovirus factor into diseases of aging and vaccine responses, and by what mechanisms? Geroscience. 2017;39:261–71.

9. Simanek AM, Dowd JB, Pawelec G, Melzer D, Dutta A, Aiello AE. Seropositivity to cytomegalovirus, inflammation, all-cause and cardiovascular disease-related mortality in the United States. PLoS One. 2011;6:e16103.

10. Wang H, Peng G, Bai J, He B, Huang K, Hu X, Liu D. Cytomegalovirusinfection and relative risk of cardiovascular disease (ischemic heart disease, stroke, and cardiovascular death): a meta-analysis of prospective studies up to 2016. J Am Heart Assoc. 2017;6:e005025.

11. Zhou YF, Leon MB, Waclawiw MA, Popma JJ, Yu ZX, Finkel T, Epstein SE. Association between prior cytomegalovirus infection and the risk of restenosis after coronary atherectomy. N Engl J Med. 1996;335:624–30.

12. Izadi M, Fazel M, Saadat SH, Nasseri MH, Ghasemi M, Dabiri H, Aryan RS, Esfahani AA, Ahmadi A, Kazemi-Saleh D, et al. Cytomegalovirus localization in atherosclerotic plaques is associated with acute coronary syndromes: report of 105 patients. Methodist Debakey Cardiovasc J. 2012;8:42–6.

13. Compton T, Kurt-Jones EA, Boehme KW, Belko J, Latz E, Golenbock DT, Finberg RW. Human cytomegalovirus activates inflammatory cytokine responses via CD14 and toll-like receptor 2. J Virol. 2003;77:4588–96.

14. Cheng J, Ke Q, Jin Z, Wang H, Kocher O, Morgan JP, Zhang J, Crumpacker CS. Cytomegalovirus infection causes an increase of arterial blood pressure. PLoS Pathog. 2009;5:e1000427.

15. Gkrania-Klotsas E, Langenberg C, Sharp SJ, Luben R, Khaw KT, Wareham NJ. Higher immunoglobulin G antibody levels against cytomegalovirus are associated with incident ischemic heart disease in the population-based EPIC-Norfolk cohort. J Infect Dis. 2012;206:1897–903.

16. Sorlie PD, Nieto FJ, Adam E, Folsom AR, Shahar E, Massing M. A prospective study of cytomegalovirus, herpes simplex virus 1, and coronary heart disease: the atherosclerosis risk in communities (ARIC) study. Arch Intern Med. 2000;160:2027–32.

17. Mehta SK, Stowe RP, Feiveson AH, Tyring SK, Pierson DL. Reactivation and shedding of cytomegalovirus in astronauts during spaceflight. J Infect Dis. 2000;182:1761–4.

18. McVoy MA, Adler SP. Immunologic evidence for frequent age-related cytomegalovirus reactivation in seropositive immunocompetent individuals. J Infect Dis. 1989;160:1–10.

19. Wertheimer AM, Bennett MS, Park B, Uhrlaub JL, Martinez C, Pulko V, Currier NL, Nikolich-Zugich D, Kaye J, Nikolich-Zugich J. Aging and cytomegalovirus infection differentially and jointly affect distinct circulating T cell subsets in humans. J Immunol. 2014;192:2143–55.

20. Weinberger B, Lazuardi L, Weiskirchner I, Keller M, Neuner C, Fischer KH, Neuman B, Wurzner R, Grubeck-Loebenstein B. Healthy aging and latent infection with CMV lead to distinct changes in CD8+ and CD4+ T-cell subsets in the elderly. Hum Immunol. 2007;68:86–90.

21. Trzonkowski P, Mysliwska J, Szmit E, Wieckiewicz J, Lukaszuk K, Brydak LB, Machala M, Mysliwski A. Association between cytomegalovirus infection, enhanced proinflammatory response and low level of anti-hemagglutinins during the anti-influenza vaccination–an impact of immunosenescence. Vaccine. 2003;21:3826–36.

22. Bucci L, Ostan R, Giampieri E, Cevenini E, Pini E, Scurti M, Vescovini R, Sansoni P, Caruso C, Mari D, et al. Immune parameters identify Italian centenarians with a longer five-year survival independent of their health and functional status. Exp Gerontol. 2014;54:14–20.

23. van de Berg PJ, Yong SL, Remmerswaal EB, van Lier RA, ten Berge IJ. Cytomegalovirus-induced effector T cells cause endothelial cell damage. Clin Vaccine Immunol. 2012;19:772–9.

24. Pachnio A, Ciaurriz M, Begum J, Lal N, Zuo J, Beggs A, Moss P. Cytomegalovirus infection leads to development of high frequencies of cytotoxic virus-specific CD4+ T cells targeted to vascular endothelium. PLoS Pathog. 2016;12:e1005832.

25. Foley RN, Parfrey PS, Sarnak MJ. Epidemiology of cardiovascular disease in chronic renal disease. J Am Soc Nephrol. 1998;9:S16–23.

26. Rayner HC, Pisoni RL, Bommer J, Canaud B, Hecking E, Locatelli F, Piera L, Bragg-Gresham JL, Feldman HI, Goodkin DA, et al. Mortality and hospitalization in haemodialysis patients in five European countries: results from the Dialysis outcomes and practice patterns study (DOPPS). Nephrol Dial Transplant. 2004;19:108–20.

27. Longenecker JC, Coresh J, Powe NR, Levey AS, Fink NE, Martin A, Klag MJ. Traditional cardiovascular disease risk factors in dialysis patients compared with the general population: the CHOICE study. J Am Soc Nephrol. 2002;13:1918–27.

28. Betjes MG, Huisman M, Weimar W, Litjens NH. Expansion of cytolytic CD4 +CD28- T cells in end-stage renal disease. Kidney Int. 2008;74:760–7.

29. Betjes MG, Litjens NH, Zietse R. Seropositivity for cytomegalovirus in patients with end-stage renal disease is strongly associated with atherosclerotic disease. Nephrol Dial Transplant. 2007;22:3298–303.

30. Zawada AM, Rogacev KS, Schirmer SH, Sester M, Bohm M, Fliser D, Heine GH. Monocyte heterogeneity in human cardiovascular disease. Immunobiology. 2012;217:1273–84.

31. Kooman JP, Kotanko P, Schols AM, Shiels PG, Stenvinkel P. Chronic kidney disease and premature ageing. Nat Rev Nephrol. 2014;10:732–42.

32. Rogacev KS, Seiler S, Zawada AM, Reichart B, Herath E, Roth D, Ulrich C, Fliser D, Heine GH. CD14++CD16+ monocytes and cardiovascular outcome in patients with chronic kidney disease. Eur Heart J. 2010;32:84–92.

33. Andersson J, Libby P, Hansson GK. Adaptive immunity and atherosclerosis. Clin Immunol. 2009;134:33–46.

34. Ammirati E, Cianflone D, Vecchio V, Banfi M, Vermi AC, De Metrio M, Grigore L, Pellegatta F, Pirillo A, Garlaschelli K, et al. Effector memory T cells are associated with atherosclerosis in humans and animal models. J Am Heart Assoc. 2012;1:27–41.

35. Vasto S, Colonna-Romano G, Larbi A, Wikby A, Caruso C, Pawelec G. Role of persistent CMV infection in configuring T cell immunity in the elderly. Immun Ageing. 2007;4:2.

36. Derhovanessian E, Maier AB, Hahnel K, Beck R, de Craen AJ, Slagboom EP, Westendorp RG, Pawelec G. Infection with cytomegalovirus but not herpes simplex virus induces the accumulation of late-differentiated CD4+ and CD8 + T-cells in humans. J Gen Virol. 2011;92:2746–56.

37. Ji YN, An L, Zhan P, Chen XH. Cytomegalovirus infection and coronary heart disease risk: a meta-analysis. Mol Biol Rep. 2012;39:6537–46.

38. Muhlestein JB, Horne BD, Carlquist JF, Madsen TE, Bair TL, Pearson RR, Anderson JL. Cytomegalovirus seropositivity and C-reactive protein have independent and combined predictive value for mortality in patients with angiographically demonstrated coronary artery disease. Circulation. 2000;102:1917–23.

39. Chiu YL, Lin CH, Sung BY, Chuang YF, Schneck JP, Kern F, Pawelec G, Wang GC. Cytotoxic polyfunctionality maturation of cytomegalovirus-pp65-specific CD4 + and CD8 + T-cell responses in older adults positively correlates with response size. Sci Rep. 2016;6:19227.

40. Savva G, Pachnio A, Kaul B, Morgan K, Huppert F, Brayne C, Moss P. Cytomegalovirus infection is associated with increased mortality in the older population. Aging Cell. 2013;12(3):381–7.

41. Stenvinkel P. Inflammation in end-stage renal failure: could it be treated? Nephrol Dial Transplant. 2002;17(Suppl 8):33–8. discussion 40

42. Blankenberg S, Rupprecht HJ, Bickel C, Espinola-Klein C, Rippin G, Hafner G, Ossendorf M, Steinhagen K, Meyer J. Cytomegalovirus infection with interleukin-6 response predicts cardiac mortality in patients with coronary artery disease. Circulation. 2001;103:2915–21.

43. Cantisan S, Torre-Cisneros J, Lara R, Zarraga S, Montejo M, Solana R. Impact of cytomegalovirus on early immunosenescence of CD8+ T lymphocytes after solid organ transplantation. J Gerontol A Biol Sci Med Sci. 2013;68:1–5.

44. Litjens NH, de Wit EA, Betjes MG. Differential effects of age, cytomegalovirus-seropositivity and end-stage renal disease (ESRD) on circulating T lymphocyte subsets. Immun Ageing. 2011;8:2.

45. Huang L, Langerak AW, Wolvers-Tettero IL, Meijers RW, Baan CC, Litjens NH, Betjes MG. End stage renal disease patients have a skewed T cell receptor Vbeta repertoire. Immun Ageing. 2015;12:28.

46. Hagiwara N, Toyoda K, Inoue T, Shimada H, Ibayashi S, Iida M, Okada Y. Lack of association between infectious burden and carotid atherosclerosis in Japanese patients. J Stroke Cerebrovasc Dis. 2007;16:145–52.

47. Sansoni P, Vescovini R, Fagnoni FF, Akbar A, Arens R, Chiu YL, Cicin-Sain L, Dechanet-Merville J, Derhovanessian E, Ferrando-Martinez S, et al. Newadvances in CMV and immunosenescence. Exp Gerontol. 2014;55:54–62.

48. Wang GC, Dash P, McCullers JA, Doherty PC, Thomas PG. T cell receptor alphabeta diversity inversely correlates with pathogen-specific antibody levels in human cytomegalovirus infection. Sci Transl Med. 2012;4:128ra142.

49. Yu HT, Youn JC, Kim JH, Seong YJ, Park SH, Kim HC, Lee WW, Park S, Shin EC. Arterial stiffness is associated with cytomegalovirus-specific senescent CD8+ T cells. J Am Heart Assoc. 2017;6:e006535.

50. Pamukcu B, Lip GY, Devitt A, Griffiths H, Shantsila E. The role of monocytes in atherosclerotic coronary artery disease. Ann Med. 2010;42:394–403.

Neuroinflammation and neurohormesis in the pathogenesis of Alzheimer's disease and Alzheimer-linked pathologies: modulation by nutritional mushrooms

Angela Trovato Salinaro[1†], Manuela Pennisi[1,4†], Rosanna Di Paola[2†], Maria Scuto[1], Rosalia Crupi[2], Maria Teresa Cambria[1], Maria Laura Ontario[1], Mario Tomasello[1], Maurizio Uva[3], Luigi Maiolino[3], Edward J. Calabrese[5], Salvatore Cuzzocrea[2] and Vittorio Calabrese[1*†]

Abstract

Human life develops and expands not only in time and space, but also in the retrograde permanent recollection and interweaving of memories. Therefore, individual human identity depends fully on a proper access to the autobiographical memory. Such access is hindered or lost under pathological conditions such as Alzheimer's disease, including recently associated oxidant pathologies, such as ocular neural degeneration occurring in glaucoma or neurosensorial degeneration occurring in Menière's disease. Oxidative stress and altered antioxidant systems have been suggested to play a role in the aetiology of major neurodegenerative disorders, and altered expression of genes sensing oxidative stress, as well as decreased cellular stress response mechanisms could synergistically contribute to the course of these oxidant disorders. Thus, the theory that low levels of stress can produce protective responses against the pathogenic processes is a frontier area of neurobiological research focal to understanding and developing therapeutic approaches to neurodegenerative disorders. Herein, we discuss cellular mechanisms underlying AD neuroinflammatory pathogenesis that are contributory to Alzheimer's disease. We describe endogenous cellular defence mechanism modulation and neurohormesis as a potentially innovative approach to therapeutics for AD and other neurodegenerative conditions that are associated with mitochondrial dysfunction and neuroinflammation. Particularly, we consider the emerging role of the inflammasome as an important component of the neuroprotective network, as well as the importance of *Coriolus* and *Hericium* nutritional mushrooms in redox stress responsive mechanisms and neuroprotection.

Keywords: Oxidative stress, Neurodegenerative disorders, Neurohormesis, Mushrooms

Background

Alzheimer's disease (AD) is a neurodegenerative progressive disorder affecting more than 15 million people worldwide and represents the most current cause of dementia in the elderly, accounting for 50–60% of all cases in Western world [1].

The pathological signs of AD are amyloid plaques containing amyloid-β (Aβ) peptide derived from transamyloid precursor protein and neurofibrillary tangles constituted by hyper phosphorylated tau protein in medial temporal lobe structures and cortical areas of the brain along with neuronal death and synapse loss [2]. It has been demonstrated that inflammation cascade is linked to neurodegenerative diseases, particularly, Alzheimer's disease (AD) [3, 4]. In order to resist to different injuries, brain cells have developed networks of responses that detect and control different forms of stress [5, 6]. These are mainly proteins, including heat shock proteins (Hsps), lipoxin A4 (LXA4), thioredoxin (Trx) and sirtuins, controlled by vitagenes, a redox-dependent complex of genes [7]. LXA4 is an endogenous eicosanoid, produced by arachidonic acid metabolism, endowed with anti-inflammatory properties in different

* Correspondence: calabres@unict.it
†Equal contributors
[1]Department of Biomedical and Biotechnological Sciences, School of Medicine, University of Catania, Via Santa Sofia 97, 95123 Catania, Italy
Full list of author information is available at the end of the article

inflammatory syndromes, such as periodontitis, nephritis, arthritis, inflammatory bowel disease. LXA4 blocks the productions of pro-inflammatory mediators including free radical oxygen and nitrogen reactive intermediates (ROS/RNS), and acts as an endogenous "braking signal" in the inflammatory process. It is generally acknowledged as "signal stop" of inflammation [8]. The discovery of agents capable of increasing LXA4 levels and subsequently Aβ uptake by phagocytic cells is increasingly being recognized as a potential therapeutic target for AD treatment. Previous studies have demonstrated that mushrooms significantly upregulate LXA4 in the brain. Mushrooms have been used in traditional medicine, for many years [9], and a long list of therapeutic properties exists that have been associated with mushroom extracts, including antitumor, immunomodulatory, antioxidant, antiviral, antibacterial, and hepatoprotective effects. Mushrooms are a rich font of polysaccharides, and many of them have been shown to stimulate host immune responses. Among the most powerful known immunostimulators, β-glucans derived from mushrooms stimulate immune cells and cytokine responses [8, 10].

Taken into account the fact that Alzheimer's disease is characterized by neurodegeneration associated with neuroinflammation, in our recent study we have shown that *Coriolus versicolor* and *Hericium erinaceus* biomass preparations have neuroprotective effects and act by modulating the inflammatory process associated with the pathology of AD, as well as regulating brain cellular stress response mechanisms [4].

There is a growing body of evidence demonstrating a link between Alzheimer's disease and glaucoma. Notably, amyloid deposits, constituted of amyloid beta (Aβ) aggregates, a characteristic feature of several neurodegenerative diseases, such as Alzheimer's, mild cognitive impairment and Parkinson's disease (PD), have been recently implicated in the pathogenesis of retinal damage, of age-related macular degeneration and glaucoma. Glaucoma is a progressive optic neuropathy characterized by gradual degeneration of neuronal tissue due to retinal ganglion cell loss, associated to visual field loss over time resulting in irreversible blindness [11, 12]. It is a leading cause of irreversible blindness estimated to affect 79.6 million people worldwide by 2020. Accumulation of Aβ characterizes glaucoma as a protein misfolding disease, suggesting a pathogenic role for oxidative stress in the pathogenesis of retinal degenerative damage associated to this ocular pathology. In particular, factors such as tissue hypoxia and disturbed protein metabolism have been identified to interact in a vicious cycle underlying the oxidative stress-driven pathogenesis of glaucoma, ultimately leading to apoptotic retina ganglion cell death [13]. Research studies have demonstrated that retinal ganglion cell (RGC) damage in glaucoma is not limited to the primary insulted neurons, but also involves neighbouring neurons. In view of these considerations glaucoma can be viewed as a neurodegenerative disease which, similarly to other neurodegenerative pathologies, i.e., Alzheimer's and Parkinson's disease, where irreversible functional deficit ensues as consequence of neuronal dysfunction and death. Interestingly, recent evidence from our laboratory have demonstrated higher levels of vitagenes Heat Shock Protein 72 (Hsp72) and Heme oxygenase (HO-1) in the blood of patients with glaucoma than in controls [14]. These changes were associated with an increased expression of Trx and sirtuin 1 in the same experimental group. Similar results have been found in another oxidant disorder impacted by a progressive degenerative damage of neurosensorial acustic system, such as Ménière's disease [15]. Ménière's disease (MD) is characterized by the triad of fluctuating hearing loss, episodic vertigo and tinnitus, and by endolymphatic hydrops found on post-mortem examination. Increasing evidence suggests that oxidative stress is involved in the development of endolymphatic hydrops and that cellular damage and apoptotic cell death might contribute to the sensorineural hearing loss found in later stages of MD [16]. Consistent with this notion, studies are presently under way in our laboratory testing the conceivable possibility that mushrooms supplementation can reverse oxidative damage, thereby affecting the clinical course of Meniere's disease pathology. Thus, modulation of endogenous cellular defense mechanisms such as the vitagene network may open to new therapeutic approaches in diseases associated with tissue damage and cell death, such as in glaucomatous or Meniere neurodegeneration [14, 15]. In this review, we specifically discuss the main neuroprotective and nutritional activities of *Coriolus* and *Hericium* mushrooms. Moreover, we will introduce the emerging role of hormesis and inflammasome as important components of neuroprotective network operating in redox-dependent brain cell stress responsive mechanisms. Our focus presently highlights the hypothesis linking oxidative stress and neurodegeneration to the AD pathogenesis, and indicate that stress responsive genes may represent an important target for novel cytoprotective strategies, as molecules inducing this defense mechanism, via nutritional and/or pharmacological approaches, can exploit the potential for antidegenerative therapeutic interventions [14].

Neurohormesis

At the core of adaptive responses at the cell and origin of biological organization is the concept of hormesis [17]. Hormesis is the expression of integrative adaptive responses that are manifest via a biphasic dose response with very specific quantitative response feature (i.e. maximum amplitude and width of the adaptive response) and induced by either a direct stimulatory response or as a modest overcompensation to a disruption of homeostasis

[18]. Detailed assessments of pre- and post-conditioning, the adaptive response in radiation, the priming response, as commonly reported in microbial and plant models, and the so-called steeling effect widely reported in the clinical psychology area, all these phenomena act via hormetic mechanisms and comprise a broadly integrated and evolutionarily based adaptive system that has been highly conserved [19]. Such hormetic dose responses provide a quantitative description of the bounds of biological plasticity [20], and a measure of the extent to which adaptive processes may be upregulated, which is especially relevant to the comprehension of protective effects induced by plant and fungal species. The hormetic concept is particularly important since it provides reliable estimates of the upper limit for the induction of potential therapeutic responses and should play a key role in the design of experimental studies and clinical trials. Hormesis, especially in vulnerable biological systems, such as the brain, is of relevant interest to the toxicological community for the dose-response model. Particularly, neurohormesis affects memory, learning and performance, as well as nutritional antioxidants and neurodegenerative responses mediated by oxidative stress in cellular models for various diseases such as AD [9, 17]. In fact, the presence of oxidative stress markers in the brains of patients with neurodegenerative diseases has been recognized which supports the rationale for neuroprotective nutritional interventions based on the action antioxidants and anti-inflammatory agents, such as polyphenols or mushrooms [7]. Neurohormesis can be applied to both polyphenol and nutritional mushroom molecular mechanisms of action. It has been, in fact, known that polyphenols and mushrooms activate the heat shock protein (Hsp) pathway, which plays a crucial role in the cellular stress response. With respect to this, for instance although there is no doubt about the protective effect of HO-1 against oxidative and nitrosative stress, on the contrary, excessive HO-1 upregulation may be toxic for cells. According to this principle, drugs, toxins and natural substances, administered at low doses can result in a positive response, while at higher concentrations promote prevalent toxic effects [17].

Role of the inflammasome

Oxidative stress is one of the main components of the pathogenesis of neurodegenerative diseases. The molecular mechanisms underlying oxidative stress include inflammation, mitochondrial dysfunction and apoptosis that culminates in neuronal death [21, 22]. Modulation of cellular stress pathways through the use of small redox active molecules represents a new approach to the study of neurologic and psychiatric pathologies [23]. In particular sulforaphane and hydroxytyrosol, as well as nutritional mushrooms are increasingly considered as possible candidates to regulate physiological pathways related with (1)

cellular stress response and vitagene networks; (2) redox imbalance/oxidative stress, (3) mitochondrial function (4) immune response and anti-neuroinflammation (5) heat shock response control, and (6) synaptic dysfunction [24]. Excessive oxidative stress levels have been correlated to AD pathogenesis, increased protein carbonylation, nitration, cysteine-oxidation, lipid peroxidation, and DNA/RNA oxidation, were revealed in brain and peripheral tissue samples from patients with AD by post-mortem studies. Increased oxidative stress can damage mitochondrial proteins. Of particular significance to the pathophysiology of main neurodegenerative disorders are findings of reduced levels of mRNA (and protein subunits) that are involved in the transfer of electrons in complex I of the electron transport chain (ETC), in AD patients. Decreased efficiency of the electron transfer process within complex I and complex IV, results in increased leakage and mono-electronic reduction of molecular oxygen to form the superoxide anion [25], with ensuing damage to proteins, lipids and DNA. As well, increasing evidence supports a role of immune activation as a prominent causative factor in the pathogenesis of a number of major neurologic and neuropsychiatric disorders [26]. Consistent with this notion, current studies have demonstrated that the inflammasome modulates neuroinflammatory processes at the initial stage, with a secondary cascade of events inclusive of oxidative stress, redox homeostasis disruption associated to mitochondrial dysfunction (Fig. 1) [27]. The inflammasome is a multiprotein complex that contains many copies of a receptor for pathogen- or damage-derived molecular patterns (Pathogen Associated Molecular Patterns, PAMPs), pro-caspases-1, and an adaptor, apoptotic speck-containing protein with a caspase activation and recruitment domain (CARD) [ASC], which induces caspase-1 maturation [28]. Active caspase-1 is responsible for rapid, lytic cell death (pyroptosis). Upon sensing PAMP or damage associated molecular pattern (DAMP), absent in melanoma 2 (AIM2) and/or PYD domains-containing protein 3 (NLRP3), inflammasomes activate caspase-8 and caspase-1, respectively, leading to both pyroptotic and apoptotic cell death [29]. Mitochondria represent major sources of DAMPs capable of triggering neuroinflammatory responses, with resulting pyroptosis, apoptosis and autophagy [30]. AIM2 is a cytoplasmic sensor that recognizes and binds the double-stranded DNA (dsDNA) of microbial or host origin. Upon binding to DNA, AIM2 assembles inflammasome complex, which induces pyroptosis and proteolytic cleavage of the proinflammatory cytokines pro-IL-1β and pro-IL-18. A wrong recognition of cytoplasmic self-DNA by AIM2 provides to the development of autoimmune and inflammatory diseases, as well as neurodegenerative disorders [31].

A direct activation link between inflammation and the pathogenesis of Alzheimer's disease has been

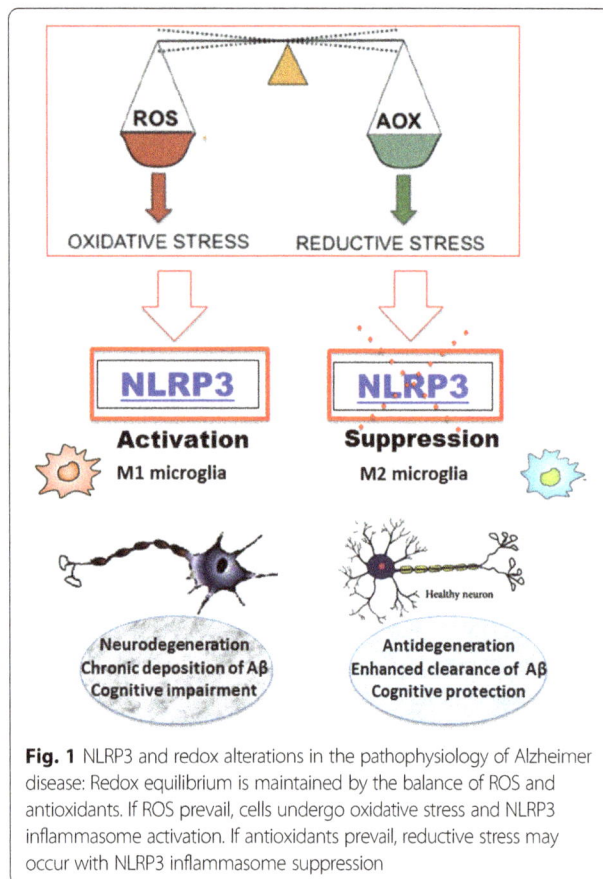

Fig. 1 NLRP3 and redox alterations in the pathophysiology of Alzheimer disease: Redox equilibrium is maintained by the balance of ROS and antioxidants. If ROS prevail, cells undergo oxidative stress and NLRP3 inflammasome activation. If antioxidants prevail, reductive stress may occur with NLRP3 inflammasome suppression

demonstrated by numerous in vitro and in vivo studies. in particular the inflammasome NLRP £ has been identified as a possible therapeutic target for the treatment of neurodegenerative diseases. This hypothesis was accredited by the observation of a deficiency of NLRP3 and caspase-1 in mice AA / PS1 (transgenic mice for chronic deposition of Ab), in which Ab deposits were reduced, resulting in an increase in M2 microglia [32]. We have provided recent evidence of a neuroprotective action of the *Hericium erinaceus* (MRLs, UK) mushroom when administered orally to rat. In the brain of rats receiving oral administration of *Hericium erinaceus*, was measured maximum expression of LXA4, an anti-inflammatory compound, in cortex and hippocampus. LXA4 upregulation was related with an increased amount of proteins, such as thioredoxin, Hsp72 and heme oxygenase-1 involved in cellular stress response [4].

Plausibly, LXA4 signalling activation and stress-responsive vitagene proteins modulation could serve as a potential therapeutic target for AD-related inflammation and neurodegenerative damage. Our results indicate that nutritional supplementation with an opportune biomass preparation from a well characterized strain of *Hericium erinaceus* or *Coriolus versicolor* can induced critical

proteins modulation involved in brain age-associated neurodegenerative diseases [33]. In view of the fact that in AD pathology, amyloid plaques accumulation (APs), composed of amyloid-beta peptide (Aβ) aggregates, and neurofibrillary tangles (NFTs) formation, composed of misfolded Tau proteins, are related with a deficit in those mechanisms participating in the induction of cyto-protective proteins (Hsps) or, more generally, cellular pathways of stress tolerance, it is conceivable to hypothesize that in these conditions, administration of *Hericium erinaceus* or *Coriolus versicolor* biomass, by enhancing the redox potential and inducing neuropro-tection through neurohormetic mechanisms such as vitagenes upregulation, may promote resilience in damaged neurons, and hence resistance to proteotoxic insults and apoptotic neurodegeneration. Consistent with this concept, restoration of normal proteostasis is crucial for neuronal survival. Our research suggests new potential strategies based on the induction of vitagene defence system as a foundamental mechanism to promote proteome homeostasis and hence withstand pathological mechanisms associated to unhealthy aging of the brain associated to neurodegenerative diseases [4].

Coriolus versicolor

The medicinal properties of mushrooms have long been known to traditional medicine (Fig. 2a, b) [34, 35]. Anti-oxidant, anti-bacterial, and anti-viral properties have been attributed to mushrooms by controlled studies [36]. It has been shown that mushrooms are capable to stimulate the immune system of the host due to the high content of β-glucans, which activate many types of immune cells and stimulate cytokine responses [37–39]. Several of these polysaccharides are currently used in East countries in association to radio and chemotherapy [40]. In addition, Cordymin, a peptide with low molecular weight (10,906 Da), with anti-inflammatory properties has been isolated from the medical mushroom *Cordyceps sinensis* [41] and from *Cordyceps militaris* [42]. This peptide significantly inhibited the polymorphonuclear cells infil-tration and IR-induced up regulation of C3 protein produced in the brain, interleukin-1β, and tumour necrosis factor-α, which had a neuroprotective effect on the ischemic brain, due to the inhibition of inflammation [34].

Although the polysaccharides derived from mush-rooms are hardly synthesizable molecules and the active molecules present in the mushrooms are still not well known, the Asian clinical practice employs preparations derived from mushrooms, including *Agaricus campestris*, *Pleurotus ostreatus* and *Coriolus versicolor* extracts [43]. Polysaccharides obtained from *coriolus versicolor* (Fig. 2a) are commercially among the best options. This mushroom is known for its medical applications, and is usually used to degrade organic contaminants such as

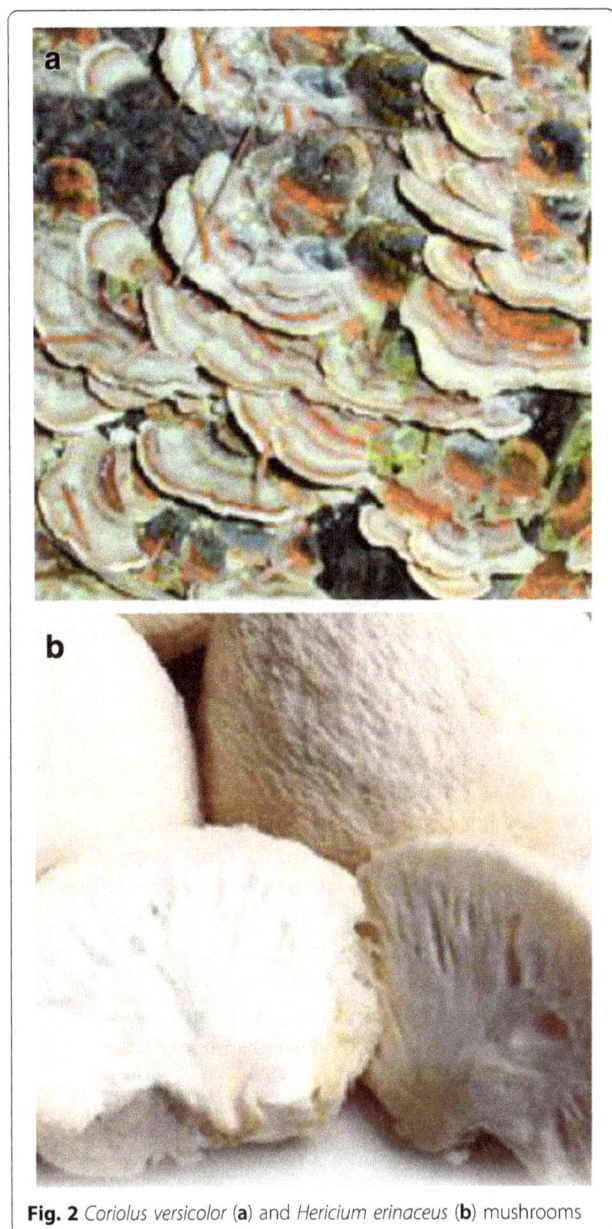

Fig. 2 *Coriolus versicolor* (**a**) and *Hericium erinaceus* (**b**) mushrooms

pentachlorophenol (PCP) [44]. Polysaccharide K or Kerstin (PSK) and polysaccharopeptide (PSP) are the main commercial preparations obtained by C *versicolor* mycelia [45]. These compounds stimulate the production of interleukin-6, interferons, immunoglobulin G, macrophages, and T-lymphocytes by enhancing the immune system against immunosuppressive effects of radiotherapy and chemotherapy. Polysaccharopeptides possess anticancer activity inhibiting the production of superoxide dismutase (SOD) and glutathione peroxidase [46]. Experimental animal and human studies have shown that oral administration of PSK and PSP controlled carcinomas [47]. It is reported that PSK produces apoptosis in HL-60 Human promyelocytic leukaemia cells through

the activation of mitochondrial and caspase-dependent pathways [48] and overexpression of proapoptotic protein Bax [49]. Of particular interest are the polysaccaropeptides produced by *Coriolus versicolor, which* are used to supplement the chemotherapy and radiotherapy of cancer and infectious diseases. Chronic inflammation favours the progression of Alzheimer's disease (AD), however identification of mechanisms able of resolving the pro-inflammatory environment stimulating AD pathology remains an area of active investigation [50, 51]. Taking into account this neurobiological rationale, our recent study, carried out to demonstrate a potential neuroprotective role of coriolus versicolor biomass preparation in neuroinflammatory pathogenesis associated with Alzheimer's disease in rat, has been undertaken to provide experimental evidence that biomass from *Coriolus* or *Hericium* regulate important redox sensitive pathways linked to cellular stress response and hence confer neuroprotection [3, 4, 52]. Lipoxin A4 (LXA4) derived from *Coriolus* is an endogenous eicosanoid capable to resolving inflammation process, acting as an endogenous "braking signal" in the inflammatory cascade. Treatment with the pro-resolving mediator aspirin-triggered lipoxin A4 (ATL), caused cognition improvement, reduced Ab levels, and enhanced phagocytic activity of microglia in Tg2576 transgenic AD mice [53]. Moreover, LXA4 levels declined with age, a finding even more evident in 3xTg-AD mice [54]. LXA4 action is regulated by the interaction with G protein-coupled receptor. N-formyl-peptide receptor 1 (FPRL1), also known as ALX (lipoxin A4 receptor) or CCR12, belongs to the formyl-peptide receptor (FPR)-related family of G protein-coupled receptors (GPCRs) that also includes FPR and FPRL2 [55, 56]. All factors able to increase Lipoxin A4 (LXA4) levels and consequently uptake of Ab by phagocytic cells are a hypothetical therapeutic target for AD. Consistent with this notion, in AD pathology, the accumulation of amyloid plaques (APs), constituted of amyloid-beta peptide (Ab) aggregates, and neurofibrillary tangles (NFTs), constituted of misfolded Tau proteins, is related to a deficiency in the activation of cytoprotective proteins (Hsps) or, more generally, of cellular stress tolerance pathways [55]. In these conditions, it is demonstrated that the administration of *Coriolus* in the brain of rats causes the maximum induction of LXA4 in cortex and hippocampus. Notably, no significant modifications in I-Kappa-B-Alpha (IkBa), Nuclear Factor Kappa B (NFkB) and cyclooxygenase-2 (COX-2) brain levels were associated with Hsps induction [4]. Furthermore, LXA4 up-regulation is related with Nrf-2 regulated vitagenes, thus increasing the content of proteins involved in cellular oxidative stress response, such as thioredoxin, Hsp72 and heme oxygenase [52]. Therefore the induction of vitagenes, could help vulnerable neurons resist proteotoxic insults and to reduce apoptotic neurodegeneration.

Hericium erinaceus

Hericium erinaceus (Fig. 2b) fruit bodies and mycelia contain an extraordinarily large quantity of structurally different bioactive and potentially bioactive components. The reported health-promoting properties of these compounds include anticarcinogenic, antibiotic, antidiabetic, antifatigue, antihypertensive, antihyperlipodemic, antisenescence, cardioprotective, nephroprotective, hepatoprotective, and neuroprotective properties and improvement of anxiety, depression and cognitive function [57]. The antioxidant activity of *Hericium erinaceus* has been observed in diabetic rat model in which the intra peritoneal (i.p.) administration of an aqueous extract of *Hericium erinaceus* (100 and 200 mg/kg body weight) resulted in a significant decrease in the serum glucose level, significant increase in the insulin level and attenuated serum lipid profiles (disorders) as compared to control rats. These findings were accompanied by increased activities in the antioxidative enzymes catalase (CAT), superoxide dismutase (SOD), and glutathione peroxidase (GSH-Px) and increased GSH (glutathione) and reduced malondialdehyde (MDA) levels in the liver, suggesting that the mechanism of the health-promoting effects seems to be the result of inhibition of ROS [58]. Endowed with different biological activities, *Hericium*-derived hericenones and erinacines, isolated from its fruiting body, stimulate nerve growth factor (NGF) synthesis in cultured astrocytes [59]. NGF influences basal forebrain cholinergic neurons modulating the activity of two enzymes, such as cholineacetyltransferase and acetyl cholinesterase. The first pathological events of Alzheimer's disease are the loss and dysfunction of cholinergic neurons. *Hericium erinaceus* administration improves cognitive dysfunction. Less, however, is known about the clinical relevance of *Hericium erinaceus* in regulating neurogenesis in the nervous system and its role in neurodegenerative disorders such as Alzheimer's disease and other types of dementia. Recently, basic and clinical studies have shown that Alzheimer's disease is closely associated with amyloid beta (Aβ)-induced neuroinflammation, responsible for, the resident macrophages of the brain, and activated microglia may then promote neuronal injury through the release of proinflammatory and cytotoxic factors, exacerbating the course of the disease [60]. A new neuroprotective strategy, like an oral administration of a biomass *Hericium* biomass preparation given for 3 month, as done in our recent study [4] can represent a therapeutic target to minimize the deleterious effects related to oxidative burden, such as that occurring in brain aging and in neurodegenerative disorders. Treatment with *Hericium erinaceus* caused a significant increase of LXA4 production in most of the brain

regions like cortex, hippocampus followed by substantia Nigra, striatum and cerebellum and in a modulated expression of cytoprotective proteins, such as Heme oxygenase 1 (HO-1), Heat Shock Protein 70 (Hsp70) and thioredoxin (TRX). These results are coherent with recent evidence obtained in mice, showing neuroprotection by *Hericium erinaceus* on Aβ 25–35 peptide-induced cognitive dysfunction [61, 62].

Conclusions

Accumulating evidence has indicated that oxidative stress and excess reactive oxygen and nitrogen intermediates play an important role in the progression of many chronic inflammatory diseases, including cardiovascular diseases, diabetes, and neurodegenerative disorders [63]. Imbalance between ROS generation and antioxidant enzyme activities will cause lipid peroxidation, nuclear and mitochondrial DNA damage and protein oxidation, resulting in brain damage and amnesia [64]. A growing number of studies have demonstrated that dietary interventions regulate mitochondrial ROS production, detoxification and oxidative damage repair. Many (but not all) of these nutritional interventions are related with extension of lifespan, or protection against diseases related with age, in mammals. Emerging nutraceuticals are today showing promise as modulators of mitochondrial redox metabolism capable of eliciting beneficial outcomes. Mushrooms, known for their strong antioxidant properties, have attracted interest due to their potential in neuroprotection, antioxidant, and anti-inflammatory effects, as well as in proteome and mitochondrial homeostasis restoration as a basic mechanism to withstand mitochondrial dysfunction-associated neuroinflammatory disorders.

Abbreviations

AD: Alzheimer's disease; AIM2: Absent in melanoma 2; ALX: Lipoxin A4 receptor; APs: Amyloid plaques; ASC: Apoptotic speck-containing protein; ATL: Aspirin triggered lipoxin A4; Aβ: Amyloid-beta peptide; CAT: Catalase; CBF: Cerebral blood flow; COX-2: Cyclooxygenase-2; *DAMP*: Damage associated molecular pattern; ETC: Electron transport chain; FPRL1: N-formyl-peptide receptor 1; GPCRs: G protein-coupled receptors; GSH: Glutathione; GSH-Px: Glutathione peroxidase; HO-1: Heme oxygenase 1; Hsp70: Heat shock protein 70; Hsp72: Heat shock protein 72; Hsps: Heat shock proteins; IkBa: I-Kappa-B-Alpha; LXA4: Lipoxin A4; MDA: Malondialdehyde; NFkB: Nuclear factor kappa B; NFTs: Neurofibrillary tangles; NGF: Nerve growth factor; NLRP3: PYD domains-containing protein 3; PCP: Pentachlorophenol; PD: Parkinson's disease; PSK: Polysaccharide K or Krestin; PSP: Polysaccharopeptide; RGC: Retinal ganglion cell; ROS: Radical oxygen species; SOD: Superoxide dismutase; *TRX*: Thioredoxin

Acknowledgements

Not applicable

Funding

Research activities in the area of dose response have been funded by the United States Air Force and ExxonMobil Foundation over a number of years. However, such funding support has not been used for the present manuscript (EJC).

Authors' contributions

"All authors had full access to the study and take responsibility for the integrity and the accuracy of the study concept and design. Drafting of the manuscript: ATS, MP, RDP, MS, RC, MTC, MLO, MT, MU, LM, EJC, SC, VC. ATS and MP equally contributed as first author. Critical revision of the manuscript for important intellectual content: VC, SC and EJC. Study supervision: VC and EJC." All authors read and approved the final manuscript.

Competing interests

The authors declare that they have no competing interests.

Author details

[1]Department of Biomedical and Biotechnological Sciences, School of Medicine, University of Catania, Via Santa Sofia 97, 95123 Catania, Italy. [2]Department of Chemical, Biological, Pharmaceutical and Environmental Sciences University of Messina, Messina, Italy. [3]Department of Medical and Surgery Sciences and Advanced Technology, University of Catania, Catania, Italy. [4]Spinal Unit, Emergency Hospital "Cannizzaro", Catania, Italy. [5]Environmental Health Sciences Division, School of Public Health, University of Massachusetts, Amherst, MA, USA.

References

1. Ziegler-Graham K, Brookmeyer R, Johnson E, Arrighi HM. Worldwide variation in the doubling time of Alzheimer's disease incidence rates. Alzheimer Dement. 2008;4(5):316–23.

2. Blennow K, Zetterberg H. Pinpointing plaques with PIB. Nat Med. 2006;12(7):753–4.

3. Calabrese V, Cornelius C, Dinkova-Kostova AT, Calabrese EJ, Mattson MP. Cellular stress responses, the hormesis paradigm, and vitagenes: novel targets for therapeutic intervention in neurodegenerative disorders. Antioxid Redox Signal. 2010;13:1763–811.

4. Trovato Salinaro A, Siracusa R, Di Paola R, Scuto M, Ontario ML, Bua O, et al. Redox modulation of cellular stress response and lipoxin A4 expression by Hericium erinaceus in rat brain: relevance to Alzheimer's disease pathogenesis. Immun Ageing. 2016;13:23.

5. Kirstein J, Morito D, Kakihana T, Sugihara M, Minnen A, Hipp MS, et al. Proteotoxic stress and ageing triggers the loss of redox homeostasis across cellular compartments. EMBO J. 2015;34:2334–49.

6. Calabrese V, Dattilo S, Petralia A, Parenti R, Pennisi M, Koverech G, et al. Analytical approaches to the diagnosis and treatment of aging and aging-related disease: redox status and proteomics. Free Radic Res. 2015;49:511–24.

7. Calabrese V, Giordano J, Signorile A, Laura Ontario M, Castorina S, De Pasquale C, et al. Major pathogenic mechanisms in vascular dementia: roles of cellular stress response and hormesis in neuroprotection. J. Neurosci Res. 2016;94:1588–603.

8. Yang F, Xie J, Wang W, Xie Y, Sun H, Jin Y, et al. Regional arterial infusion with lipoxin A4 attenuates experimental severe acute pancreatitis. PLoS One. 2014;9:108525.

9. Calabrese V, Giordano J, Ruggieri M, Berritta D, Trovato A, Ontario ML, et al. Hormesis, cellular stress response, and redox homeostasis in autism spectrum disorders. J Neurosci Res. 2016;94:1488–98.

10. Hawkins KE, DeMars KM, Singh J, Yang C, Cho HS, Frankowski JC, et al. Neurovascular protection by post-ischemic intravenous injections of the lipoxin A4 receptor agonist, BML-111, in a rat model of ischemic stroke. J Neurochem. 2014;129:130–42.

11. Cesareo M, Martucci A, Ciuffoletti E, Mancino R, Cerulli A, Sorge RP, et al. Association between Alzheimer's disease and glaucoma: a study based on Heidelberg retinal tomography and frequency doubling technology Perimetry. Front Neurosci. 2015;9:479.

12. Tham YC, Li X, Wong TY, Quigley HA, Aung T, Cheng CY. Global prevalence of glaucoma and projections of glaucoma burden through 2040: a systematic review and meta-analysis. Ophthalmology. 2014;121:2081–90.

13. Carelli V, La Morgia C, Valentino ML, Barboni P, Ross-Cisneros FN, Sadun AA. Retinal ganglion cell neurodegeneration in mitochondrial inherited disorders. Biochim Biophys Acta. 2009:518–28.

14. Trovato Salinaro A, Cornelius C, Koverech G, Koverech A, Scuto M, Lodato F, Fronte V, Muccilli V, Reibaldi M, Longo A, Uva MG, Calabrese V. Cellular stress response, redox status, and vitagenes in glaucoma: a systemic oxidant disorder linked to Alzheimer's disease. Front Pharmacol. 2014;5:129. https://doi.org/10.3389/fphar.2014.00129.

15. Calabrese V, Cornelius C, Maiolino L, Luca M, Chiaramonte R, Toscano MA, Serra A. Oxidative stress, redox homeostasis and cellular stress response in Ménière's disease: role of vitagenes. Neurochem Res. 2010;35:2208–17.

16. Requena T, Cabrera S, Martín-Sierra C, Price SD, Lysakowski A, Lopez-Escamez JA. Identification of two novel mutations in FAM136A and DTNA genes in autosomal-dominant familial Meniere's disease. Hum Mol Genet. 2015;24:1119–26.

17. Calabrese EJ, Mattson MP. How does hormesis impact biology, toxicology, and medicine? NPJ Aging Mech Dis. 2017;3:13.

18. Calabrese EJ, Baldwin LA. The frequency of U-shaped dose responses in the toxicological literature. Toxicol Sci. 2001;62:330–8.

19. Calabrese EJ, Bachmann KA, Bailer AJ, Bolger PM, Borak J, Cai L, et al. Biological stress response terminology: integrating the concepts of adaptive response and preconditioning stress within a hormetic dose-response framework. Toxicol App Pharmacol. 2007;222:122–8.

20. Calabrese EJ, Mattson MP. Hormesis provides a generalized quantitative estimate of biological plasticity. J Cell Commun Sign. 2011;5:25–38.

21. Lim JH, Gerhart-Hines Z, Dominy JE, Lee Y, Kim S, Tabata M, et al. Oleic acid stimulates complete oxidation of fatty acids through protein Kinase A-dependent activation of SIRT1-PGC1 alpha complex. J Biol Chem. 2013;288:7117–26.

22. Guest J, Garg M, Bilgin A, Grant R. Relationship between central and peripheral fatty acids in humans. Lipids Health Dis. 2013;12:30–7.

23. Liu Z, Zhou T, Ziegler AC, Dimitrion P, Zuo L. Oxidative stress in neurodegenerative diseases: from molecular mechanisms to clinical applications. Oxidative Med Cell Longev. 2017;23:45–55.

24. Patel S, Goyal A. Recent developments in mushrooms as anti-cancer therapeutics: a review. 3. Biotech. 2012;2:1–15.

25. Talalay P, Zimmerman AW. Reply to Scahill: behavioral outcome measures in autism. Proc Natl Acad Sci U S A. 2015;112:E350–E.

26. Hroudova J, Singh N, Fisar Z. Mitochondrial dysfunctions in neurodegenerative diseases: relevance to Alzheimer's disease. Biomed Res Int. 2014;56:89–99.

27. Morris G, Berk M. The many roads to mitochondrial dysfunction in neuroimmune and neuropsychiatric disorders. BMC Med. 2015;13:34–47

28. Kim YK, Shin JS, Nahm MH. NOD-like receptors in infection, immunity, and diseases. Yonsei Med J. 2016;57:5–14.

29. Davis BK, Wen HT, Ting JPY. The Inflammasome NLRs in immunity, inflammation, and associated diseases. Annu Rev Immunol. 2011;29:707–35.

30. Aachoui Y, Sagulenko V, Miao EA, Stacey KJ. Inflammasome-mediated pyroptotic and apoptotic cell death, and defense against infection. Curr Opin Microbiol. 2013;16:319–26.

31. Bosch ME, Kielian T. Neuroinflammatory paradigms in lysosomal storage diseases. Front Neurosci-Switz. 2015;9:33–46.

32. Gadani SP, Walsh JT, Lukens JR, Kipnis J. Dealing with danger in the CNS: the response of the immune system to injury. Neuron. 2015;87:47–62.

33. Heneka MT. Inflammasome activation and innate immunity in Alzheimer's disease. Brain Pathol. 2017;27:220–2.

34. Cornelius C, Graziano A, Calabrese EJ, Calabrese V. Hormesis and vitagenes in aging and longevity: mitochondrial control and hormonal regulation. Horm Mol Biol Clin Investig. 2013;16:73–89.

35. Wang D, Calabrese EJ, Lian B, Lin Z, Calabrese V. Hormesis as a mechanistic approach to understanding herbal treatments in traditional Chinese medicine. Pharmacol Ther. 2017. https://doi.org/10.1016/j.pharmthera.2017.10.013. Nov 8. pii: S0163-7258(17)30263-2.

36. Elsayed EA, El Enshasy H, Wadaan MA, Aziz R. Mushrooms: a potential natural source of anti-inflammatory compounds for medical applications. Mediat Inflamm. 2014;2014:835–41.

37. Paterson RR, Lima N. Biomedical effects of mushrooms with emphasis on pure compounds. Biom J. 2014;37:357–68.

38. Komura DL, Ruthes AC, Carbonero ER, Gorin PA, Iacomini M. Water-soluble polysaccharides from Pleurotus ostreatus var. florida mycelial biomass. Int J Biol Macromol. 2014;70:354–9.

39. Wasser SP. Medicinal mushroom science: current perspectives, advances, evidences, and challenges. Biom J. 2014;37:345–56.

40. Lindequist U, Kim HW, Tiralongo E, Van Griensven L. Medicinal mushrooms. Evid Based Complement Alternat Med. 2014;12:1–2.

41. Xu T, Beelman RB, Lambert JD. The cancer preventive effects of edible mushrooms. Anti Cancer Agents Med Chem. 2012;12:1255–63.

42. Wang J, Liu YM, Cao W, Yao KW, Liu ZQ, Guo JY. Anti-inflammation and antioxidant effect of Cordymin, a peptide purified from the medicinal mushroom Cordyceps sinensis, in middle cerebral artery occlusion-induced focal cerebral ischemia in rats. Metab Brain Dis. 2012;27:159–65.

43. Wong JH, Ng TB, Wang H, Sze SC, Zhang KY, Li Q, et al. Cordymin, an antifungal peptide from the medicinal fungus Cordyceps militaris. Phytomedicine. 2011;18:387–92.

44. Cui J, Goh KK, Archer R, Singh H. Characterisation and bioactivity of protein-bound polysaccharides from submerged-culture fermentation of Coriolus versicolor Wr-74 and ATCC-20545 strains. J Ind Microbiol. 2007;34:393–402.

45. Trovato SA, Pennisi M, Crupi R, Di Paola R, Alario A, Modafferi S, Di Rosa G, Fernandes T, Signorile A, Maiolino L, Cuzzocrea S, Calabrese V. Neuroinflammation and mitochondrial dysfunction in the pathogenesis of Alzheimer's disease: modulation by Coriolus Versicolor (Yun-Zhi) nutritional mushroom. J Neurol Neuromed. 2017;2:19–28.

46. Cui J, Chisti Y. Polysaccharopeptides of Coriolus versicolor: physiological activity, uses, and production. Biotechnol Adv. 2003;21:109–22.

47. Ng TB. A review of research on the protein-bound polysaccharide (polysaccharopeptide, PSP) from the mushroom Coriolus versicolor (Basidiomycetes: Polyporaceae). Gen Pharmacol. 1998;30:1–4.

48. Hirahara N, Edamatsu T, Fujieda A, Fujioka M, Wada T, Tajima Y. Protein-bound polysaccharide-K induces apoptosis via mitochondria and p38 mitogen-activated protein kinase-dependent pathways in HL-60 promyelomonocytic leukemia cells. Oncol Rep. 2013;30:99–104.

49. Ho CY, Kim CF, Leung KN, Fung KP, Tse TF, Chan H, et al. Coriolus versicolor (Yunzhi) extract attenuates growth of human leukemia xenografts and induces apoptosis through the mitochondrial pathway. Oncol Rep. 2006;16:609–16.

50. Figueiredo-Pereira ME, Rockwell P, Schmidt-Glenewinkel T, Serrano P. Neuroinflammation and J2 prostaglandins: linking impairment of the ubiquitin-proteasome pathway and mitochondria to neurodegeneration. Front Mol Neurosci. 2015;7

51. Joshi YB, Pratico D. The 5-lipoxygenase pathway: oxidative and inflammatory contributions to the Alzheimer's disease phenotype. Front Cell Neurosci. 2015; 8:436. https://doi.org/10.3389/fncel.2014.00436.

52. Trovato Salinaro A, Siracusa R, Di Paola R, Scuto M, Fronte V, Koverech G, Luca M, Serra A, Toscano MA, Petralia A, Cuzzocrea S, Calabrese V. Redox modulation of cellular stress response and lipoxin A4 expression by Coriolus versicolor in rat brain: relevance to Alzheimer's disease pathogenesis. Neurotoxicology. 2016;53:350–8.

53. Dunn HC, Ager RR, Baglietto-Vargas D, Cheng D, Kitazawa M, Cribbs DH, et al. Restoration of lipoxin A4 signaling reduces Alzheimer's disease-like pathology in the 3xTg-AD mouse model. J Alzheimers Dis. 2015;43:893–903.

54. Gangemi S, Pescara L, D'Urbano E, Basile G, Nicita-Mauro V, Davi G, et al. Aging is characterized by a profound reduction in anti-inflammatory lipoxin A4 levels. Exp Gerontol. 2005;40:612–4.

55. Le Y, Murphy PM, Wang JM. Formyl-peptide receptors revisited. Trends Immunol. 2002;23(11):541–8.

56. Chiang N, Serhan CN, Dahlen SE, Drazen JM, Hay DW, Rovati GE, et al. The lipoxin receptor ALX: potent ligand-specific and stereoselective actions in vivo. Pharm Rev. 2006;58:463–87.

57. Friedman M. Chemistry, nutrition, and health-promoting properties of Hericium erinaceus (Lion's mane) mushroom fruiting bodies and mycelia and their bioactive compounds. J Agric Food Chem. 2015;63:7108–23.

58. Liang B, Guo ZD, Xie F, Zhao AN. Antihyperglycemic and antihyperlipidemic activities of aqueous extract of Hericium ein experimental diabetic rats. BMC Complement Altern Med. 2013;13:253. https://doi.org/10.1186/1472-6882-13-253.

59. Lai CL, Lin RT, Liou LM, Liu CK. The role of event-related potentials in cognitive decline in Alzheimer's disease. Clin Neurophysiol. 2010;121:194–9.

60. Mori K, Inatomi S, Ouchi K, Azumi Y, Tuchida T. Improving effects of the mushroom Yamabushitake (Hericium erinaceus) on mild cognitive impairment: a double-blind placebo-controlled clinical trial. Phytother Res. 2009;23:367–72.

61. Wu J, Wang AT, Min Z, Xiong YJ, Yan QY, Zhang JP, et al. Lipoxin A(4) inhibits the production of proinflammatory cytokines induced by beta-amyloid in vitro and in vivo. Biochem Biophys Res Commun. 2011;408:382–7.

62. McGeer PL, McGeer EG. Innate immunity, local inflammation, and degenerative disease. Sci Aging Knowl Environ. 2002;3:23–32.

63. Nakamura T, Cho DH, Lipton SA. Redox regulation of protein misfolding, mitochondrial dysfunction, synaptic damage, and cell death in neurodegenerative diseases. Exp Neurol. 2012;238:12–21.

64. Biasibetti R, Tramontina AC, Costa AP, Dutra MF, Quincozes-Santos A, Nardin P, et al. Green tea (−)epigallocatechin-3-gallate reverses oxidative stress and reduces acetylcholinesterase activity in a streptozotocin-induced model of dementia. Behav Brain Res. 2013;236:186–93.

23

Immunosenescence and lymphomagenesis

Salvatrice Mancuso[1][*], Melania Carlisi[2], Marco Santoro[2], Mariasanta Napolitano[1], Simona Raso[2] and Sergio Siragusa[1]

Abstract

One of the most important determinants of aging-related changes is a complex biological process emerged recently and called "immunosenescence". Immunosenescence refers to the inability of an aging immune system to produce an appropriate and effective response to challenge. This immune dysregulation may manifest as increased susceptibility to infection, cancer, autoimmune disease, and vaccine failure. At present, the relationship between immunosenescence and lymphoma in elderly patients is not defined in a satisfactory way.

This review presents a brief overview of the interplay between aging, cancer and lymphoma, and the key topic of immunosenescence is addressed in the context of two main lymphoma groups, namely Non Hodgkin Lymphoma (NHL) and Hodgkin Lymphoma (HL). Epstein Barr Virus (EBV) plays a central role in the onset of neoplastic lymphoproliferation associated with immunological changes in aging, although the pathophysiology varies vastly among different disease entities. The interaction between immune dysfunction, immunosenescence and Epstein Barr Virus (EBV) infection appears to differ between NHL and HL, as well as between NHL subtypes.

Keywords: Lymphoma, Lymphomagenesis, Immunosenescence, Ageing, Cancer

Background

Immunosenescence is a peculiar remodeling of the immune system, caused by aging, associated with a wide variety of alterations of immune functions. Mounting biological evidence supports the potential clinical relevance and impact of immunosenescence [1, 2]. Indeed, it is has been implicated in pathophysiology of dementia, frailty, cardiovascular diseases, and it is cause of increased susceptibility to infectious disease, autoimmunity and cancer. Hematological malignancies and lymphoma are diseases that typically affect the elderly, with a median age for the most common lymphoma type, Diffuse Large B-cell Lymphoma (DLBCL), of > 70 years at diagnosis [3]. With the profound changes in demographic profiles of western countries and a steadily rising life expectancy, the number of elder patients with lymphoma is increasing [4, 5].

Although the risk of developing these neoplasms is higher in individuals with inherited predisposition or subjected to environmental risk factors, most cases cannot be associated with identifiable underlying conditions. In fact, lymphomagenesis is proven to be a molecularly complex process resulting in a broad category of different lymphoproliferative disorders. On the basis of histologic features, the pathogenetic events involved in disease initiation and/or progression may vary significantly [6].

Information regarding global burden of immunosenescence in lymphomagenesis is limited and requires a detailed understanding by the type of lymphoma considered, because the mechanism might vary in different specific cases [7].

This review aims to summarize the current state of understanding about the role of immunosenescence and development of lymphoma in older age.

We conducted a systematic research on PubMed, without filtering the results by date, language, or article type. Several studies have shown the potential to address the problem; however, no reports were found of studies in which clinically relevant relationships between the development of lymphoma and the complex underlying immunosenescence were elucidated.

Aging, cancer and immunosenescence
Age-related changes and cancer

It is commonly accepted that aging is the main risk factor for major chronic diseases such as cardiovascular diseases, cancer and neurodegenerative diseases [8].

* Correspondence: salvatrice.mancuso@unipa.it
[1]Haematology, Biomedical Department of Internal Medicine and Medical Specialties, University of Palermo, Palermo, Italy
Full list of author information is available at the end of the article

Recently, nine candidate hallmarks of aging were described in relation to genetic, epigenetic and environmental events [Table 1] [9, 10]. The resulting aging process and the aging phenotype, characterized by loss of fitness, create a favorable condition for aberrant neoplastic proliferation [11]. The strong association between cancer and age is supported by epidemiological data, indicating an increased incidence of malignancies in elderly patients. Indeed, about 55% of tumors affect subjects who are over 65 years of age https://seer.cancer.gov/archive/csr/1975_2005/. Aging reflects the sum of all changes accumulating with time by effect of genetic and environmental causes [12, 13]. The more prolonged exposure to carcinogens in older people and the increase in mutational load, epigenetic gene silencing, telomere dysfunction, unrestricted replicative potential, altered stromal milieu, apoptosis evasion, all contribute to an altered environment that promotes neoplastic proliferation [14–17].

Biological basis of immunosenescence

Among the spectrum of hallmarks, the changes of the immune response during aging now emerge as an expanding field of research, supported by copious experimental data [18]. Immunosenescence is a complex biological process that occurs in both the innate and adaptive components of the immune system [19]. Most of the effector functions of neutrophils, monocyte/macrophage lineage and natural killer (NK) cells decrease, concomitantly with a basal activation state [20–22]. Chronic antigenic stimulation probably underlies the marked changes in the adaptive immune system [23]. The ultimate consequence is a shift from loss of diversity of the T-cell receptor (TCR) repertoire to an increase in number of exhausted CD28$^-$ T cells, and profound functional changes in CD4 T cell subpopulations [8, 24, 25]. Together, these alterations of the innate and adaptive immunity favor the gradual development of a state of chronic inflammatory process called "inflammaging" [26, 27]. It is not perfectly clear if the state of slightly raised inflammatory mediators is really part of immunosenescence or an independent phenomenon

Table 1 The hallmarks of aging

Genomic instability
Telomer attrition
Epigenetic alterations
Loss of proteostasis
Deregulated nutrient-sensing
Mitochondrial dysfunction
Cellular senescence
Stem cell exhaustion
Altered intercellular communication

with additive effects on morbidity and mortality [28, 29]. To this regard, a basic characteristic of the immune system is plasticity, the capability of immune cells to undergo modification and adapt to different situations [30]. There is limited knowledge on whether immunosenescence is really associated with detrimental clinical outcomes or whether changes in immune parameters of older people reflect adaptive responses to the clinical and immunological history of the subject [31–33]. Therefore, it is necessary to reconsider some conclusions on the basis of many disparate findings in the literature. Against certain generalizations related to immunosenescence, context-dependent immune ageing processes need to be identified, with a detailed understanding of those diseases that are of major health interest [34].

Immunosenescence and defects in cancer protection

It is well known that both the innate and the adaptive immune system protect the host against carcinogenesis by a process called "immunosurveillance". By means of this process, the immune cells identify and eliminate cancerous cells before tumor develops [35]. In some cases, the functional ability of immunosurveillance cannot prevent the tumors from escaping and growing because the pressure exerted by the immune system can select many variants of resistant tumor cells. Immunosenescence can be considered as an additional factor which further promotes the tumor's escape mechanism [36].

Dysregulated function of the immune system affecting older people involves both innate and adaptive parts, with many mechanisms sharing molecular pathways implicated in the carcinogenesis process [37]. Among age-related alterations, the impairment of apoptotic cell death and the immunosuppressive role of some cytokines, such as interleukin-10 (IL-10) and transforming growth factor-β (TGF-β) which increasing in the elderly, could be relevant in the relationship between ageing and risk of tumor development [38, 39]. Therefore, immunosenescence may be linked to immune tolerance and contribute to an increased incidence of cancer with age.

Some evidence suggests that tumor-induced immunosuppression, through active mechanisms that can avoid or evade immune attack, might be more effective in ageing. Regarding the Fas ligand/Fas receptor (FasL/FasR) mechanism, the increased FasR expression observed in aged leukocytes might facilitate the immune escape of tumors expressing FasL [40]. A further example is the release of immunosuppressive cytokines by tumor cells such as TGF- β, IL-10 and others, that can suppress T cell responses and, in old subjects, may synergize with immunosuppressive cytokines overproduced by aged leukocytes [38].

Immunosenescence and non-Hodgkin lymphoma

Non-Hodgkin lymphoma and aging

The current available data focuses on B cell Non Hodgkin Lymphomas (NHL), which represent more than 90% of lymphoid neoplasms worldwide [41]. They are a heterogeneous group of clonal tumors of mature B cells that have distinctive clinical and biological behaviors [42–44]. NHL subtypes tend to mimic stages of normal B cell differentiation so that they can be classified according to the corresponding normal stage. In the context of NHL, a stepwise increase in the incidence of DLBCL over the last 20 years has been observed, particularly for patients older than 65 years [45]. The current increase in life expectancy naturally results in a higher number of elderly patients. Between lymphoma and aging, a complex interplay can be described [46]. B cell NHLs develop by a multistep process closely related to normal B cell counterpart that can be favored with aging [47]. Many potential factors can play a role in lymphomagenesis in the elders. As with all other cancer types, chronological ageing is associated with the accumulation of DNA damage particularly in stem cells [48]. Recently, significant large scale studies by whole-exome sequencing data have reported age-related clonal hematopoiesis, with somatic mutations in genes that are recurrently mutated in hematological neoplasms [49–51]. Also, epigenetic abnormalities that have a role in lymphoma development as in leukemia can accumulate with aging [52].

Immunosenescence, chronic infection and lymphomagenesis in non-Hodgkin lymphoma of the elderly

In addition to abnormal genetic events, also age-related impairment in cancer protection is expected to promote B cell lymphomagenesis. The phenotype called "immunosenescence" is associated with a complex dysfunction that increases sensitivity to infections. Chronic infection with Cytomegalovirus (CMV) and EBV in the elderly caused by restricted T cell response can alter the B cell immune repertoire, leading to infection-linked diseases as well as some types of lymphoma [53]. It is known how B lymphomagenesis can be driven by microbial pathogens through chronic antigenic stimulation, and several examples are available in this regard. Some lymphotropic oncogenic viruses, EBV, Human-Herpesvirus-8 (HHV8), Human T-lymphotropic virus HTLV1) are directly responsible for lymphoid cell neoplastic transformation and are causative agents of different histologic entities, with varying aggressiveness. Other pathogens, indirectly via chronic inflammation of the mucosa-associated lymphoid tissue (MALT), have been associated with MALT Marginal Zone Lymphoma in various organs: Helicobacter pyloric, Campylobacter jejeuni, Chlamydia psittaci and Borrelia burgdorferi [54, 55]. Also, a causal relationship between Hepatitis C Virus (HCV) and NHL has been demonstrated and the most plausible molecular mechanism is lymphoma development by continuous antigenic stimulation. However, an increased incidence of NHL hystotypes linked to infections in the elderly has not been reported. A specific provisional entity in 2008's World Health Organization (WHO) classification of tumors of hematopoietic and lymphoid tissue has been described as "EBV-positive DLBCL of the elderly" (EBV-DLBCL-E) [56, 57]. This lymphoproliferative disease occurs in absence of any primary or secondary immune deficiency and tends to have a post germinative center (GC)-phenotype and a poor prognosis [58]. The possible pathogenetic mechanism is lymphoma development as a consequence of immunosenescence and as part of the normal aging process, with a reduction in T cell repertoire. Immune modification can facilitate a second genetic event favored by EBV chronic infection in genetically instable B cell compartment. EBV-positive DLBCL thus represents a significant proof of the complex interplay between immunosenescence and lymphoma, and supports the leading role played by viruses in this setting. In 2016's updated WHO classification of lymphoid neoplasia, this entity is now recognized as definite and the term "elderly" has been substituted by "not otherwise specified" (NOS) in such that these lymphomas can be present in younger patients as well [59]. In this patient group, EBV-positive DLBCLs usually have a positive outcome in contrast to EBV-DLBCL-E [60]. Nevertheless, EBV-DLBCL-E is a relatively rare lymphoid malignancy (< 5% in Western countries) and cannot explain the increased incidence of B-NHL in older patients.

Diffuse large B cell lymphoma and aging-related molecular changes

Few studies have investigated whether a signature of aging can be seen in B cell NHL. Histopathologic features of DLBCL do not differ between age groups. However, studies of gene expression profiling (GEP) have described a higher frequency of activated B cell (ABC) DLBCL subtype in the elderly together with an increased B-cell lymphoma-2 (BCL2) expression and more genomic abnormalities [61–63]. These specificities can provide a basic understanding of the biological and clinical characteristics as well as the worst prognosis of DBCL in older patients.

Potential molecular alterations based on age in DLBCL patients have been described. Beheshti et al. identified significant age-related molecular changes after examining global transcriptome DLBCL data from The Cancer Genome Atlas, and striking transcriptional differences were associated with decreased metabolism and telomere dysfunction. The greatest functional changes occurring in older populations were related to key genes that strongly regulate the immune system [64]. These molecular factors influence tumor size and tumor progression in older DLBCL patients, but it is not clear if these findings may improve our understanding of lymphomagenesis as well as the role of immunosenescence.

Immunosenescence and Hodgkin's lymphoma
Epidemiology and biology of Hodgkin lymphoma
Classical Hodgkin Lymphomas (cHL) are unusual B cell-derived malignancies and the majority of them manifest clinically in young adults, even though a bimodal age curve is described, with a second peak later in life. They account for 30% of all lymphomas. In contrast with NHL, their absolute incidence has not apparently changed and no increase has been observed in aged population [65, 66].

Neoplastic tissues include rare malignant Hodgkin and Reed-Stenberg (HRS) cells within an extensive but ineffective inflammatory/immune cell infiltrate composed of macrophages, eosinophils, mast cells and T cells [67]. Although HRS cells have lost expression of certain B cell surface proteins and, particularly, B cell receptors, they do not die by apoptosis, so alternative pathways for survival and growth are exploited [68]. Key strategies leverage different mechanisms, such as nuclear factor kappa-light-chain-enhancer of activated B cells (NF-κB) signaling, Janus kinase/signal transducers and activators of transcription (JAK/STAT) pathway, AP-1 transcription factor, tumor necrosis factor (TNF) receptor family protein expression but latest data support the major role of immune evasion [69–72]. Malignant HRS cells escape immune attack using multiple stratagems, including enhanced PD-1 signalling, secretion of soluble factors with inhibitory effects such as IL-10 and recruitment of abundant immunosuppressive C-C chemokine receptor type 4 regulatory T-cells (CCR4 Tregs) [73–75]. These features are highly informative for the position of immunosurveillance to tumor cells in cHL pathogenesis.

Epstein-Barr virus and lymphomagenesis of Hodgkin lymphoma in the elderly
The biology and origin of cHL can be related to the oncogenic role of EBV [57]. EBV is a human virus, etiologically linked to a significantly wide range of lymphoproliferative diseases of B, T and NK cells. The role of EBV as growth-transforming agent is not linked to a single and simple oncogenic mechanism, but to a complex interplay between different patterns of viral gene expression, cellular genetic changes and immunity of the host. cHL is one of the major B cell malignancy types linked to EBV although it can occur in EBV-positive and negative form, both in apparently immunocompetent subjects [76]. But virus-specific immune surveillance should not be viewed as secondary. Indeed, immune impairment enhances lymphoma risk and the incidence of lymphoma and proportion of cHL cases that are EBV-positive are increased in Human Immunodeficiency Virus (HIV)-infected individuals. Furthermore, the proportion of cHL cases associated to EBV varies significantly with age and is more prevalent in older adults. The cases arising in the elderly appear as a different disease compared to cHL in young patients [77]. There are more patients who are found in advanced stages with B-symptoms and poor performance status, outlining a different pattern of histology subtypes with mixed cellularity that appear more evident if compared with younger individuals. EBV-associated disease was recognized as a poor prognostic factor and was also associated with an advanced-stage lymphoma [78]. The peak of cHL in adults may be attributed, at least partially, to senescence of EBV immunity and to an increased viral load. The prominent role of immunosenescence compared to other aging-related factors can explain why the increase in incidence of diffuse large B cell lymphoma over the last decades due to aging population has not been reflected in the incidence of cHL, which appears to stay constant [79]. cHL of the elderly, because of morphological features and association with EBV, is probably similar to cHL during HIV infection. In HIV-infected people, the incidence of cHL is 10-fold higher than in the general population, and the development of HIV-related cHL is not dependent on profound T-cell depletion, but only a modest impairment of CD4 lymphocytes is sufficient to elevate EBV viral load in the B cell system [80]. Indeed, after the introduction of Highly Active Antiretroviral Therapy (HAART) in the treatment of HIV infection, cHL incidence among HIV–infected cohorts has slightly increased [81, 82]. These common features between lymphomagenesis of cHL in older patients and in HIV-infected subjects reflect many similarities between biology of immunosenescence in aging and residual immunological defects in treated HIV infection [83]. Indeed, long-term therapy with HAART is associated with an increased risk of complications with degenerative nature and of cancer types that are similar to those observed among the elderly [84].

Other links between immunosenescence and lymphoma in the elderly
In addition to the role of immunosenescence in the pathogenesis of lymphomas, still little is known about the interactions between aging immune system changes and other aspects of lymphoma biology as well as lymphoma management. Recently, some reports have emerged on the possible role of immunosenescence in the progression of cancer; furthermore, immunosenescence-associated changes are exacerbated by chemotherapy. Older patients' immune background could play a critical role for higher

risk of infections as a side effect of chemotherapy. Immunosenescence might, therefore, contribute to negative outcomes in patients with lymphoma and could be a target for therapy.

Finally, whether, or to what extent, immunosenescence plays a role in response or toxicity to anti-neoplastic therapy with immune checkpoint inhibitors is still a matter of debate, representing a relevant unmet need.

Conclusion

The phenomenon of immunosenescence plays an essential, but poorly defined, role in the development of lymphoma. Older people are a heterogeneous portion of population that experiences various degrees of ageing and immune system remodeling. In addition, the mechanism of lymphomagenesis might vary by the type of lymphoma considered. In this setting, impairment of immune functions can predispose to development of lymphoma related to oncovirus infection, through reduced ability to clear infectious agents, chronic antigenic stimulation, lymphoma growth, immune evasion. EBV plays a central role in the onset of neoplastic lymphoproliferation, associated with immunological changes in aging. Current clinical and epidemiological findings, confirmed by molecular evidence, have generally revealed the oncogenic role of EBV only in a small size sample of lymphoma subtypes of elderly: EBV-DLBCL-E and cHL [85–87].

Since aging, as well as immunosenescence, is heterogeneous, both inter-individually and intra-individually, the assessment of this decline should be done individually and adapted not solely on chronological age. Currently, aging assessment is clinical and based upon a geriatric evaluation [88–90]. The challenging question is to find key biomarkers of immunaging that can help to better estimate the role of the aging phenotype and to include a measure of immunosenescence in studies by collecting data on elderly patients with cHL and EBV-DLBCL [91]. Thus far, of all the age-associated immune parameters found to be informative, it is not possible to select those that are crucial for clinical relevance.

Looking to the future, the new understanding of immunosenescence will have an impact on the treatment of lymphomas to further individualize therapy. Lastly, for research agenda, HIV-infected patients receiving HAART provide a model for a better understanding of how immune dysfunction with limited immune deficiency can promote lymphoma development [92].

Abbreviations
(ABC) subtype: Activated B cell subtype; (GC)-phenotype: Germinative center phenotype; BCL2: B-cell lymphoma-2; CCR4 Tregs: C-C chemokine receptor type 4 regulatory T-cells; cHL: Classical Hodgkin Lymphomas; CMV: Cytomegalovirus; DLBCL: Diffuse Large B-cell Lymphoma; DLBCL, NOS: Diffuse Large B-cell Lymphoma, not otherwise specified; EBV: Epstein Barr Virus; EBV-DLBCL-E: EBV-positive DLBCL of the elderly; FasL: Fas ligand; FasR: Fas receptor; GEP: Gene expression profiling; HAART: Highly Active Antiretroviral Therapy; HCV: Hepatitis C Virus; HHV8: Human-Herpesvirus-8; HIV: Human Immunodeficiency Virus; HL: Hodgkin lymphoma; HRS cells: Hodgkin and Reed-Stenberg; HTLV1: Human T-lymphotropic virus; IL-10: Interleukin-10; JAK/STAT: Janus kinase/signal transducers and activators of transcription; MALT: Mucosa-associated lymphoid tissue; NF-κB: Nuclear factor kappa-light-chain-enhancer of activated B cells; NHL: Non Hodgkin lymphoma; NK cells: Natural killer cells; TCR: T-cell receptor; TGF-β: Transforming growth factor-β; TNF: Tumor necrosis factor; WHO: World Health Organization

Acknowledgements
Francesco Moscato, University of Glasgow, revised English language. The University of Palermo (IT), Doctoral Course of Experimental Oncology and Surgery, Cycle XXXII support Melania Carlisi, PhDst, for this research. The University of Palermo (IT), Doctoral Course of Experimental Oncology and Surgery, Cycle XXXIII support Marco Santoro, PhDst, for this research. The University of Palermo (IT), Doctoral Course of Experimental Oncology and Surgery, Cycle XXXIII support Simona Raso, PhDst, for this research.

Authors' contributions
SM contributed to conception and design, designed the review, carried out the literature research, and manuscript preparation. MC carried out the manuscript editing and manuscript review. All authors read and approved the final manuscript.

Competing interests
The authors declare that they have no competing interests.

Author details
[1]Haematology, Biomedical Department of Internal Medicine and Medical Specialties, University of Palermo, Palermo, Italy. [2]Department of Surgical, Oncological and Stomatological Disciplines, University of Palermo, Palermo, Italy.

References
1. Caruso C, Accardi G, Virruso C, Candore G. Sex, gender and immunosenescence: a key to understand the different lifespan between men and women? Immun Ageing. 2013;10(1):20.
2. Accardi G, Caruso C. Immune-inflammatory responses in the elderly: an update. Immun Ageing. 2018;15:11.
3. Thieblemont C, Coiffier B. Lymphoma in older patients. J Clin Oncol. 2007; 25(14):1916–23.
4. Edwards BK, Brown ML, Wingo PA, Howe HL, Ward E, Ries LA, et al. Annual report to the nation on the status of cancer, 1975-2002, featuring population-based trends in cancer treatment. J Natl Cancer Inst. 2005;97(19): 1407–27.
5. Morton LM, Wang SS, Devesa SS, Hartge P, Weisenburger DD, Linet MS. Lymphoma incidence patterns by WHO subtype in the United States, 1992-2001. Blood 2006;107(1):265–276.
6. Morton LM, Slager SL, Cerhan JR, Wang SS, Vajdic CM, Skibola CF, et al. Etiologic heterogeneity among non-Hodgkin lymphoma subtypes: the InterLymph non-Hodgkin lymphoma subtypes project. J Natl Cancer Inst Monogr. 2014;2014(48):130–44.
7. Sarkozy C, Salles G, Falandry C. The biology of aging and lymphoma: a complex interplay. Curr Oncol Rep. 2015;17(7):32.

8. Fülöp T, Dupuis G, Witkowski JM, Larbi A. The role of Immunosenescence in the development of age-related diseases. Rev Investig Clin. 2016;68(2):84–91.

9. López-Otín C, Blasco MA, Partridge L, Serrano M, Kroemer G. The Hallmarks of Agin. Cell. 2013;153(6):1194–217.

10. Faragher R, Frasca D, Remarque E, Pawelec G, ImAginE Consortium. Better immunity in later life: a position paper. Age (Dordr). 2014;36(3):9619.

11. Campisi J. Cancer and ageing: rival demons? Nat Rev Cancer. 2003;3(5):339–49.

12. Finkel T, Serrano M, Blasco MA. The common biology of cancer and ageing. Nature. 2007;448(7155):767–74.

13. Falandry C, Bonnefoy M, Freyer G, Gilson E. Biology of cancer and aging: a complex association with cellular senescence. J Clin Oncol. 2014;32(24):2604–1.

14. Malaguarnera L, Cristaldi E, Malaguarnera M. The role of immunity in elderly cancer. Crit Rev Oncol Hematol. 2010;74(1):40–60.

15. Wang J, Geiger H, Rudolph KL. Immunoaging induced by hematopoietic stem cell aging. Curr Opin Immunol. 2011;23(4):532–6.

16. Song Z, Wang J, Guachalla LM, Terszowski G, Rodewald HR, Ju Z, Rudolph KL. Alterations of the systemic environment are the primary cause of impaired B and T lymphopoiesis in telomere-dysfunctional mice. Blood. 2010;115(8):1481–9.

17. Ju Z, Jiang H, Jaworski M, Rathinam C, Gompf A, Klein C, Trumpp A, Rudolph KL. Telomere dysfunction induces environmental alterations limiting hematopoietic stem cell function and engraftment. Nat Med. 2007;13(6):742–7.

18. Franceschi C, Bonafè M, Valensin S. Human immunosenescence: the prevailing of innate immunity, the failing of clonotypic immunity, and the filling of immunological space. Vaccine. 2000;18(16):1717–20.

19. Castelo-Branco C, Soveral I. The immune system and aging: a review. Gynecol Endocrinol. 2014;30(1):16–22.

20. Montgomery RR, Shaw AC. Paradoxical changes in innate immunity in aging: recent progress and new directions. J Leukoc Biol. 2015;98(6):937–4.

21. Drew W, Wilson DV, Sapey E. Inflammation and neutrophil immunosenescence in health and disease: Targeted treatments to improve clinical outcomes in the elderly. Exp Gerontol. 2017;105:70–7.

22. Linton PJ, Thoman ML. Immunosenescence in monocytes, macrophages, and dendritic cells: lessons learned from the lung and heart. Immunol Lett. 2014;162(1 Pt B):290–7.

23. Fülöp T, Larbi A, Pawelec G. Human T cell aging and the impact of persistent viral infections. Front Immunol. 2013;4:271.

24. Palmer DB. The effect of age on thymic function. Front Immunol. 2013;4:316.

25. Hadrup SR, Strindhall J, Køllgaard T, Seremet T, Johansson B, Pawelec G, thor Straten P, Wikby A. Longitudinal studies of clonally expanded CD8 T cells reveal a repertoire shrinkage predicting mortality and an increased number of dysfunctional cytomegalovirus-specific T cells in the very elderly. J Immunol. 2006;176(4):2645–53.

26. Franceschi C, Bonafè M, Valensin S, Olivieri F, De Luca M, Ottaviani E, De Benedictis G. Inflamm-aging. An evolutionary perspective on immunosenescence. Ann N Y Acad Sci. 2000;908:244–54.

27. Fulop T, Dupuis G, Baehl S, Le Page A, Bourgade K, Frost E, et al. From inflamm-aging to immune-paralysis: a slippery slope during aging for immune-adaptation. Biogerontology. 2016;17(1):147–57.

28. Goto M. Inflammaging (inflammation + aging): a driving force for human aging based on an evolutionarily antagonistic pleiotropy theory? Biosci Trends. 2008;2(6):218–30.

29. Pawelec G, Goldeck D, Derhovanessian E. Inflammation, ageing and chronic disease. Curr Opin Immunol. 2014;29:23–8.

30. Grignolio A, Mishto M, Faria AM, Garagnani P, Franceschi C, Tieri P. Towards a liquid self: how time, geography, and life experiences reshape the biological identity. Front Immunol. 2014;5:153.

31. Nilsson BO, Ernerudh J, Johansson B, Evrin PE, Löfgren S, Ferguson FG, Wikby A. Morbidity does not influence the T-cell immune risk phenotype in the elderly: findings in the Swedish NONA immune study using sample selection protocols. Mech Ageing Dev. 2003;124(4):469–76.

32. Hakim FT, Gress RE. Immunosenescence: deficits in adaptive immunity in the elderly. Tissue Antigens. 2007;70(3):179–89.

33. Shanley DP, Aw D, Manley NR, Palmer DB. An evolutionary perspective on the mechanisms of immunosenescence. Trends Immunol. 2009;30(7):374–81.

34. Pawelec G. Does the human immune system ever really become "senescent"? F1000Res. 2017;6.

35. Koebel CM, Vermi W, Swann JB, Zerafa N, Rodig SJ, Old LJ, Smyth MJ, Schreiber RD. Adaptive immunity maintains occult cancer in an equilibrium state. Nature. 2007;450(7171):903–7.

36. Kim R, Emi M, Tanabe K. Cancer immunoediting from immune surveillance to immune escape. Immunology. 2007;121(1):1–1.

37. Fulop T, Larbi A, Witkowski JM, Kotb R, Hirokawa K, Pawelec G. Immunosenescence and cancer. Crit Rev Oncog. 2013;18(6):489–513.

38. Zhou D, Chrest FJ, Adler W, Munster A, Winchurch RA. Increased production of TGF-beta and II-6 by aged spleen cells. Immunol Lett. 1993;36(1):7–11.

39. Hanahan D, Weinberg RA. The hallmarks of cancer. Cell. 2000;100(1):57–70.

40. Walker PR, Saas P, Dietrich PY. Role of Fas ligand (CD95L) in immune escape: the tumor cell strikes back. J Immunol. 1997;158(10):4521–4.

41. Skrabek P, Turner D, Seftel M. Epidemiology of non-Hodgkin lymphoma. Transfus Apher Sci. 2013;49(2):133–8.

42. Balague Ponz O, Ott G, Hasserjian RP, Elenitoba-Johnson KS, de Leval L, de Jong D. Commentary on the WHO classification of tumors of lymphoid tissues (2008): aggressive B-cell lymphomas. J Hematop. 2009;2(2):83–7.

43. Martelli M, Ferreri AJ, Agostinelli C, Di Rocco A, Pfreundschuh M, Pileri SA. Diffuse large B-cell lymphoma. Crit Rev Oncol Hematol. 2013;87(2):146–71.

44. Puvvada S, Kendrick S, Rimsza L. Molecular classification, pathway addiction, and therapeutic targeting in diffuse large B cell lymphoma. Cancer Genet. 2013;206(7–8):257–65.

45. Sarkozy C, Coiffier B. Diffuse large B-cell lymphoma in the elderly: a review of potential difficulties. Clin Cancer Res. 2013;19(7):1660–9.

46. Klapper W, Kreuz M, Kohler CW, Burkhardt B, Szczepanowski M, Salaverria I, et al. Molecular Mechanisms in Malignant Lymphomas Network Project of the Deutsche Krebshilfe. Patient age at diagnosis is associated with the molecular characteristics of diffuse large B-cell lymphoma. Blood. 2012; 119(8):1882–7.

47. Lenz G, Nagel I, Siebert R, Roschke AV, Sanger W, Wright GW, et al. Aberrant immunoglobulin class switch recombination and switch translocations in activated B cell-like diffuse large B cell lymphoma. J Exp Med. 2007;204(3):633–43.

48. Morrison SJ, Wandycz AM, Akashi K, Globerson A, Weissman IL. The aging of hematopoietic stem cells. Nat Med. 1996;2(9):1011–6.

49. Porter CC, Baturin D, Choudhary R, DeGregori J. Relative fitness of hematopoietic progenitors influences leukemia progression. Leukemia. 2011; 25(5):891–5.

50. Genovese G, Kähler AK, Handsaker RE, Lindberg J, Rose SA, Bakhoum SF, et al. Clonal hematopoiesis and blood-cancer risk inferred from blood DNA sequence. N Engl J Med. 2014;371(26):2477–87.

51. Bowman RL, Busque L, Levine RL. Clonal hematopoiesis and evolution to hematopoietic malignancies. Cell Stem Cell. 2018;22(2):157–70.

52. Wada T, Koyama D, Kikuchi J, Honda H, Furukawa Y. Overexpression of the shortest isoform of histone demethylase LSD1 primes hematopoietic stem cells for malignant transformation. Blood. 2015;125(24):3731–46.

53. Weltevrede M, Eilers M, de Melker HE, van Baarle D. Cytomegalovirus persistence and T-cell immunosenescence in people aged fifty and older: a systematic review. Exp Gerontol. 2016 May;77:87–95.

54. Suarez F, Lortholary O, Hermine O, Lecuit M. Infection-associated lymphomas derived from marginal zone B cells: a model of antigen-driven lymphoproliferation. Blood. 2006;107(8):3034–44.

55. Zucca E, Bertoni F, Vannata B, Cavalli F. Emerging role of infectious etiologies in the pathogenesis of marginal zone B-cell lymphomas. Clin Cancer Res. 2014;20(20):5207–16.

56. Campo E, Swerdlow SH, Harris NL, Pileri S, Stein H, Jaffe ES. The 2008 WHO classification of lymphoid neoplasms and beyond: evolving concepts and practical applications. Blood. 2011;117(19):5019–32.

57. Shannon-Lowe C, Rickinson AB, Bell AI. Epstein-Barr virus-associated lymphomas. Philos Trans R Soc Lond B Biol Sci. 2017;372(1732). https://doi.org/10.1098/rstb.2016.0271.

58. Castillo JJ, Beltran BE, Miranda RN, Young KH, Chavez JC, Sotomayor EM. EBV-positive diffuse large B-cell lymphoma of the elderly: 2016 update on diagnosis, risk-stratification, and management. Am J Hematol. 2016;91(5):529–37.

59. Swerdlow SH, Campo E, Pileri SA, Harris NL, Stein H, Siebert R, et al. The 2016 revision of the World Health Organization classification of lymphoid neoplasms. Blood. 2016;127(20):2375–90.

60. Nicolae A, Pittaluga S, Abdullah S, Steinberg SM, Pham TA, Davies-Hill T, et al. EBV-positive large B-cell lymphomas in young patients: a nodal lymphoma with evidence for a tolerogenic immune environment. Blood. 2015;126(7):863–72.

61. Rosenwald A, Wright G, Chan WC, Connors JM, Campo E, Fisher RI, et al. Lymphoma/Leukemia Molecular Profiling Project. The use of molecular profiling to predict survival after chemotherapy for diffuse large-B-cell lymphoma. N Engl J Med. 2002;346(25):1937–47.

62. Mareschal S, Lanic H, Ruminy P, Bastard C, Tilly H, Jardin F. The proportion of activated B-cell like subtype among de novo diffuse large B-cell lymphoma increases with age. Haematologica. 2011;96(12):1888–90.

63. Dubois S, Viailly PJ, Mareschal S, Bohers E, Bertrand P, Ruminy P, et al. Next-generation sequencing in diffuse large B-cell lymphoma highlights molecular divergence and therapeutic opportunities: a LYSA study. Clin Cancer Res. 2016;22(12):2919–28.

64. Beheshti A, Neuberg D, McDonald JT, Vanderburg CR, Evens AM. The impact of age and sex in DLBCL: systems biology analyses identify distinct molecular changes and signaling networks. Cancer Inform. 2015;14:141–8.

65. Parkin DM, Muir CS. Cancer incidence in five continents. Comparability and quality of data. IARC Sci Publ. 1992;120:45–173.

66. Taylor PR, Angus B, Owen JP, Proctor SJ. Hodgkin's disease: a population-adjusted clinical epidemiology study (PACE) of management at presentation. Northern Region Lymphoma Group. QJM. 1998;91(2):131–9.

67. Mathas S, Hartmann S, Küppers R. Hodgkin lymphoma: pathology and biology. Semin Hematol. 2016;53(3):139–47.

68. Schwering I, Bräuninger A, Klein U, Jungnickel B, Tinguely M, Diehl V, et al. Loss of the B-lineage-specific gene expression program in Hodgkin and reed-Sternberg cells of Hodgkin lymphoma. Blood. 2003 Feb;101(4):1505–12.

69. Weniger MA, Küppers R. NF-κB deregulation in Hodgkin lymphoma. Semin Cancer Biol. 2016;39:32–9.

70. Joos S, Küpper M, Ohl S, von Bonin F, Mechtersheimer G, Bentz M, et al. Genomic imbalances including amplification of the tyrosine kinase gene JAK2 in CD30+ Hodgkin cells. Cancer Res. 2000;60(3):549–52.

71. Mathas S, Hinz M, Anagnostopoulos I, Krappmann D, Lietz A, Jundt F, et al. Aberrantly expressed c-Jun and JunB are a hallmark of Hodgkin lymphoma cells, stimulate proliferation and synergize with NF-kappa B. EMBO J. 2002; 21(15):4104–13.

72. Aldinucci D, Celegato M, Casagrande N. Microenvironmental interactions in classical Hodgkin lymphoma and their role in promoting tumor growth, immune escape and drug resistance. Cancer Lett. 2016;380(1):243–52.

73. Gordon SR, Maute RL, Dulken BW, Hutter G, George BM, McCracken MN, et al. PD-1 expression by tumour-associated macrophages inhibits phagocytosis and tumour immunity. Nature. 2017;545(7655):495–9.

74. Skinnider BF, Mak TW. The role of cytokines in classical Hodgkin lymphoma. Blood. 2002;99(12):4283–97.

75. Ishida T, Ishii T, Inagaki A, Yano H, Komatsu H, Iida S, Inagaki H, Ueda R. Specific recruitment of CC chemokine receptor 4-positive regulatory T cells In Hodgkin lymphoma fosters immune privilege. Cancer Res. 2006;66(11): 5716–22.

76. Glaser SL, Lin RJ, Stewart SL, Ambinder RF, Jarrett RF, Brousset P, et al. Epstein-Barr virus-associated Hodgkin's disease: epidemiologic characteristics in international data. Int J Cancer. 1997;70(4):375–82.

77. Erdkamp FL, Breed WP, Bosch LJ, Wijnen JT, Blijham GB. Hodgkin disease in the elderly. A registry-based analysis. Cancer. 1992;70(4):830–4.

78. Asano N, Yamamoto K, Tamaru J, Oyama T, Ishida F, Ohshima K, et al. Age-related Epstein-Barr virus (EBV)–associated B-cell lymphoproliferative disorders: comparison with EBV-positive classic Hodgkin lymphoma in elderly patients. Blood. 2009;113(12):2629–36.

79. Proctor SJ, Wilkinson J, Sieniawski M. Hodgkin lymphoma in the elderly: a clinical review of treatment and outcome, past, present and future. Crit Rev Oncol Hematol. 2009;71(3):222–32.

80. Cesarman E. Pathology of lymphoma in HIV. Curr Opin Oncol. 2013;25(5): 487–94.

81. Carroll V, Garzino-Demo A. HIV-associated lymphoma in the era of combination antiretroviral therapy: shifting the immunological landscape. Pathog Dis. 2015;73(7).

82. Clifford GM, Polesel J, Rickenbach M, Dal Maso L, Keiser O, Kofler A, Swiss HIV Cohort, et al. Cancer risk in the Swiss HIV cohort study: associations with immunodeficiency, smoking, and highly active antiretroviral therapy. J Natl Cancer Inst. 2005;97(6):425–32.

83. Fülöp T, Herbein G, Cossarizza A, Witkowski JM, Frost E, Dupuis G, Pawelec G, Larbi A. Cellular Senescence, Immunosenescence and HIV. Interdiscip Top Gerontol Geriatr. 2017;42:28–46.

84. Hart BB, Nordell AD, Okulicz JF, Palfreeman A, Horban A, Kedem E, et al. INSIGHT SMART and ESPRIT Groups. Inflammation-related morbidity and mortality among HIV-positive adults: how extensive is it? J Acquir Immune Defic Syndr. 2018;77(1):1–7.

85. Engert A, Ballova V, Haverkamp H, Pfistner B, Josting A, Dühmke E, Müller-Hermelink K, Diehl V, German Hodgkin's Study Group. Hodgkin's lymphoma in elderly patients: a comprehensive retrospective analysis from the German Hodgkin's study group. J Clin Oncol. 2005;23(22):5052–60.

86. Jarrett RF, Stark GL, White J, Angus B, Alexander FE, Krajewski AS, Scotland and Newcastle Epidemiology of Hodgkin Disease Study Group, et al. Impact of tumor Epstein-Barr virus status on presenting features and outcome in age-defined subgroups of patients with classic Hodgkin lymphoma: a population-based study. Blood. 2005;106(7):2444–51.

87. Evens AM, Helenowski I, Ramsdale E, Nabhan C, Karmali R, Hanson B, et al. A retrospective multicenter analysis of elderly Hodgkin lymphoma: outcomes and prognostic factors in the modern era. Blood. 2012;119(3):692–5.

88. Kenis C, Bron D, Libert Y, Decoster L, Van Puyvelde K, Scalliet P, et al. Relevance of a systematic geriatric screening and assessment in older patients with cancer: results of a prospective multicentric study. Ann Oncol. 2013;24(5):1306–12.

89. Wildiers H, Heeren P, Puts M, Topinkova E, Janssen-Heijnen ML, Extermann M, et al. International Society of Geriatric Oncology consensus on geriatric assessment in older patients with cancer. J Clin Oncol. 2014;32(24):2595–603.

90. Tucci A, Martelli M, Rigacci L, Riccomagno P, Cabras MG, Salvi F, et al. Comprehensive geriatric assessment is an essential tool to support treatment decisions in elderly patients with diffuse large B-cell lymphoma: a prospective multicenter evaluation in 173 patients by the lymphoma Italian Foundation (FIL). Leuk Lymphoma. 2015;56(4):921–6.

91. Falandry C, Gilson E, Rudolph KL. Are aging biomarkers clinically relevant in oncogeriatrics? Crit Rev Oncol Hematol. 2013;85(3):257–65.

92. Wong NS, Chan KCW, Cheung EKH, Wong KH, Lee SS. Immune recovery of middle-aged HIV patients following antiretroviral therapy: an observational cohort study. Medicine (Baltimore). 2017;96(28):e7493.

24

NK cells of the oldest seniors represent constant and resistant to stimulation high expression of cellular protective proteins SIRT1 and HSP70

Lucyna Kaszubowska[1*], Jerzy Foerster[2], Jan Jacek Kaczor[3], Daria Schetz[4], Tomasz Jerzy Ślebioda[1] and Zbigniew Kmieć[1]

Abstract

Background: Natural killer cells (NK cells) are cytotoxic lymphocytes of innate immunity that reveal some immunoregulatory properties, however, their role in the process of ageing is not completely understood. The study aimed to analyze the expression of proteins involved in cellular stress response: sirtuin 1 (SIRT1), heat shock protein 70 (HSP70) and manganese superoxide dismutase (SOD2) in human NK cells with reference to the process of ageing. Non-stimulated and stimulated with IL-2, LPS or PMA with ionomycin cells originated from peripheral blood samples of: seniors aged over 85 ('the oldest'; $n = 25$; 88.5 ± 0.5 years, mean $\pm$ SEM), seniors aged under 85 ('the old'; $n = 30$; 75.6 ± 0.9 years) and the young ($n = 31$; 20.9 ± 0.3 years). The relationships between the levels of expression of cellular protective proteins in the studied population were also analyzed. The concentrations of carbonyl groups and 8-isoprostanes, markers of oxidative stress, in both stimulated and non-stimulated cultured NK cells were measured to assess the level of the oxidative stress in the cells.

Results: The oldest seniors varied from the other age groups by significantly higher expression of SIRT1 and HSP70 both in non-stimulated and stimulated NK cells. These cells also appeared to be resistant to further stimulations with IL-2, LPS or PMA with ionomycin. Highly positive correlations between SIRT1 and intracellular HSP70 in both stimulated and non-stimulated NK cells were observed. SOD2 presented low expression in non-stimulated cells, whereas its sensitivity to stimulation increased with age of donors. High positive correlations between SOD2 and surface HSP70 were observed. We found that the markers of oxidative stress in NK cells did not change with ageing.

Conclusions: The oldest seniors revealed well developed adaptive stress response in NK cells with increased, constant levels of SIRT1 and intracellular HSP70. They presented also very high positive correlations between expression of these cellular protective proteins both in stimulated and non-stimulated cells. These phenomena may contribute to the long lifespan of this group of elderly. Interestingly, in NK cells SOD2 revealed a distinct role in cellular stress response since it showed sensitivity to stimulation increasing with age of participants. These observations provide novel data concerning the role of NK cells in the process of ageing.

Keywords: NK cells, Ageing, Adaptive stress response, SIRT1, HSP70, SOD2, Isoprostanes, Carbonyl groups, Oxidative stress, Innate immunity

* Correspondence: lkras@gumed.edu.pl
[1]Department of Histology, Medical University of Gdańsk, Dębinki 1, 80-211 Gdańsk, Poland
Full list of author information is available at the end of the article

Background

Natural killer cells (NK cells) are cytotoxic lymphocytes of innate immune system. They are cytotoxic ILCs1 (innate lymphoid cells type 1) crucial for immune response against viral infection and tumor cells [1, 2] but demonstrate also some immunoregulatory activities by secretion of cytokines and chemokines [3, 4]. They may adjust to the alterations of the cellular environment and develop a type of antigen-specific immunological memory exposing characteristics of both innate and adaptive immunity [5, 6]. After activation by cytokines such as IL-2, IL-12, IL-15 and IL-18 in different combinations or target cell challenge they secrete a range of cytokines, e.g. TNF, IFN-γ, IL-5, IL-10, IL-13, GM-CSF and chemokines IL-8, MIP-1α, MIP-1β and RANTES [7–9].

Interleukin 2 is one of the key NK cell cytokines required for the survival, proliferation and activation of MKK/ERK pathway, which was shown to be necessary for the activation of NK cells, IFN-γ secretion, CD25 and CD69 expression and enhanced cytotoxic function [10].

NK cells can be also activated by lipopolysaccharide (LPS), a component of the outer membrane of Gram-negative bacteria [11, 12]. LPS is recognized by Toll-like receptors 4 (TLR4) which play a crucial role in innate immunity and are expressed also on the surface of NK cells [13, 14]. TLR4 interacts by binding lipid A, a part of LPS molecule what results in activation of NF-κB pathway and expression of genes coding for proinflammatory cytokines, e.g. TNF, IL-1, IL-6, GM-CSF and chemokines, e.g. IL-8, RANTES, MIP-1α, MCP-1 [15, 16].

Phorbol 12-myristate 13-acetate (PMA) is a protein kinase C (PKC) activator used for a strong and unspecific stimulation of NK cells. Ionomycin (Ca^{2+} ionophore A23187) is a calcium ion channel opening antibiotic that mimicks the action of inositol triphosphate (IP3) and increases intracellular cytoplasmic free Ca^{2+} concentration by causing an influx of calcium ions from the extracellular space into cell cytoplasm [17]. Ca^{2+}-PKC pathway is involved in the phosphorylation of STAT4 which binds to numerous sequences in the genome including promoters of proinflammatory cytokine genes such as IFN-γ and TNF [18]. PMA with ionomycin are used for short (1-6 h) cell stimulation to induce the expression of cytokines, e.g. IFN-γ [19–21] and for both short [19] and longer (up to 48 h) cell stimulations to analyze profiles of gene and protein expression [22, 23].

Ageing is associated with the progressive increase in the proinflammatory status caused by the general decrease in the capacity to cope with a variety of stress factors and impairment of regulatory mechanisms concerning cytokine secretion. In ageing increased serum level of IL-6 and TNF, elevated level of C reactive protein and decreased concentration of anti-inflammatory cytokine IL-10 have been often reported [24]. These phenomena have been described as "inflamm-aging" [25]. However, ageing is also characterized by the increase of oxidative stress due to the redox imbalance caused by discrepancy between the amount of reactive oxygen species (ROS) generation and the activity of anti-oxidative mechanisms [26]. Thus, the theory of oxidation-inflammation was proposed as the main cause of ageing and the new term "oxi-inflamm-aging" was introduced to accentuate the relation between the redox state and functional capacity of the ageing immune system [27].

Adaptive stress response of cells and organisms to an intracellular or extracellular moderate stress is referred to the term hormesis used in toxicology to reflect a dose response to drugs, toxins or some natural substances. Low doses of these substances may elicit a positive response regarding adaptation to or protection from the stress agents, whereas at higher concentrations the same substances reveal toxic effects [28, 29]. The cellular adaptive response usually contributes to the synthesis of various stress resistance proteins, such as heat shock proteins, sirtuins, heme oxygenase and thioredoxin system [29].

SIRT1 is a redox sensitive protein that protects cells against cellular senescence caused by oxidative stress [30]. It is a (NAD$^+$) - dependent deacetylase that targets a variety of transcription factors, including FOXO1, 3 and 4, p53, NF-κB, PGC-1 and HSF-1. These factors control cellular stress adaptive responses which can then modulate the lifespan [31]. Expression of chaperons that protect cells against cellular stress is under control of heat shock factor-1 (HSF1), which is activated within minutes after appearing of the stress agent [32–34]. The presence of HSF-1 in the stress regulatory network indicates the central role of protein homeostasis in SIRT1-mediated cellular protection [35]. Manganese superoxide dismutase (SOD2) is a major mitochondrial enzymatic antioxidant which is under control of FOXO1, FOXO3a, FOXO4 and NF-κB transcription factors activated in cellular stress adaptive responses [36, 37].

The changes in the expression of SIRT1 in PBMCs [38] or HSP70 in granulocytes [39] or monocytes and lymphocytes [40, 41] have been described in the process of ageing. However, there are no studies regarding this phenomenon in NK cells, lymphocytes associated with healthy ageing and longevity [42, 43]. Therefore, the aim of our study was to analyze the expression of the proteins involved in cellular stress response: sirtuin 1, heat shock protein 70 and manganese superoxide dismutase in both non-stimulated and stimulated with IL-2, LPS and PMA with ionomycin human NK cells of the young, seniors under 85 and the oldest seniors aged over 85. We studied both the influence of the process of stimulation on the level of cellular protective proteins and the potential relationships between these proteins in the process of ageing. The levels of oxidative stress markers were also measured both in stimulated and control (non-stimulated) NK cells.

Methods

Participants

Eighty six volunteers aged between 19 and 94 years (62 women and 24 men) participated in this study. The exclusion criteria included: CRP > 5 mg/L, cancer, autoimmune disease, diabetes, infection, use of immunosuppressive drugs, glucocorticoids or non-steroid anti-inflammatory drugs (NSAID). Absence of dementia was assessed using the "Mini Mental State Examination" and only seniors with the score above 23 points were qualified to the study [44]. All senior volunteers underwent a geriatric assessment. The Katz's index of independence in "Activities of Daily Living" (ADL) was used and only seniors with 5-6 points were enrolled to the study [45]. Senior volunteers were recruited among inhabitants of local retirement homes whereas young volunteers were students of Medical University of Gdańsk, Poland. The participants were subdivided into 3 age groups: young (range 19-24 years), old (seniors aged under 85; range 65-84 years) and the oldest (seniors at the age over 85; range 85-94 years). The characteristics of the study population are shown in Table 1. All volunteers signed informed consent and the study received approval from Ethical Committee of Medical University of Gdańsk, Poland (No 225/2010). An immunological characteristics of the study population was described earlier [46].

Preparation of peripheral blood mononuclear cell cultures

Peripheral blood mononuclear cells (PBMCs) were isolated from venous blood samples collected in tubes with EDTA by conventional ficoll-uropoline density gradient centrifugation. PBMCs were then washed and resuspended in RPMI1640 medium supplemented with 5% FBS, penicillin (100 U/ml) – streptomycin (100 μg/ml) and 2-mercaptoethanol (5×10^{-5} M) (all purchased from Sigma - Aldrich, Saint Louis, MO, USA). Cells (5×10^5 / 0.5 ml) were cultured for 48 h in the absence (control) or presence of IL-2 (100 U/ml) (BD Biosciences, San Jose, CA, USA), LPS (1 μg/ml) or PMA (50 ng/ml) and ionomycin (500 ng/ml, all purchased from Sigma-Aldrich). PBMCs treated in this way were studied for the expression of SIRT1, SOD2 and HSP70 (surface and intracellular). The intracellular expression of TNF and IFN-γ, was studied in PBMCs (5×10^5 / 0.5 ml) cultured in the absence (control) or presence of IL-2 (100 U/ml) (BD Biosciences, San Jose, CA, USA), LPS (1 μg/ml) (Sigma-Aldrich, Saint Louis, MO, USA) or PMA (50 ng/

Table 1 Characteristics of the study population

Parameter	Young	Old	Oldest
Number	31	30	25
Age (yr)	20.9 ± 0.3	75.6 ± 0.9	88.5 ± 0.5
Sex (F/M)	22/9	20/10	20/5
Smoking status			
Current smoker	6	3	1
Ex-smoker	3	3	0
Nonsmoker	22	24	24
Weight (kg)	$59.8 \pm 1.7^{a,b}$	68.7 ± 2.0^a	68.4 ± 2.3^b
BMI (Body Mass Index)	$20.4 \pm 0.4^{a,b}$	25.6 ± 0.6^a	26.5 ± 0.9^b
Total cholesterol (mg/dL)	170.5 ± 5.6^a	193.6 ± 8.3^a	184.1 ± 9.4
HDL – cholesterol (mg/dL)	$58.7 \pm 2.6^{a,b}$	47.3 ± 2.3^a	43.7 ± 2.2^b
LDL – cholesterol (mg/dL)	96.1 ± 4.3^a	123.3 ± 7.3^a	113.7 ± 6.9
Triglyceride (mg/dL)	$78.3 \pm 8.2^{a,b}$	114.8 ± 11.2^a	133.0 ± 14.8^b
Glucose (mg/dL)	89.35 ± 1.33	94.4 ± 3.3	91.36 ± 3.4
Creatinine (mg/dL)	0.86 ± 0.03^b	0.87 ± 0.04^c	$1.05 \pm 0.05^{b,c}$
Uric acid (mg/dL)	4.95 ± 0.21^b	5.37 ± 0.28	6.22 ± 0.36^b

All data are presented as means ± SEM. Statistically significant differences between age groups are marked with:
[a] young vs old
[b] young vs oldest
[c] old vs oldest

ml) and ionomycin (500 ng/ml) (Sigma - Aldrich, Saint Louis, MO, USA) for 5 h. Simultaneously, Golgi Stop reagent (0.5 μl / well in 0.5 ml of medium, BD Biosciences, San Jose, CA, USA) was added to PBMC cultures (5×10^5 / 0.5 ml) to stop extracellular export of cytokines. Then PBMCs were collected and washed with 1 ml of BD Staining Buffer.

Staining of surface and intracellular antigens for flow cytometry

PBMCs (2.5×10^5 cells) were aliquoted into flow cytometry tubes and CD3-FITC-conjugated (0.125 μg/ml; clone UCHT1) (BD Biosciences, San Jose, CA, USA) or CD3-PE-Cy7-conjugated (0.125 μg/ml; clone SK7) (BD Biosciences, San Jose, CA, USA), CD56-APC-conjugated (0.6 μg/ml; clone NCAM16.2) (BD Biosciences, San Jose, CA, USA) and Hsp70-PE-conjugated (1 μg/ml; clone N27F34) (Abcam, Cambridge, England) monoclonal antibodies were added for cell surface antigen staining. After 30 min of incubation in the dark at room temperature 2 ml of BD FACS Lysing Solution was added and samples were incubated for subsequent 10 min in the same conditions. Then cells were washed twice with 1 ml of BD Staining Buffer (PBS without Ca^{2+} and Mg^{2+}, 1% FBS, 0.09% sodium azide) and resuspended in 0.25 ml of Fixation/Permeabilization Solution for 20 min at 4 °C following manufacturer's protocol (BD Cytofix/Cytoperm Fixation/Permeabilization Kit).

Cells were washed twice with 1 ml of BD Perm/Wash buffer and relevant volumes of MnSOD-FITC-conjugated (1 μg/ml; clone MnS-1) (eBioscience, San Diego, CA, USA), Hsp70-PE-conjugated (1 μg/ml; clone N27F34) (Abcam, Cambridge, England), SIRT1-Alexa Fluor 488 – conjugated (1 μg/ml; clone 19A7AB4) (Abcam, Cambridge, England), TNF-PE-Cy7- conjugated (0.125 μg/ml; clone MAb11) (BD Biosciences, San Jose, CA, USA) or IFN-γ-PE-conjugated (0.125 μg/ml; clone 4S.B3) (BD Biosciences, San Jose, CA, USA) monoclonal antibodies were added for staining of intracellular antigens following the manufacturer's instructions. After 30 min of incubation in the dark at room temperature cells were washed twice with 1 ml of BD Perm/Wash buffer and resuspeded in Staining Buffer prior to flow cytometric analysis. Samples were run on a BD FACSCalibur flow cytometer equipped with argon-ion laser (488 nm) and data were evaluated with BD CellQuest Pro software (BD Biosciences, San Jose, CA, USA) after collecting 10,000 gated events (lymphocytes). Peripheral blood lymphocytes were gated using forward (FSC) and side scatter (SSC) parameters. NK cells were identified in the CD3-negative region based on the expression of CD56 surface marker and defined as CD3-CD56+ cells. NK cell subset, gated on CD3-CD56+ cells, was further analyzed for the frequency of cells expressing the particular cellular protective protein (SIRT1, HSP70, SOD2) or cytokine (TNF and IFN-γ). Relevant isotype controls for both surface and intracellular staining were also used.

Separation of NK cells for measurement of protein carbonyl groups and 8-isoprostane concentrations in cell lysates

NK cells (CD3$^-$CD56$^+$) were isolated from PBMCs by negative selection with the use of Human NK Cell Enrichment Kit and EasySep Magnet (Stemcell Technologies, Vancouver, Canada). PBMCs were incubated with EasySep Human NK Cell Enrichment Cocktail (a suspension of monoclonal antibodies bound in bispecific Tetrameric Antibody Complexes (TAC) directed against cell surface antigens on human blood cells: CD3, CD4, CD14, CD19, CD20, CD36, CD66b, CD123, HLA-DR, glycophorin A and dextran for 10 min, then vortexed for 30 s and incubated with EasySep D Magnetic Particles (a suspension of magnetic dextran iron particles) for subsequent 5 min. Then cells were resuspended in 2.5 ml of recommended medium (PBS with 2% FBS and 1 mM EDTA, Ca^{2+} and Mg^{2+} free), mixed gently and placed into the magnet. After 2.5 min the desired fraction was poured off into a new tube. Aliquots of the cell fractions were stained with relevant volumes of CD56-PE- and CD3-PerCP-conjugated monoclonal antibodies (BD Biosciences, San Jose, CA, USA). After 30 min of incubation

in the dark at room temperature cells were washed with 2 ml of BD CellWASH solution and finally 0.5 ml of BD CellFIX solution was added. Samples were stored at 4 °C up to 24 h until analyzed by flow cytometry to check the purity of the enriched NK cell fractions and all showed almost 95% purity.

Then, NK cell extracts were prepared with the use of Mammalian Cell & Tissue Extraction Kit (BioVision Research Products, Mountain View, CA, USA) following the manufacturer's protocol. The total protein concentration of samples was estimated with Bradford assay (Sigma - Aldrich, Saint Louis, MO, USA). Cell lysates were stored at – 70 °C for further analysis. The content of protein carbonyl groups in NK cell extracts was determined with the BioCell PC Test Kit, an enzyme-linked immunosorbent assay (BioCell, Auckland, New Zealand). Samples were provided for ELISA procedure following the manufacturer's instructions. Absorbances were measured at 450 nm with Bio-Rad plate reader. A standard curve reflecting absorbances of the increasing concentrations of protein carbonyls in the supplied oxidized protein standards was made and used to determine the concentration of carbonyl groups in the analyzed samples. Data in the study are expressed as nanomoles of carbonyl groups per mg of cellular extract protein (nmol/mg).

The concentration of 8-isoprostanes in NK cell extracts was determined with the 8-Isoprostane ELISA Kit (Cayman Chemical, Ann Arbor, MI, USA). Samples were provided for ELISA procedure following manufacturer's instructions. Cell lysates were supplied in the presence of 0.005% BHT. Absorbances were measured at 405 nm with Bio-Rad plate reader. A standard curve was made with the use of 8-Isoprostane ELISA Standard provided with the kit and the concentrations of 8-isoprostanes in the analyzed samples were evaluated. Data in the study present the total 8-isoprostane content in NK cell lysates expressed as pg/ml.

Statistics

All data are expressed as means ± SEM. Normality of data distribution was analyzed by Shapiro-Wilk test. ANOVA test for normal distribution and Kruskal-Wallis test for non-parametric distribution were used to compare experimental data. The multiple comparisons were performed with Tukey's post-hoc test for normal distribution and Dunn's post-hoc test for non –parametric distribution. Paired Student's t-test for normal distribution and Wilcoxon signed-rank test for non-parametric distribution were used to compare two related samples. Student's t test for normal distribution and Mann-Whitney U test for non-parametric distribution were used to compare two independent samples. The Spearman correlation coefficient (R) was applied to present the strength of the relationship between variables

(Statistica, version 12; Statsoft, Tulsa, OK, USA). Differences and correlations with $p < 0.05$ were considered as statistically significant.

Results

Expression of SIRT1 and HSP70^{intracellular} in non- stimulated and stimulated NK cells of the seniors and the young

The gating strategy performed for flow cytometric analysis of NK cells is demonstrated in Fig. 1. Flow cytometry data were analyzed and presented in two ways, i.e. as the percentage of NK cells showing the expression of the studied protein (% of positive cells) and mean fluorescence intensity (MFI) measured in the samples.

In the group of the oldest seniors 20% of NK cells independently on the presence or absence of stimulation revealed increased intracellular expression of SIRT1 (range $19.98 \pm 5.77\%$ – $21.82 \pm 5.56\%$). It was significantly lower in the group of seniors under 85 (range $1.37 \pm 0.77\%$ – $2.22 \pm 1.33\%$) and in the young (range $0.64 \pm 0.24\%$ – $2.64 \pm 0.8\%$) in all studied conditions

(Fig. 2a). In contrast to NK cells of the younger subjects, NK cells of the oldest seniors were not sensitive to any type of the applied method of stimulation (Fig. 2a, b). In the young, NK cells were sensitive to stimulation with IL-2 and PMA with ionomycin (Fig. 2a, b). In the elderly under 85, NK lymphocytes were sensitive to IL-2 (Fig. 2a) or IL-2 and LPS (Fig. 2b), although in general the incubation with LPS revealed rather a limited influence on the expression level of SIRT1 in the cells (Fig. 2a, b).

It was also noteworthy that nearly 40% of NK cells of the oldest seniors showed increased expression of HSP70^{intracellular} in all studied samples (range $35.6 \pm 6.8\%$ - $41.7 \pm 6.28\%$) on the contrary to NK cells of the old (range 6.87 ± 2.37 – $13.61 \pm 2.76\%$) and the young (range $3.28 \pm 0.77\%$ - $12.32 \pm 1.34\%$) (Fig. 2c). Out of the studied stimulating agents only PMA with ionomycin increased HSP70^{intracellular} expression in NK cells of the oldest subjects (Fig. 2d). Similarly to SIRT1, the expression of HSP70^{intracellular} in NK cells of the young and the old was sensitive to stimulation with IL-2 and PMA with ionomycin, whereas the effect of LPS was very limited (Fig. 2c, d).

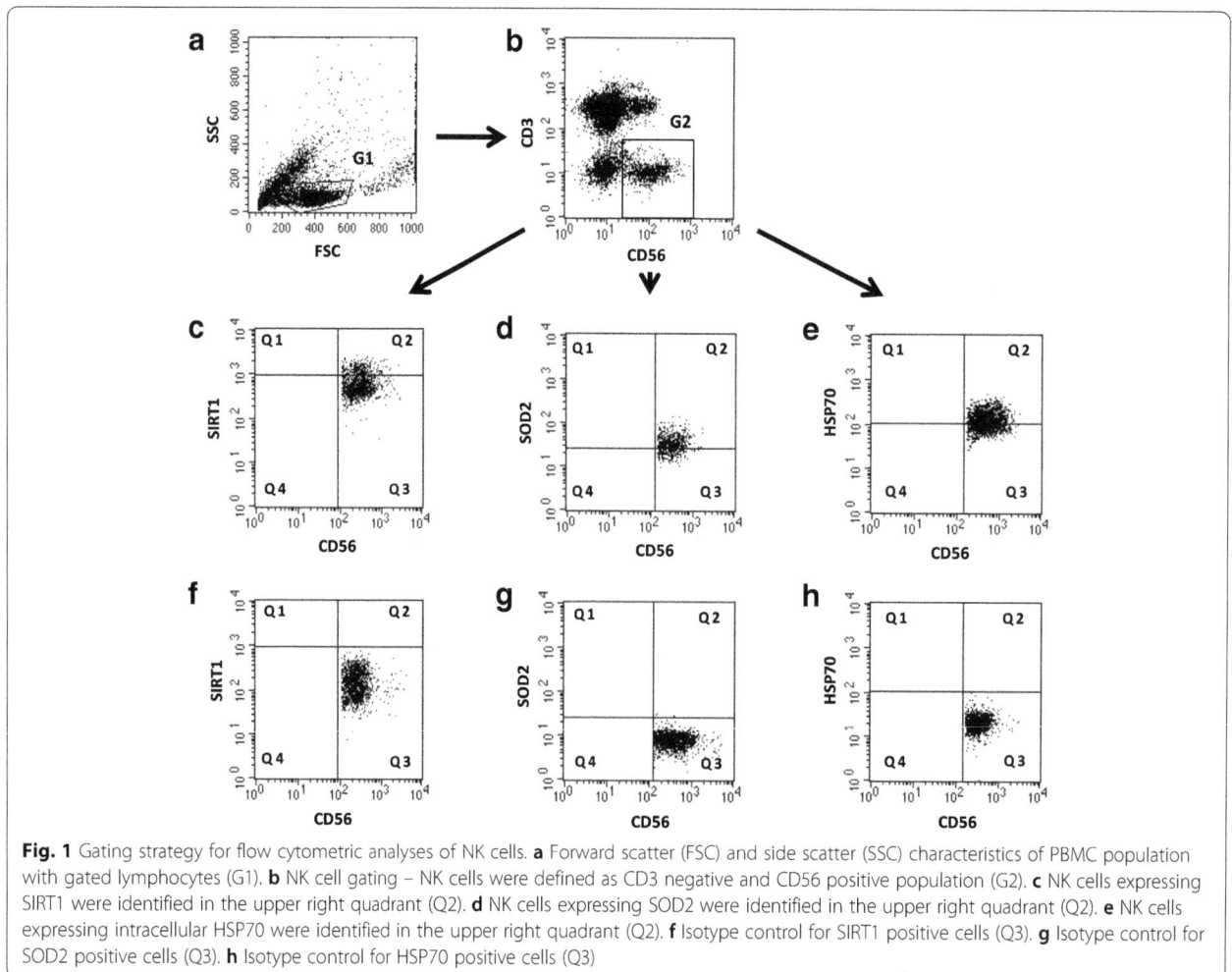

Fig. 1 Gating strategy for flow cytometric analyses of NK cells. **a** Forward scatter (FSC) and side scatter (SSC) characteristics of PBMC population with gated lymphocytes (G1). **b** NK cell gating – NK cells were defined as CD3 negative and CD56 positive population (G2). **c** NK cells expressing SIRT1 were identified in the upper right quadrant (Q2). **d** NK cells expressing SOD2 were identified in the upper right quadrant (Q2). **e** NK cells expressing intracellular HSP70 were identified in the upper right quadrant (Q2). **f** Isotype control for SIRT1 positive cells (Q3). **g** Isotype control for SOD2 positive cells (Q3). **h** Isotype control for HSP70 positive cells (Q3)

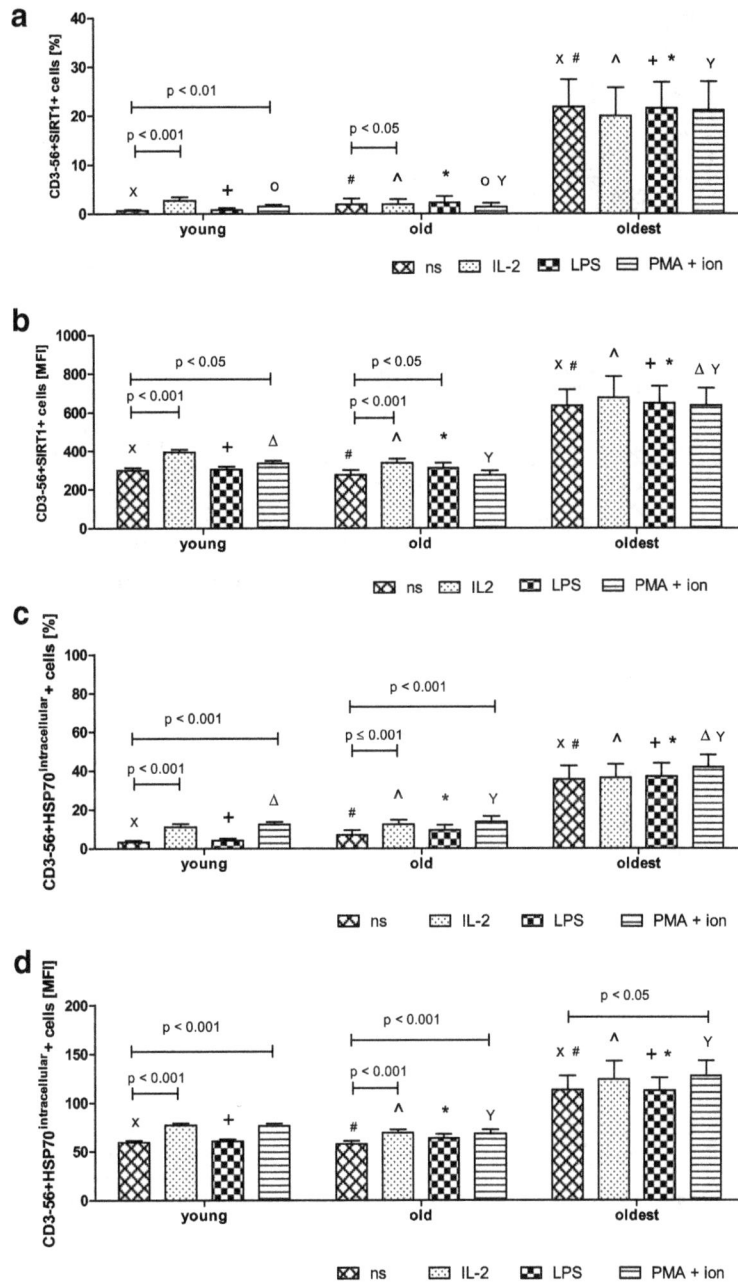

Fig. 2 Expression of SIRT1 and intracellular HSP70 in non-stimulated and stimulated NK cells of the young, the old aged under 85 and the oldest seniors (aged over 85). Data are presented as means ± SEM and show expression of the studied proteins in NK cells demonstrated as percentages of cells with the expression of a particular protein (%) or mean fluorescence intensity (MFI). The same symbols over bars (^{X}, $^+$, ^{o}, $^\#$, $^\wedge$, $^\Delta$, ^{Y}) denote statistically significant differences between similarly treated NK cells of different age groups (i.e. young vs old; young vs oldest or old vs oldest). Horizontal lines above paired bars denote statistically significant differences between treated and untreated NK cells of the same age group (i.e. non-stimulated vs stimulated with IL-2, LPS or PMA with ionomycin). **a** Expression of SIRT1 (%): ^{X}, $^\#$, $^\wedge$, $^+$, *, $^Y p < 0.001$; $^o p \leq 0.01$. **b** Expression of SIRT1 (MFI): $^\#$, $^+$, *, $^Y p < 0.001$; $^\wedge$, $^X p < 0.01$; $^\Delta p < 0.05$. **c** Expression of HSP70^{intracellular} (%): ^{X}, $^+$, $^Y p < 0.001$; $^\#$, *, $^\Delta p < 0.01$; $^\wedge p < 0.05$. **d** Expression of HSP70^{intracellular} (MFI): $^\#$, $^+$, ^{Y}, $^* p \leq 0.001$; ^{X}, $^\wedge p \leq 0.01$

Expression of SOD2 and HSP70^{surface} in non-stimulated and stimulated NK cells of the seniors and the young

The intracellular expression of the other cytoprotective protein SOD2 revealed a different pattern compared to the expression of SIRT1 and HSP70^{intracellular}. The NK cells of the oldest seniors appeared to be the most sensitive to the stimulation. We observed a significant increase in SOD2 expression after stimulation with IL-2 (twofold) and PMA with ionomycin (nearly fourfold) compared to non-stimulated cells (13.8 ± 2.69%) (Fig. 3a).

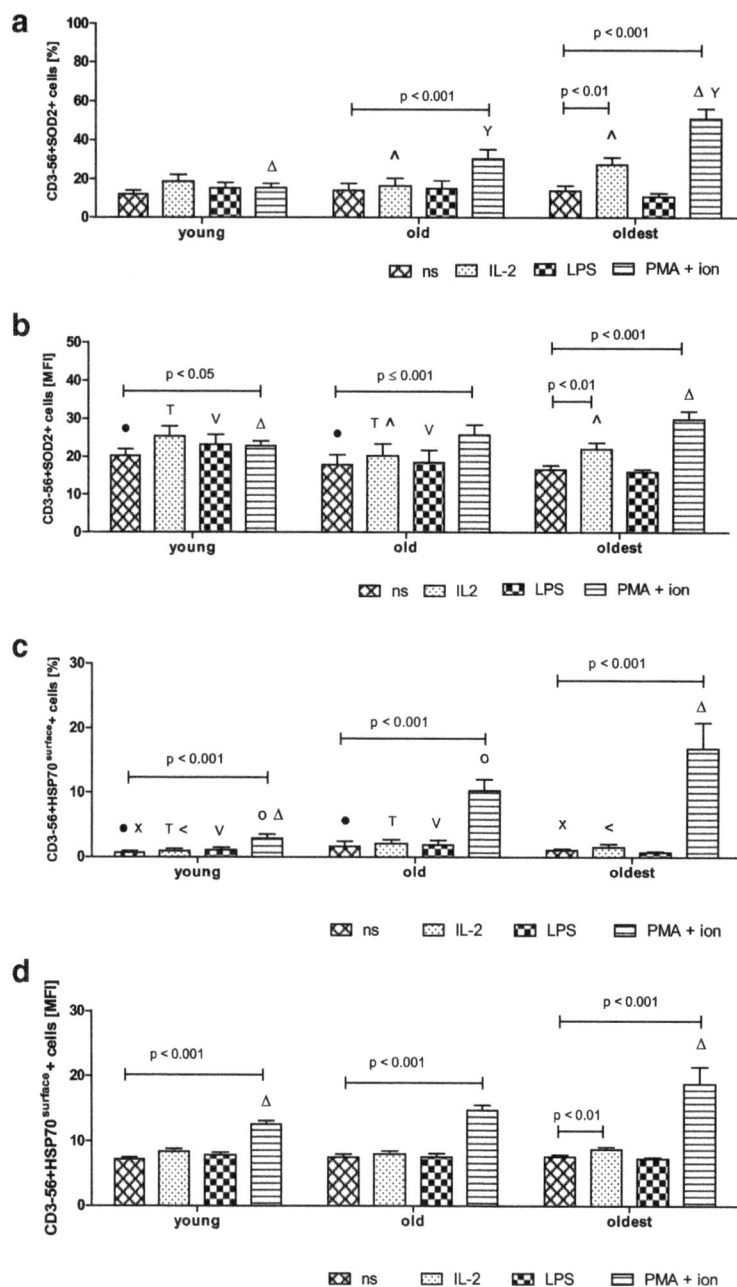

Fig. 3 Expression of SOD2 and surface HSP70 in non-stimulated and stimulated NK cells of the young, the old aged under 85 and the oldest seniors (aged over 85). Data are presented as means ± SEM and concern expression of the studied proteins in NK cells demonstrated as percentages of cells with expression of a particular protein (%) or mean fluorescence intensity (MFI). The same symbols over bars $^{X, <, \bullet, T, \circ, V,}$ $^{\wedge, \Delta, Y}$ denote statistically significant differences between similarly treated NK cells of different age groups (i.e. young vs old; young vs oldest or old vs oldest). Horizontal lines above paired bars denote statistically significant differences between treated and untreated NK cells of the same age group (i.e. non-stimulated vs stimulated with IL-2, LPS or PMA with ionomycin). **a** Expression of SOD2 (%): $^{\Delta}p < 0.001$; $^{\wedge, Y}p < 0.01$. **b** Expression of SOD2 (MFI): $^{T, \wedge, V}p < 0.01$; $^{\Delta, \bullet}p < 0.05$. **c** Expression of HSP70^{surface} (%): $^{X, \circ, \Delta}p < 0.001$; $^{T, <, V, \bullet}p < 0.01$. **d** Expression of HSP70^{surface} (MFI): $^{\Delta}p \leq 0.001$

In the elderly below 85 years NK cells were sensitive to the stimulation with PMA with ionomycin and revealed twofold increase in SOD2 expression compared to non-stimulated cells (14.0 ± 3.54%). In NK cells of the young, however, we did not observe any alterations in SOD2 expression after stimulation (Fig. 3a). These results were also confirmed by the measurements of the mean fluorescence intensity (MFI) (Fig. 3b). The only differences between these two analyses concerned the young subjects as NK cells of the young stimulated with PMA and ionomycin showed a significant increase in the expression level of SOD2 in the analysis of MFI (Fig. 3b).

The extracellular HSP70 (HSP70^{surface}) was expressed in NK cells of all age groups after stimulation at a very low level, comparable to resting NK cells, except for NK cells stimulated with PMA and ionomycin (Fig. 3c). The combination of these two agents increased the expression of HSP70^{surface} in all studied age groups: in the young fourfold, in the old sixfold and in the oldest nearly sixteen-fold compared to the level in non-stimulated cells; i.e. $0.66 \pm 0.27\%$ in the young, $1.65 \pm 0.76\%$ in the old and $1.07 \pm 0.21\%$ in the oldest (Fig. 3c). Similar results were obtained after the analysis of MFI parameter specific for the studied groups. This method revealed additionally the susceptibility of NK cells of the oldest seniors to the stimulation with IL-2 (Fig. 3d). LPS did not influence significantly the expression level of SOD2 and HSP70^{surface} (Fig. 3a-d).

Expression of TNF and IFN-γ in non-stimulated and stimulated NK cells of the seniors and the young

The expression of TNF in NK cells of all studied age groups increased significantly after stimulation with PMA and ionomycin; i.e. in the young nearly elevenfold and in the old and the oldest fourfold in relation to the level of non-stimulated cells (respectively $0.19 \pm 0.04\%$, $0.24 \pm 0.05\%$ and $0.37 \pm 0.06\%$,) (Fig. 4a). The similar results for all age groups were obtained after analysis of MFI in the studied samples (Fig. 4b).

The expression of IFN-γ in NK cells of all age groups increased after their stimulation with IL-2 and PMA with ionomycin compared to the low level detectable in non-stimulated cells, i.e. $1.47 \pm 0.13\%$ in the young, $2.74 \pm 0.7\%$ in the old and $4.5 \pm 0.95\%$ in the oldest. In the young the expression of IFN-γ increased sixfold after stimulation with PMA and ionomycin, in the old 1.5-fold after stimulation with IL-2 and twelvefold after stimulation with PMA and ionomycin, in the oldest 1.33-fold after stimulation with IL-2 and nearly fivefold after stimulation with PMA and ionomycin (Fig. 4c). The results of MFI analysis were comparable to data presenting the percentages of cells with the expression of the studied protein in all age groups. In the young, however, a significant increase in the expression of IFN-γ was observed additionally after stimulation with IL-2 (Fig. 4d). Similarly to the other studied proteins, LPS did not affect the expression level of TNF or IFN-γ (Fig. 4a-d).

Concentration of protein carbonyl groups and 8-isoprostanes in NK cell extracts from non-stimulated and stimulated NK cells of the seniors and the young

The highest concentration of carbonyl groups in the cultured NK cells was observed in the young (range $0.49 \pm 0.03 - 0.53 \pm 0.04$). It was significantly higher compared to the old (range $0.33 \pm 0.04 - 0.34 \pm 0.03$, except for non-stimulated cells) and the oldest (range $0.28 \pm 0.04 - 0.33 \pm 0.06$). Analysis of the related samples, i.e. non-stimulated vs stimulated showed that the process of NK cell stimulation did not influence the level of oxidative stress in these cells, as there were no significant changes in the concentration of carbonyl groups after applied treatments in the studied age groups (Fig. 5a).

Similar results were obtained after the analysis of the concentrations of 8-isoprostanes in NK cell extracts. The highest concentration of 8-isoprostanes was observed in the young in most of the analyzed samples (range $70.00 \pm 5.77 - 83.85 \pm 6.86$). It was significantly higher compared to the oldest (range $48.48 \pm 3.86 - 54.36 \pm 3.5$), except for samples treated with LPS. However, there were no significant differences between concentration of 8-isoprostanes in NK cell extracts of the young and the old or old and the oldest, except for senior cells treated with combination of PMA and ionomycin (old vs oldest) (Fig. 5b). The analysis of the related samples, i.e. non-stimulated vs stimulated showed that process of NK cell stimulation did not influence the level of oxidative stress in these cells, as there were no significant changes in the concentration of 8-isoprostanes after applied treatments in the studied age groups. The only significant difference was observed between non-stimulated and LPS-stimulated NK cells of the young (Fig. 5b).

Relationships between the analyzed parameters of NK cells stimulated in the same conditions within the studied age groups

Some relationships between expression levels of the analyzed cellular protective proteins, cytokines and concentrations of carbonyl groups and 8-isoprostanes in NK cells of the studied population were observed. Interestingly, very high positive correlations between SIRT1 and HSP70^{intracellular} in all NK cell samples, i.e. non-stimulated or treated with IL-2, LPS or PMA with ionomycin were noted. Low positive correlations were found also between the expression of SIRT1 and: (i) TNF (in all applied conditions), (ii) IFN-γ (in all conditions except for PMA + ionomycin), (iii) SOD2 (in samples stimulated with IL-2 and PMA with ionomycin) and HSP70^{surface} (in cells stimulated with IL-2) (Table 2).

The expression of HSP70^{intracellular} revealed relationships similar to these of SIRT1. Low positive correlations were found between the expression of this protein and: (i) TNF (in all applied conditions), (ii) IFN-γ (in all conditions except for PMA + ionomycin), (iii) SOD2 in samples stimulated with IL-2 and PMA + ionomycin and (iv) HSP70^{surface} (in cells stimulated with IL-2) (Table 2).

HSP70^{surface} expression correlated with: (i) SOD2 (moderate to high correlation in all applied conditions), (ii) TNF (in all applied conditions except for non-

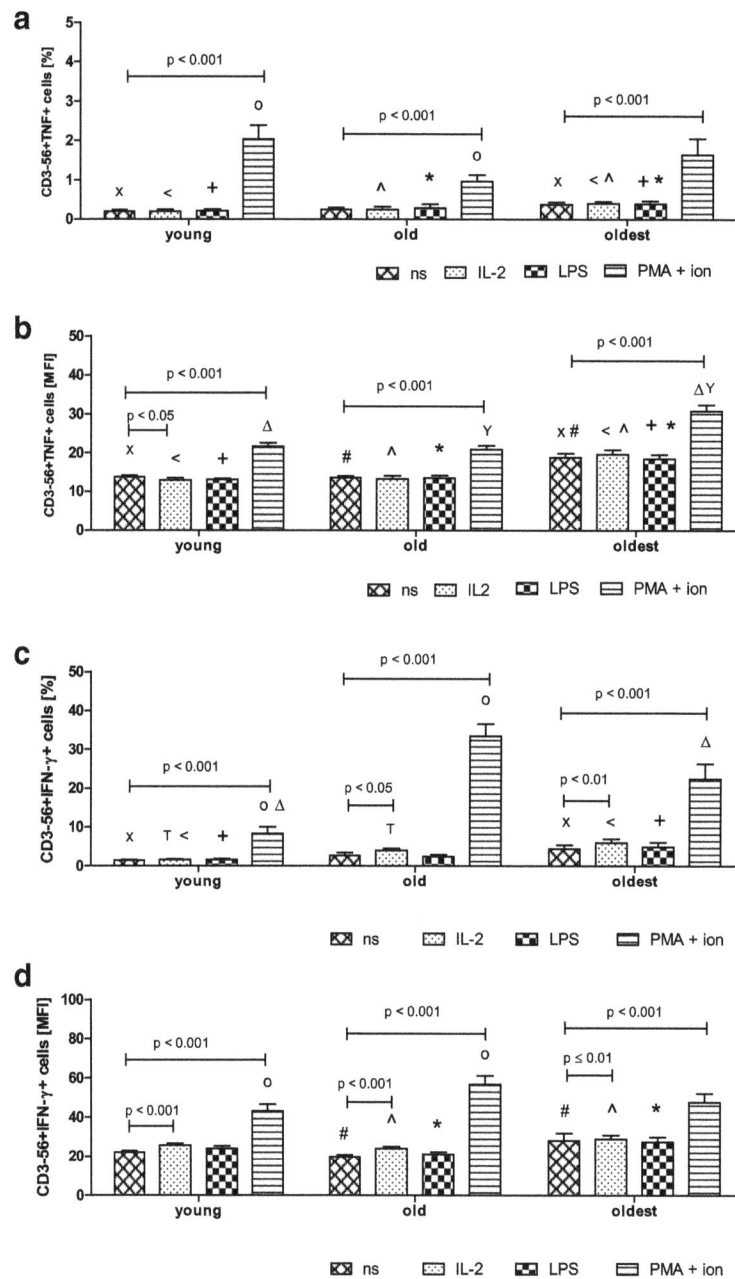

Fig. 4 Expression of TNF and IFN-γ in non-stimulated and stimulated NK cells of the young, the old aged under 85 and the oldest seniors (aged over 85). Data are presented as means ± SEM and concern expression of the studied proteins in NK cells demonstrated as percentages of cells with expression of a particular protein (%) or mean fluorescence intensity (MFI). The same symbols over bars $^{X, <, T, \circ, \wedge, \Delta, +, *, \#, Y}$ denote statistically significant differences between similarly treated NK cells of different age groups (i.e. young vs old; young vs oldest or old vs oldest). Horizontal lines above paired bars denote statistically significant differences between treated and untreated NK cells of the same age group (i.e. non-stimulated vs stimulated with IL-2, LPS or PMA with ionomycin): **a** Expression of TNF (%): $^{\wedge, <}$ $p \leq 0.001$; *, $^{X}p < 0.01$; $^{\circ,+}p < 0.05$. **b** Expression of TNF (MFI): $^{X, \#, <, \wedge, +, *, \Delta, Y}p < 0.001$. **c** Expression of IFN-γ (%): $^{<, \circ}$ $p < 0.001$; $^{\Delta, X, T}p < 0.01$; $^{+}p < 0.05$ **d** Expression of IFN-γ (MFI): $^{\#, *, \circ}$ $p \leq 0.01$; $^{\wedge}$ $p < 0.05$

stimulated NK cells) and (iii) IFN-γ (in cells stimulated with LPS). The expression of TNF correlated with: (i) SOD2 (in cells stimulated with PMA and ionomycin) and (ii) IFN-γ (in non-stimulated cells and cells treated with IL-2 and LPS). Low positive correlation was

observed also between IFN-γ and SOD2 in cells stimulated with LPS (Table 2).

Some relationships were also observed between concentration of carbonyl groups or 8-isoprostanes and the other studied parameters. Carbonyl groups revealed

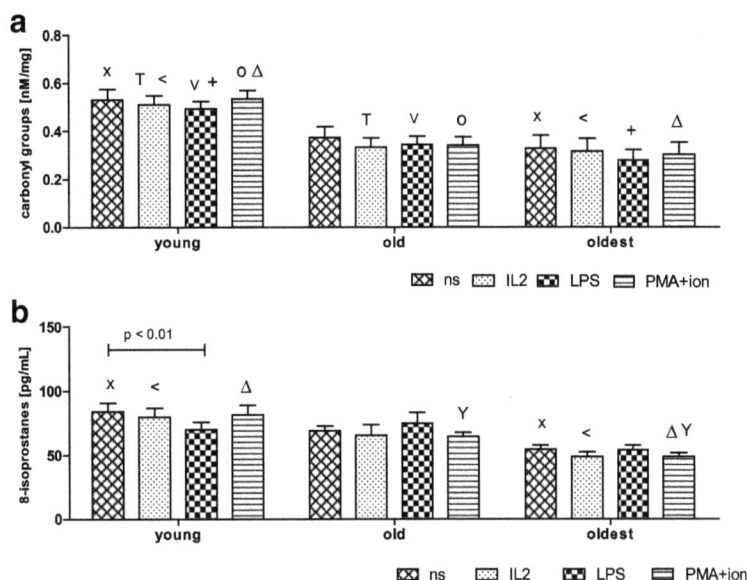

Fig. 5 Concentration of protein carbonyl groups and 8-isoprostanes in cell extracts prepared from non-stimulated and stimulated NK cells of the young, the old aged under 85 and the oldest (aged over 85). Data are presented as means ± SEM. The same symbols over bars $^{X}, ^{<}, ^{T}, ^{o}, ^{\Delta}, ^{V}, ^{+}$ denote statistically significant differences between similarly treated NK cells of different age groups (i.e. young vs old; young vs oldest or old vs oldest). Horizontal lines above paired bars denote statistically significant differences between treated and untreated NK cells of the same age group (i.e. non-stimulated vs stimulated with IL-2, LPS or PMA with ionomycin). **a** The concentration of protein carbonyl groups in cell extracts of NK cells expressed as nmol/mg protein: $^{\Delta}, ^{+}, ^{o}p \leq 0.01$; $^{X}, ^{T}, ^{<}, ^{V}p < 0.05$. **b.** The concentration of 8-isoprostanes in cell extracts of NK cells expressed as pg/mL: $^{<}, ^{\Delta}, ^{X}p \leq 0.001$; $^{Y}p < 0.05$

weak, negative correlations with: (i) SOD2 (in cells stimulated with PMA and ionomycin), (ii) HSP70[intracellular] (in non-stimulated and stimulated with PMA and ionomycin cells) and IFN-γ (in cells stimulated with LPS). Similarly, 8-isoprostanes showed weak, negative correlations with: (i) SIRT1 (in cells stimulated with LPS), (ii) HSP70[intracellular] (in non-stimulated cells), TNF (in non-stimulated and stimulated with IL-2 cells) (Table 2).

Relationships observed between the age and the analyzed parameters studied in non-stimulated and stimulated NK cells

Remarkably, the expression of SIRT1 and HSP70[intracellular-] showed similar positive correlations with age in all studied variants, except for the NK cells stimulated with IL-2. The expression of TNF revealed rather low to moderate positive correlations with age in all applied experimental conditions. Interestingly, the levels of both carbonyl groups and 8-isoprostanes in NK cells correlated negatively with age in non-stimulated cells and in all variants of stimulation except for LPS in tests concerning 8-isoprostanes (Table 3).

Discussion

The main finding of this study is that NK cells of the oldest seniors cultured for 2 days reveal high, constant level of stress response proteins expression, i.e. SIRT1

and HSP70 compared to seniors aged under 85 and the young people. Interestingly, the level of expression of SIRT1 and HSP70 in the oldest seniors did not change after stimulation of NK cells with various types of stimuli such as IL-2, LPS or PMA with ionomycin. On the contrary, the process of NK cell stimulation influenced significantly the expression level of SOD2 in the elderly, increasing with age of donors. The study shows also numerous correlations between the expression of cellular protective proteins in both stimulated and non-stimulated (control) NK cells and age of the study participants. Then, we provide some novel data concerning the influence of NK cell stimulation on the level of oxidative stress in these cells.

The study population was characterized by a slight increase in BMI observed in seniors, but the statistically significant differences were observed only between the young and both groups of seniors. The old and oldest participants did not differ significantly. These observations corresponded to the findings of the other authors who found that an increase in BMI was associated with ageing [47]. Then, the biochemical parameters of blood samples revealed some differences between age groups but they still remained within normal ranges [48]. These data support clinically reported good health of participants.

The results presented in the study correspond to our earlier observations concerning expression of cellular

Table 2 Correlation analysis of the study population

Parameter	Stimulation type	Compared parameter (after stimulation in the same conditions)						
		SOD2	SIRT1	HSP70^{intr}	HSP70^{surf}	TNF	IFN-γ	Carbonyl groups
SIRT1	none	ns						
	IL-2	0.222						
	LPS	ns						
	PMA/ion	0.231						
HSP70^{intr}	none	ns	0.967					
	IL-2	0.235	0.957					
	LPS	ns	0.975					
	PMA/ion	0.315	0.926					
HSP70^{surf}	none	0.694	ns	ns				
	IL-2	0.825	0.232	0.287				
	LPS	0.747	ns	ns				
	PMA/ion	0.652	ns	ns				
TNF	none	ns	0.406	0.445	ns			
	IL-2	ns	0.313	0.354	0.375			
	LPS	ns	0.390	0.403	0.276			
	PMA/ion	0.461	0.435	0.421	0.446			
IFN-γ	none	ns	0.415	0.464	ns	0.361		
	IL-2	ns	0.424	0.451	ns	0.301		
	LPS	0.257	0.371	0.421	0.369	0.368		
	PMA/ion	ns	ns	ns	ns	ns		
Carbonyl groups	none	ns	ns	−0.315	ns	ns	ns	
	IL-2	ns	ns	ns	ns	ns	ns	
	LPS	ns	ns	ns	ns	ns	− 0.346	
	PMA/ion	−0.313	ns	−0.33	ns	ns	ns	
8-Isoprostanes	none	ns	ns	−0.407	ns	−0.416	ns	ns
	IL-2	ns	ns	ns	ns	−0.437	ns	ns
	LPS	ns	−0.438	ns	ns	ns	ns	ns
	PMA/ion	ns	ns	ns	ns	ns	ns	ns

All values are presented as statistically significant ($p < 0.05$) Spearman's correlation coefficients (R). 'ns' denotes statistically not significant. '*HSP70^{intr}*' intracellular HSP70, '*HSP70^{surf}*' surface HSP70, '*PMA/ion*' PMA + ionomycin

Table 3 Correlation analysis of the study population: age vs the analyzed parameters

	Stimulation type	Compared parameter							
		SOD2	SIRT1	HSP70^{intr}	HSP70^{surf}	TNF	IFN-γ	Carbonyl groups	8-isoprostanes
Age	none	−0.225	0.301	0.300	ns	0.44	ns	−0.423	−0.584
	IL-2	ns	ns	ns	ns	0.478	0.242	−0.385	−0.685
	LPS	ns	0.417	0.409	ns	0.53	ns	−0.491	ns
	PMA/ion	ns	0.273	0.219	0.409	0.379	ns	−0.44	−0.555

All values are presented as statistically significant ($p < 0.05$) Spearman's correlation coefficients (R). 'ns' denotes statistically not significant. '*HSP70^{intr}*' - intracellular HSP70; '*HSP70^{surf}*' - surface HSP70; '*PMA/ion*' – PMA + ionomycin

protective proteins in NK cells analyzed shortly after blood sample collection [46]. It is noteworthy that non-stimulated NK cells of the oldest seniors both briefly after isolation and after culturing for 48 h presented significantly higher expression levels of both SIRT1 and HSP70^{intracellular} compared to seniors under 85 and the young. Interestingly, in NK cells cultured for 48 h the expression of SIRT1 was even higher compared to freshly analyzed cells [46]. This might have been caused by the cell culture-induced state of oxidative stress [49, 50]. Our data concerning SIRT1 expression corresponded to the level of oxidative stress we found in cells cultured in vitro and freshly isolated ones [46].

On the contrary to SIRT1, the increased expression of HSP70^{intracellular} was higher in freshly isolated NK cells in contrast to the cultured ones [46]. This phenomenon may result from different characteristics of transcription patterns of both *SIRT1* and *HSP72* genes resulting from particular signaling pathways being under control of distinct transcription factors [30, 32, 33, 51]. Expression of chaperons that protect cells against cellular stress is under control of heat shock factor-1 (HSF1), which is activated within minutes after appearance of the stress factor, e.g. increase in temperature. The following increase in mRNA expression was observed within 6 h after triggering of cellular stress signaling pathway [32–34]. Kinetics of *SIRT1* gene expression is different as SIRT1 was detected within 24 h [52, 53] or 48-96 h after exposure to a stress factor [54, 55].

Interestingly, the expression of both SIRT1 and HSP70 in NK cells of the oldest did not change independently on the type of a stimulatory agent. On the contrary, in the young and elderly under 85, NK cells were sensitive to stimulation with IL-2 and PMA with ionomycin. These observations may suggest the role of hormesis in the process of ageing. Increasing levels of markers of oxidative stress and proinflammatory state are characteristics of the process of immunosenescence and can activate an adaptive stress response that may positively affect the lifespan [56]. Heat shock proteins and sirtuins are both involved in cellular adaptive response [29]. E.g. Wang et al. showed in endothelial progenitor cells that SIRT1 protein level increased in response to oxidative stress [53].

Intriguingly, the expression level of SOD2 in cultured, non-stimulated NK cells was quite low and comparable for all age groups. NK cells of the oldest seniors revealed, however, the highest sensitivity to stimulation compared to the other age groups. We observed higher expression of SOD2 in freshly isolated cells [46] and lower in cultured ones and this increase in SOD2 expression might have been caused by the change of cellular environment during process of NK cell isolation. This characteristic pattern of SOD2 expression can result from specific kinetics of *SOD2* gene transcription. The increase in mRNA synthesis is observed within 1-2 h after stimulation, the peak of synthesis occurs 4 - 6 h after stimulation and then SOD2 gene expression decreases [57, 58].

The pattern of surface HSP70 expression resembled to some extent that of SOD2. It was quite low in non-stimulated NK cells and differed only slightly between age groups presenting higher expression in seniors. NK cells of the oldest revealed the highest sensitivity to stimulation compared to the other age groups. According to Multhoff and colleagues, the commercially available antibodies are not able to distinguish integrated in the cell membrane HSP70 proteins but they rather detect HSP70 bound to TLR receptors on the cell surface [59]. Interestingly, in our studies lower and higher levels of HSP70^{surface} seemed to correspond to lower (in cultured) and higher (in freshly isolated) levels of HSP70^{intracellular} expression [46]. However, the accurate analysis of the origin of the extracellular HSP70 was out of scope of the presented study.

NK cells cultured for 48 h without stimulation showed very low level of TNF expression, comparable between the young and the old and slightly higher in the oldest. In all age groups NK cells were sensitive to stimulation with PMA and ionomycin. Increased production of proinflammatory cytokines in the process of ageing in mononuclear cells was observed earlier [60]. It was related to the proinflammatory state that accompanies the process of ageing, illustrated by the CRP values increasing with age [41]. This increase was also noted in the studied population but it did not exceed the normal range [46].

Similarly, cultured NK cells showed low, comparable levels of IFN-γ in the young and the old and higher expression in the oldest. This expression increased then significantly after activation; i.e. stimulation with PMA and ionomycin in all age groups. The weaker increase, but also significant in comparison to the young was observed after stimulation with IL-2 in the old and especially in the oldest seniors. These results are in line with observations described by Hayhoe et al. who showed significantly raised level of IFN-γ expression in NK cells of individuals aged more than 60 years compared to younger counterparts [61]. However, Krishnaraj reported diminished in the elderly secretion of IFN-γ after stimulation of NK cells with IL-2 for 18 h in comparison to the young but this deficiency appeared to be overcome by prolonged stimulation with IL-2 (7-day culture) [62]. Le Garff-Tavernier and colleagues noticed impaired production of IFN-γ in non-stimulated NK cells of the older subjects, but activated with IL-2 NK cells of the oldest seniors showed recovering of NK-cell function [43].

The process of ageing is accompanied by the increased levels of oxidative stress [63]. In this context, we obtained interesting results concerning the level of oxidative stress in NK cells which corresponded to our previous results regarding freshly isolated cells [46]. The highest concentrations of both carbonyl groups and 8-isoprostanes in NK cells were observed in the young and they differed significantly from the oldest. In spite of significant differences between the concentrations of carbonyl groups, their levels did not exceed normal ranges found in cell lysates, i.e. 1.3 nmol/mg in MRC-5-fibroblasts [64], and human plasma, i.e. 1.83 ± 0.4 nmol/mg [65], although they were definitely higher than in freshly isolated cells. Given the background from the meta-analysis of data concerning the measurement of 8-isoprostanes in different tissues and with the use of various methods, we found that results we obtained in both the young and the oldest were still within the normal range as depending on the tissue they might differ enormously. Erve and coworkers estimated that on average, the concentration of 8-isoprostanes detected in the plasma was 39.5 ± 36.2 pg/mL [66]. Thus, we could conclude that in spite of some differences between age groups in the level of markers of oxidative stress, i.e. carbonyl groups or 8-isoprostanes, they were still within the normal range. The most intriguing in this study was the lower level of markers of oxidative stress in the group of seniors, especially in the oldest, in the context of "Oxidative Stress Theory of Aging" [67]. However, Ristow and Zarse noted that ROS production within the mitochondria could cause an adaptive response and generate increased stress resistance which could result in a long-term reduction of oxidative stress. This type of retrograde response was named mitohormesis [68]. Then, Ristow and Schmeisser found that ROS can act as essential signaling molecules to promote metabolic health and longevity [69].

As we found no differences between the non-stimulated and stimulated samples (except NK cells treated with LPS in the young), we could draw the conclusion that different methods of NK cell activation did not influence the level of oxidative stress in the cells. When we compared our results from the present study with data obtained in freshly isolated cells, we also noted, that the levels of oxidative stress in NK cells cultivated 48 h in vitro were higher compared to the levels detected in freshly isolated cells [46]. These data might suggest that cell culture increased the level of oxidative stress in cultivated cells and this phenomenon was discussed by Professor Barry Halliwell [50]. However, the increased concentrations of carbonyl groups or isoprostanes remained within the normal range [64–66]. In this context, results concerning the elevated expression levels of cellular protective proteins, i.e. SIRT1 and HSP70, in

the oldest, but not in the old or the young seemed to be even more interesting, because all the cells were cultured in the same conditions.

The present data related to the analysis of the relationships between the compared parameters corresponded to the results of our earlier study performed on freshly isolated NK cells [46]. Interestingly, positive correlations between two cellular protective proteins, i.e. SIRT1 and HSP70^{intracellular} were very high in cultured, both stimulated and non-stimulated NK cells. These relationships may corroborate the specific role of cellular protective proteins, involved in hormetic adaptive response [29]. Then, they correspond to results demonstrated by Westerheide et al., showing that SIRT1 directly deacetylates HSF1 (heat shock factor 1) and activates the cellular stress response [35]. The relationships between other protective proteins, i.e. SIRT1 and SOD2 showed rather low correlations in cells stimulated with IL-2 and PMA with ionomycin. Expression of SOD2 is under control of transcription factors of the FOXO family that promote the expression of stress response genes. SIRT1 activates several transcription factors of this family and some relationships between these two proteins have been reported [36, 56, 70].

We found rather low correlation coefficients between the expression of cellular protective proteins and cytokines in NK cells. The correlations were observed between SIRT1 and TNF (in all applied conditions) and between SIRT1 and IFN-γ (in all applied conditions except for PMA + ionomycin). NF-κB is a transcription factor responsible for the inflammatory response, which regulates expression of proinflammatory cytokines, e.g. IL-1, IL-6, TNF [15]. There is a regulatory loop between the expression of a cellular protective protein SIRT1 and the activity of transcription factor NF-κB, so that some relationships between SIRT1 and TNF have been reported [71, 72]. Of note, the synthesis of IFN-γ is under control of different transcription factors than TNF and subjected to the other mechanisms of regulation [73].

Interestingly, HSP70^{surface} revealed moderate to high positive correlation with SOD2. The expression of both proteins is controlled indirectly by SIRT1 so some positive feedback loops may also exist [35, 36, 56, 70]. Rather low positive correlations were observed also between HSP70^{surface} and TNF in all stimulated samples. These relationships may illustrate the proinflammatory state in activated NK cells characterized by increased level of TNF in response to increased level of surface HSP70.

Most of the analyzed parameters correlated with age, i.e. cellular protective proteins (SIRT1 and HSP70) and cytokines (TNF and IFN-γ) positively indicating their increase with age and markers of oxidative stress (carbonyl groups and 8-isoprostanes) negatively, showing their decrease with age. Our results correspond to data of the other groups concerning the increase in expression of SIRT1 in serum samples [74] and HSP70 in PBMCs [40] in the process of healthy ageing. They are also comparable with our previous results regarding the raise of concentration of proinflammatory cytokines; i.e. TNF and IL-6 in sera of the elderly [75]. The negative correlation between the level of oxidative stress and age seems to be surprising but it corresponds to conclusions presented by Ristow and Zarse concerning decrease in the level of oxidative stress resulting from cellular stress adaptive response to increased ROS formation in the process of ageing [68].

The advantage of our study is that although some relationships were already described earlier, i.e. between SIRT1 and HSP70, they concerned cell lines or animal models [35, 76]. We showed these relationships in cells isolated directly from human blood samples of participants recruited from different age groups. Moreover, we have demonstrated age-related changes in a specific population of lymphocytes, NK cells, which have yet not been studied regarding involvement of cellular protective proteins in the process of ageing.

Conclusions

Our study provides new data concerning ageing of the human immune system and the role of NK cells in this process. We analyzed NK cells isolated from peripheral blood samples of different age groups. The cells were subjected to various types of stimulation to compare their influence on the expression of both cellular protective proteins involved in the adaptive stress response and cytokines, secreted by NK cells after activation. It was found that NK cells of the oldest seniors, aged over 85, presented constant, resistant to further stimulation, increased level of cellular protective proteins involved in stress response, i.e. SIRT1 and HSP70. We also observed very high positive correlations between SIRT1 and HSP70^{intracellular} in cultured, both stimulated and non-stimulated NK cells, suggestive of a specific role of these proteins in cellular adaptive response. On the contrary, SOD2 did not present the high, constant expression level in NK cells but revealed susceptibility to stimulation increasing with the age of participants. High positive correlations between SOD2 and HSP70^{surface} expression indicated a distinct role of SOD2 in cellular stress response in ageing process. Moreover, NK cells, of seniors did not show an increased level of oxidative stress markers such as isoprostanes and carbonyl groups.

In summary, our novel data show that NK cells of the oldest seniors reveal increased adaptation to stress response, a phenomenon that may contribute to the long lifespan of this group of the elderly.

Abbreviations

ADL: Activities of daily living; CRP: C reactive protein; ERK: Extracellular signal-regulated kinase; FOXO: Forkhead transcription factor class O; GM-CSF: Granulocyte macrophage colony - stimulating factor; HSF: Heat shock factor; HSP: Heat shock protein; MCP: Macrophage chemoattractant protein; MFI: Mean fluorescence intensity; MIP: Macrophage inflammatory protein; MKK: Mitogen - activated protein kinase kinase; MMSE: Mini mental state examination; NF-κB: Nuclear factor kappa-light-chain-enhancer of activated B cells; NSAID: Non-steroid anti-inflammatory drug; PGC: Peroxisome proliferator - activated receptor gamma coactivator; PKC: Protein kinase C; PMA: Phorbol myristate acetate; RANTES: Regulated on activation, normal T cell expressed and secreted; SIRT: Sirtuin; SOD: Superoxide dismutase; STAT: Signal transducer and activator of transcription; TAC: Tetrameric antibody complexes; TLR: Toll-like receptor

Acknowledgements
Not applicable.

Funding
This study was supported by grant N N404 597640 from the National Science Centre (NCN, Poland) and by ST-12 internal funds of the Medical University of Gdańsk, Poland.

Authors' contributions
LK conceived the project, performed flow cytometry experiments, analyzed and interpreted the data and wrote the manuscript, JF qualified young and old subjects to the project and participated with DS and TŚ in project development, JJK performed measurements of carbonyl groups and isoprostanes, ZK supervised the project performance, analyzed the data and prepared with LK the final version of the article. All authors approved the final version of the manuscript.

Competing interests
The authors declare that they have no competing interests.

Author details
[1]Department of Histology, Medical University of Gdańsk, Dębinki 1, 80-211 Gdańsk, Poland. [2]Department of Social and Clinical Gerontology, Medical University of Gdańsk, Dębinki 1, 80-211 Gdańsk, Poland. [3]Department of Bioenergetics and Physiology of Exercise, Medical University of Gdańsk, Dębinki 1, 80-211 Gdańsk, Poland. [4]Department of Pharmacology, Medical University of Gdańsk, Dębowa 23, 80-204 Gdańsk, Poland.

References
1. Artis D, Spits H. The biology of innate lymphoid cells. Nature. 2015;517:293–301.
2. Cording S, Medvedovic J, Aychek T, Eberl G. Innate lymphoid cells in defense, immunopathology and immunotherapy. Nat Immunol. 2016;17:755–7.
3. Bryceson YT, Chiang SCC, Darmanin S, Fauriat C, Schlums H, Theorell J, Wood SM. Molecular mechanisms of natural killer cell activation. J Innate Immun. 2011;3:216–26.
4. Hazeldine J, Lord JM. The impact of ageing on natural killer cell function and potential consequences for health in older adults. Ageing Res Rev. 2013;12:1069–78.
5. Sun JC, Ugolini S, Vivier E. Immunological memory within the innate immune system. EMBO J. 2014;33:1295–303.
6. Vivier E, Raulet DH, Moretta A, Caligiuri MA, Zitvogel L, Lanier LL, Yokoyama WM, Ugolini S. Innate or adaptive immunity? The example of natural killer cells. Science. 2011;331:44–9.

7. De Maria A, Bozzano F, Cantoni C, Moretta L. Revisiting human natural killer cell subset function revealed cytolytic CD56(dim)CD16+ NK cells as rapid producers of abundant IFN-gamma on activation. Proc Natl Acad Sci U S A. 2011;108:728–32.

8. Fauriat C, Long EO, Ljunggren HG, Bryceson YT. Regulation of human NK-cell cytokine and chemokine production by target cell recognition. Blood. 2010;115:2167–76.

9. Mariani E, Meneghetti A, Neri S, Ravaglia G, Forti P, Cattini L, Facchini A. Chemokine production by natural killer cells from nonagenarians. Eur J Immunol. 2002;32:1524–9.

10. Yu TK, Caudell EG, Smid C, Grimm EA. IL-2 activation of NK cells: involvement of MKK1/2/ERK but not p38 kinase pathway. J Immunol. 2000;164:6244–51.

11. Goodier MR, Londei M. Lipopolysaccharide stimulates the proliferation of human CD56+CD3- NK cells: a regulatory role of monocytes and IL-10. J Immunol. 2000;165:139–47.

12. Varma TK, Lin CY, Toliver-Kinsky TE, Sherwood ER. Endotoxin-induced gamma interferon production: contributing cell types and key regulatory factors. Clin Diagn Lab Immunol. 2002;9:530–43.

13. Mian MF, Lauzon NM, Andrews DW, Lichty BD, Ashkar AA. FimH can directly activate human and murine natural killer cells via TLR4. Mol Ther. 2010;18:1379–88.

14. O'Connor GM, Hart OM, Gardiner CM. Putting the natural killer cell in its place. Immunology. 2006;117:1–10.

15. Bonizzi G, Karin M. The two NF-κB activation pathways and their role in innate and adaptive immunity. Trends Immunol. 2004;25:280–8.

16. Tamai R, Asai Y, Hashimoto M, Fukase K, Kusumoto S, Ishida H, Kiso M, Ogawa T. Cell activation by monosaccharide lipid a analogues utilizing toll-like receptor 4. Immunology. 2003;110:66–72.

17. Chopra RK, Nagel JE, Chrest FJ, Adler WH. Impaired phorbol ester and calcium ionophore induced proliferation of T cells from old humans. Clin Exp Immunol. 1987;70:456–62.

18. Good SR, Thieu VT, Mathur AN, Yu Q, Stritesky GL, Yeh N, O'Malley JT, Perumal NB, Kaplan MH. Temporal induction pattern of STAT4 target genes defines potential for Th1 lineage-specific programming. J Immunol. 2009;183:3839–47.

19. Chang HC, Guarente L. SIRT1 and other sirtuins in metabolism. Trends Endocrinol Metab. 2014;25:138–45.

20. Elpek KG, Rubinstein MP, Bellemare-Pelletier A, Goldrath AW, Turley SJ. Mature natural killer cells with phenotypic and functional alterations accumulate upon sustained stimulation with IL-15/IL-15Ralpha complexes. Proc Natl Acad Sci U S A. 2010;107:21647–52.

21. Kaszubowska L, Dettlaff-Pokora A, Hak L, Szarynska M, Ryba M, Mysliwska J, Mysliwski A. Successful ageing of nonagenarians is related to the sensitivity of NK cells to activation. J Physiol Pharmacol. 2008;59(Suppl 9):187–99.

22. Liu Z, Kharmate G, Patterson E, Khan MM. Role of H1 receptors in histamine-mediated up- regulation of STAT4 phosphorylation. Int Immunopharmacol. 2006;6:485–93.

23. Wendt K, Wilk E, Buyny S, Buer J, Schmidt RE, Jacobs R. Gene and protein characteristics reflect functional diversity of CD56dim and CD56bright NK cells. J Leukoc Biol. 2006;80:1529–41.

24. Bueno V, Sant'Anna OA, Lord JM. Ageing and myeloid-derived suppressor cells: possible involvement in immunosenescence and age-related disease. Age (Dordr). 2014;36:9729.

25. Franceschi C, Bonafe M, Valensin S, Olivieri F, De Luca M, Ottaviani E, De Benedictis G. Inflamm-aging. An evolutionary perspective on immunosenescence. Ann N Y Acad Sci. 2000;908:244–54.

26. Barja G. Free radicals and aging. Trends Neurosci. 2004;27:595–600.

27. De la Fuente M, Miquel J. An update of the oxidation-inflammation theory of aging: the involvement of the immune system in oxi-inflamm-aging. Curr Pharm Des. 2009;15:3003–26.

28. Calabrese EJ, Baldwin LA. Defining hormesis. Hum Exp Toxicol. 2002;21:91–7.

29. Calabrese V, Cornelius C, Dinkova-Kostova AT, Iavicoli I, Di Paola R, Koverech A, Cuzzocrea S, Rizzarelli E, Calabrese EJ. Cellular stress responses, hormetic phytochemicals and vitagenes in aging and longevity. Biochim Biophys Acta. 2012;1822:753–83.

30. Hwang JW, Yao H, Caito S, Sundar IK, Rahman I. Redox regulation of SIRT1 in inflammation and cellular senescence. Free Radic Biol Med. 2013;61:95–110.

31. Saunders LR, Verdin E. Stress response and aging. Science. 2009;323:1021–2.

32. Hensen SM, Heldens L, Van Genesen ST, Pruijn GJ, Lubsen NH. A delayed antioxidant response in heat-stressed cells expressing a non-DNA binding HSF1 mutant. Cell Stress Chaperones. 2013;18:455–73.

33. Östling P, Björk JK, Roos-Mattjus P, Mezger V, Sistonen L. Heat shock factor 2 (HSF2) contributes to inducible expression of hsp genes through interplay with HSF1. J Biol Chem. 2007;282:7077–86.

34. Rossi A, Trotta E, Brandi R, Arisi I, Coccia M, Santoro MG. AIRAP, a new human heat shock gene regulated by heat shock factor 1. J Biol Chem. 2010;285:13607–15.

35. Westerheide SD, Anckar J, Stevens SM Jr, Sistonen L, Morimoto RI. Stress-inducible regulation of heat shock factor 1 by the deacetylase SIRT1. Science. 2009;323:1063–6.

36. Hori YS, Kuno A, Hosoda R, Horio Y. Regulation of FOXOs and p53 by SIRT1 modulators under oxidative stress. PLoS One. 2013;8:e73875.

37. Morgan MJ, Liu Z. Crosstalk of reactive oxygen species and NF-κB signaling. Cell Res. 2011;21:103–15.

38. Owczarz M, Budzinska M, Domaszewska-Szostek A, Borkowska J, Polosak J, Gewartowska M, Slusarczyk P, Puzianowska-Kuznicka M. miR-34a and miR-9 are overexpressed and SIRT genes are downregulated in peripheral blood mononuclear cells of aging humans. Exp Biol Med. 2017;242:1453–61.

39. Kovalenko EI, Boyko AA, Semenkov VF, Lutsenko GV, Grechikhina MV, Kanevskiy LM, Azhikina TL, Telford WG, Sapozhnikov AM. ROS production, intracellular HSP70 levels and their relationship in human neutrophils: effects of age. Oncotarget. 2014;5:11800–12.

40. Njemini R, Bautmans I, Lambert M, Demanet C, Mets T. Heat shock proteins and chemokine/cytokine secretion profile in ageing and inflammation. Mech Ageing Dev. 2007;128:450–4.

41. Singh T, Newman AB. Inflammatory markers in population studies of ageing. Ageing Res Rev. 2011;10:319–29.

42. Gayoso I, Sanchez-Correa B, Campos C, Alonso C, Pera A, Casado JG, Morgado S, Tarazona R, Solana R. Immunosenescence of human natural killer cells. J Innate Immun. 2011;3:337–43.

43. Le Garff-Tavernier M, Beziat V, Decocq J, Siguret V, Gandjbakhch F, Pautas E, Debré P, Merle-Beral H, Vieillard V. Human NK cells display major phenotypic and functional changes over the lifespan. Aging Cell. 2010;9:527–35.

44. Folstein MF, Folstein SE, McHugh PR. "Mini-mental state". A practical method for grading the cognitive state of patients for the clinician. J Psychiatr Res. 1975;12:189–98.

45. Katz S, Ford AB, Moskowitz RW, Jackson BA, Jaffe MW. Studies of illness in the aged. The index of ADL: a standardized measure of biological and psychosocial function. JAMA. 1963;185:914–9.

46. Kaszubowska L, Foerster J, Kaczor JJ, Schetz D, Ślebioda TJ, Kmieć Z. Expression of cellular protective proteins SIRT1, HSP70 and SOD2 correlates with age and is significantly higher in NK cells of the oldest seniors. Immun Ageing. 2017;14:3.

47. Hajek A, König HH. The longitudinal association between informal caregiving and body mass index in the second half of life: findings of the German ageing survey. Public Health. 2017;151:81–6.

48. Merck Manual Professional Version. Normal Laboratory Values. http://www.merckmanuals.com/en-pr/professional/appendixes/normal-laboratory-values/blood-tests-normal-values. Accessed 30 Jan 2018.

49. Halliwell B. Biochemistry of oxidative stress. Biochem Soc Trans. 2007;35:1147–50.

50. Halliwell B. Oxidative stress in cell culture: an under-appreciated problem? FEBS Lett. 2003;540:3–6.

51. Chen X, Lu Y, Zhang Z, Wang J, Yang H, Liu G. Intercellular interplay between Sirt1 signalling and cell metabolism in immune cell biology. Immunology. 2015;145:455–67.

52. Kauppinen A, Suuronen T, Ojala J, Kaarniranta K, Salminen A. Antagonistic crosstalk between NF- kB and SIRT1 in the regulation of inflammation and metabolic disorders. Cell Signal. 2013;25:1939–48.

53. Wang YQ, Cao Q, Wang F, Huang LY, Sang TT, Liu F, Chen SY. SIRT1 protects against oxidative stress-induced endothelial progenitor cells apoptosis by inhibiting FOXO3a via FOXO3a ubiquitination and degradation. J Cell Physiol. 2015;230:2098–107.

54. Belloni L, Pollicino T, De Nicola F, Guerrieri F, Raffa G, Fanciulli M, Raimondo G, Levrero M. Nuclear HBx binds the HBV minichromosome and modifies the epigenetic regulation of cccDNA function. Proc Natl Acad Sci U S A. 2009;106:19975–9.

55. Yun JM, Chien A, Jialal I, Devaraj S. Resveratrol up-regulates SIRT1 and inhibits cellular oxidative stress in the diabetic milieu: mechanistic insights. J Nutr Biochem. 2012;23:699–705.

56. Merksamer PI, Liu Y, He W, Hirschey MD, Chen D, Verdin E. The sirtuins, oxidative stress and aging: an emerging link. Aging. 2013;5:144–50.

57. Kamiński MM, Röth D, Sass S, Sauer SW, Krammer PH, Gülow K. Manganese superoxide dismutase: a regulator of T cell activation-induced oxidative signaling and cell death. Biochim Biophys Acta. 1823;2012:1041–52.

58. Kaszubowska L, Wierzbicki PM, Karsznia S, Damska M, Ślebioda TJ, Foerster J, Kmieć Z. Optimal reference genes for qPCR in resting and activated human NK cells–flow cytometric data correspond to qPCR gene expression analysis. J Immunol Methods. 2015;422:125–9.

59. Multhoff G, Hightower LE. Distinguishing integral and receptor-bound heat shock protein 70 (Hsp70) on the cell surface by Hsp70-specific antibodies. Cell Stress Chaperones. 2011;16:251–5.

60. Fagiolo U, Cossarizza A, Scala E, Fanales-Belasio E, Ortolani C, Cozzi E, Monti D, Franceschi C, Paganelli R. Increased cytokine production in mononuclear cells of healthy elderly people. Eur J Immunol. 1993;23:2375–8.

61. Hayhoe RP, Henson SM, Akbar AN, Palmer DB. Variation of human natural killer cell phenotypes with age: identification of a unique KLRG1-negative subset. Hum Immunol. 2010;71:676–81.

62. Krishnaraj R. Senescence and cytokines modulate the NK cell expression. Mech Ageing Dev. 1997;96:89–101.

63. Cui H, Kong Y, Zhang H. Oxidative stress, mitochondrial dysfunction, and aging. J Signal Transduct. 2012. https://doi.org/10.1155/2012/646354.

64. Sitte N, Merker K, Grune T. Proteasome-dependent degradation of oxidized proteins in MRC-5 fibroblasts. FEBS Lett. 1998;440:399–402.

65. Adams S, Green P, Claxton R, Simcox S, Williams MV, Walsh K, Leeuwenburgh C. Reactive carbonyl formation by oxidative and non-oxidative pathways. Front Biosci. 2001;6:A17–24.

66. Van 't Erve TJ, Kadiiska MB, London SJ, Mason RP. Classifying oxidative stress by F2-isoprostane levels across human diseases: a meta-analysis. Redox Biol. 2017;12:582–99.

67. Hagen TM. Oxidative stress, redox imbalance, and the aging process. Antioxid Redox Signal. 2003;5:503–6.

68. Ristow M, Zarse K. How increased oxidative stress promotes longevity and metabolic health: the concept of mitochondrial hormesis (mitohormesis). Exp Gerontol. 2010;45:410–8.

69. Ristow M, Schmeisser S. Extending life span by increasing oxidative stress. Free Radic Biol Med. 2011;51:327–36.

70. Brunet A, Sweeney LB, Sturgill JF, Chua KF, Greer PL, Lin Y, Tran H, Ross SE, Mostoslavsky R, Cohen HY, Hu LS, Cheng HL, Jedrychowski MP, Gygi SP, Sinclair DA, Alt FW, Greenberg ME. Stress-dependent regulation of FOXO transcription factors by the SIRT1 deacetylase. Science. 2004;303:2011–5.

71. Katto J, Engel N, Abbas W, Herbein G, Mahlknecht U. Transcription factor NFκB regulates the expression of the histone deacetylase SIRT1. Clin Epigenetics. 2013;5:11.

72. Yang H, Zhang W, Pan H, Feldser HG, Lainez E, Miller C, Leung S, Zhong Z, Zhao H, Sweitzer S, Considine T, Riera T, Suri V, White B, Ellis JL, Vlasuk GP, Loh C. SIRT1 activators suppress inflammatory responses through promotion of p65 deacetylation and inhibition of NF-κB activity. PLoS One. 2012;7:e46364.

73. Nakayama A, Kawasaki H, Jin C, Munekata E, Taira K, Yokoyama KK. Transcriptional regulation of interferon gamma gene by p300 co-activator. Nucleic Acids Res Suppl. 2001;1:89–90.

74. Kilic U, Gok O, Erenberk U, Dundaroz MR, Torun E, Kucukardali Y, Elibol-Can B, Uysal O, Dundar T. A remarkable age-related increase in SIRT1 protein expression against oxidative stress in elderly: SIRT1 gene variants and longevity in human. PLoS One. 2015;10:e0117954.

75. Kaszubowska L, Kaczor JJ, Hak L, Dettlaff-Pokora A, Szarynska M, Kmiec Z. Sensitivity of natural killer cells to activation in the process of ageing is related to the oxidative and inflammatory status of the elderly. J Physiol Pharmacol. 2011;62:101–9.

76. Liu DJ, Hammer D, Komlos D, Chen KY, Firestein BL, Liu AY. SIRT1 knockdown promotes neural differentiation and attenuates the heat shock response. J Cell Physiol. 2014;229:1224–35.

Crocetin attenuates inflammation and amyloid-β accumulation in APPsw transgenic mice

Jin Zhang[†], Yuchao Wang[*†], Xueshuang Dong and Jianghua Liu

Abstract

Background: Crocetin, an agent derived from saffron, has multiple pharmacological properties, such as neuroprotective, anti-oxidant, and anti-inflammatory actions. These properties might benefit the treatment of Alzheimer's disease (AD). In the present study, we tested whether crocetin attenuates inflammation and amyloid-β (Aβ) accumulation in APPsw transgenic mice, AD mouse models. Cell viability and the levels of Aβ40 and Aβ42 in HeLa cells stably transfected with Swedish mutant APP751 were evaluated. Mice with Swedish mutant APP751 transgene were used as transgenic mouse models of AD, and were orally administrated with crocetin. Aβ protein and inflammatory cytokines were measured with ELISA. NF-κB and P53 were measured with western blot assay. Learning and memory were analyzed with Morris water maze and novel object recognition tests.

Results: Crocetin significantly reduced Aβ40 and Aβ42 secretion in Hela cells without effecting cell viability. In AD transgenic mice, crocetin significantly reduced the pro-inflammatory cytokines and enhanced anti-inflammatory cytokine in plasma, suppressed NF-κB activation and P53 expression in the hippocampus, decreased Aβ in various brain areas, and improved learning and memory deficits.

Conclusion: Crocetin improves Aβ accumulation-induced learning and memory deficit in AD transgenic mice, probably due to its anti-inflammatory and anti-apoptotic functions.

Keywords: Crocetin, Alzheimer's disease (AD), Aβ accumulation, NF-κB, P53

Background

Alzheimer's disease (AD) is a progressive age-related neurodegenerative disorder that heavily affects the hippocampus and the cerebral cortex. Its major manifestations include progressive cognitive deficits, alterations of personality, and behavioral disturbances [1–3]. Accumulation of toxic amyloid beta (Aβ) plaques in extracellular spaces and neurofibrillary tangles in neurons are the most important neuropathological hallmarks of AD [1].

Substantial evidence demonstrates the involvement of inflammatory reaction in AD [4, 5]. For instance, Aβ amyloids within the central nervous system are able to activate microglia, followed by initiation of a pro-inflammatory cascade that in turn induces the release of potentially neurotoxic substances, including cytokines, chemokines,

reactive oxygen and nitrogen species, and various proteolytic enzymes, ultimately results in neurodegeneration [5, 6]. Moreover, activation of microglia may lead to accumulation of Aβ and formation of neurofibrillary tangles [6, 7]. Reversely, epidemiological observations also show that patients receiving various non-steroidal anti-inflammatory drugs (NSAIDs) for diverse systemic inflammatory disorders have a lower incidence and prevalence of AD [8]. Based on these findings, one of current strategies is to use anti-inflammatory drugs to down-regulate the inflammation in AD. Although long-term use of NSAIDs consistently reduces the relative risk of AD, it often incurs undesirable side-effects on the gastrointestinal tract, liver, kidney, and heart, etc. [9–11]. On the contrary, some natural herbal alternatives possessing anti-inflammatory property while having the least adverse effects may provide ideal therapeutic benefits to neurodegenerative diseases, including AD.

* Correspondence: mingyueweixiao123@163.com
[†]Jin Zhang and Yuchao Wang contributed equally to this work.
Department of Neurology, Daqing Oilfield General Hospitals, No. 9 Zhongkang Road, Daqing 163001, China

Crocetin, a natural apocarotenoid dicarboxylic acid and a derivative from saffron, has been known to exert multiple benefits, such as, anti-cancer, anti-oxidant [12], anti-inflammatory [13], anti-apoptotic [14], and neuroprotective effects [15]. Crocetin has been reported to inhibit Aβ fibrillization and stabilize Aβ oligomers [16]. However, crocetin's anti-inflammatory effect against Aβ accumulation and cognitive deficit in AD mouse models has not yet been investigated.

In this study, we investigated the effect of crocetin on Aβ production, learning and memory function, inflammation and apoptosis-related protein expressions in APPsw transgenic mouse AD models. Our results support that crocetin might have therapeutic potentials for AD.

Results

Crocetin reduced Aβ secretion in both in vitro and in vivo conditions

We tested whether crocetin affects the production of Aβ42 and Aβ40. To analyze production of Aβ42 and Aβ40, we used Hela cells as an in vitro model, and transfected these cells with plasmids containing DNA of APPsw. First, we examined toxic effects of crocetin on Hela cells, and found that exposure of 10, 20, and 40 μM crocetin to the Hela cells transfected with APPsw up to 8 h did not reduce cell viability (Fig. 1a). When the exposure duration increased to 24 h, no obvious change of cell viability could be found (Additional file 1: Figure S1A). Please note that crocetin exposure for 24 h did not affect cell viability significantly in control Hela cells as well (Additional file 1: Figure S1B). After incubation of successfully transfected Hela cells with concentrations of crocetin for 8 h, the levels of both Aβ42 (Fig. 1b) and Aβ40 (Fig. 1c) in culture medium were decreased in a concentration-dependent manner. The data indicate that crocetin reduces secretion of Aβ42 and Aβ40, and this effect is not due to loss of Aβ42 and Aβ40 producing cells. Further study shows that crocetin treatment for

24 h had no effect on APP protein expressions in the Hela cells transfected with APPsw (Additional file 1: Figure S1C).

We next utilized APP-SW transgenic mice as an AD model [17]. Crocetin (10 and 30 mg/kg/day) and saline was administered to adult transgenic mice (9 months old) for 6 months. We confirmed that 15 months old transgenic mice exhibited higher levels of insoluble Aβs in the hippocampus (Fig. 2a), the cerebral cortex (Fig. 2b), and the cerebellum (Fig. 2c), than wild-type mice. Crocetin at the dosage of 30 mg/kg/day ($n = 6$), but not 10 mg/kg/day ($n = 10$), reduced the levels of insoluble Aβs in the hippocampus, the cerebral cortex and the cerebellum (Fig. 2a, b and c), compared with the transgenic mice, received administration of saline only (control; $n = 10$). The data provide in vivo evidence showing that crocetin is capable of decreasing secretion of insoluble Aβs, consistent with our in vitro data shown in Fig. 1.

Crocetin improved learning and memory in transgenic AD mouse models

We next employed Morris Water Maze to test whether crocetin improves deficits in the acquisition and retrieval of memory in transgenic AD mouse models. We observed that the time wild-type mice (WT) spent in finding the escaping platform gradually decreased with training trials, while the transgenic mice lost this trend (Fig. 3a). Interestingly, long-term administration of crocetin (10 and 30 mg/kg/day) improved the performance of transgenic mice during training sessions (Fig. 3a). After the training sessions, the escaping platform was removed, and we recorded the time the mice spent in the target quarter where the escaping platform had existed. As illustrated in Fig. 3b, after chronic administration of crocetin at 30 mg/kg/day, but not 10 mg/kg/day, transgenic mice lingered longer in the target quarter. Therefore,

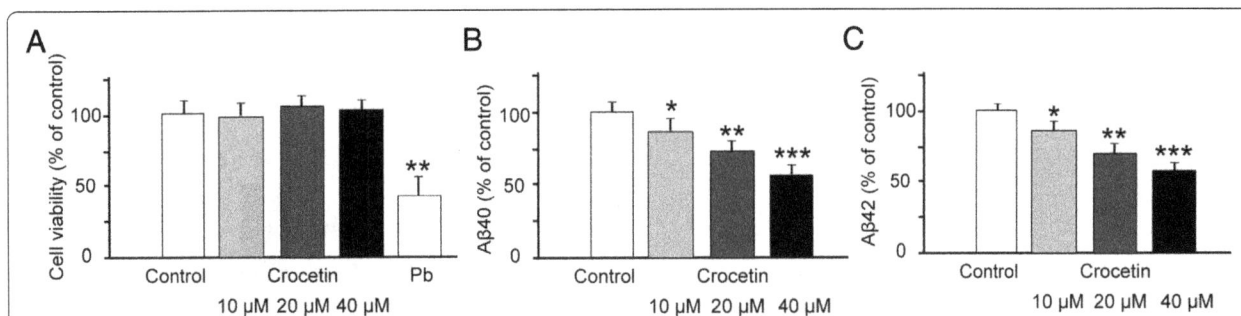

Fig. 1 Effect of crocetin on cell viability and the levels of Aβ42 and Aβ40 in APPsw-transfected cells. Cells were treated with crocetin at the indicated concentrations for 8 h. Pb (80 mg/L) was employed as a positive control. Cell viability was measured using MTT assay, and the levels of Aβ42 and Aβ40 in cultured medium were measured using a sandwich ELISA. Crocetin did not affect the viability of APPsw-transfected cells (a), but reduced the levels of Aβ40 (b) and Aβ42 (c) in a dose-dependent manner. ($n = 4$) * $p < 0.05$; ** $p < 0.01$; *** $p < 0.001$

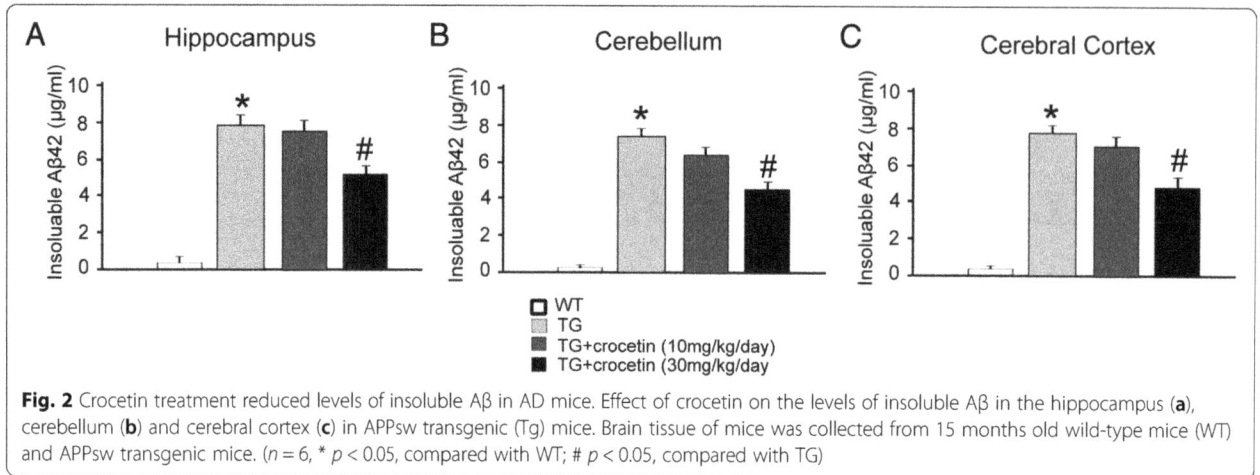

Fig. 2 Crocetin treatment reduced levels of insoluble Aβ in AD mice. Effect of crocetin on the levels of insoluble Aβ in the hippocampus (**a**), cerebellum (**b**) and cerebral cortex (**c**) in APPsw transgenic (Tg) mice. Brain tissue of mice was collected from 15 months old wild-type mice (WT) and APPsw transgenic mice. ($n = 6$, * $p < 0.05$, compared with WT; # $p < 0.05$, compared with TG)

chronic administration of crocetin improved memory acquisition and retrieval in AD mice.

To further confirm the benefits of crocetin to cognitive deficits in AD mouse model, we performed novel object recognition task, another behavioral paradigm to evaluate cognitive function [18]. In this task, the mice were exposed to two identical objects, then one object was replaced by a novel object. If the mice memorized the familiar objects well, they will explore the novel object more than the familiar one. The wild-type mice showed > 80% time exploring novel object (memory index), while APPsw transgenic mice showed less than 40% time exploring novel object, representing memory deficits (Fig. 4). After receiving chronic administration of crocetin (30 mg/kg/day), the transgenic mice explored the novel object longer than transgenic mice received saline treatment (Fig. 4). Consistent with our findings in Morris water maze, the novel object recognition test further supports the notion that crocetin improves cognitive function in AD mouse models.

Crocetin inhibited apoptosis-related protein expressions and inflammatory reaction in transgenic AD mouse models

As inflammation is a major cause of amyloid plaque deposition, we hypothesize that crocetin may counteract this process by reversing inflammatory reaction in the hippocampus. We did observe that NF-κB-p65 were increased in transgenic mice, and crocetin (30 mg/kg/day) dramatically attenuated the increase in transgenic mice (Fig. 5a, b). Interestingly, we also observed that the transgenic mice exhibited elevated p53 levels in the hippocampus, which may suggest the existence of enhanced apoptosis; while crocetin reversed this alteration (Fig. 5a, c). Of note, Aβ plaques were decreased after crocetin treatment in the AD mice (Additional file 1: Figure S2).

We also examined the levels of pro-inflammatory cytokines, including TNF-α, IL-1β, IL-8, and IL-6 in plasma to test whether crocetin attenuates inflammatory reaction in the transgenic AD mouse models (Fig. 6a-d). In the transgenic mice, the levels of these cytokines were tens of folds higher than wild-type mice (Fig. 6), while

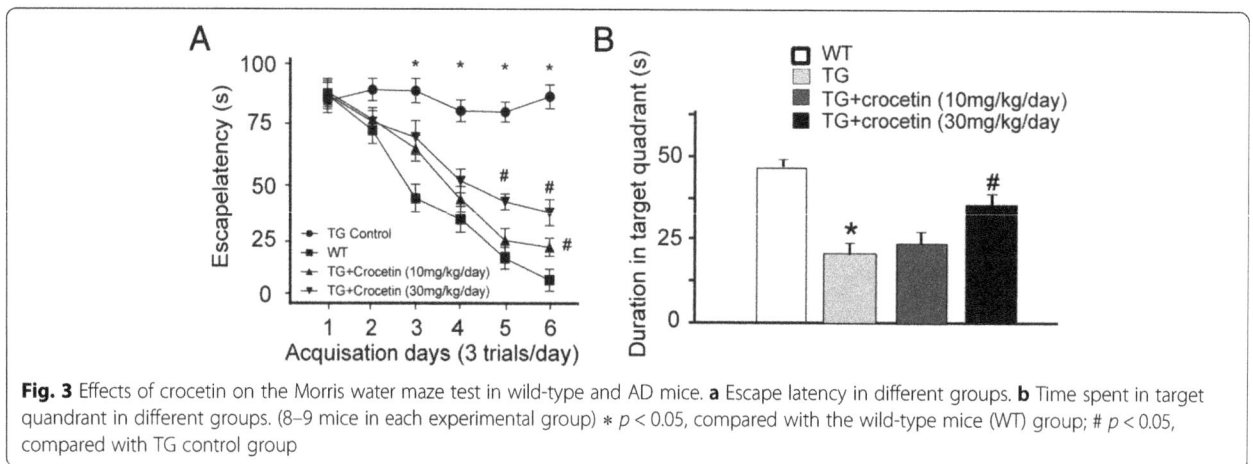

Fig. 3 Effects of crocetin on the Morris water maze test in wild-type and AD mice. **a** Escape latency in different groups. **b** Time spent in target quandrant in different groups. (8–9 mice in each experimental group) * $p < 0.05$, compared with the wild-type mice (WT) group; # $p < 0.05$, compared with TG control group

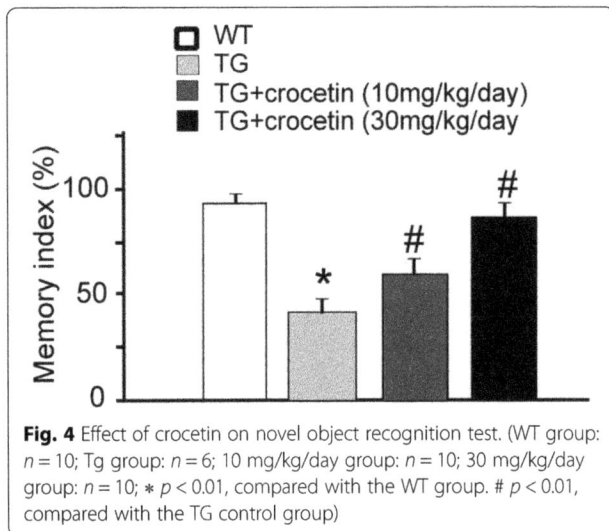

Fig. 4 Effect of crocetin on novel object recognition test. (WT group: n = 10; Tg group: n = 6; 10 mg/kg/day group: n = 10; 30 mg/kg/day group: n = 10; * p < 0.01, compared with the WT group. # p < 0.01, compared with the TG control group)

crocetin (10 and 30 mg/kg/day) reduced the levels of these pro-inflammatory cytokines by 30–40%. Also, IL-10 levels, as an anti-inflammatory cytokine, were increased in the transgenic AD mice, while crocetin treatment further enhanced IL-10 levels (Fig. 6e).

The data in Figs. 5 and 6 suggest that crocetin attenuates inflammatory reactions in APPsw transgenic mice.

Discussion

As previously reported [17], we observed that the transgenic mice carry a human familial AD gene (amyloid precursor protein with the "Swedish" double mutation, and display age-related Aβ plaque (Fig. 2), quantifiable inflammatory response (Figs. 5 and 6), and memory deficits (Figs. 3 and 4), confirming that the transgenic mice can be valid AD models. Given that crocetin has multiple pharmacological targets [19], potential mechanisms underlying crocetin treatment of AD may be multifactorial. In the present study, we demonstrated that oral

administration of crocetin significantly reduced insoluble Aβ, and improve learning and memory in transgenic AD mouse models. Moreover, crocetin treatment significantly attenuated the production of plasma pro-inflammatory cytokines and reversed upregulation of NF-κB P65 subunit and P53 in the hippocampus of the AD mouse models. These results indicated that crocetin improves learning and memory deficit in AD mice probably due to its modulation of multiple processes, including neuroinflammation, peripheral inflammation.

Crocetin (30 mg/kg) treatment significantly lowered both insoluble Aβ42 and soluble Aβ40 in vitro (Fig. 1), and overall insoluble amyloid in different brain areas in aged transgenic AD mice (Fig. 2). These findings were consistent with previous observations showing that crocetin improves insoluble Aβ degradation [20] and inhibit Aβ fibrillization [16]. The behavioral benefits of crocetin to AD transgenic mice (Figs. 3 and 4) are also consistent with previously reported therapeutic efficacy of saffron in memory deficits seen in AD patients [21, 22]. Our results suggest that crocetin could be an important component in saffron that possesses therapeutic values for AD.

Immune system has modulatory effect on learning and memory. Chronic inflammation in AD, featured by elevated TNF-α, IL-1β, and IL-6, may play critical roles in deterioration of learning and memory [4, 5, 23, 24]. Crocetin is a potent anti-inflammatory compound, at least partially due to its NSAID-mimetic nature, including inhibition of inflammatory cytokines [25], induction of nitric oxide synthase (iNOS) [26], and generation of NF-κB [27]. We observed that crocetin (30 mg/kg/day) was effective in significantly lowering plasma levels of pro-inflammatory cytokines, such as TNF-α, IL-1β, IL-6 and IL-8, while it increased the anti-inflammatory cytokine IL-10. At this dose, the AD transgenic mice showed improvement in learning and memory. These results suggest that the beneficial

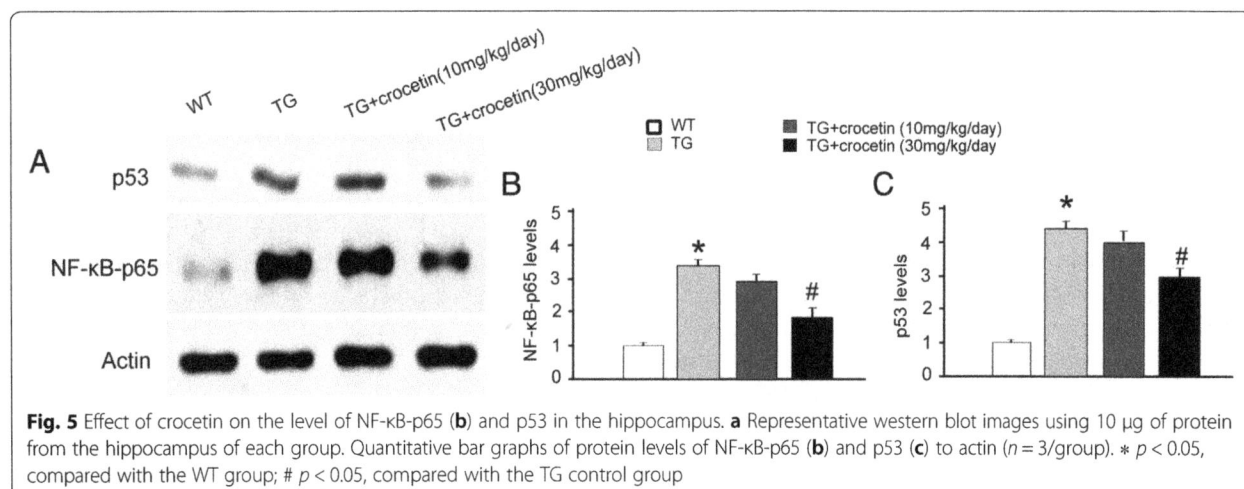

Fig. 5 Effect of crocetin on the level of NF-κB-p65 (b) and p53 in the hippocampus. a Representative western blot images using 10 μg of protein from the hippocampus of each group. Quantitative bar graphs of protein levels of NF-κB-p65 (b) and p53 (c) to actin (n = 3/group). * p < 0.05, compared with the WT group; # p < 0.05, compared with the TG control group

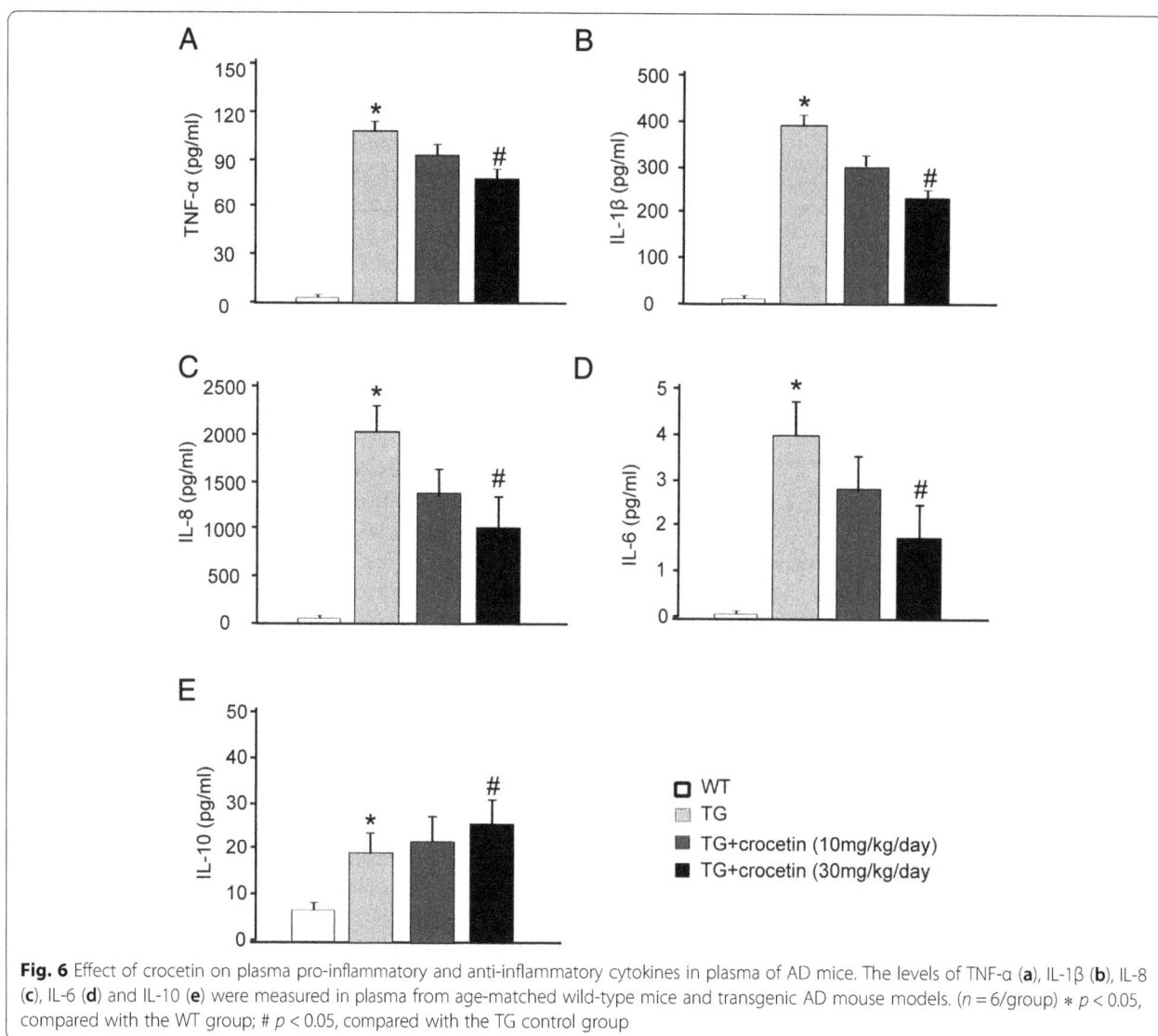

Fig. 6 Effect of crocetin on plasma pro-inflammatory and anti-inflammatory cytokines in plasma of AD mice. The levels of TNF-α (**a**), IL-1β (**b**), IL-8 (**c**), IL-6 (**d**) and IL-10 (**e**) were measured in plasma from age-matched wild-type mice and transgenic AD mouse models. ($n = 6$/group) $*$ $p < 0.05$, compared with the WT group; # $p < 0.05$, compared with the TG control group

effects of crocetin on learning and memory could correlate with its anti-inflammatory reaction.

p53, a transcription factor, controls many vital cellular pathways, including apoptosis. Upregulation of p53 has been associated with neuron death in chronic neurodegenerative diseases, including AD [28, 29]. Moreover, intervention of signal transduction pathways associated with p53-induced neuron death has been shown to maintain neuronal viability and restore cognitive function in AD [29, 30]. The results that crocetin inhibited p53 in the hippocampus of AD mice support that crocetin may have anti-apoptotic and neuroprotective effects.

NF-κB, a multifunctional transcription factor, is not only an important target in the brain for controlling neuroinflammation, but also an essential survival factor in response to a variety of stress stimuli that usually cause in neuron death [31]. Our data in Fig. 5 were consistent with previous research, showing that NF-κB activation in the

brain was enhanced in AD animal models and patients [32]. However, treatment of crocetin decreased NF-κB p65 subunit, suggesting that crocetin could modulate NF-κB-mediated cellular signaling pathways, such as, neuro-inflammation and neurotoxicity, and could ultimately improve learning and memory deficits in AD mice.

Above all, crocetin at the dosages that effectively reverse pathophysiology of AD has good bioavailability and adequate safety, as demonstrated in previous studies, showing that crocetin is permeable to blood brain barrier following oral administration, is relatively nontoxic, and has minimal side-effects at doses even greater than the doses we used in our experiments [26, 33, 34].

Conclusions

In summary, crocetin has multiple beneficial effects on AD. It significantly reduced Aβ secretion both in vitro and in vivo. In transgenic AD mouse models, crocetin significantly reduced the pro-inflammatory cytokines and enhanced the anti-inflammatory cytokine in the plasma, suppressed NF-kB activation and p53 expression in the hippocampus, decreased overall insoluble Aβ in the hippocampus, cerebral cortex, and cerebellum, and reversed learning and memory deficits in transgenic AD mice. Therefore, crocetin may have therapeutic potential for AD.

Methods

Cell culture

HeLa cells were maintained in Dulbecco's modified Eagle medium (DMEM, Thermo Fisher Scientific, Waltham, MA, USA) supplemented with 10% fetal bovine serum (GibcoTM, Thermo Fisher Scientific, USA) containing 100 units/mL penicillin, 100 μg/mL streptomycin, under a humidified atmosphere of 5% CO_2 at 37 °C. Two days later, APP751 carrying the Swedish mutation (APPsw) was transfected into Hela cells with BioT (Bioland Scientific LLC, Paramount, CA) according to the manufacturer's instructions.

Cell viability measurement

Cell viability was analyzed by MTT assay with Vybrant™ MTT cell proliferation assay kit (Thermo Fisher Scientific, USA) following manufacturer's instruction. Cells at 80% confluence in a 96-well plate were incubated with crocetin (dissolved in PBS) at the desired concentration for 8 h. Control cells were incubated in DMEM medium containing equal volume of saline. Then, cells were incubated with Vybrant™ MTT solution for 1 h at 37 °C. The absorbance at 570 nm was detected using a microplate reader (Bio-Rad, Hercules, CA, USA).

Aβ peptide assay

Cells cultured in a 35 mm dish with a confluence of 80% were incubated with crocetin at concentrations of 10–40 μM for 8 h in serum-free DMEM medium. The conditioned medium was analyzed using a sandwich enzyme-linked immunosorbent assay (ELISA; Invitrogen, CA, USA) specific for Aβ40 or Aβ42 following the manufacturer's instruction.

Animals and drug administration

All animal care and experimental protocols were approved by Institute of Animal care and use committee and Office of Laboratory Animal Welfare in University of Daqing Oilfield General Hospital. Nine months old male C57/BL6 wild type (WT) mice and male APPsw transgenic mice with C57/BL6 background were used in this study. All animals were housed at 22 ± 2 °C, and relative humidity of 45–75% with 12 h light–dark cycle, and water and food were provided ad libitum.

Crocetin was dissolved in saline, and was orally administered to APPsw transgenic AD mice once a day at doses of 0, 10, and 30 mg/kg for 6 months. Age and sex matched wild type C57 mice were administered with same volume of saline under the same paradigm.

In vivo insoluble Aβ42 detection

For in vivo detection of insoluble Aβ42 peptides in the brain, the transgenic and wild type mice that had undergone behavior tests were anesthetized and decapitated at the age of 15 months. The hippocampus, cerebellum and cerebral cortex were dissected, and the tissue samples were immersed in Tris-buffer solution (20 mM Tris; 137 mM NaCl; pH 7.4) at 10% (w/v), and homogenized. Then tissue homogenates were added to formic acid, centrifuged at 100,000 g for 1 h at 4 °C, then neutralized with formic acid neutralization buffer (1 M Tris base, 0.5 M Na_2HPO_4, 0.05% NaN_3). Insoluble Aβ42 levels were determined using the same sandwich ELISA kit used for in vitro detection.

Morris water maze test

Morris water maze was used to test spatial learning and memory, including memory acquisition and retention [35, 36]. The water maze consists of a circular pool (120 cm in diameter and 60 cm in depth), filled with water at 24–26 °C to a depth of 40 cm. An invisible escape platform with a diameter of 8 cm, was submerged approximately 1 cm below the water surface in the center of the designated quadrant of the pool. Briefly, acquisition phase was conducted for 6 consecutive days by putting each mouse in the pool to find the platform for a total of three trials per day with a 1 h inter-trial interval. The amount of time the mouse spent to find the hidden platform (escape latency) was recorded. The retention phase was conducted in the seventh day. The platform was removed and mice were given 120 s to freely explore the pool. The total duration of time spent in the target quadrant that had contained the escape platform during the acquisition phase was measured.

Novel object recognition test

Novel object recognition test was used for memory assessment [18]. Briefly, mice were placed into a square-shaped arena and were accustomed to two identical (familiar) objects for 10 min. On the following day, one of familiar objects was replaced by a novel object, mice were placed in the same arena and were allowed to explore freely for 5 min. The amount of time taken to explore each object was measured, and the memory index was calculated according to the following equation: memory index (%) = (exploring time for novel object/total exploring time for objects) × 100.

Western blot analysis

Following behavioral tests, the hippocampus was collected. Protein was extracted in RIPA lysis and extraction buffer (Thermo Fisher Scientific, USA) following the manufacturer's instruction. The protein concentration was measured with a BCA protein assay kit (Beyotime Biotechnology, China). 10 μg total protein was used for standard western blot. Primary antibodies: rabbit polyclonal anti-P53 (1:500), rabbit polyclonal anti-NF-κB-p65 (1:500), and mouse anti-β-actin (1:10,000), were purchased from Abcam (Shanghai, China). Secondary horseradish peroxidase-conjugated antibodies and Pierce™ western blotting substrate (Thermo Fisher Scientific, Shanghai, China) were used to visualize p53, NF-κB-p65, and β-actin. Band density was processed by imaging quantification. Ratios of the band density for the proteins of interest to that for β-actin were calculated.

ELISA assay

Whole blood from mice was collected with EDTA-treated tubes. Blood cells are removed from plasma by centrifugation for 10 min at 2,000 g. The resulting supernatant was collected for ELISA assay. TNF-α, IL-1β, IL-6, IL-8 and IL-10 in plasma were measured using mouse ELISA kits (Thermo Fisher Scientific, Shanghai, China), according to manufacturer's instruction. Protein levels were expressed as pg/μg of total proteins determined over an albumin standard curve.

Statistical analysis

Data are presented as mean ± SD. Statistical significance was determined by one-way ANOVA with Dunnett's or Tukey's post-tests using the GraphPad Prism® 5 software. P values of less than 0.05 were considered statistically significant.

Abbreviations

AD: Alzheimer's disease; Aβ: Amyloid-β

Acknowledgements

Not applicable.

Funding

Not applicable.

Authors' contributions

Jin Zhang, Yuchao Wang, Xueshuang Dong, Jianghua Liu performed the experiments, analyzed and interpreted the data; Jin Zhang, Yuchao Wang were major contributor in writing the manuscript; All authors read and approved the final manuscript.

Competing interests

The authors declare that they have no competing interests.

References

1. Masters CL, Bateman R, Blennow K, Rowe CC, Sperling RA, Cummings JL. Alzheimer's disease. Nat Rev Dis Primers. 2015;1:15056.
2. Kumar A, Singh A, Ekavali. A review on Alzheimer's disease pathophysiology and its management: an update. Pharmacol Rep. 2015;67:195–203.
3. Scheltens P, Blennow K, Breteler MM, de Strooper B, Frisoni GB, Salloway S, Van der Flier WM. Alzheimer's disease. Lancet. 2016;388:505–17.
4. Rogers J, Shen Y. A perspective on inflammation in Alzheimer's disease. Ann N Y Acad Sci. 2000;924:132–5.
5. Wyss-Coray T, Rogers J. Inflammation in Alzheimer disease-a brief review of the basic science and clinical literature. Cold Spring Harb Perspect Med. 2012;2:a006346.
6. Van Eldik LJ, Carrillo MC, Cole PE, Feuerbach D, Greenberg BD, Hendrix JA, Kennedy M, Kozauer N, Margolin RA, Molinuevo JL, et al. The roles of inflammation and immune mechanisms in Alzheimer's disease. Alzheimers Dement (N Y). 2016;2:99–109.
7. Hickman SE, Allison EK, El Khoury J. Microglial dysfunction and defective beta-amyloid clearance pathways in aging Alzheimer's disease mice. J Neurosci. 2008;28:8354–60.
8. Miguel-Alvarez M, Santos-Lozano A, Sanchis-Gomar F, Fiuza-Luces C, Pareja-Galeano H, Garatachea N, Lucia A. Non-steroidal anti-inflammatory drugs as a treatment for Alzheimer's disease: a systematic review and meta-analysis of treatment effect. Drugs Aging. 2015;32:139–47.
9. Bjorkman DJ. Current status of nonsteroidal anti-inflammatory drug (NSAID) use in the United States: risk factors and frequency of complications. Am J Med. 1999;107:3S–8S discussion S-10S.
10. Catella-Lawson F, McAdam B, Morrison BW, Kapoor S, Kujubu D, Antes L, Lasseter KC, Quan H, Gertz BJ, FitzGerald GA. Effects of specific inhibition of cyclooxygenase-2 on sodium balance, hemodynamics, and vasoactive eicosanoids. J Pharmacol Exp Ther. 1999;289:735–41.
11. Grosser T, Ricciotti E, FitzGerald GA. The cardiovascular pharmacology of nonsteroidal anti-inflammatory drugs. Trends Pharmacol Sci. 2017;38:733–48.
12. Yoshino F, Yoshida A, Umigai N, Kubo K, Lee MC. Crocetin reduces the oxidative stress induced reactive oxygen species in the stroke-prone spontaneously hypertensive rats (SHRSPs) brain. J Clin Biochem Nutr. 2011;49:182–7.
13. Nam KN, Park YM, Jung HJ, Lee JY, Min BD, Park SU, Jung WS, Cho KH, Park JH, Kang I, et al. Anti-inflammatory effects of crocin and crocetin in rat brain microglial cells. Eur J Pharmacol. 2010;648:110–6.
14. Xiang M, Yang M, Zhou C, Liu J, Li W, Qian Z. Crocetin prevents AGEs-induced vascular endothelial cell apoptosis. Pharmacol Res. 2006;54:268–74.
15. Tashakori-Sabzevar F, Hosseinzadeh H, Motamedshariaty VS, Movassaghi AR, Mohajeri SA. Crocetin attenuates spatial learning dysfunction and hippocampal injury in a model of vascular dementia. Curr Neurovasc Res. 2013;10:325–34.
16. Ahn JH, Hu Y, Hernandez M, Kim JR. Crocetin inhibits beta-amyloid fibrillization and stabilizes beta-amyloid oligomers. Biochem Biophys Res Commun. 2011;414:79–83.
17. Chun YS, Kim J, Chung S, Khorombi E, Naidoo D, Nthambeleni R, Harding N, Maharaj V, Fouche G, Yang HO. Protective roles of Monsonia angustifolia and its active compounds in experimental models of Alzheimer's disease. J Agric Food Chem. 2017;65:3133–40.
18. Leger M, Quiedeville A, Bouet V, Haelewyn B, Boulouard M, Schumann-Bard P, Freret T. Object recognition test in mice. Nat Protoc. 2013;8:2531–7.
19. Rameshrad M, Razavi BM, Hosseinzadeh H. Saffron and its derivatives, crocin, crocetin and safranal: a patent review. Expert Opin Ther Pat. 2018;28:147-165.
20. Tiribuzi R, Crispoltoni L, Chiurchiu V, Casella A, Montecchiani C, Del Pino AM, Maccarrone M, Palmerini CA, Caltagirone C, Kawarai T, et al. Trans-crocetin improves amyloid-beta degradation in monocytes from Alzheimer's disease patients. J Neurol Sci. 2017;372:408–12.
21. Akhondzadeh S, Sabet MS, Harirchian MH, Togha M, Cheraghmakani H, Razeghi S, Hejazi S, Yousefi MH, Alimardani R, Jamshidi A, et al. Saffron in the treatment of patients with mild to moderate Alzheimer's disease: a 16-week, randomized and placebo-controlled trial. J Clin Pharm Ther. 2010;35:581–8.
22. Akhondzadeh S, Shafiee Sabet M, Harirchian MH, Togha M, Cheraghmakani H, Razeghi S, Hejazi SS, Yousefi MH, Alimardani R, Jamshidi A, et al. A 22-week, multicenter, randomized, double-blind controlled trial of Crocus sativus in the treatment of mild-to-moderate Alzheimer's disease. Psychopharmacology. 2010;207:637–43.

23. Khemka VK, Ganguly A, Bagchi D, Ghosh A, Bir A, Biswas A, Chattopadhyay S, Chakrabarti S. Raised serum proinflammatory cytokines in Alzheimer's disease with depression. Aging Dis. 2014;5:170–6.

24. Rubio-Perez JM, Morillas-Ruiz JM. Serum cytokine profile in Alzheimer's disease patients after ingestion of an antioxidant beverage. CNS Neurol Disord Drug Targets. 2013;12:1233–41.

25. Hosseinzadeh H, Nassiri-Asl M. Avicenna's (Ibn Sina) the canon of medicine and saffron (Crocus sativus): a review. Phytother Res. 2013;27:475–83.

26. Yang R, Tan X, Thomas AM, Shen J, Qureshi N, Morrison DC, Van Way CW 3rd. Crocetin inhibits mRNA expression for tumor necrosis factor-alpha, interleukin-1beta, and inducible nitric oxide synthase in hemorrhagic shock. JPEN J Parenter Enteral Nutr. 2006;30:297–301.

27. Song L, Kang C, Sun Y, Huang W, Liu W, Qian Z. Crocetin inhibits lipopolysaccharide-induced inflammatory response in human umbilical vein endothelial cells. Cell Physiol Biochem. 2016;40:443–52.

28. Morrison RS, Kinoshita Y. The role of p53 in neuronal cell death. Cell Death Differ. 2000;7:868–79.

29. Szybinska A, Lesniak W. P53 dysfunction in neurodegenerative diseases - the cause or effect of pathological changes? Aging Dis. 2017;8:506–18.

30. Chang JR, Ghafouri M, Mukerjee R, Bagashev A, Chabrashvili T, Sawaya BE. Role of p53 in neurodegenerative diseases. Neurodegener Dis. 2012;9:68–80.

31. Shih RH, Wang CY, Yang CM. NF-kappaB signaling pathways in neurological inflammation: a mini review. Front Mol Neurosci. 2015;8:77.

32. Hong JT. NF-kB as a mediator of brain inflammation in AD. CNS Neurol Disord Drug Targets. 2017. https://doi.org/10.2174/1871527316666170807130011.

33. Ahmad AS, Ansari MA, Ahmad M, Saleem S, Yousuf S, Hoda MN, Islam F. Neuroprotection by crocetin in a hemi-parkinsonian rat model. Pharmacol Biochem Behav. 2005;81:805–13.

34. Hosseini A, Razavi BM, Hosseinzadeh H. Pharmacokinetic properties of saffron and its active components. Eur J Drug Metab Pharmacokinet. 2018;43:383–390.

35. Morris R. Developments of a water-maze procedure for studying spatial learning in the rat. J Neurosci Methods. 1984;11:47–60.

36. Bromley-Brits K, Deng Y, Song W. Morris water maze test for learning and memory deficits in Alzheimer's disease model mice. J Vis Exp. 2011;53:2920.

26

Ageing: from inflammation to cancer

Giulia C. Leonardi[1†], Giulia Accardi[2†], Roberto Monastero[3], Ferdinando Nicoletti[1] and Massimo Libra[1*]

Abstract

Ageing is the major risk factor for cancer development. Hallmark of the ageing process is represented by inflammaging, which is a chronic and systemic low-grade inflammatory process. Inflammation is also a hallmark of cancer and is widely recognized to influence all cancer stages from cell transformation to metastasis. Therefore, inflammaging may represent the biological phenomena able to couple ageing process with cancer development. Here we review the molecular and cellular pathway involved in age-related chronic inflammation along with its potential triggers and their connection with cancer development.

Keywords: Ageing, Cancer, DAMPs, Inflammation, Microbiota, MiRna, Obesity, Senescence

Background
Inflammation, inflammaging and cancer

Ageing is a nearly universal biological process characterized, in multicellular organisms, by the progressive loss of cells functions and tissues renewal due to complex, heterogeneous and dynamic mechanisms and affected by several genetic, epigenetic, environmental and fortuitous factors [1, 2]. The term "inflammaging" is used to define the systemic and sterile (in the absence of infection) low-grade chronic inflammation status that is nowadays considered a central biological mainstay of the ageing process [3, 4]. Indeed, inflammation is a beneficial process as an acute, transient immune response to harmful conditions but with ageing there is a reduction in the capability to endure with antigenic, chemical, physical and nutritional triggers and it becomes chronic and of low grade, leading to tissues dysfunction and degeneration [5, 6].

Numerous evidences show how apparently different age-related pathologies, including cancer, cardiovascular diseases and type 2 diabetes reveal a common inflammatory background [7, 8]. Epidemiological studies demonstrate the relationship between increased levels of inflammatory mediators like Interleukin(IL)-6 or C-reactive protein (CRP) to multiple age-related diseases [9]. In fact, inflammaging is characterized by the establishment of a systemic proinflammatory state with increased level of circulating interleukins such as IL-6, IL-1 and Tumor Necrosi Factor(TNF)-α and inflammatory markers, such as CRP [6]. This results from the activation of signalling networks critical to inflammation, such as those regulated by the Nuclear Factor (NF)-kB transcription factor, along with a variety of different sources of the inflammatory stimuli triggering and sustaining inflammaging, such as senescent cells, the meta-inflammation, the gut microbiota and nutrition [10–12].

In the nineteenth century Rudolph Virchow was the first to hypothesize a connection between inflammation and cancer, but only in the last two decades researchers have produced striking evidences on the role played by the inflammatory process in promoting cancer [13, 14]. Indeed, not only cancer can arise on sites of chronic inflammation but also a pro-inflammatory microenvironment, supported by inflammatory cells and mediators, is an essential component of cancer and one of its hallmarks [15–17].

Chronic inflammation is, thus, associated with all stages of cancer development increasing its risk, supporting cancer initiation, promoting cancer progression, and supporting metastatic diffusion [10]. Recently, it has been demonstrated that preventive treatment with anti-inflammatory drugs like aspirin reduce the incidence and mortality for colorectal cancer [18]. This leads the way to the potential preventive and therapeutic role of the modulation of cancer-associated inflammatory microenvironment [19].

The aim of this review is to explore the role of the main actors contributing in the development of inflammaging and cancer.

---

* Correspondence: m.libra@unict.it
†Equal contributors
[1]Department of Biomedical and Biotechnological Sciences, Pathology and Oncology Section, University of Catania, Catania, Italy
Full list of author information is available at the end of the article

Sources and modulators of inflammaging

The ageing and the inflammaging act at different levels of complexity involving several tissues and organs as well as the immune system and our associated ecosystems (gut microbiota). All of these factors are thought to contribute to the systemic inflammatory state, through the imbalance of pro-inflammatory and/or anti-inflammatory mediators (Fig. 1) [6, 20].

Immunosenescence

In the elderly, many alterations of innate and acquired immunity have been described and viewed as deleterious, hence the term immunosenescence. Immunosenescence is a complex process involving multiple reorganizational and developmentally regulated changes, rather than simple unidirectional decline of complete immune function. On the other hand, some immunological parameters are commonly notably reduced in the elderly, and reciprocally good function is tightly correlated to health status. Whereas innate immunity is relatively well preserved in elderly, acquired immunity is more susceptible due to both the functional decline associated with the passage of time, and to antigen burden to which an individual has been exposed during lifetime. This chronic antigenic stress, which affects the immune system throughout life with a progressive activation of macrophages and related cells contributes to determine an inflammatory status. Our immune system is quite efficient in fighting acute infections in young people, but not particularly efficient in responding to chronic stimuli, especially when they occur late in life. This leads to an increased production of inflammatory mediators associated with the presence of chronic infections [8, 20, 21].

Cellular senescence

Cellular senescence is characterized by a state of permanent cell-cycle arrest due to exposure to stressful stimuli such as telomere erosion, oncogene activation, oxygen free radicals (ROS), chemicals and ionizing radiation [22] Therefore, cellular senescence is widely considered a tumor suppressing mechanism but growing evidences link this process to hyperplastic and degenerative diseases through chronic inflammation [23, 24]. In fact, senescent cells despite their growth arrest are metabolically and transcriptionally active and set up a specific crosstalk with their microenvironment elicited by the synthesis of a wide number of secretory protein [25, 26]. This phenotype is called "senescence-associated secretory phenotype" (SASP) and is considered a key process for our current understanding on the link between cellular senescence, inflammation and cancer development [24, 27].

Replicative senescence in normal cell is due to critical telomere erosion that activates DNA damage response and persistent p53 activation with cell cycle arrest [28, 29]. Severely damaged DNA (e.g. double strands break) and oncogene activation or loss of tumor suppressor induce cellular senescence through p53 activation accompanied by p21 expression [28–32]. DNA damage can also activate p16, which is a second barrier to prevent growth of transformed cells through senescence [33].

Once established, senescent cells gradually develop the secretory phenotype largely mediated by the transcription factors (NF)-kB and CCAAT/enhancer-binding protein beta (C/EBPb) induced by the upregulation of DNA damage response effectors like NBS1, ATM and CHK2 [34–36]. SASP associated secretory proteins include cytokines (most notably IL-1α, IL-1β, IL-6, and IL-8), numerous chemokines

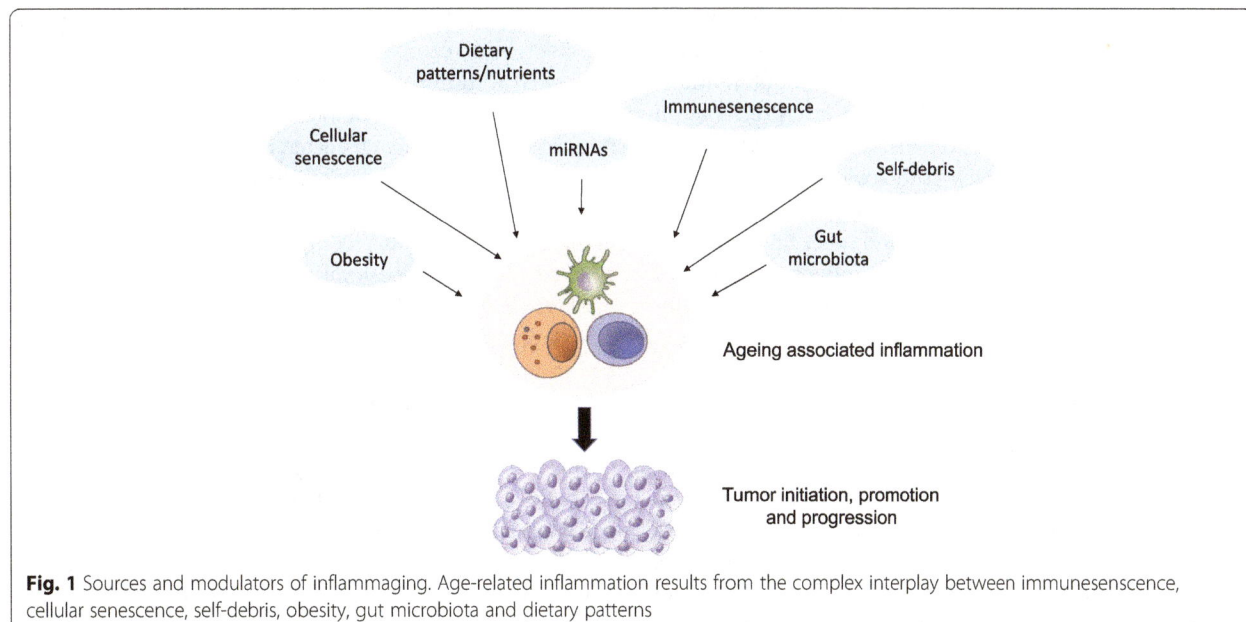

Fig. 1 Sources and modulators of inflammaging. Age-related inflammation results from the complex interplay between immunesenscence, cellular senescence, self-debris, obesity, gut microbiota and dietary patterns

(chemoattractants and macrophage inflammatory proteins), growth factors [hepatocyte growth factor (HGF), transforming growth factor(TGF)-β, granulocyte-macrophage colony stimulating factor (GM-CSF)] and matrix-remodelling enzymes [37, 38]. Importantly, SASP expression profile varies among different tissues and different triggers but IL-6 and IL-8 are highly conserved and have a major role in maintaining the SASP in senescent cells [37, 38]. Moreover, the paracrine signalling operated through SASP has been demonstrated to induce senescence in surrounding cells therefore propagating this process throughout the tissue [39–41]. Overall SASP-associated mediators cooperate to establish a pro-inflammatory environment and to recruit immune cells into the senescent tissue. This inflammatory state along with the immune cells infiltration surrounding senescent cells removes the damaged and transformed cells [42]. However, it has been demonstrated that senescent cells increase with age, and this can be interpreted either as an effect of reduced clearance ability (and so senescent cells gradually accumulate) and/or because aged individuals generate senescent cells faster than their immune system can handle [23]. The accumulation of senescent cells, typical of ageing tissues, is therefore associated with an altered microenvironment orchestrated by the activation of NF-kB pro-inflammatory program (i.e. increased pro-inflammatory cytokines, extracellular degrading enzymes, growth factors). In vitro and in vivo studies have demonstrated that this process not only alters the normal tissue and structure function but, importantly, can stimulate the growth of nearby malignant cells exerting a positive selection on cancer-initiating cells and stimulating cancer progression [24, 43, 44].

In addition to SASP, another type of senescence associated inflammatory response (SIR) has been described. It shares few genes expression features with SASP and is mainly a cell autonomous mechanism with a small number of secreted factors and with no recruitment of immune cells to the senescent tissue. SIR can be interpreted as an intermediate state between homeostasis and overt inflammation, associated with many pathological conditions (e.g. obesity, type 2 diabetes, dyslipidaemia). It is still unclear why some senescent cells start SIR and other SASP but this two phenotypes may represent a continuous spectrum of an inflammatory process, where SIR arises first and later evolve into SASP [27].

Self-debris triggers of inflammaging

Ageing is associated with a progressive accumulation of damaged macromolecules and cells (self-debris) due to increased production and/or inadequate elimination. These waste products derive from cellular and metabolic process and are released as a consequence of cell/organelle injury. Importantly, self-debris can mimic bacterial products and can activate the innate immunity as endogenous danger-associated molecular patterns (DAMPs). Hence, damaged cellular and organelle components, ROS and metabolites (e.g. ATP, fatty acids, urate crystals, ceramides, cardiolipin, amyloid, succinate, per-oxidized lipids, advanced glycation end-products, altered N-glycans and HMGB1) are recognized by innate immunity receptors [45, 46]. Toll-like receptor family (TLR), intracellular NOD-like receptors (NLRs) and cytosolic DNA sensors initiate a reaction that leads to the upregulation of inflammation associated pathway and mediators. In particular TLRs stimulate inflammation through Myd88-mediated NF-kB and activator protein 1(AP-1) activation. DAMPs derived activation of NLRs (particularly Nlrp3) leads to the inflammasome assembly and consecutive secretion of several proinflammatory mediators. As self-debris accumulates, the innate immune response to DAMPs become chronic and maladaptive leading to inflammaging [47].

Gut microbiota

The bacterial population of the gut microbiota (GM) represents the largest number and concentration of microbes of the human body and it has been demonstrated to take part in many physiological and pathological processes [48, 49]. The homeostasis of this ecosystem composed by microbiota, the gut associated lymphoid tissue (GALT) and the intestinal mucosa is strictly dependent on a physiological low-grade inflammation that secures its symbiotic feature [50].

Ageing is associated with changes in the microbial composition of gut microbiota with an increasing presence of *Bacteroides* in the elderly compared to the higher presence of *Firmicutes* in younger adults [51]. Several studies have also showed the correlation between microbial diversity, frailty scores and environmental factors- such as dietary pattern- in elderly individuals [51–53]. In this context, the alteration in gut microbiota composition seems to be also intrinsically connected with the aged sustained alteration in gastrointestinal tract (e.g. reduction of intestinal motility, poor dentition, modification of salivary characteristics) [54]. Importantly, the modification of gut microbiota in elderly can facilitate the onset of dysbiosis and the prevalence of pathogenic species in the intestinal microbial composition and this has been associated with increased level of systemic pro-inflammatory markers (IL-6, IL-8, TNF-α, CRP) [51–53]. The association between gut dysbiosis and cancer is, therefore, not only limited to a direct pathogenic role exerted by specific bacteria on the intestinal epithelium but it is also linked to an overall derangement of this ecosystem that has systemic consequences through inflammatory pathways [49, 55].

Finally, a variety of sources are responsible for triggering and maintaining inflammaging at local and systemic level and it is thought that aged-associated change in gut microbiota can represent an important trigger of the inflammaging processes and the associated pro-tumorigenic state.

The striking role played by the gut microbiota in health maintenance as well as in the development of different pathologic conditions is leading to the development of preventive and therapeutic approach using the modulation of the gut microbial community [49, 56, 57]. As the ageing gut microbiota is increasingly recognized as a fundamental player in in the ageing process, being a source of systemic chronic inflammation, it is intriguing to elucidate the role of its potential modulation on ageing.

Obesity, nutrition and metaflammation

Ageing is associated in many people, particularly in Western countries, with an increase in visceral fat that leads to obesity along with insulin resistance [58]. Moreover, epidemiological data suggest a significant association between increased body mass index and several types of cancer, such us pancreatic cancer, prostate cancer, colon cancer, post-menopausal breast cancer and many others [59, 60]. Even though the molecular links between obesity and cancer are not yet completely elucidated, it is now widely accepted that obesity itself is responsible for a chronic inflammatory state [61]. Obesity-induced inflammation can be described as metaflammation: a low-grade, chronic inflammatory state orchestrated by metabolic cells in response to an excess of nutrients and energy [5]. An important feature of obese inflammation is that it originates from metabolic signals and within metabolic cells such as the adipocyte. Indeed the exposure to excessive levels of nutrients, in particular of glucose and free fatty acids, induces a stress activation that in turn triggers inflammatory intracellular signalling pathways.

The major intracellular contributors to the induction of inflammation in metabolic tissues are represented by c-jun N-terminal kinase (JNK), inhibitor of κ kinase (IKK), and protein kinase R (PKR) [62]. These kinases ultimately regulate the downstream transcriptional programs activation of transcription factors AP-1, NF-κB, and interferon regulatory factor (IRF), resulting in increased expression of pro-inflammatory cytokines such as TNF-α, C-C motif chemokine ligand (CCL)2, or IL-1β, IL-6 [59, 62]. Over time, this low-grade inflammation may induce the recruitment and activation of many immune cells, such as macrophages, mast cells, and various T cell populations, driving the adipose tissue toward a modified environment resulting in a stronger pro-inflammatory response [59]. The inflammation induced by nutrient excess is maintained with no resolution and the inflammatory pathways continue to reinforce each other, from metabolic cell signals of distress to immune cell responses [62].

A large body of evidence indicates that both quantitative and qualitative characteristics of nutrition have a profound effect on the development of a pro-inflammatory carcinogenic environment [63]. As a consequence, nutrition influences the incidence, natural progression and therapeutic

response of malignant diseases, both in humans and in preclinical animal models through modulation of chronic inflammation [64]. Beyond the undeniable links among quantitative overnutrition, obesity, inflammation and elevated cancer risk, epidemiological studies have linked cancer to qualitative disequilibria in food composition [63].

The Western-type diet, which is high in red meat, high-fat dairy products, refined grains, and simple carbohydrates, has been associated with higher levels of CRP and IL-6. The Mediterranean diet and more in general diets high in fruit and vegetable intake have been associated with lower levels of inflammation [65–69]. Several researches have also associated specific nutrients with different level of inflammatory markers. The impact of different nutrients on the systemic body inflammation has been experimentally condensed into one-dimensional numeric values. The "dietary inflammatory index" (DII) weights each major macronutrient and multiple micronutrients on the basis of their general proinflammatory effects, as measured, for example, by assessment of C-reactive protein in serum [63]. This index significantly correlates with the risk of developing postmenopausal breast cancer, colorectal cancer, lung cancer in smokers, non-Hodgkin lymphoma, bladder cancer, and nasopharyngeal carcinoma [70–75].

Among the different factors that can modulate ageing inflammaging and metaflammation nutritional intervention plays a critical and interesting role. The reduction of obesity through bariatric surgery is associated with a decrease in cancer mortality [76]. Several animal cancer models have shown a significant impact of the fasting and feeding cycles in cancer growth and in particular starvation and low caloric diets seem to play the greater role through immunomodulation and anti-inflammatory effects [64]. Moreover, specific dietary patterns, all sharing a prevalent plant-based diet, seem to greatly impact longevity in different population through the interaction between nutrients and nutrient-sensing pathways such as those regulated by IGF1 [77, 78]. In this context and from a preventing standpoints experimental and epidemiological studies have often demonstrated the potential role of polyphenols containing food in the prevention of neurodegenerative diseases and cancer, particularly modulating cellular stress response pathways associated with inflammaging [79–81]. Given the evidence discussed above it appears plausible to attempt dietary interventions or to provide food supplements to promote long-term and systemic modulation of chronic low-grade inflammation process (in the form of inflammageing and metaflammation), in an anticancer perspective strategies and towards the enhancement of health status of the elderly population [7, 82].

In this context, an important role is played by epigenetic modulation of gene expression where microRNAs are among the main players. MicroRNAs (miRs) are small, non-coding RNAs involved in the regulation of transcriptional and translational processes and represent one of the most abundant classes of regulatory molecules [83]. miR regulation entails both repressing and activating gene expression, by interacting with complementary sequences in coding and non-coding regions of their mRNA targets [84]. The specificity of miRs targeting is low and a single miR can target hundreds of mRNAs. However, a group of miRs can regulate complex biological processes, including inflammaging, cellular senescence and tumorigenesis, by acting in a coordinated fashion on pathways of functionally related genes [85, 86]. Moreover, an increasing number of studies has shown that environmental factors, including diet, cigarette smoke, stress, virus can modulate miRs expression and activity. Thus, miRs are able to couple environmental exposure to specific human phenotype and disease through gene expression modulation [87, 88].

MicroRNAs are also involved in the ageing process. In particular, mir-21, mir-146a and mir-126 participate in the regulation of the NF-kB activated pathways that is central in cellular senescence, inflammaging and cancer development [89]. Moreover, an interesting aspect emerging from microRNAs studies is that centenarians may have a different miRs profile [90]. Several preclinical and clinical studies in different age-associated disease, including cancer, show that miRs can represent not only an early diagnostic markers but also an important tool for risk-based patients' stratification [91, 92]. Furthermore, taken together these evidences support that miRs modulation might a be a potential tool to interfere with those pathways involved in the ageing process and in age associated diseases including cancer.

Conclusions

Age is the most important risk factor for cancer development and the increase in life expectancy will heighten both medical and social consequence of this and other age-related disease.

The complexity of the ageing process and its players has been progressively unrevealed by the thorough effort operated by researchers leading to the comprehension that inflammation represent the common milieu of the ageing process and age-related pathologies. Cronic antigen load, cellular senescence, self-debris damage response, gut microbiota, metaflammation and miRs all together influence and foster inflammaging but how they interact and what is their relative weight is still to be elucidated.

The deep comprehension of the processes involved in inflammaging will open the possibility for therapeutic interventions leading to an increased control of age-associated disease and ultimately to a healthier ageing.

Abbreviations
ATM: ataxia-teleangectasia mutated gene; C/EBPb: CCAAT/enhancer-binding protein beta; CRP: C-reactive protein; DAMPs: danger-associated molecular patterns; DNA: deoxyribonucleic acid; GALT: gut associated lymphoid tissue; GM: gut microbiota; GM-CSF: granulocyte-macrophage colony stimulating factor; HGF: hepatocyte growth factor; HMGB1: High Mobility Group Box 1 protein; IKK: inhibitor of κ kinase; IL-1: interleukin 1; IL-6: interleukin 6; IL-8: interleukin 8; IRF: interferon regulatory factor; JNK: c-jun N-terminal kinase; miRs: microRNAs; NF-κB: nuclear factor kappa-light-chain-enhancer of activated B cells; PKR: protein kinase R; ROS: oxygen free radicals; SASP: senescence-associated secretory phenotype; SIR: senescence associated inflammatory response; TGF-β: Transforming growth factor-beta; TLR: toll-like receptor family; TNF-α: tumor necrosis factor α

Acknowledgements
None

Funding
Not applicable

Authors' contributions
GCL and GA wrote the paper. All authors edited the paper and approved its final version.

Competing interests
The authors declare they have no competing interests.

Author details
[1]Department of Biomedical and Biotechnological Sciences, Pathology and Oncology Section, University of Catania, Catania, Italy. [2]Department of Pathobiology and Medical Biotechnologies, Immunosenescence and Ageing Group, University of Palermo, Palermo, Italy. [3]Department of Experimental Biomedicine and Clinical Neurosciences, Neurology Section, University of Palermo, Palermo, Italy.

References
1. López-Otín C, Blasco MA, Partridge L, Serrano M, Kroemer G. The hallmarks of ageing. Cell. 2013;153:1194–217.
2. Accardi G, Caruso C. Updates in pathobiology: causality and chance in ageing, age-related diseases and longevity. In: Accardi G, Caruso C, editors. Updates in pathobiology: causality and chance in ageing, age-related diseases and longevity. Palermo: university press; 2017. p. 13–23.
3. Franceschi C, Bonafè M, Valensin S, Olivieri F, De Luca M, Ottaviani E, De Benedictis G. Inflamm-ageing: an evolutionary perspective on immunosenescence. Ann N Y Acad Sci. 2000;908:244–54.
4. Franceschi C. Inflammaging as a major characteristic of old people: can it be prevented or cured? Nutr Rev. 2007;65:173–6.
5. Medzhitov R. Origin and physiological roles of inflammation. Nature. 2008; 454:428–35.
6. Cevenini E, Monti D, Franceschi C. Inflamm-ageing. Curr Opin Clin Nutr Metab Care. 2013;16(1):14–20.
7. Franceschi C, Capri M, Monti D, Giunta S, Olivieri F, Sevini F, Panourgia MP, Invidia L, Celani L, Scurti M, Cevenini E, Castellani GC, Salvioli S. Inflamm-ageing and antiinflamm-ageing: a systemic perspective on ageing and longevity emerged from studies in humans. Mech Ageing Dev. 2007;128:92–105.

8. Vasto S, Candore G, Balistreri CR, Caruso M, Colonna-Romano G, Grimaldi MP, Listi F, Nuzzo D, Lio D, Caruso C. Inflammatory networks in ageing, age-related diseases and longevity. Mech Ageing Dev. 2007;128(1):83–91.

9. Kiecolt-Glaser JK, Preacher KJ, MacCallum RC, Atkinson C, Malarkey WB, Glaser R. Chronic stress and age-related increases in the proinflammatory cytokine IL-6. Proc Natl Acad Sci U S A. 2003;100:9090–5.

10. Karin M. Nuclear factor-κB in cancer development and progression. Nature. 2006;441:431–6.

11. Tieri P, Termanini A, Bellavista E, Salvioli S, Capri M, Franceschi C. Charting the NF-kB pathway interactome map. PLoS One. 2012;7:32678.

12. Salminen A, Huuskonen J, Ojala J, Kauppinen A, Kaarniranta K, Suuronen T. Activation of innate immunity system during ageing: NF-kB signaling is the molecular culprit of inflamm-ageing. Ageing Res Rev. 2008;7:83–105.

13. Balkwill F, Mantovani A. Inflammation and cancer: back to Virchow? Lancet. 2001;357:539–45.

14. Mantovani A, Allavena P, Sica A, Balkwill F. Cancer-related inflammation. Nature. 2008;454:436–44.

15. Coussens LM, Werb Z. Inflammation and cancer. Nature. 2002;420:860–7.

16. Hanahan D, Weinberg RA. Hallmarks of cancer: the next generation. Cell. 2011;144:646–74.

17. Vasto S, Carruba G, Lio D, Colonna-Romano G, Di Bona D, Candore G, Caruso C. Inflammation, ageing and cancer. Mech Ageing Dev. 2009;130(1–2):40–5.

18. Chia WK, Ali R, Toh HC. Aspirin as adjuvant therapy for colorectal cancer-reinterpreting paradigms. Nat Rev Clin Oncol. 2012;9:561–70.

19. Baldassano S, Accardi G, Vasto S. Beta-glucans and cancer: the influence of inflammation and gut peptide. Eur J Med Chem. 2017; https://doi.org/10.1016/j.ejmech.2017.09.013.

20. Cevenini E, Caruso C, Candore G, Capri M, Nuzzo D, Duro G, Rizzo C, Colonna-Romano G, Lio D, di Carlo D, Palmas MG, Scurti M, Pini E, Franceschi C, Vasto S. Age-related inflammation: the contribution of different organs, tissues and systems. How to face it for therapeutic approaches. Curr Pharm Des. 2010;16:609–18.

21. Caruso C, Accardi G, Virruso C, Candore G. Sex, gender and immunosenescence: a key to understand the different lifespan between men and women? Immun Ageing. 2013;10(Suppl 1):20.

22. Muñoz-Espín D, Serrano M. Cellular senescence: from physiology to pathology. Nat Rev Mol Cell Biol. 2014;15:482–96.

23. Campisi J, d'Adda di Fagagna F. Cellular senescence: when bad things happen to good cells. Nat Rev Mol Cell Biol. 2007;8:729–40.

24. Krtolica A, Parrinello S, Lockett S, Desprez PY, Campisi J. Senescent fibroblasts promote epithelial cell growth and tumorigenesis: a link between cancer and aging. Proc Natl Acad Sci U S A. 2001;98:12072–7.

25. Rodier F, Coppé JP, Patil CK, Hoeijmakers WA, Muñoz DP, Raza SR, Freund A, Campeau E, Davalos AR, Campisi J. Persistent DNA. Damage signalling triggers senescence-associated inflammatory cytokine secretion. Nat Cell Biol. 2009;11:973–9.

26. Kuilman T, Peeper DS. Senescence-messaging secretome: SMS-ing cellular stress. Nat Rev Cancer. 2009;9:81–94.

27. Pribluda A, Elyada E, Wiener Z, Hamza H, Goldstein RE, Biton M, Burstain I, Morgenstern Y, Brachya G, Billauer H, Biton S, Snir-Alkalay I, Vucic D, Schlereth K, Mernberger M, Stiewe T, Oren M, Alitalo K, Pikarsky E, Ben-Neriah YA. Senescence-inflammatory switch from cancer-inhibitory to cancer-promoting mechanism. Cancer Cell. 2013;24:242–56.

28. d'Adda di Fagagna F, Reaper PM, Clay-Farrace L, Fiegler H, Carr P, Von Zglinicki T, Saretzki G, Carter NP, Jackson SP. A DNA damage checkpoint response in telomere-initiated senescence. Nature. 2003;426:194–8.

29. Herbig U, Jobling WA, Chen BP, Chen DJ, Sedivy J. Telomere shortening triggers senescence of human cells through a pathway involving ATM, p53, and p21(CIP1), but not p16(INK4a). Mol Cell. 2004;14:501–13.

30. DiLeonardo A, Linke SP, Clarkin K, Wahl GMDNA. Damage triggers a prolonged p53-dependent G1 arrest and long-term induction of Cip1 in normal human fibroblasts. Genes Dev. 1994;8:2540–51.

31. Michaloglou C, Vredeveld LC, Soengas MS, Denoyelle C, Kuilman T, van der Horst CM, Majoor DM, Shay JW, Mooi WJ. Peeper DS. BRAFE600-associated senescence- like cell cycle arrest of human nevi. Nature. 2005;436:720–4.

32. Lin AW, Barradas M, Stone JC, van Aelst L, Serrano M, Lowe SW. Premature senescence involving p53 and p16 is activated in response to constitutive MEK/ MAPK mitogenic signaling. Genes Dev. 1998;12:3008–19.

33. Jacobs JJ, de Lange T. Significant role for p16(INK4a) in p53-independent telomere-directed senescence. Curr Biol. 2004;14:2302–8.

34. Rodier F, Muñoz DP, Teachenor R, Chu V, Le O, Bhaumik D, Coppé JP, Campeau E, Beauséjour CM, Kim SH, Davalos AR, Campisi J. DNA-SCARS: distinct nuclear structures that sustain damage-induced senescence growth arrest and inflammatory cytokine secretion. J Cell Sci. 2011;124:68–81.

35. Chien Y, Scuoppo C, Wang X, Fang X, Balgley B, Bolden JE, Premsrirut P, Luo W, Chicas A, Lee CS, Kogan SC, Lowe SW. Control of the senescence-associated secretory phenotype by NF-kappaB promotes senescence and enhances chemosensitivity. Genes Dev. 2011;25:2125–36.

36. Salminen A, Kauppinen A, Kaarniranta K. Emerging role of NF-kappaB signaling in the induction of senescence-associated secretory phenotype (SASP). Cell Signal. 2012;24:835–45.

37. Coppe JP, Desprez PY, Krtolica A, Campisi J. The senescence-associated secretory phenotype: the dark side of tumor suppression. Annu Rev Pathol. 2010;5:99–118.

38. Acosta JC, O'Loghlen A, Banito A, Guijarro MV, Augert A, Raguz S, Fumagalli M, Da Costa M, Brown C, Popov N, Takatsu Y, Melamed J, d'Adda di Fagagna F, Bernard D, Hernando E, Gil J. Chemokine signaling via the CXCR2 receptor reinforces senescence. Cell. 2008;133:1006–18.

39. Acosta JC, Banito A, Wuestefeld T, Georgilis A, Janich P, Morton JP, Athineos D, Kang TW, Lasitschka F, Andrulis M, Pascual G, Morris KJ, Khan S, Jin H, Dharmalingam G, Snijders AP, Carroll T, Capper D, Pritchard C, Inman GJ, Longerich T, Sansom OJ, Benitah SA, Zender L, Gil JA. Complex secretory program orchestrated by the inflammasome controls paracrine senescence. Nat Cell Biol. 2013;15:978–90.

40. Campisi J. Senescent cells, tumor suppression and organismal aging: good citizens, bad neighbors. Cell. 2005;120:513–22.

41. Hubackova S, Krejcikova K, Bartek J, Hodny Z. IL1- and TGFbeta-Nox4 signaling, oxidative stress and DNA damage response are shared features of replicative, oncogene-induced, and drug-induced paracrine 'bystander senescence'. Aging. 2012;4:932–51.

42. Xue W, Zender L, Miething C, Dickins RA, Hernando E, Krizhanovsky V, Cordon-Cardo C, Lowe SW. Senescence and tumour clearance is triggered by p53 restoration in murine liver carcinomas. Nature. 2007;445:656–60.

43. Bavik C, Coleman I, Dean JP, Knudsen B, Plymate S, Nelson PS. The gene expression program of prostate fibroblast senescence modulates neoplastic epithelial cell proliferation through paracrine mechanisms. Cancer Res. 2006;66:794–802.

44. Coppe JP, Kauser K, Campisi J, Beausejour CM. Secretion of vascular endothelial growth factor by primary human fibroblasts at senescence. J Biol Chem. 2006;281:29568–74.

45. Dall'Olio F, Vanhooren V, Chen CC, Slagboom PE, Wuhrer M, Franceschi CN. Glycomic biomarkers of biological aging and longevity: a link with inflammaging. Ageing Res Rev. 2013;12(Suppl 2):685–98.

46. Feldman N, Rotter-Maskowitz A, Okun EDAMP. As mediators of sterile inflammation in aging- related pathologies. Ageing Res Rev. 2015;24:29–39.

47. Franceschi C, Campisi J. Chronic inflammation (inflammaging) and its potential contribution to age-associated diseases. J Gerontol A Biol Sci Med Sci. 2014;69(Suppl 1):4–9.

48. O'Hara AM, Shanahan F. The gut flora as a forgotten organ. EMBO Rep. 2006;7:688–93.

49. Sekirov I, Russell SL, Antunes LCM, Finlay BB. Gut microbiota in health and disease. Physiol Rev. 2010;90:859–904.

50. Noverr MC, Huffnagle GB. Does the microbiota regulate immune responses outside the gut? Trends Microbiol. 2004;12:562–8.

51. O'Toole PW, Jeffery IB. Gut microbiota and aging. Science. 2015;350:1214–5.

52. Claesson MJ, Jeffery IB, Conde S, Power SE, O'Connor EM, Cusack S, Harris HM, Coakley M, Lakshminarayanan B, O'Sullivan O, Fitzgerald GF, Deane J, O'Connor M, Harnedy N, O'Connor K, O'Mahony D, van Sinderen D, Wallace M, Brennan L, Stanton C, Marchesi JR, Fitzgerald AP, Shanahan F, Hill C, Ross RP, O'Toole PW. Gut microbiota composition correlates with diet and health in the elderly. Nature. 2012;488:178–84.

53. Ticinesi A, Milani C, Lauretani F, Nouvenne A, Mancabelli L, Lugli GA, Turroni F, Duranti S, Mangifesta M, Viappiani A, Ferrario C, Maggio M, Ventura M, Meschi T. Gut microbiota composition is associated with polypharmacy in elderly hospitalized patients. Sci Rep. 2017;7(1):11102.

54. Lovat LB. Age related changes in gut physiology and nutritional status. Gut. 1996;38:306–9.

55. Li Y, Kundu P, Seow SW, de Matos CT, Aronsson L, Chin KC, Karre K, Pettersson S, Greicius G. Gut microbiota accelerate tumor growth via c-jun and STAT3 phosphorylation in APCMin/+ mice. Carcinogenesis. 2012;33(6):1231–8.

56. Banna GL, Torino F, Marletta F, Santagati M, Salemi R, Cannarozzo E, Falzone L, Ferraù F, Libra M. Lactobacillus rhamnosus GG: an overview to explore the rationale of its use in cancer. Front Pharmacol. 2017;8:603.

57. Przemska-Kosicka A, Childs CE, Enani S, Maidens C, Dong H, Dayel IB, Tuohy K, Todd S, Gosney MA, Yaqoob P. Effect of a synbiotic on the response to seasonal influenza vaccination is strongly influenced by degree of immunosenescence. Immun Ageing. 2016;13:6.

58. Ahima RS. Connecting obesity, aging and diabetes. Nat Med. 2009;15:996–7.

59. Khandekar MJ, Cohen P, Spiegelman BM. Molecular mechanisms of cancer development in obesity. Nat Rev Cancer. 2011;11:886–95.

60. Renehan AG, Tyson M, Egger M, Heller RF, Zwahlen M. Body-mass index and incidence of cancer: a systematic review and meta-analysis of prospective observational studies. Lancet. 2008;371:569–78.

61. Hotamisligil GS. Inflammation and metabolic disorders. Nature. 2006;444:860–7.

62. Gregor MF, Hotamisligil GS. Inflammatory mechanisms in obesity. Annu Rev Immunol. 2011;29:415–45.

63. Shivappa N, Steck SE, Hurley TG, Hussey JR, Hébert JR. Designing and developing a literature-derived, population-based dietary inflammatory index. Public Health Nutr. 2014;17:1689–96.

64. Zitvogel L, Pietrocola F, Kroemer G. Nutrition, inflammation and cancer. Nat Immunol. 2017;18(8):843–50.

65. Chrysohoou C, Panagiotakos DB, Pitsavos C, Das UN, Stefanadis C. Adherence to the Mediterranean diet attenuates inflammation and coagulation process in healthy adults: the ATTICA study. J Am Coll Cardiol. 2004;44:152–8.

66. Esposito K, Marfella R, Ciotola M, Di Palo C, Giugliano F, Giugliano G, D'Armiento M, D'Andrea F, Giugliano D. Effect of a Mediterranean-style diet on endothelial dysfunction and markers of vascular inflammation in the metabolic syndrome: a randomized trial. JAMA. 2004;292:1440–6.

67. Esmaillzadeh A, Kimiagar M, Mehrabi Y, Azadbakht L, FB H, Willett WC. Fruit and vegetable intakes, C-reactive protein, and the metabolic syndrome. Am J Clin Nutr. 2006;84:1489–97.

68. Ferrucci L, Cherubini A, Bandinelli S, Bartali B, Corsi A, Lauretani F, Martin A, Andres-Lacueva C, Senin U, Guralnik JM. Relationship of plasma polyunsaturated fatty acids to circulating inflammatory markers. J Clin Endocrinol Metab. 2006;9:439–46.

69. Carruba G, Cocciadiferro L, Di Cristina A, Granata OM, Dolcemascolo C, Campisi I, Zarcone M, Cinquegrani M, Traina A. Nutrition, aging and cancer: lessons from dietary intervention studies. Immun Ageing. 2016;13:13.

70. Shivappa N, Hébert JR, Taborelli M, Montella M, Libra M, Zucchetto A, Crispo A, Grimaldi M, La Vecchia C, Serraino D, Polesel J. Dietary inflammatory index and non-Hodgkin lymphoma risk in an Italian case-control study. Cancer Causes Control. 2017;28(Suppl 7):791–9.

71. Shivappa N, Hébert JR, Rosato V, Rossi M, Libra M, Montella M, Serraino D, La Vecchia C. Dietary inflammatory index and risk of bladder cancer in a large Italian case-control study. Urology. 2017;100:84–9.

72. Shivappa N, Hébert JR, Zucchetto A, Montella M, Libra M, Garavello W, Rossi M, La Vecchia C, Serraino D. Increased risk of nasopharyngeal carcinoma with increasing levels of diet-associated inflammation in an Italian case-control study. Nutr Cancer. 2016;68(Suppl 7):1123–30.

73. Harmon BE, Wirth MD, Boushey CJ, Wilkens LR, Draluck E, Shivappa N, Steck SE, Hofseth L, Haiman CA, Le Marchand L, Hébert JR. The dietary inflammatory index is associated with colorectal cancer risk in the multiethnic cohort. J Nutr. 2017;147:430–8.

74. Hodge AM, Bassett JK, Shivappa N, Hébert JR, English DR, Giles GG, Severi G. Dietary inflammatory index, Mediterranean diet score, and lung cancer: a prospective study. Cancer Causes Control. 2016;27:907–17.

75. Shivappa N, Blair CK, Prizment AE, Jacobs DR, Hebert JR. Prospective study of the dietary inflammatory index and risk of breast cancer in postmenopausal women. Mol Nutr Food Res. 2016;61:5.

76. Sjöström L, Gummesson A, Sjöström CD, Narbro K, Peltonen M, Wedel H, Bengtsson C, Bouchard C, Carlsson B, Dahlgren S, Jacobson P, Karason K, Karlsson J, Larsson B, Lindroos AK, Lönroth H, Näslund I, Olbers T, Stenlöf K, Torgerson J, Carlsson LM. Swedish obese subjects study. Effects of bariatric surgery on cancer incidence in obese patients in Sweden (Swedish obese subjects study): a prospective, controlled intervention trial. Lancet Oncol. 2009;10:653–62.

77. Aiello A, Accardi G, Candore G, Gambino CM, Mirisola M, Taormina G, Virruso C, Caruso C. Nutrient sensing pathways as therapeutic targets for healthy ageing. Expert Opin Ther Targets. 2017;21(Suppl 4):371–80.

78. Davinelli S, Willcox DC, Scapagnini G. Extending healthy ageing: nutrient sensitive pathway and centenarian population. Immun Ageing. 2012;9:9.

79. Scapagnini G, Davinelli S, Kaneko T, Koverech G, Koverech A, Calabrese EJ, Calabrese V. Dose response biology of resveratrol in obesity. J Cell Commun Signal. 2014;8(Suppl 4):385–91.

80. Davinelli S, Maes M, Corbi G, Zarrelli A, Willcox DC, Scapagnini G. Dietary phytochemicals and neuro-inflammaging: from mechanistic insights to translational challenges. Immun Ageing. 2016;13:16.

81. Pandima DK, Rajavel T, Daglia M, Nabavi SF, Bishayee A, Nabavi SM. Targeting miRNAs by polyphenols: novel therapeutic strategy for cancer. Semin Cancer Biol. 2017;46:146–57.

82. Augustin LS, Libra M, Crispo A, Grimaldi M, De Laurentiis M, Rinaldo M, D'Aiuto M, Catalano F, Banna G, Ferrau' F, Rossello R, Serraino D, Bidoli E, Massarut S, Thomas G, Gatti D, Cavalcanti E, Pinto M, Riccardi G, Vidgen E, Kendall CW, Jenkins DJ, Ciliberto G, Montella M. Low glycemic index diet, exercise and vitamin D to reduce breast cancer recurrence (DEDiCa): design of a clinical trial. BMC Cancer. 2017;17(Suppl 1):69.

83. Park K, Kim KB. miRTar hunter: a prediction system for identifying human microRNA target sites. Molecules and Cells. 2013;35:195–201.

84. Breving K, Esquela-Kerscher A. The complexities of microRNA regulation: mirandering around the rules. Int J Biochem Cell Biol. 2010;42:1316–29.

85. Schroen B, Heymans S. Small but smart– microRNAs in the centre of inflammatory processes during cardiovascular diseases, the metabolic syndrome, and ageing. Cardiovasc Res. 2012;93:605–13.

86. Schwarzenbach H, Nishida N, Calin GA, Pantel K. Clinical relevance of circulating cell-free microRNAs in cancer. Nat Rev Clin Oncol. 2014;11:145–56.

87. Qiu C, Chen G, Cui Q. Towards the understanding of microRNA and environmental factor interactions and their relationships to human diseases. Sci Rep. 2012;2:318.

88. Vrijens K, Bollati V, Nawrot TS. MicroRNAs as potential signatures of environmental exposure or effect: a systematic review. Environ Health Perspect. 2015;123(Suppl 5):399–411.

89. Olivieri F, Rippo MR, Monsurrò V, Salvioli S, Capri M, Procopio AD, Franceschi C. MicroRNAs linking inflamm-aging, cellular senescence and cancer. Ageing Res Rev. 2013;12:1056–68.

90. Olivieri F, Spazzafumo L, Santini G, Lazzarini R, Albertini MC, Rippo MR, Galeazzi R, Abbatecola AM, Marcheselli F, Monti D, Ostan R, Cevenini E, Antonicelli R, Franceschi C, Procopio AD. Age-related differences in the expression of circulating microRNAs: miR-21 as a new circulating marker of inflammaging. Mech Ageing Dev. 2012;133:675–85.

91. Falzone L, Candido S, Salemi R, Basile MS, Scalisi A, McCubrey JA, Torino F, Signorelli SS, Montella M, Libra M. Computational identification of microRNAs associated to both epithelial to mesenchymal transition and NGAL/MMP-9 pathways in bladder cancer. Oncotarget. 2016;7(Suppl 45):72758–66.

92. Schulte C, Zeller T. microRNA-based diagnostics and therapy in cardiovascular disease-summing up the facts. Cardiovasc Diagn Ther. 2015;5(Suppl 1):17–36.

27

The association of high sensitivity C-reactive protein and incident Alzheimer disease in patients 60 years and older: The HUNT study, Norway

Jessica Mira Gabin[1*], Ingvild Saltvedt[2,3], Kristian Tambs[4^] and Jostein Holmen[1]

Abstract

Background: With ageing, long-standing inflammation can be destructive, contributing to development of several disorders, among these Alzheimer's disease (AD). C-reactive protein (CRP) is a relatively stable peripheral inflammatory marker, but in previous studies the association between highly sensitive CRP (hsCRP) and AD have shown inconsistent results. This study examines the association between AD and hsCRP in blood samples taken up to 15 years prior to the diagnoses of 52 persons with AD amongst a total of 2150 persons ≥60 years of age.

Results: Data from Norway's Nord-Trøndelag Health Study (HUNT 2) and the Health and Memory Study (HMS) were linked. The participants had an average age of 73 years, and diagnosed with AD up to 15 years [mean 8.0 (±3.9)] following hsCRP measurement. Logistic regression models showed an adverse association between hsCRP and AD in participants aged 60-70.5 (odds ratio: 2.37, 95% CI: 1.01-5.58). Conversely, in participants aged 70.6-94, there was an inverse association between hsCRP and AD (odds ratio: 0.39, 95% CI: 0.19-0.84). When applying multivariate models the findings were significant in individuals diagnosed 0.4-7 years after the hsCRP was measured; and attenuated when AD was diagnosed more than seven years following hsCRP measurement.

Conclusions: Our study is in line with previous studies indicating a shift in the association between hsCRP and AD by age: in adults (60-70.5 years) there is an adverse association, while in seniors (>70.6 years) there is an inverse association. If our findings can be replicated, a focus on why a more active peripheral immune response may have a protective role in individuals ≥70 years should be further examined.

Keywords: Epidemiology, Low-grade inflammation, High sensitivity C-reactive protein, Alzheimer disease

Background

Pre-clinical and clinical studies have shown that the immune system contributes and drives Alzheimer disease (AD) pathogenesis [1]. Inflammatory proteins found outside of the brain have also been shown to be elevated in patients with AD [2]. With ageing, long-standing inflammation can be destructive, contributing to development of several disorders [3, 4].

A minor elevation in inflammatory markers in blood is termed low-grade inflammation, where the body is constantly under very mild chronic elevation, but not to the extent of acute inflammation [5]. Low grade inflammation is recognized as an important contributor to the pathophysiology of hypertension, to the initiation and progression of atherosclerosis and the development of cardiovascular disease (CVD) [6]. C-reactive protein (CRP) is a relatively stable peripheral inflammatory marker that has been used as a marker of low-grade inflammation, and the highly sensitive assay (hsCRP) has been shown to be moderately elevated in acute myocardial infarction, coronary artery disease, metabolic syndrome, neurodegenerative diseases, and hypertension

* Correspondence: jessica.gabin@ntnu.no
Kristian Tambs Deceased 18 June 2017
^Deceased
[1]HUNT Research Centre, Department of Public Health and Nursing, Norwegian University of Science and Technology (NTNU), Forskningsveien 2, 7600 Levanger, Norway
Full list of author information is available at the end of the article

[7–10]. Since several CVD have been shown to share risk factors for developing dementia, a number of studies have examined whether there is an association between low-grade peripheral inflammation and AD [11, 12]. However, previous epidemiological studies examining hsCRP and AD revealed conflicting findings. Studies examining hsCRP during midlife showed adverse associations, where moderate elevations of hsCRP were increased in persons who developed AD later in life [13]. In contrast, studies examining older participants published that higher plasma levels of hsCRP was associated with a lower risk for AD and all-cause dementia, and authors questioned whether this could be attributed to a genetic phenotype for successful aging [14, 15]. Some studies examining gene expression have shown down-regulation of immune response genes in brain regions of cognitively impaired oldest-old persons and up-regulation in cognitively intact individuals of same age [16, 17]. Locascio et al. found that low levels of hsCRP were associated with more rapid progression of illness, whereas Nilsson et al. found that although CRP was overall lower in persons with AD, elevated CRP was associated with shorter survival time [18, 19]. Other studies show the opposite, that high hsCRP levels were associated with cognitive decline [2, 13, 20, 21]. However, previous studies were based on relatively small samples and short observation time.

In Nord-Trøndelag County, Norway, a large population based health study (the HUNT Study) combined with a registry of patients with dementia, provide data suitable for long follow-up time. The aim of this study was therefore to examine the association between hsCRP and AD in blood samples taken up to 15 years prior to the AD diagnosis amongst HUNT Study participants in Nord Trøndelag County over the age of 60 years.

Methods
Study population and data collection
The HUNT Study is a voluntary health survey offered to all residents in Nord-Trøndelag County (N~130,000). The region is approximately the size of Wales, rural, and located in central Norway. The HUNT Study consists of three population-based cohorts examining in total 125,000 residents during the span of three decades; HUNT 1 (1984-1986); HUNT 2 (1995-1997) and HUNT 3 (2006-2008). The HUNT Study has examined a large number of public health issues, like somatic and mental illnesses, quality of life, social factors, life style and other health determinants. The general methods for data collection were similar in all three HUNT surveys: several questionnaires, clinical measurements and collection of blood and urine samples. Participant's age was obtained from the national population registry. History of myocardial infarction (MI), stroke, angina, diabetes mellitus

(DM), smoking, and subjective health status were self-reported by participants. Clinical measurements were conducted in survey stations following standardized protocols. Pulse, systolic and diastolic blood pressure were measured three times using a Dinamap 845XT (Critikon) based on oscillometry. Body mass index (BMI) was based on height and weight measured with the participants wearing light clothes without shoes: height to the nearest centimeter and weight to the nearest half kilogram. Blood samples measuring non-fasting glucose, creatinine, triglycerides, and cholesterol used in the present study were collected at the health survey stations and transported to the biobank in well-described methods, that are published in detail previously [22, 23].

hsCRP measurement
During HUNT 2 ($n = 65,237$) hsCRP measurement was measured in a subsample. For practical reasons, participants from four neighboring municipalities around the biochemical laboratory assaying hsCRP were selected randomly, and 9993 had their hsCRP measured (Fig. 1). The present study selected participants who had their hsCRP measured, returned the two main HUNT 2 questionnaires ($n = 8766$), and did not have prevalent dementia at time of survey participation ($n = 8760$). As hsCRP values can rise during active systemic infections or in acute inflammatory processes, we included only participants with hsCRP values less than 10 ($n = 8391$). Finally, we included only participants aged 60 and over ($n = 2585$) who had complete covariate data, which resulted in 2150 individuals who encompass the study sample. Non-fasting serum was stored at negative 80 degrees Celsius and measured two years after serum collection. The analysis were performed at a biomedical laboratory using the CRP (Latex) US (Hoffman-La Roche AG, Switzerland) standard assay for CRP analysis. Assay reproducibility was tested by the assay provider (Hitachi/Roche) and has run within [% coefficient of variation (CV) 0.43-1.34] and between days (%CV 2.51-5.70), in addition to running a method comparison ($r = 0.996$) [24].

Dementia ascertainment
The Health and Memory Study of Nord-Trøndelag (the HMS Study) collected retrospectively data on individuals with dementia from the two regional hospitals between 1995 and 2010. Additionally, residents in all nursing homes in the region were examined for dementia between 2010 and 2011and ascertained by clinicians. The data collection has been more extensively described previously [25]. Briefly, two panels encompass the HMS study: a hospital and a nursing home panel. Ascertainment was uniform amongst panels and evaluated by clinicians confirming ICD-10 diagnostic criteria for AD,

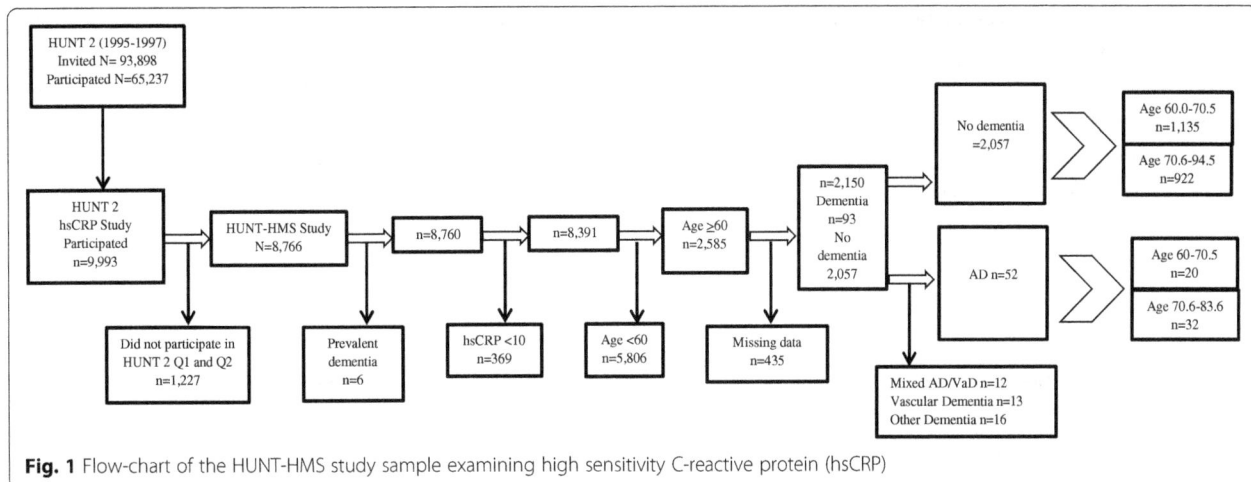

Fig. 1 Flow-chart of the HUNT-HMS study sample examining high sensitivity C-reactive protein (hsCRP)

vascular dementia (VaD), and a mixture of these (mixed AD/VaD) based on clinical examination, patient and caregiver history and diagnostic imaging. Time of diagnosis was determined at assessment by clinicians and, if unknown, based on the initial documented examination date. The eleven-digit personal identification number given to each Norwegian resident linked the participants in HUNT 2 and individuals diagnosed with dementia in the HMS Study. Ninety-three HMS participants had hsCRP values less than ten and complete covariate data, of which 52 were diagnosed with AD; and are the focus of the present study. An additional 13 individuals were diagnosed with VaD, 12 mixed AD/VaD, and 16 with dementia of other causes.

Data analysis

Participant's age was used as a continuous variable in analyses. Supplemental analyses were used to examine a significant interaction effect and created by dichotomizing participants >60 in equal groups <70.6 and ≥70.6. Level of education was categorized according to primary (seven years or less), secondary (seven to nine years), and upper secondary education (>ten years). The average of the second and third blood pressure measurement was used in analyses. Non-fasting glucose, cholesterol, triglycerides and creatinine were scored as continuous variables. The independent-samples t-test and Pearson's chi squared were used to compare the means between groups for continuous and categorical variables, and Mann-Whitney (MW) for comparisons between cases and non-cases examining hsCRP levels and potential covariates. HsCRP was examined in analyses as a continuous variable. The values of hsCRP were positively skewed and log transformations were used in all analyses and were less skewed; but neither distributions were normal. We used binary logistic models to estimate odds ratios (OR) with 95% confidence intervals (CI) for the

associations of hsCRP to the incidence of AD, all-cause dementia, and non-AD dementia. Four sets of logistic regression models were performed for each endpoint in a hierarchy. Effect modification was examined by testing the statistical significance for age x hsCRP and sex x hsCRP in multivariable models. Additional analyses were performed to examine whether time to ascertainment influenced the association by splitting the sample equally in two according to the number of years to diagnosis from baseline. All statistical analyses were performed using SPSS, version 24.

Results

The participants in the present study had an average age of 73 years and were diagnosed with AD up to 15 years [mean 8.0 (±3.9)] following hsCRP measurement. The characteristics of the study sample are shown in Table 1. Mean hsCRP are shown in their original values. Levels of hsCRP were significantly lower in the AD group ≥70.6 than in the reference group. Except from the age and sex differences, there were no significant differences between the study groups regarding other biomarkers, education, and history of MI, angina, stroke or DM.

Multiple logistic regression analyses were performed for the total sample; and repeated separately for age groups 60- 70.5, and ages greater than or equal to 70.6 at the time of HUNT 2. The results for hsCRP in the total sample are shown in the upper part of Table 2 (1), in the sample aged 60-70.5 (2), and aged greater and equal to 70.6 in the lower portion (3). Results for total dementia, mixed AD/VaD, and VaD are presented in Table 3. There was no association between hsCRP and the risk of developing AD in the total sample, but there were significant age interactions in multivariate analyses. Additional analyses were performed with age dichotomized according to median age; and results of logistic regression analyses are shown in sections (2) and (3) of

Table 1 Characteristics of participants with no dementia ($n = 2057$) and participants with Alzheimer disease ($n = 52$) at the time of HUNT2 (baseline)

HUNT 2 (1995-1997)	No dementia	Alzheimer disease	P value[a]
Total study population, n	2057	52	
Sex, Female, n (%)	1120 (54.4)	34 (65.4)	.02
Age at HUNT 2 (1995-1997), mean (SD)	70.37 (6.87)	72.28 (5.18)	.01
Time to debut, years, mean (SD)	0	8.01 (3.92)	
Education, n (%)			.40
Primary	1251 (60.8)	35 (67.3)	
Completed secondary	578 (28.1)	12 (23.0)	
Completed upper secondary	228 (11.1)	5 (9.6)	
High sensitivity C-reactive protein (hsCRP),(<3 mg/dl) mean (SD)	2.17 (2.03)	1.95 (1.90)	.25
<70.6	$n = 1135$	$n = 20$	
hsCRP, mean (SD)	2.13 (2.05)	2.77 (1.93)	.08
≥70.6	$n = 922$	$n = 32$	
hsCRP, mean (SD)	2.23 (2.01)	1.44 (1.71)	.00
Creatinine (53-115 µmol/L), mean (SD)	90.91 (16.25)	87.73 (12.74)	.16
Cholesterol (3.5-6.5 mmol/L), mean (SD)	6.54 (1.22)	6.63 (1.97)	.60
Triglycerides (0.6-1.8 mmol/L), mean (SD)	1.90 (1.02)	2.03 (1.25)	.38
Non-fasting blood glucose (4.0-5.9 mmol/L), mean (SD)	5.90 (1.86)	5.80 (1.22)	.68
Body Mass Index (kg/m^2) mean (SD)	27.12 (4.15)	26.87 (4.02)	.67
Pulse (beats/min), mean (SD)	72.01 (13.21)	71.48 (12.73)	.78
Systolic BP (mmHg), mean (SD)	151.81 (22.91)	157.40 (22.31)	.08
Diastolic BP (mmHg), mean (SD)	85.03 (12.74)	85.85 (13.63)	.65
Diabetes Mellitus, n (%)	133 (6.5)	2 (3.8)	.45
Myocardial Infarction, n (%)	173 (8.4)	2 (3.8)	.24
Angina Pectoris, n (%)	258 (12.5)	5 (9.6)	.53
Stroke, n (%)	85 (4.1)	1 (1.9)	.43
Daily Smoker, ever, n (%)	1191 (57.9)	27 (52.0)	.16
Subjective health status			.27
Poor, n (%)	48 (2.3)	1 (1.9)	
Not so good, n (%)	757 (36.8)	18 (34.6)	
Good, n (%)	1129 (54.9)	33 (63.5)	
Very good, n (%)	123 (6.0)		

[a]P-values are derived from t tests for continuous variables and x^2 tests for the binary variables

Table 2. In participants between 60 and 70.5, an adverse association was observed between hsCRP and AD. Conversely, in participants between 70.6 and 94, there was an inverse association between hsCRP and AD. Additional adjustment for all covariates did not change the finding.

Additional analyses were performed and presented in Table 2 (4-9) examining whether the number of years to AD onset from baseline influenced the association between hsCRP and AD. A similar adverse trend was observed amongst the sample diagnosed 0.4 to 7 years following hsCRP measurement. Amongst those 60-70.5, the adverse association between hsCRP and AD was attenuated and did not retain significance. An opposite trend was observed amongst those ≥70.6, where an inverse association was observed in participants diagnosed up to seven years later. The inverse association between hsCRP and AD amongst those diagnosed with AD seven-15 years later was attenuated and did not retain significance.

Discussion

The main finding of our study was that hsCRP levels were adversely associated with participants aged between 60 and 70.5, and inversely associated with developing AD in participants aged ≥70.6. When applying

Table 2 Multiple logistic regression analyses on the association of hsCRP and Alzheimer disease (AD)

	AD	NC[a]	Debut AD 0.4-7 years later		NC[a]	Debut AD 7-15 years later		NC[a]
(1) Age ≥60[b]	n = 2150	52	(4) Age ≥ 60	n = 2150	23	(7) Age ≥ 60	n = 2150	29
Model 1[c]	.77 (.47-1.26)		Model 1	.80 (.39-1.67)		Model 1	.84 (.41-1.71)	
Model 2[d]	.75 (.46-1.24)		Model 2	.82 (.39-1.73)		Model 2	.80 (.39-1.64)	
Model 3[e]	.78 (.47-1.32)		Model 3	.86 (.39-1.86)		Model 3	.83 (.39-1.75)	
Model 4[f]	.82 (.49-1.38)		Model 4	.93 (.42-2.04)		Model 4	.83 (.39-1.77)	
hsCRP*Age	.93 (.87-.99)		hsCRP*Age	.88 (.80-.97)		hsCRP*Age	.59 (.70-4.70)	
hsCRP*Sex	.90 (.31-2.64)		hsCRP*Sex	1.24 (.27-5.73)		hsCRP*Sex	2.40 (.37-15.71)	
(2) Age 60-70.5[b]	n = 1176	20	(5) Age 60-70.5	n = 1176	6	(8) Age 60-70.5	n = 1176	14
Model 1	1.85 (.89-3.85)		Model 1	4.20 (1.05-16.77)		Model 1	1.31 (.50-3.39)	
Model 2	1.83 (.85-3.93)		Model 2	5.77 (1.32-25.35)		Model 2	1.12 (.41-3.02)	
Model 3	2.34 (1.02-5.35)		Model 3	11.32 (2.01-63.67)		Model 3	1.29 (.44-3.80)	
Model 4	2.37 (1.01-5.58)		Model 4	14.20 (1.80- 112.22)		Model 4	1.29 (.42-3.96)	
hsCRP*Age	1.10 (.82-1.46)		hsCRP*Age	1.07 (.59-1.95)		hsCRP*Age	1.58 (1.03-2.42)	
hsCRP*Sex	2.40 (.37-15.71)		hsCRP*Sex	9.02 (.15-552.04)		hsCRP*Sex	1.67 (.48-5.78)	
(3) Age 70.6-94[b]	n = 974	32	(6) Age 70.6-94	n = 974	17	(9) Age 70.6-94	n = 974	15
Model 1	.36 (.18-.74)		Model 1	.35 (.13-.93)		Model 1	.48 (.16-1.46)	
Model 2	.36 (.18-.73)		Model 2	.33 (.13-.89)		Model 2	.50 (.16-1.5)	
Model 3	.35 (.17-.74)		Model 3	.31 (.11-.84)		Model 3	.53 (.17-1.68)	
Model 4	.39 (.19-.84)		Model 4	.34 (.12-.96)		Model 4	.54 (.16-1.81)	
hsCRP*Age	.93 (.77-1.13)		hsCRP*Age	.77 (.58-1.03)		hsCRP*Age	1.07 (.82-1.39)	
hsCRP*Sex	.65 (.14-2.99)		hsCRP*Sex	.64 (.08-4.97)		hsCRP*Sex	1.54 (.08-30.13)	

Results of the total sample (age ≥ 60) are shown in the upper left section (1), in age group 60-70.5 in middle left section (2) and in age group >70.6 in lower left section (3). Section 4-9 show analyses according to time from baseline (HUNT 2) to debut of AD, in different age groups
[a]Number of dementia cases
[b]Age when examined in HUNT 2
[c]Model 1: log transformed high specificity C-reactive protein (hsCRP)
[d]Model 2: hsCRP, age, sex, education
[e]Model 3: hsCRP, age, sex, education, cholesterol, triglycerides, non-fasting blood glucose, creatinine, body mass index, pulse
[f]Model 4: SBP, age, sex, education, cholesterol, triglycerides, non-fasting blood glucose, glomerular filtration rate, body mass index, pulse, history of myocardial infarction, diabetes mellitus, angina, stroke, smoking, subjective health status

multivariate models the findings were significant in individuals diagnosed only 0.4-7 years after the hsCRP was measured; and attenuated when AD was diagnosed more than seven years following hsCRP measurement.

Our findings support previous studies that report contrast findings when considering age. As in previous studies, participants in the younger age bracket (60-70.5) advocated that high hsCRP was associated with an increased risk of AD [13]. In oldest participants, our findings support previous studies reporting an inverse association between hsCRP and AD [14, 15, 18, 19, 26–30].

Our study had a number of strengths in comparison with earlier studies, as a large number of subjects over the age of 60 had a follow-up time of up to 16 years. In addition, the prospective study design allowed for extensive control for numerous chronic conditions. Also, the utilized hsCRP assay has been shown to be a peripheral biomarker with high assertion. Our study should, however, be interpreted with some limitations. The HUNT Study participants are mostly Caucasian and the

population is well educated, and results may not apply to all ethnicities or social demographics. The sample sizes in stratified analyses were relatively small. Although efforts were made to identify participants diagnosed with dementia in the region during 1995–2011 by performing hospital record searches and examining nursing home residents, we had no access to data from individuals with dementia who were under the care of their general practitioner, and these will appear as false-negatives in the data set. However, the proportion of false-negatives to true-negatives in the non-case group is quite low because the prevalence of dementia is, after all, low. Therefore, the contamination of the non-case group will not be substantial, and the effect estimates will be little more than inconsequential. Lastly, the prescription registry was not linked with the current study, and we cannot exclude that medication had an influence on hsCRP values, as it has been known that NSAIDs and lipid lowering medication such as statins reduce hsCRP values [31].

Table 3 Complete analysis using logistic regression in examining the association of log transformed high sensitivity C reactive protein (hsCRP) and dementia

	Total Dementia	NC[a]	Combined AD, Mixed AD and Vascular Dementia	NC[a]	Alzheimer Disease	NC[a]	Mixed AD and Vascular Dementia	NC[a]
(1) Study sample N = 7758	HUNT 2	102	HUNT 2	84	HUNT 2	55	HUNT 2	29
Model 1[b]	1.55 (1.13-2.12)		1.57 (1.11-2.21)		1.23 (.79-1.90)		2.41 (1.37-4.25)	
Model 2[c]	1.02 (.72-1.44)		1.01 (.69-1.49)		.74 (.45-1.22)		1.71 (.92-3.19)	
Model 3[d]	1.03 (.71-1.48)		1.02 (.68-1.52)		.79 (.47-1.31)		1.60 (.84-3.06)	
Model 4[e]	1.01 (.70-1.45)		1.02 (.68-1.54)		.81 (.48-1.35)		1.55 (.80-2.97)	
hsCRP*Age	.98 (.95-1.00)		.98 (.95-1.01)		.98 (.94-1.02)		.98 (.93-1.03)	
hsCRP*Sex	.83 (.40-1.72)		.86 (.38-1.93)		.93 (.32-2.69)		.56 (.16-2.03)	
(2) <60[f] N = 5608		9		7		3		4
Model 1	2.12 (.77-5.85)		1.83 (.57-5.90)		.08 (.00-3.71)		6.00 (1.29-28.00)	
Model 2	1.75 (.59-5.24)		1.40 (.39-5.04)		.06 (.00-2.96)		5.39 (.93-31.18)	
Model 3	2.43 (.79-7.47)		1.87 (.50-7.03)		.06 (.00-7.13)		5.26 (.82-33.72)	
Model 4	1.88 (.58-6.14)		1.53 (.37-6.25)		.05 (.00-8.31)		5.14 (.71-37.45)	
hsCRP*Age	1.06 (.90-1.26)		1.38 (1.01-1.90)		1.00 (.61-1.66)		.86 (.23-3.27)	
hsCRP*Sex	.24 (.02-2.69)		.96 (.56-1.63)				.06 (.00-10.03)	
(3) ≥60[f] N = 2150		93		77		52		25
Model 1	.90 (.62-1.29)		.92 (.62-1.37)		.77 (.47-1.26)		1.33 (.68-2.59)	
Model 2	.89 (.62-1.28)		.91 (.61-1.36)		.75 (.46-1.24)		1.31 (.67-2.58)	
Model 3	.98 (.57-1.67)		.90 (.59-1.37)		.78 (.47-1.32)		1.19 (.46-3.09)	
Model 4	.88 (.60-1.29)		.92 (.61-1.41)		.82 (.49-1.38)		1.21 (.59-2.48)	
hsCRP*Age	.96 (.91-1.01)		.95 (.90-1.01)		.93 (.97-.99)		1.01 (.91-1.11)	
hsCRP*Sex	.99 (.46-2.12)		.92 (.39-2.14)		.90 (.31-2.64)		.77 (.19-3.17)	

[a]Number of dementia cases
[b]Model 1: log transformed high specificity C-reactive protein (hsCRP)
[c]Model 2: hsCRP, age, sex, education
[d]Model 3: hsCRP, age, sex, education, cholesterol, triglycerides, non-fasting blood glucose, creatinine, body mass index, pulse
[e]Model 4: SBP, age, sex, education, cholesterol, triglycerides, non-fasting blood glucose, glomerular filtration rate, body mass index, pulse, history of myocardial infarction, diabetes mellitus, angina, stroke, smoking, subjective health status
[f]Age when examined in HUNT 2

One challenge of the present study is to understand why hsCRP are in contrast when examining age of the participant during the years hsCRP is observed until the AD onset. It is questionable whether lower hsCRP values provides protection from AD, or if it is the result of the neuropathology in older at-risk individuals. A recent meta-analysis of CRP in persons with AD discussed whether CRP levels could be different in different stages of the disease trajectory. The authors speculated whether CRP is decreased in mild or moderate AD, and increased in the following severe stage [32]. Dementia disorders are progressive and fatal disorders, as the blood samples obtained were an average of 8 years prior to diagnosis, it must be assumed that these were taken before AD developed or in very early stages. The results in this study appear to be more dependent on the age of the participant.

There have been a number of studies examining how immune responses can be affected by the pathophysiology of AD. Advances in neuroimmunology have shown

that the molecular innate immune response is dysfunctional in AD [33]. The body's immune response in AD responds to an aggregation of amyloid-β (Aβ) peptides in the endoplasmic reticulum (ER) that causes stress and activation of the unfolded protein response (UPR) [34]. UPR aims to alleviate stress and minor elevations of systemic inflammatory markers, reflects the presence of stressed cells. In circumstances of chronic or prolonged ER stress, sensors responsible for binding to misfolded proteins change from acting pro-protective to pro-apoptotic [35]. It has been postulated that the molecular mechanisms involved in the innate immune response are disrupting UPR functioning and can be involved in the pathogenesis of AD [34]. Although the precise molecular pathways of neuroinflammation remain unclear, a gene expression study found inflammatory changes in the aging brain regarded as age-dependent [17]. Interestingly, the period between the sixth and seventh decade was observed to undergo robust gene expression changes.

It is known that clinical AD is preceded by decades of a prodromal phase. During this asymptomatic phase, systemic changes are known to be occurring. To examine whether our findings were influenced by ascertainment time, samples were split by the number of years participants developed AD following hsCRP measurement, see Table 2 (sections 4-9). There was a stronger association in participants who were diagnosed up to seven years later in comparison with those who were diagnosed seven to 15 years later. However, sample sizes in these stratified analyses were small and it is questionable whether the finding is a true association or the result of preclinical AD. Although, participants with dementia were ascertained in both nursing home and residential settings, it is perhaps speculative to say that nursing home participants were in a more severe stage than those at home, as there can be many other factors determining whether a Norwegian resident needs placement in nursing care. For example, those living in secluded areas, and often alone are demanding admission to a nursing home facility sooner than residents living at home with help from family and regardless of the stage severity. It is therefore difficult to distinguish strictly on this basis. Therefore, we examined stage severity using years to onset. Since the hsCRP marker was taken an approximately 8 years prior to diagnosis, it is most likely these participants were not exhibiting cognitive decline or at most, mild cognitive impairment.

Finally, low-grade inflammation is defined as being a state where the body is constantly under very mild chronic inflammation but not to the extent of acute inflammation. Minor elevation in inflammatory markers are measured in blood with inflammatory markers, such as hsCRP. Defining a precise cut-off between these two states is difficult, but many previous studies define a hsCRP under 10 with low-grade inflammation; and values above this as clinically significant inflammatory states [5]. The American Heart Association have suggested that cut points of hsCRP below 1 mg/l, between 1 and 3 mg/l, and greater than 3 mg/l can be used to find those at lower, average, and high relative risk for CVD events [36]. Replication of our data will strengthen the existing evidence whether similar cut points of hsCRP, in addition to a panel of other inflammatory markers, such as interleukins, should be considered clinically relevant when monitoring patients at risk for dementia.

Conclusions

Our study is in line with previous studies indicating a shift in the association between hsCRP and AD by age: in adults (60-70.5 years) there is an adverse association, while in seniors (>70.6 years) there is an inverse association. Regardless that the nature of the association remains unclear, our data and data from preclinical and clinical studies have established the immune system-mediated actions contribute and drive AD pathogenesis [1]. Continued research in persons at risk is needed to advance the role inflammation has in AD. If our findings can be replicated, future intervention studies should assess whether medical treatment of low-grade inflammation will reduce incidence of AD. More studies are needed to further examine why a more active peripheral immune response may have a protective role in individuals ≥70 years.

Abbreviations

AD: Alzheimer disease; Aβ: Amyloid beta; BMI: Body mass index; CI: Confidence interval; CRP: C reactive protein; CV: Coefficient of variation; DM: Diabetes mellitus; ER: Endoplasmic reticulum; HMS: Health and Memory Study of Nord-Trøndelag (1995–2010); hsCRP: High specificity C reactive protein; HUNT 1: Helse Undersøkelse Nord-Trøndelag (1984–1986); HUNT 2: Helse Undersøkelse Nord-Trøndelag (1995–1997); HUNT 3: Helse Undersøkelse Nord-Trøndelag (2006-2008); ICD-10: International Classification of Diseases, Tenth Revision; MI: Myocardial infarction; MW: Mann Whitney; NSAIDs: Non steroidal anti inflammatory drugs; OR: Odds ratio; T2D: Type two diabetes mellitus; UPR: Unfolded protein response; VaD: Vascular dementia

Acknowledgements

We thank the HUNT-HMS study participants and their caregivers.

Funding

ExtraStiftelsen and the Norwegian Health Association are the study's funding sources, and they had no other role in the HUNT-HMS Study. The corresponding author had full access to all data in the study and had final responsibility for the decision to submit for publication. The HUNT Study is a collaborative effort of the Faculty of Medicine and Health Sciences at the Norwegian University of Science and Technology (NTNU), the Norwegian Institute of Public Health, the Nord-Trøndelag County Council, and the Central Norwegian Regional Health Authority. The HMS Study was funded by the Norwegian Institue of Public Health, the NTNU, Nord-Trøndelag Hospital Trust, and Innlandet Hospital Trust.

Authors' contributions

JG, IS, and KT designed the HMS Study, and JH was co-principal investigator of both the HUNT 1 and HUNT 2 studies. JH led data collection. IS oversaw the dementia panel. JMG analyzed the patient data with assistance from JH and KT. JMG interpreted the data and drafted the manuscript. All authors read and approved the final manuscript.

Competing interests

The authors declare that they have no competing interests.

Author details

[1]HUNT Research Centre, Department of Public Health and Nursing, Norwegian University of Science and Technology (NTNU), Forskningsveien 2, 7600 Levanger, Norway. [2]Department of Neuromedicine and Movement science, NTNU, the Faculty of Medicine and Health, Post Office Box 8905, 7491 Trondheim, Norway. [3]Department of Geriatrics, St. Olav University Hospital, Post Office Box 3250, 7006 Trondheim, Norway. [4]Division of Mental Health, Norwegian Institute of Public Health, Post Office Box 4404, Nydalen, 0403 Oslo, Norway.

References

1. Heppner FL, Ransohoff RM, Becher B. Immune attack: the role of inflammation in Alzheimer disease. Nat Rev Neurosci. 2015;16(6):358–72.
2. Engelhart MJ, et al. Inflammatory proteins in plasma and the risk of dementia: the rotterdam study. Arch Neurol. 2004;61(5):668–72.
3. Paine NJ, et al. Induced mild systemic inflammation is associated with impaired ability to improve cognitive task performance by practice. Psychophysiology. 2015;52(3):333–41.
4. Vanltallie TB. Alzheimer's disease: innate immunity gone awry? Metabolism. 2017;69s:S41–s49.
5. Eklund CM. Proinflammatory cytokines in CRP baseline regulation. Adv Clin Chem. 2009;48:111–36.
6. Nosalski R, et al. Novel immune mechanisms in hypertension and cardiovascular risk. Curr Cardiovasc Risk Rep. 2017;11(4):12.
7. Devaraj S, Siegel D, Jialal I. Statin therapy in metabolic syndrome and hypertension post-JUPITER: what is the value of CRP? Curr Atheroscler Rep. 2011;13(1):31–42.
8. Matusik P, et al. Do we know enough about the immune pathogenesis of acute coronary syndromes to improve clinical practice? Thromb Haemost. 2012;108(3):443–56.
9. Kushner I, Rzewnicki D, Samols D. What does minor elevation of C-reactive protein signify? Am J Med. 2006;119(2):166. e17-28
10. Woloshin S, Schwartz LM. Distribution of C-reactive protein values in the United States. N Engl J Med. 2005;352(15):1611–3.
11. Heneka MT, et al. Neuroinflammation in Alzheimer's disease. Lancet Neurol. 2015;14(4):388–405.
12. Michaud M, et al. Proinflammatory cytokines, aging, and age-related diseases. J Am Med Dir Assoc. 2013;14(12):877–82.
13. Schmidt R, et al. Early inflammation and dementia: a 25-year follow-up of the Honolulu-Asia aging study. Ann Neurol. 2002;52(2):168–74.
14. van Himbergen TM, et al. Biomarkers for insulin resistance and inflammation and the risk for all-cause dementia and alzheimer disease: results from the Framingham heart study. Arch Neurol. 2012;69(5):594–600.
15. Silverman JM, et al. C-reactive protein and familial risk for dementia: a phenotype for successful cognitive aging. Neurology. 2012;79(11):1116–23.
16. Katsel P, Tan W, Haroutunian V. Gain in brain immunity in the oldest-old differentiates cognitively normal from demented individuals. PLoS One. 2009;4(10):e7642.
17. Berchtold NC, et al. Gene expression changes in the course of normal brain aging are sexually dimorphic. Proc Natl Acad Sci U S A. 2008;105(40):15605–10.
18. Locascio JJ, et al. Plasma amyloid beta-protein and C-reactive protein in relation to the rate of progression of Alzheimer disease. Arch Neurol. 2008;65(6):776–85.
19. Nilsson K, Gustafson L, Hultberg B. C-reactive protein level is decreased in patients with Alzheimer's disease and related to cognitive function and survival time. Clin Biochem. 2011;44(14-15):1205–8.
20. Yaffe K, et al. Inflammatory markers and cognition in well-functioning African-American and white elders. Neurology. 2003;61(1):76–80.
21. Teunissen CE, et al. Inflammation markers in relation to cognition in a healthy aging population. J Neuroimmunol. 2003;134(1-2):142–50.
22. Krokstad S, et al. Cohort profile: the HUNT study. International Journal of Epidemiology: Norway; 2012.
23. Holmen J, et al. The Nord-Trøndelag health study 1995-97 (HUNT 2): objectives, contents, methods and participation. Norsk Epidemiologi. 2003;13(1):19–32.
24. Laugsand LE, et al. Insomnia and high-sensitivity C-reactive protein: the HUNT study, Norway. Psychosom Med. 2012;74(5):543–53.
25. Bergh S, et al. Cohort Profile: The Health and Memory Study (HMS): a dementia cohort linked to the HUNT study in Norway. Int J Epidemiol. 2014; 43(6):1759-68. doi: 10.1093/ije/dyu007. Epub 2014 Feb 12.
26. Yarchoan M, et al. Association of plasma C-reactive protein levels with the diagnosis of Alzheimer's disease. J Neurol Sci. 2013;333(1-2):9–12.
27. O'Bryant SE, et al. Decreased C-reactive protein levels in Alzheimer disease. J Geriatr Psychiatry Neurol. 2010;23(1):49–53.
28. Sundelof J, et al. Systemic inflammation and the risk of Alzheimer's disease and dementia: a prospective population-based study. J Alzheimers Dis. 2009;18(1):79–87.
29. Tan ZS, et al. Inflammatory markers and the risk of Alzheimer disease: the Framingham study. Neurology. 2007;68(22):1902–8.
30. Wichmann MA, et al. Long-term systemic inflammation and cognitive impairment in a population-based cohort. J Am Geriatr Soc. 2014;62(9):1683–91.
31. Asher J, Houston M. Statins and C-reactive protein levels. J Clin Hypertens (Greenwich). 2007;9(8):622–8.
32. Gong C, et al. A meta-analysis of C-reactive protein in patients with Alzheimer's disease. Am J Alzheimers Dis Other Demen. 2016;31(3):194–200.
33. Rivest S. Regulation of innate immune responses in the brain. Nat Rev Immunol. 2009;9(6):429–39.
34. Bernales S, Soto MM, McCullagh E. Unfolded protein stress in the endoplasmic reticulum and mitochondria: a role in neurodegeneration. Front Aging Neurosci. 2012;4:5.
35. Jager R, et al. The unfolded protein response at the crossroads of cellular life and death during endoplasmic reticulum stress. Biol Cell. 2012;104(5):259–70.
36. Torres JL, Ridker PM. High sensitivity C-reactive protein in clinical practice. Am Heart Hosp J. 2003;1(3):207–11.

Association of immunoglobulin GM allotypes with longevity in long-living individuals from Southern Italy

Annibale A. Puca[1,2], Anna Ferrario[2], Anna Maciag[2], Giulia Accardi[3], Anna Aiello[3], Caterina Maria Gambino[3], Giuseppina Candore[3], Calogero Caruso[3*], Aryan M. Namboodiri[4] and Janardan P. Pandey[4]

Abstract

Background: The aim of this study was to analyse the role of GM allotypes, i.e. the hereditary antigenic determinants expressed on immunoglobulin polypeptide chains, in the attainment of longevity. The role played by immunoglobulin allotypes in the control of immune responses is well known as well as the role of an efficient immune response in longevity achievement. So, it is conceivable that particular GM allotypes may contribute to the generation of an efficient immune response that supports successful ageing, hence longevity.

Methods: In order to show if GM allotypes play a role in the achievement of longevity, we typed the DNA of 95 Long-living individuals (LLIs) and 96 young control individuals (YCs) from South Italy for GM3/17 and GM23+/− alleles.

Results: To demonstrate the role of GM allotypes in the attainment of longevity we compared genotype and allele frequencies of GM allotypes between LLIs and YCs. A global chi-square test (3 × 2) shows that the distribution of genotypes at the GM 3/17 locus is highly significantly different in LLIs from that observed in YCs ($p < 0.0001$). The 2 × 2 chi-square test shows that the carriers of the GM3 allele contribute to this highly significant difference. Accordingly, GM3 allele is significantly overrepresented in LLIs. No significant differences were instead observed regarding GM23 allele.

Conclusion: These preliminary results show that GM3 allotype is significantly overrepresented in LLIs. To best of our knowledge, this is the first study performed to assess the role of GM allotypes in longevity. So, it should be necessary to verify the data in a larger sample of individuals to confirm GM role in the attainment of longevity.

Keywords: GM allotypes, HMCV, HSV-1, Immune response, Longevity

Background

The term allotype refers to any genetic variant of a protein. However, in immunology it is used for hereditary antigenic determinants expressed on immunoglobulin polypeptide chains, i.e. the genetic markers of γ chains (GM). GM allotypes are encoded by autosomal codominant alleles that follow Mendelian laws of heredity on immunoglobulin heavy chain γ1, γ2 and γ3 genes [1]. The role played by immunoglobulin allotypes in the control of immune responses was recognized 46 years ago

[2]. Several studies have clearly shown that immune response to many infectious agents, vaccines, and auto-antigens is associated with particular GM allotypes [3]. Moreover, the well-known differences in the frequencies of GM allotypes among different ethnic groups, and the strong linkage disequilibrium within a given ethnic group, suggest that Darwinian selection over many generations, i.e. selection by major infectious diseases, has played a role in the maintenance of polymorphisms of IGHG genes, of which some are common and others are rare [3].

On the other hand, the role of an efficient immune response in the attainment of longevity is well known [4]; hence it is reasonable to hypothesize an association of GM allotypes with longevity. Using hypothesis driven candidate gene approaches, numerous studies have

* Correspondence: Calogero.caruso@unipa.it; calogero.caruso@unipa.it
[3]Department of Pathobiology and Medical Biotechnologies, University of Palermo, Corso Tukory 211, 90134 Palermo, Italy
Full list of author information is available at the end of the article

identified particular GM genes as risk factors for many malignant, infectious, and autoimmune diseases, but most of these findings have not been confirmed or refuted by the genome-wide association studies (GWAS) [3]. In addition, GWAS on longevity have not demonstrated associations of these genotypes with longevity. In fact, although most GM alleles are common within an ethnic group (some with gene frequency > 70%), they are not being evaluated in the GWAS of longevity, because these determinants are not included in the commonly employed genotyping platforms. In fact, since GM allotypes were not typed in the haplotype map (HapMap) project, they cannot be imputed. Even in the 1000 Genomes project, the coverage of this region is very low, resulting in poor quality of imputation [5].

Therefore, a candidate gene approach is necessary for evaluating the possible role played by GM genes in the attainment of longevity. So, in this paper we have analysed, by classic case control study, the distribution GM allotypes in longevous people and controls from Southern Italy. To this end, we analysed the frequencies of GM3 and GM17 determinants (arginine to lysine replacement) expressed in the constant heavy (CH)1 region of IgG1 heavy chain, and GM23- and GM23+ determinants (valine to methionine replacement) in the fragment crystallisable region (Fc) of IgG2 heavy chain [1, 3].

Results

In order to demonstrate the role of GM allotypes in the attainment of longevity and to strengthen previous results suggesting that genetic factors involved in immune responses may play a key role in longevity, we compared genotype and allele frequencies of GM allotypes between LLIs and YCs.

The genotype frequency distributions of GM3/17 genotypes and alleles are presented in Tables 1 and 2, respectively. A global chi-square test (3 × 2) shows that the distribution of the three genotypes at the GM 3/17 locus is highly significantly different in LLIs from that observed in YCs ($p < 0.0001$). The 2 × 2 chi-square test shows that the carriers of the GM3 allele contribute to this highly significant difference. Accordingly, GM3 allele is significantly overrepresented in LLIs (Table 2) (OR = 2.13; $P = 0.0003$).

Since it is well known that immune system ages differently in males and females [6], we analysed data separately for men and women. Results show that GM3 allele is significantly associated with longevity in both the sexes (data not shown).

The genotype frequency distributions of GM23 genotypes and alleles are presented in Tables 3 and 4, respectively. No significant differences were found for the distribution of GM23 genotypes and alleles between LLIs

Table 1 GM 3/17 genotypes in 95 Long-living individuals (LLIs) and Controls (YCs)

	LLI s	YCs	Chi square	P
GM 3/3	48	17	18.99	0.00001
Rest	47	70		
Total	95	87		
	LLI	Controls	Chi square	P
GM 3/17	37	57	12.83	0.0003
Rest	58	30		
Total	95	87		
	LLI	Controls	Chi square	P
GM 17/17	10	13	0.802	0.3704
Rest	85	74		
Total	95	87		

3/3 genotype OR (C.I. 2.16–8.18) = 4.21 ($P < 0.00001$)

and YCs. Also, analysing data according to sexes, no significant differences were found in both males and females (data not shown).

Discussion

The LLIs, i.e. those approaching 100 years of age, are a model of successful ageing. The exceptional longevity of LLIs is to some extent genetically guided, as emphasized by the family clustering of extreme longevity and the reduced mortality of the centenarian siblings compared to age-related elderly [7]. Longevity genes can be discovered by genetic association studies or GWAS conducted on LLIs [7, 8]. These kinds of studies identify the gene variants that have been selected by the demographic pressure and, therefore, are somehow significant for human health. The identification of these genetic variants is important since they could represent potential targets for fighting ageing-related diseases. Several research groups are working on genes involved in oxidative stress, in lipid and glucose metabolism, in immune-inflammatory responses, in DNA damage and in repair, in nutrient sensing pathways. Many results have been obtained in association studies of candidate genes, but other results are still in conflict. In particular, to date, the majority of GWAS, that rely on large population sets for multiple testing and power issues, have only confirmed the decreased

Table 2 GM 3/17 Alleles in Long-living individuals (LLIs) and Controls (YCs)

	N = 190		N = 174		OR	C.I.	p
	LLIs		YCs				
	+	%	+	%			
3	133	70	91	52	2.13	1.38–3.27	=0.0003
17	57	30	83	48			

Significance of distribution by chi square test (2 × 2) $p = 0.0005$

Table 3 GM 23 genotypes in Long-living individuals (LLIs) and Controls (YCs)

	N = 96			N = 92		
	LLIs			YCs		
	+	−	%	+	−	%
23 −/−	20	76	20.8	18	74	19.6
23 +/−	38	58	39.6	39	53	42.4
23 +/+	38	58	39.6	35	57	38.0

Significance of distribution by chi square test (2 × 6) p = NS

frequency of detrimental alleles of apolipoprotein E (APOE) and the increase of protective alleles of forkhead box O3A (FOXO3A) with some exceptions [7–10].

In the present paper we have analysed, by a classic case control study, the distribution of GM allotypes, in longevous people and controls from Southern Italy. Data show that GM3 allotype is significantly overrepresented in LLIs. To the best of our knowledge, no study has evaluated GM allotype role in human longevity. Since the distribution of GM allotypes in the population under study is not known, a note of caution must be taken into account, because of the relatively small sample sizes of LLIs and controls. However, a study performed on the sheep several years ago reported an influence of IgG3 allotypes in ageing of sheep. These findings, showing the role played by GM allotypes in other animal species, fit ours [11].

A study by de Vries et al. [12] is relevant to our findings. Descendants of Dutch colonists, who emigrated to Surinam and survived epidemics of typhoid and yellow fever with a total mortality of about 60%, were tested for different polymorphisms, including GM allotypes, whose frequencies were compared with those of Dutch control sample. Several polymorphisms, including GM allotypes, were shown to influence the chance for survival, indicating selection through genetic control of immune response to pathogens. Another example of such selection is the longevity associated variant of Bactericidal/Permeability-increasing (BPI) Family B member 4 (BPIFB4), which belong to a family of proteins, BPI and lipid transfer protein (LTP), involved in the activation of toll-like receptor(TLR)-4 in the innate immune response [13].

Table 4 GM 23 Alleles in Long-living individuals (LLIs) and Controls (YCs)

	N = 192		N = 184	
	LLIs		Controls	
	+	%	+	%
23 +	114	59.4	109	59.2
23 -	78	40.6	75	40.8

Significance of distribution by chi square test (2 × 2) p = N.S

So, it is conceivable that particular GM allotypes may contribute to the generation of a dynamic immune response that supports successful ageing, hence longevity, whereas certain other allotype combinations may produce suboptimal levels of immunity and reduced life span.

In particular, GM allotypes have been shown to be involved in the immunological control of viruses, including herpes simplex virus(HSV)-1 and human cytomegalovirus (HCMV) [14, 15]. Herpes viruses, such as HCMV and HSV-1, have been associated with a variety of health problems, including cognitive decline, and overall mortality in the elderly [16–19]. Accordingly, recent data show that effective control of herpes viruses is impaired during healthy ageing, most probably due to loss of cellular control of early viral reactivation [20–22].

Recently, an interplay between particular GM and cluster of designation(CD)16A alleles in the outcome of HSV-1 infection has been demonstrated. The CD16A-158 V/V genotype associates with an asymptomatic course of HSV-1 infection only in homozygotes for the GM3 allele. Additional studies to determine the mechanism underlying this association showed that CD16A-158 V and GM3 alleles epistatically enhanced the antibody-dependent cell-mediated cytotoxicity (ADCC) against opsonized HSV-1-infected fibroblasts [14].

Concerning HCMV, in different populations it has been demonstrated the association of human IgG1 allotypes with immune response to the virus and some kinds of cancer thought to be associated with HCMV [23, 24]. More interestingly, in another Southern Italy population, GM17/17 (the alternative allele of GM3) was associated with the risk of developing HCMV symptomatic infection [15]. It is well known the role of chronic infections from herpes viruses, in particular from HCMV, in the impairment of immune responses of elderly people, hence contributing to immunosenescence [25, 26]. Accordingly, the severity of many infections is higher in the elderly compared to younger adults and infectious diseases are frequently associated with frailty and death. Reciprocally, an immune good function is tightly correlated to health status and longevity [4, 27–29].

On the other hand, our immune system is known to be quite efficient in fighting acute infections in young people, but not particularly efficient in responding to chronic stimuli, especially when they occur late in life. This leads to an increased production of inflammatory mediators. So, this chronic antigenic stress contributes to determine an inflammatory status called inflamm-ageing, responsible for age-related diseases. Reciprocally, the control of inflamm-ageing is associated with longevity [4, 30–33]. Accordingly, an efficient control of Herpes Virus chronic infections by GM allotypes might contribute to observed association with longevity through a decrease of inflammatory status.

Several mechanisms have been proposed to explain the role played by GM allotypes in the control of virus infections. IgG allotypes might modulate avidity of the interaction of IgG with Fcγ receptor (FcγR), so influencing the efficacy of immune response. In addition, they might modulate the strength of ADCC, thus involving cells of innate response such as natural killer (NK) cells [2, 3].

Conclusion

This is the first report implicating GM allotypes in longevity. It needs to be replicated in an independent and larger multi-ethnic study population. However, it has been reported that the association with longevity of other genes related to control of immune response as human leukocyte antigens (HLA) and killer immunoglobulin-like receptors (KIR), is population specific, being heavily affected by the population-specific genetic and environmental history [34]. On the other hand, it is also possible that there are other life span-associated loci on chromosome 14q32 (where the GM genes are located), distinct from GM, whose alleles are in significant linkage disequilibrium with those of the GM loci. This putative linkage disequilibrium could give rise to the associations observe.

Methods

We genotyped 96 Long-living individuals (LLIs) (40 female, mean age 96.7, age-range 91–104; 56 male, mean age 93.6, age range 90–104 years) and 96 young control individuals (YCs) (66 female, mean age 31.9, age-range 20–44; and 30 male, mean age 35.2, age range 23–45 years) already recruited as part of the Southern Italian Centenarian Study [35]. The LLIs were thoroughly investigated for demographic characteristics, medical history (past and present diseases), level of independence and cognitive status. All subjects donated blood samples for DNA study and gave written informed consent to the study, which was approved by Ethical Committee of Salerno University. All methods were performed in accordance with the relevant guidelines and regulations. The study was conducted in accordance with the ethical principles that have their origins in the Declaration of Helsinki.

DNA was obtained from peripheral blood leukocytes by the salting-out technique and stored until the use. For the determination of GM3 and GM17 allotypes (A to G substitution), a direct DNA sequencing method, Sanger sequencing, was used. The DNA segment encoding the CH1 region of γ1 chain was amplified by polymerase chain reaction (PCR) according to Balbìn et al., [36] using the following primers: 5' CCCCTGGCA CCCTCCTCCAA 3' and 5' GCCCTGGACTGGGG CTGCAT 3'. The purified double-stranded PCR product (364 bp) was subjected to automated DNA sequencing

on an ABI PRISM 3730xl DNA Analyzer. IgG2 markers GM 23– and 23+ (a G to A substitution in the Fc of the γ2 chain) were genotyped by a nested PCR-restriction fragment length polymorphism(RFLP) method [37]. IgG3 markers GM5 and GM21 were not typed, because TaqMan genotyping assays for the IgG3 allotypes are not yet available. Due to technical problems, it was not possible to type for GM3/17 one LLI and nine YCs and fror GM23 four YCs. Because of almost absolute linkage disequilibrium at GM loci within an ethnic group, subjects positive for the IgG1 allotypes GM3 and GM17 are most likely positive for the IgG3 allotypes GM5 and GM21 (Pandey, unpublished observations).

Allele and genotype frequencies among groups were estimated by gene counting. The different chi-squares tests were used to detect significant changes in genetic variables between groups where appropriate. Standard odds ratios (OR) with 95% confidence interval (CI) were calculated.

Abbreviations

ADCC: Antibody-dependent cell-mediated cytotoxicity; APOE: Apolipoprotein E; BPIFB4: Bactericidal/Permeability-increasing Family B member 4; CD: Cluster of designation; CH: Constant heavy; CI: Confidence interval; Fc: Fragment crystallisable region; FcγR: Fcγ receptor; FOXO3A: Forkhead box O3A; GM: Genetic markers of γ chains; GWAS: Genome-wide association studies; HapMap: Haplotype map; HCMV: Human cytomegalovirus; HLA: Human leukocyte antigen; HSV: Herpes simplex virus; KIR: Killer immunoglobulin-like receptor; LLI: Long-living individual; LTP: Lipid transfer protein; NK: Natural killer; OR: Odd ratios; PCR: Polymerase chain reaction; RFLP: Restriction fragment length polymorphism; TLR: Toll-like receptor; Yc: Young control individual

Acknowledgements

Not applicable.

Funding

This work was supported by grant he study was supported by Cariplo Foundation (n.2016–0874) and by Italian Ministry of Health (Ricerca Corrente, RF-2011-02348194) to A.P. and by grant of Italian Ministry of University (PRIN: progetti di ricerca di rilevante interesse nazionale – Bando 2015 Prot 20157ATSLF "Discovery of molecular and genetic/epigenetic signatures underlying resistance to age-related diseases and comorbidities") to AP, CC and GC. GA, AA are fellows of this project.

Authors' contributions

CC, AAP and JPP designed the study. AMN and JPP performed the experiments. AAP, AF and AM recruited the subjects and selected the sample. Statistical analysis was performed by CC, AA and JPP. GA, CMG and GC drafted the manuscript. CC, AAP and JPP revised the manuscript. All authors approved the final version of this manuscript.

Competing interests

Prof. Caruso is the Editor in Chief of Immunity & Ageing, Dr. Accardi is member of the Editorial Board. The other authors declare that they have no competing interests.

Author details

[1]Department of Medicine and Surgery, University of Salerno, Baronissi, Italy. [2]IRCCS MultiMedica, Milan, Italy. [3]Department of Pathobiology and Medical Biotechnologies, University of Palermo, Corso Tukory 211, 90134 Palermo, Italy. [4]Department of Microbiology and Immunology, Medical University of South Carolina, Charleston, SC 29425, USA.

References

1. Oxelius VA, Pandey JP. Human immunoglobulin constant heavy G chain (IGHG) (Fcγ) (GM) genes, defining innate variants of IgG molecules and B cells, have impact on disease and therapy. Clin Immunol. 2013;149: 475–86.
2. Lieberman R, Stiffel C, Asofsky R, Mouton D, Biozzi G, Benacerraf B. Genetic factors controlling anti-sheep erythrocyte antibody response and immunoglobulin synthesis in backcross and F2 progeny of mice genetically selected for "high" or "low" antibody synthesis. J Exp Med. 1972;136:790–8.
3. Pandey JP, Li Z. The forgotten tale of immunoglobulin allotypes in cancer risk and treatment. Exp Hematol Oncol. 2013;2:6.
4. Accardi G, Caruso C. Immune-inflammatory responses in the elderly: an update. Immun Ageing. 2018;15:11.
5. Pandey JP, Namboodiri AM, Nietert PJ, Yoshimura R, Hori H. Immunoglobulin genotypes and cognitive functions in schizophrenia. Immunogenetics. 2018;70:67–72.
6. Caruso C, Accardi G, Virruso C, Candore G. Sex, gender and immunosenescence: a key to understand the different lifespan between men and women? Immun Ageing. 2013;10:20.
7. Puca AA, Spinelli C, Accardi G, Villa F, Caruso C. Centenarians as a model to discover genetic and epigenetic signatures of healthy ageing. Mech Ageing Dev. 2018;174:95–102.
8. Ferrario A, Villa F, Malovini A, Araniti F, Puca AA. The application of genetics approaches to the study of exceptional longevity in humans: potential and limitations. Immun Ageing. 2012;9:7.
9. Bae H, Gurinovich A, Malovini A, Atzmon G, Andersen SL, Villa F, Barzilai N, Puca A, Perls TT, Sebastiani P. Effects of FOXO3 polymorphisms on survival to extreme longevity in four centenarian studies. J Gerontol A Biol Sci Med Sci. 2018;73:1439–47.
10. Sebastiani P, Gurinovich A, Bae H, Andersen S, Malovini A, Atzmon G, Villa F, Kraja AT, Ben-Avraham D, Barzilai N, Puca A, Perls TT. Four genome-wide association studies identify new extreme longevity variants. J Gerontol A Biol Sci Med Sci. 2017;72:1453–64.
11. Carapelli R, Rando A, Iannelli D, Scala F, Chiofalo I. Age influenced IgG3 allotype in sheep. Immunol Lett. 1982;(6):301–4.
12. de Vries RR, Meera Khan P, Bernini LF, van Loghem E, van Rood JJ. Genetic control of survival in epidemics. J Immunogenet. 1979;6:271–87.
13. Villa F, Carrizzo A, Spinelli CC, Ferrario A, Malovini A, Maciąg A, Damato A, Auricchio A, Spinetti G, Sangalli E, Dang Z, Madonna M, Ambrosio M, Sitia L, Bigini P, Calì G, Schreiber S, Perls T, Fucile S, Mulas F, Nebel A, Bellazzi R, Madeddu P, Vecchione C, Puca AA. Genetic analysis reveals a longevity-associated protein modulating endothelial function and angiogenesis. Circ Res. 2015;117:333–45.
14. Moraru M, Black LE, Muntasell A, Portero F, López-Botet M, Reyburn HT, Pandey JP, Vilches C. NK cell and Ig interplay in defense against herpes simplex virus type 1: epistatic interaction of CD16A and IgG1 Allotypes of variable affinities modulates antibody-dependent cellular cytotoxicity and susceptibility to clinical reactivation. J Immunol. 2015; 195:1676–84.
15. Di Bona D, Accardi G, Aiello A, Bilancia M, Candore G, Colomba C, Caruso C, Duro G, Gambino CM, Macchia L, Pandey JP. Association between γ marker, human leucocyte antigens and killer immunoglobulin-like receptors and the natural course of human cytomegalovirus infection: a pilot study performed in a Sicilian population. Immunology. 2018;153:523–31.
16. Siscovick DS, Schwartz SM, Corey L, Grayston JT, Ashley R, Wang SP, Psaty BM, Tracy RP, Kuller LH, Kronmal RA. Chlamydia pneumoniae, herpes simplex virus type 1, and cytomegalovirus and incident myocardial infarction and coronary heart disease death in older adults: the cardiovascular health study. Circulation. 2000;102:2335–40.
17. Savva GM, Pachnio A, Kaul B, Morgan K, Huppert FA, Brayne C, Moss PA. Medical Research Council cognitive function and ageing study. Cytomegalovirus infection is associated with increased mortality in the older population. Aging Cell. 2013;12:381–7.
18. Monastero R, Caruso C, Vasto S. Alzheimer's disease and infections, where we stand and where we go. Immun Ageing. 2014;11:26.
19. Barnes LL, Capuano AW, Aiello AE, Turner AD, Yolken RH, Torrey EF, Bennett DA. Cytomegalovirus infection and risk of Alzheimer disease in older black and white individuals. J Infect Dis. 2015;211:230–7.
20. Solana R, Tarazona R, Aiello AE, Akbar AN, Appay V, Beswick M, Bosch JA, Campos C, Cantisán S, Cicin-Sain L, Derhovanessian E, Ferrando-Martínez S, Frasca D, Fülöp T, Govind S, Grubeck-Loebenstein B, Hill A, Hurme M, Kern F, Larbi A, López-Botet M, Maier AB, McElhaney JE, Moss P, Naumova E, Nikolich-Zugich J, Pera A, Rector JL, Riddell N, Sanchez-Correa B, Sansoni P, Sauce D, van Lier R, Wang GC, Wills MR, Zieliński M, Pawelec G. CMV and Immunosenescence: from basics to clinics. Immun Ageing. 2012;9:23.
21. Itzhaki RF. Herpes simplex virus type 1 and Alzheimer's disease: increasing evidence for a major role of the virus. Front Aging Neurosci. 2014;6:202.
22. Parry HM, Zuo J, Frumento G, Mirajkar N, Inman C, Edwards E, Griffiths M, Pratt G, Moss P. Cytomegalovirus viral load within blood increases markedly in healthy people over the age of 70 years. Immun Ageing. 2016;13:1.
23. Pandey JP. Immunoglobulin GM genes, cytomegalovirus Immunoevasion, and the risk of glioma, neuroblastoma, and breast Cancer. Front Oncol. 2014;4:236.
24. Pandey JP, Kistner-Griffin E, Radwan FF, Kaur N, Namboodiri AM, Black L, Butler MA, Carreón T, Ruder AM. Immunoglobulin genes influence the magnitude of humoral immunity to cytomegalovirus glycoprotein B. J Infect Dis. 2014;210:1823–6.
25. Pawelec G, Akbar A, Caruso C, Effros R, Grubeck-Loebenstein B, Wikby A. Is immunosenescence infectious? Trends Immunol. 2004;25:406–10.
26. Pawelec G, Akbar A, Caruso C, Grubeck-Loebenstein B, Solana R, Wikby A. Human immunosenescence: is it infectious? Immunol Rev. 2005;205: 257–68.
27. Vasto S, Caruso C. Immunity & Ageing: a new journal looking at ageing from an immunological point of view. Immun Ageing. 2004;1:1.
28. Caruso C, Vasto S. Immunity and aging. In: Ratcliffe, MJH. (Editor in Chief), Encyclopedia of Immunobiology, 2016, Vol. 5, pp. 127–132. Oxford: Academic Press.
29. Rubino G, Bulati M, Aiello A, Aprile S, Gambino CM, Gervasi F, Caruso C, Accardi G. Sicilian centenarian offspring are more resistant to immune ageing. Aging Clin Exp Res. 2018, [Epub ahead of print].
30. Vasto S, Candore G, Balistreri CR, Caruso M, Colonna-Romano G, Grimaldi MP, Listi F, Nuzzo D, Lio D, Caruso C. Inflammatory networks in ageing, age-related diseases and longevity. Mech Ageing Dev. 2007; 128:83–91.
31. Cevenini E, Caruso C, Candore G, Capri M, Nuzzo D, Duro G, Rizzo C, Colonna-Romano G, Lio D, Di Carlo D, Palmas MG, Scurti M, Pini E, Franceschi C, Vasto S. Age-related inflammation: the contribution of different organs, tissues and systems. How to face it for therapeutic approaches. Curr Pharm Des. 2010;16:609–18.
32. Candore G, Caruso C, Colonna-Romano G. Inflammation, genetic background and longevity. Biogerontology. 2010;11:565–73.
33. Leonardi GC, Accardi G, Monastero R, Nicoletti F, Libra M. Ageing: from inflammation to cancer. Immun Ageing. 2018;15:1.
34. Listì F, Caruso C, Colonna-Romano G, Lio D, Nuzzo D, Candore G. HLA and KIR frequencies in Sicilian centenarians. Rejuvenation Res. 2010;13: 314–8.
35. Anselmi CV, Malovini A, Roncarati R, Novelli V, Villa F, Condorelli G, Bellazzi R, Puca AA. Association of the FOXO3A locus with extreme longevity in a southern Italian centenarian study. Rejuvenation Res. 2009;12:95–104.
36. Balbín M, Grubb A, Abrahamson M, Grubb R. Determination of allotypes G1m (f) and G1m(z) at the genomic level by subclass-specific amplification of DNA and use of allele-specific probes. Exp Clin Immunogenet. 1991;8:88–95.
37. Pandey JP, Namboodiri AM, Luo Y, Wu Y, Elston RC, Thomas DL, Rosen HR, Goedert JJ. Genetic markers of IgG influence the outcome of infection with hepatitis C virus. J Infect Dis. 2008;198:1334–6.

Permissions

List of Contributors

Helen M. Parry, Jianmin Zuo, Guido Frumento, Charlotte Inman and Guy Pratt
Institute of Immunology and Immunotherapy, University of Birmingham, Vincent Drive, Birmingham B15 2TT, UK

Paul Moss
Institute of Immunology and Immunotherapy, University of Birmingham, Vincent Drive, Birmingham B15 2TT, UK
University Hospitals NHS Foundation Trust, Birmingham, UK

Emma Edwards
Institute of Immunology and Immunotherapy, University of Birmingham, Vincent Drive, Birmingham B15 2TT, UK
Charles Darwin Building, Henwick Grove, University of Worcester, Worcester WR2 6AJ, UK

Nikhil Mirajkar
University of Birmingham Medical and Dental School, Vincent Drive, Birmingham B15 2TT, UK

Mike Griffiths
West Midlands Regional Genetics Laboratories, Birmingham Women's NHS Foundation Trust, Mindelsohn Way, Edgbaston, Birmingham B15 2TG, UK

Andre Talvani
Department of Biological Sciences, Federal University of Ouro Preto, Ouro Preto, Minas Gerais, Brazil
Post-graduation Program in Biological Sciences/NUPEB, Federal University of Ouro Preto, Ouro Preto, Minas Gerais, Brazil
Post-graduation Program in Health and Nutrition, Federal University of Ouro Preto, Ouro Preto, Minas Gerais, Brazil
Post-graduation in Ecology of Tropical Biomas, Federal University of Ouro Preto, Ouro Preto, Minas Gerais, Brazil
Laboratory of the Immunobiology of Inflammation, Federal University of Ouro Preto, Ouro Preto, Minas Gerais, Brazil

Aline Priscila Batista
Post-graduation Program in Biological Sciences/NUPEB, Federal University of Ouro Preto, Ouro Preto, Minas Gerais, Brazil

Silvana Mara Turbino Luz Ribeiro, Laís Roquete Lopes, Guilherme de Paula Costa, Vivian Paulino Figueiredo and Deena Shrestha
Post-graduation Program in Biological Sciences/NUPEB, Federal University of Ouro Preto, Ouro Preto, Minas Gerais, Brazil
Laboratory of the Immunobiology of Inflammation, Federal University of Ouro Preto, Ouro Preto, Minas Gerais, Brazil

Fernando Luiz Pereira de Oliveira
Post-graduation Program in Health and Nutrition, Federal University of Ouro Preto, Ouro Preto, Minas Gerais, Brazil
Department of Statistics, Federal University of Ouro Preto, Ouro Preto, Minas Gerais, Brazil

Roney Luiz de Carvalho Nicolato
Clinical Analyses Laboratory of the Pharmacy School, Federal University of Ouro Preto, Ouro Preto, Minas Gerais, Brazil

Juliana Assis Silva Gomes
Department of Morphology, Federal University of Minas Gerais, Belo Horizonte, Minas Gerais, Brazil

Giuseppe Carruba, Cecilia Dolcemascolo, Ildegarda Campisi and Maurizio Zarcone
Division of Research and Internationalization, ARNAS-Civico Di Cristina e Benfratelli, Palermo, Italy

Letizia Cocciadiferro, Antonietta Di Cristina and Maria Cinquegrani
Research Laboratories Dr. Nicola Locorotondo, Palermo, Italy

Orazia M. Granata
Clinical Pathology, "G. DI Cristina" Pediatric Hospital ARNAS-Civico Di Cristina e Benfratelli, Palermo, Italy

Adele Traina
The Diana Project, National Cancer Institute, Milan, Italy

Michela Ferrucci
Department of Translational Research and New Technologies in Medicine and Surgery, University of Pisa, Pisa, Italy

Francesco Fornai
Department of Translational Research and New Technologies in Medicine and Surgery, University of Pisa, Pisa, Italy
I.R.C.C.S. Neuromed, Pozzilli, IS, Italy

Albino Carrizzo, Maurizio Forte, Mariateresa Ambrosio, Antonio Damato, Francesca Biagioni and Carla Busceti
I.R.C.C.S. Neuromed, Pozzilli, IS, Italy

Carmine Vecchione
I.R.C.C.S. Neuromed, Pozzilli, IS, Italy
Department of Medicine and Surgery, University of Salerno, Via S. Allende, Baronissi, SA 84081, Italy

Annibale A. Puca
Vascular Physiopathology Unit, I.R.C.C.S. Multimedica, Milan, Italy
Department of Medicine and Surgery, University of Salerno, Via S. Allende, Baronissi, SA 84081, Italy

Gabriela Silveira-Nunes and Ana Maria Caetano Faria
Departamento de Bioquímica e Imunologia, Instituto de Ciências Biológicas, Universidade Federal de Minas Gerais, Avenida Antônio Carlos 6627, Belo Horizonte, Minas Gerais 31270-901, Brazil

Elaine Speziali, Andréa Teixeira-Carvalho, Danielle M. Vitelli-Avelar, Renato Sathler-Avelar, Maria Luiza Silva, Daniel Gonçalves Chaves, Glenda Meira Cardoso and Olindo Assis Martins-Filho
Laboratório de Biomarcadores de Diagnóstico e Monitoração, Centro de Pesquisas René Rachou, FIOCRUZ, Belo Horizonte, Brazil

Eric Bassetti Soares, Silvana Maria Elói-Santos, Rosângela Teixeira and Dulciene Magalhães Queiroz
Laboratório de Biomarcadores de Diagnóstico e Monitoração, Centro de Pesquisas René Rachou, FIOCRUZ, Belo Horizonte, Brazil
Faculdade de Medicina, Universidade Federal de Minas Gerais, Belo Horizonte, Brazil

Vanessa Peruhype-Magalhães
Laboratório de Biomarcadores de Diagnóstico e Monitoração, Centro de Pesquisas René Rachou, FIOCRUZ, Belo Horizonte, Brazil
Laboratório de Imunologia Celular e Molecular, Centro de Pesquisas René Rachou, FIOCRUZ, Belo Horizonte, Brazil
Laboratório de Pesquisas Clínicas, Centro de Pesquisas René Rachou, FIOCRUZ, Belo Horizonte, Brazil

Taciana Figueiredo-Soares
Faculdade de Medicina, Universidade Federal de Minas Gerais, Belo Horizonte, Brazil
Maternidade Odete Valadares/Fundação Hospitalar do Estado de Minas Gerais (FHEMIG), Belo Horizonte, Brazil

Rodrigo Corrêa-Oliveira
Laboratório de Imunologia Celular e Molecular, Centro de Pesquisas René Rachou, FIOCRUZ, Belo Horizonte, Brazil

Gustavo Eustáquio Brito-Melo
Departamento de Farmácia, Universidade Federal dos Vales do Jequitinhonha e Mucuri, Diamantina, Minas Gerais, Brazil

Judith Lechner, Mei Chen, Ruth E. Hogg, Levente Toth, Giuliana Silvestri, Usha Chakravarthy and Heping Xu
The Wellcome-Wolfson Institute of Experimental Medicine, Queen's University Belfast, 97 Lisburn Road, Belfast BT9 7BL, UK

Emanuela Galliera
Department of Biomedical, Surgical and Oral Science, Università degli Studi di Milano, Milan, Italy
IRCCS Galeazzi Orthopaedic Institute, Milan, Italy

Monica Gioia Marazzi
Department of Biomedical Sciences for Health, Università degli Studi di Milano, Milan, Italy

Massimiliano M. Corsi Romanelli
Department of Biomedical Sciences for Health, Università degli Studi di Milano, Milan, Italy
U.O.C SMEL-1 Patologia Clinica IRCCS Policlinico San Donato, San Donato, Milan, Italy

Carmine Gazzaruso, Pietro Gallotti and Adriana Coppola
Internal Medicin, Diabetes, Vascular and Endocrine-Mtabolical Disease Unit and the Centre of Applied Clinical Research (Ce.R.C.A), Clinical Institute Betato Matteo, Vigevano, Italy

Tiziana Montalcini and Arturo Pujia
Clinical Nutrition Unit, Department of Medical and Surgical Science, University Magna Grecia of Catanzaro, Catanzaro, Italy

E. Vianello, E. Dozio and L. Tacchini
Department of Biomedical Sciences for Health, Chair of Clinical Pathology, Università degli Studi di Milano, via Luigi Mangiagalli 31, 20133 Milan, Italy

M. M. Corsi Romanelli
Department of Biomedical Sciences for Health, Chair of Clinical Pathology, Università degli Studi di Milano, via Luigi Mangiagalli 31, 20133 Milan, Italy
Laboratory Medicine Operative Unit-1, Clinical Pathology, I.R.C.C.S. Policlinico San Donato Milanese, Milan, Italy

S. Trimarchi
Department of Biomedical Sciences for Health, Chair of Clinical Pathology, Università degli Studi di Milano, via Luigi Mangiagalli 31, 20133 Milan, Italy
Thoracic Aortic Research Center, I.R.C.C.S. Policlinico San Donato, San Donato Milanese, Milan, Italy

A. Barassi
Department of Health Sciences, Università degli Studi di Milano, Milan, Italy

G. Sammarco
Laboratory Medicine Operative Unit-1, Clinical Pathology, I.R.C.C.S. Policlinico San Donato Milanese, Milan, Italy

M. M. Marrocco-Trischitta
Thoracic Aortic Research Center, I.R.C.C.S. Policlinico San Donato, San Donato Milanese, Milan, Italy

Sven Magnus Hector and Kelly Allen
Department of Ophthalmology, Zealand University Hospital, Vestermarksvej 23, DK-4000 Roskilde, Denmark

Marie Krogh Nielsen, Yousif Subhi and Torben Lykke Sørensen
Department of Ophthalmology, Zealand University Hospital, Vestermarksvej 23, DK-4000 Roskilde, Denmark
Faculty of Health and Medical Sciences, University of Copenhagen, Copenhagen, Denmark

Sergio Davinelli, Graziamaria Corbi and Giovanni Scapagnini
Department of Medicine and Health Sciences, School of Medicine, University of Molise, Campobasso, Italy

Michael Maes
IMPACT Research Center, Deakin University, Geelong, Australia
Department of Psychiatry, Faculty of Medicine, Chulalongkorn University, Bangkok, Thailand

Armando Zarrelli
Department of Chemical Sciences, University of Naples "Federico II", Complesso Universitario Monte S. Angelo, Naples, Italy

Donald Craig Willcox
Department of Human Welfare, Okinawa International University, Okinawa, Japan
Department of Geriatric Medicine, John A. Burns School of Medicine, University of Hawaii, Honolulu, USA

Manuela Zlamy and Verena Jeller
Department of Pediatrics, Medical University Innsbruck, Innsbruck, Austria

Giovanni Almanzar, Matthias Eyrich and Martina Prelog
Department of Pediatrics, University Hospital Wuerzburg, University of Wuerzburg, Josef-Schneider-Str. 2, 97080 Wuerzburg, Germany

Walther Parson
Institute of Legal Medicine, Medical University Innsbruck, Innsbruck, Austria
Penn State Eberly College of Science, University Park, PA, USA

Christian Schmidt
Department of Haematology and Oncology, University of Greifswald, Greifswald, Germany

Johannes Leierer
Department of Internal Medicine, Medical University Innsbruck, Innsbruck, Austria

Birgit Weinberger
Institute for Biomedical Aging Research, University of Innsbruck, Innsbruck, Austria

Karin Unsinn
Department of Radiology, Medical University Innsbruck, Innsbruck, Austria

Reinhard Würzner
Department of Hygiene and Medical Microbiology, Medical University Innsbruck, Innsbruck, Austria

David Pavlicek, Simona Capossela, Alessandro Bertolo and Jivko Stoyanov
Biomedical Laboratories, Swiss Paraplegic Research, Guido A. Zäch Strasse 4, 6207, Nottwil, Switzerland

Jörg Krebs and Jürgen Pannek
Swiss Paraplegic Centre, Guido A. Zäch Strasse 1, 6207, Nottwil, Switzerland

Britta Engelhardt
Theodor Kocher Institute, University of Bern, Freiestrasse 1, 3012 Bern, Switzerland

Barbara Schober-Halper, Marlene Hofmann, Stefan Oesen and Bernhard Franzke
Research Platform Active Ageing, University of Vienna, Althanstraße 14, 1090 Vienna, Austria

Barbara Wessner
Research Platform Active Ageing, University of Vienna, Althanstraße 14, 1090 Vienna, Austria
Department of Sports and Exercise Physiology, Centre for Sport Science and University Sports, University of Vienna, Auf der Schmelz 6, 1150 Vienna, Austria

Karl-Heinz Wagner
Research Platform Active Ageing, University of Vienna, Althanstraße 14, 1090 Vienna, Austria
Department of Nutritional Sciences, Faculty of Life Sciences, University of Vienna, Althanstraße 14, 1090 Vienna, Austria

Thomas Wolf and Norbert Bachl
Department of Sports and Exercise Physiology, Centre for Sport Science and University Sports, University of Vienna, Auf der Schmelz 6, 1150 Vienna, Austria

Eva-Maria Strasser and Michael Quittan
Karl Landsteiner Institute for Remobilization and Functional Health/Institute for Physical Medicine and Rehabilitation, Kaiser Franz Joseph Hospital, Social Medical Centre - South, Kundratstrasse 3, 1100 Vienna, Austria

Lutz Hamann, Jasmin Bustami and Ralf R. Schumann
Institute for Microbiology and Hygiene, Charité University Medical Center Berlin, Rahel-Hirsch-Weg 3, 10117 Berlin, Germany

Leonid Iakoubov
Cellecta Inc, Mountain View, CA, USA

Malgorzata Szwed
Department of Human Epigenetics, Mossakowski Medical Research Centre, Polish Academy of Sciences, Warsaw, Poland

Monika Puzianowska-Kuznicka
Department of Human Epigenetics, Mossakowski Medical Research Centre, Polish Academy of Sciences, Warsaw, Poland
Department of Geriatrics and Gerontology, Medical Centre of Postgraduate Education, Warsaw, Poland

Malgorzata Mossakowska
Polsenior Project, International Institute of Molecular and Cell Biology, Warsaw, Poland

Lucyna Kaszubowska, Tomasz Jerzy Ślebioda and Zbigniew Kmieć
Department of Histology, Medical University of Gdańsk, Dębinki 1, Gdańsk PL-80-211, Poland

Jerzy Foerster
Department of Social and Clinical Gerontology, Medical University of Gdańsk, Dębinki 1, Gdańsk PL-80-211, Poland

Jan Jacek Kaczor
Department of Physiotherapy, Gdansk University of Physical Education and Sport, Górskiego 1, Gdańsk PL-80-336, Poland

Daria Schetz
Department of Clinical Toxicology, Medical University of Gdańsk, Kartuska 4/6, Gdańsk PL-80-104, Poland

Giulia Accardi, Anna Aiello, Caterina Maria Gambino, Calogero Caruso and Giuseppina Candore
Sezione di Patologia generale del Dipartimento di Biopatologia e Biotecnologie Mediche (DIBIMED), Università di Palermo, Corso Tukory 211, 90134 Palermo, Italy

Valeria Gargano, Santo Caracappa, Sandra Marineo and Gesualdo Vesco
Istituto Zooprofilattico Sperimentale della Sicilia, Via Gino Marinuzzi 3, 90129 Palermo, Italy

Ciriaco Carru and Angelo Zinellu
Dipartimento di Scienze Biomediche, Università di Sassari, Viale San Pietro 43/b, 07100 Sassari, Italy

Maurizio Zarcone
UOC Epidemiologia Clinica con registro tumori di Palermo e provincia, AOUP "Paolo Giaccone", Palermo, c/o Dipartimento di Scienze per la promozione della salute e materno infantile "G. D'Alessandro", Università di Palermo, Via del Vespro 133, 90131 Palermo, Italy

Federica Belluzzo
Dipartimento BioMedico di Medicina Interna e Specialistica (Di.Bi.M.I.S.), Università di Palermo, Palermo, Italy

Gabriele Di Lorenzo
Dipartimento BioMedico di Medicina Interna e Specialistica (Di.Bi.M.I.S.), Università di Palermo, Palermo, Italy
Dipartimento BioMedico di Medicina Interna e Specialistica (Di.Bi.M.I.S), Via del Vespro, 141, 90127 Palermo, Italy

Danilo Di Bona and Luigi Macchia
Department of Allergy, Clinical Immunology, Emergency Medicine, and Transplants, University of Bari, Bari, Italy

Kathleen G. Lanzer, Tres Cookenham, William W. Reiley and Marcia A. Blackman
Trudeau Institute, 154 Algonquin Avenue, Saranac Lake, NY 12983, USA

Ye Ding, Jingyi Ren, Hongqiang Yu and Yanmin Zhou
Department of Implantology, School and Hospital of Stomatology, Jilin University, Qinghua Road 1500, Chaoyang District, Changchun 130021, China

Weixian Yu
Key laboratory of Mechanism of Tooth Development and Jaw Bone Remodeling and Regeneration in Jilin Province, Qinghua Road 1500, Chaoyang District, Changchun 130021, China

Giuseppe Giugliano
Hypertension Research Center; Department of Advanced Biomedical Sciences, Federico II University, Naples, Italy

Alessia Salemme
Federico II University, Naples, Italy

Sara De Longis and Raffaele Izzo
Hypertension Research Center; Department of Translational Medical Sciences, Federico II University, via Pansini 5, 80131 Naples, Italy

Marialuisa Perrotta, Valentina D'Angelosante and Alessandro Landolfi
Department of Angiocardioneurology and Translational Medicine, IRCCS Neuromed, Pozzilli, Isernia, Italy

Valentina Trimarco
Hypertension Research Center; Department of Neurosciences, Federico II University, Naples, Italy

Feng-Jung Yang
Graduate Institute of Clinical Medicine, College of Medicine, National Taiwan University, Taipei, Taiwan
Department of Internal Medicine, National Taiwan University Hospital Yun Lin Branch, Douliu, Taiwan

Yen-Ling Chiu
Graduate Institute of Clinical Medicine, College of Medicine, National Taiwan University, Taipei, Taiwan
Department of Internal Medicine, Far Eastern Memorial Hospital, New Taipei City, Taiwan

Graduate Program in Biomedical Informatics, Yuan Ze University, Taoyuan City, Taiwan

Hung-Yuan Chen, I-Yu Chen, Chien-Sheng Wu, Wan-Chuan Tsai, Yu-Sen Peng and Shih-Ping Hsu
Department of Internal Medicine, Far Eastern Memorial Hospital, New Taipei City, Taiwan

Kai-Hsiang Shu and Fang-Yun Lay
Department of Internal Medicine, Far Eastern Memorial Hospital, New Taipei City, Taiwan
Graduate Institute of Immunology, College of Medicine, National Taiwan University, Taipei, Taiwan

Yi-Fang Chuang
Institute of Public Health, School of Medicine, National Yang Ming University, Taipei, Taiwan

Chih-Kang Chiang
Department of Medicine, National Taiwan University Hospital, Taipei, Taiwan

George Wang
Biology of Healthy Aging Program, Division of Geriatric Medicine and Gerontology, Johns Hopkins University School of Medicine, Baltimore, MD, USA

Angela Trovato Salinaro, Maria Scuto, Maria Teresa Cambria, Maria Laura Ontario, Mario Tomasello and Vittorio Calabrese
Department of Biomedical and Biotechnological Sciences, School of Medicine, University of Catania, Via Santa Sofia 97, 95123 Catania, Italy

Manuela Pennisi
Department of Biomedical and Biotechnological Sciences, School of Medicine, University of Catania, Via Santa Sofia 97, 95123 Catania, Italy
Spinal Unit, Emergency Hospital "Cannizzaro", Catania, Italy

Rosanna Di Paola, Rosalia Crupi and Salvatore Cuzzocrea
Department of Chemical, Biological, Pharmaceutical and Environmental Sciences University of Messina, Messina, Italy

Maurizio Uva and Luigi Maiolino
Department of Medical and Surgery Sciences and Advanced Technology, University of Catania, Catania, Italy

Edward J. Calabrese
Environmental Health Sciences Division, School of Public Health, University of Massachusetts, Amherst, MA, USA

Salvatrice Mancuso, Mariasanta Napolitano and Sergio Siragusa
Haematology, Biomedical Department of Internal Medicine and Medical Specialties, University of Palermo, Palermo, Italy

Melania Carlisi, Marco Santoro and Simona Raso
Department of Surgical, Oncological and Stomatological Disciplines, University of Palermo, Palermo, Italy

Lucyna Kaszubowska, Tomasz Jerzy Ślebioda and Zbigniew Kmieć
Department of Histology, Medical University of Gdańsk, Dębinki 1, 80-211 Gdańsk, Poland

Jerzy Foerster
Department of Social and Clinical Gerontology, Medical University of Gdańsk, Dębinki 1, 80-211 Gdańsk, Poland

Jan Jacek Kaczor
Department of Bioenergetics and Physiology of Exercise, Medical University of Gdańsk, Dębinki 1, 80-211 Gdańsk, Poland

Daria Schetz
Department of Pharmacology, Medical University of Gdańsk, Dębowa 23, 80-204 Gdańsk, Poland

Jin Zhang, Yuchao Wang, Xueshuang Dong and Jianghua Liu
Department of Neurology, Daqing Oilfield General Hospitals, No. 9 Zhongkang Road, Daqing 163001, China

Giulia C. Leonardi, Ferdinando Nicoletti and Massimo Libra
Department of Biomedical and Biotechnological Sciences, Pathology and Oncology Section, University of Catania, Catania, Italy

Giulia Accardi
Department of Pathobiology and Medical Biotechnologies, Immunosenescence and Ageing Group, University of Palermo, Palermo, Italy

Roberto Monastero
Department of Experimental Biomedicine and Clinical Neurosciences, Neurology Section, University of Palermo, Palermo, Italy

Jessica Mira Gabin and Jostein Holmen
HUNT Research Centre, Department of Public Health and Nursing, Norwegian University of Science and Technology (NTNU), Forskningsveien 2, 7600 Levanger, Norway

Ingvild Saltvedt
Department of Neuromedicine and Movement science, NTNU, the Faculty of Medicine and Health, 7491 Trondheim, Norway
Department of Geriatrics, St. Olav University Hospital, 7 006 Trondheim, Norway

Kristian Tambs
Division of Mental Health, Norwegian Institute of Public Health, Nydalen, 0403 Oslo, Norway

Annibale A. Puca
Department of Medicine and Surgery, University of Salerno, Baronissi, Italy
IRCCS MultiMedica, Milan, Italy

Anna Ferrario and Anna Maciag
IRCCS MultiMedica, Milan, Italy

Giulia Accardi, Anna Aiello, Caterina Maria Gambino, Giuseppina Candore and Calogero Caruso
Department of Pathobiology and Medical Biotechnologies, University of Palermo, Corso Tukory 211, 90134 Palermo, Italy

Aryan M. Namboodiri and Janardan P. Pandey
Department of Microbiology and Immunology, Medical University of South Carolina, Charleston, SC 29425, USA

Index

A

Active Ageing, 128-129, 136-137

Acute Aortic Dissection, 70, 74

Adipokines, 15, 58-60, 62, 66-67, 162

Allergic Conjunctivitis, 164, 166, 169-170

Allergic Disease, 138

Allergic Rhinitis, 164, 167, 169-170

Angiogenesis, 17, 27, 31, 35, 75, 269

Antagonistic, 18, 143, 224, 240

Aortic Stiffening, 71

Apolipoprotein, 27, 29, 267-268

Atherosclerosis, 12, 16-17, 20, 27, 29-30, 33-35, 68, 71, 74, 83, 92, 98, 110, 140, 200, 202-204, 208-210, 257

B

Bone Densitometry, 58

Bone Morphogenetic Protein 2, 11, 17

C

Calcium, 70, 72, 74, 196, 202, 204, 206, 208, 227, 240

Cardiovascular Disease, 9, 17, 19, 26-27, 33-34, 50-51, 56, 59, 68, 70, 74, 137-139, 201-204, 208-210, 256-257

Cardiovascular Risk, 11, 17, 19-20, 26, 33-35, 83, 162, 200, 209, 264

Cellular Immunity, 1

Cellular Protective Protein, 229, 238

Choroidal Neovascularization, 57, 75, 77, 82-83

Chronic Inflammation, 37, 56, 76, 86, 96, 126, 128, 143-144, 169, 190, 207, 215, 221, 245, 250-251, 255, 263

Coronary Bypass Surgery, 71

Coronary Vasospasm, 70

Cytokine, 12, 14, 16-17, 32, 36-39, 41, 43-48, 53, 57, 68, 76, 82, 86, 91, 96, 111, 113, 116, 119, 124, 127, 145-146, 151-152, 155, 160, 165, 167, 171, 179, 186-187, 203, 207, 212, 214, 227, 229, 245, 247, 249, 255

Cytolytic Activity, 145

Cytomegalovirus, 1, 5, 7, 9-10, 48, 101-102, 111-114, 116, 119, 126-127, 166, 169-170, 184, 202, 209-210, 221, 223-224, 267-269

Cytomegalovirus Viral, 1, 5, 269

D

Dietary Intervention, 18, 20, 22, 24-25, 94, 158, 160, 256

Dietary Phytochemical, 95

E

Elastic Band Resistance, 128, 131, 137-138

Endothelial Cell, 31, 70, 76, 97, 99, 210, 248

Endothelial Damage, 70, 209

Endothelial Dysfunction, 30, 34, 70, 73, 256

Endothelial Tunica, 71

Epigenome, 18-19, 25

F

Fracture Risk, 58-59, 62, 64-65, 67

G

Gene Expression, 17-19, 24, 26, 47, 88-89, 97-98, 129, 131, 134, 163, 184, 221, 223, 225, 237, 241, 253-254, 258, 262, 264

Glycation, 58-59, 64, 67-69, 200, 252

H

Herpesvirus, 1, 9, 202, 221, 223

Homeostasis, 12, 17, 20, 24, 47, 57, 70, 86-87, 101, 107-108, 111-113, 127, 129, 132, 137-138, 145, 156, 164, 183-184, 194, 198, 203, 205, 209, 212-214, 217, 227, 252

Host Immunity, 1

Hypertension, 12, 27, 30, 34, 50-51, 56, 68, 71, 74, 79, 99, 131-132, 136, 138, 140-141, 157, 193-196, 198-201, 257, 264

I

Immune Frailty, 114-115, 122, 125

Immune System, 10, 12, 17, 36, 43, 45-48, 75-76, 84-85, 96, 98, 101-102, 110-111, 114-115, 125-127, 129, 139, 142-144, 146, 156-157, 163, 165-166, 170, 172, 203-205, 214, 219-220, 227, 245, 266-267

Inflammatory Protein, 27, 29, 239

Influenza Virus, 172 176, 178, 180-183

Innate Immunity, 6, 27-28, 33-35, 37, 47-48, 57, 145, 153, 217-218, 224, 226, 251-252, 255, 264

Isothiocyanate, 77, 82

L

Life Expectancy, 12, 18, 58, 84, 114, 125, 129, 219, 221, 254

Lymphocyte, 10, 38, 47-48, 75-76, 82, 104-106, 112, 117, 120, 130, 139, 143, 148-149, 157, 164, 170, 181-183, 210

M

Macular Degeneration, 33, 35, 49, 56-57, 75, 82-83, 143, 212

Magnesium, 70, 74

Matrix Metalloprotease, 27, 31

Memory Impairment, 185, 188-192

Mononuclear Cell, 131, 228

Myocardial Infarction, 17, 19, 26-27, 30-31, 33-34, 207-208, 260-263

N

Neovascular, 35, 49, 51, 56-57, 75-77, 79-83

Neurodegenerative Disorder, 85

Neutrophil, 28, 31, 75-76, 78-83, 119-120, 132, 224

Nutraceutical Effect, 158

O

Obesity, 11-18, 20, 26, 59, 62, 67-69, 128-129, 131-132, 158, 161-162, 250-253, 256

Osteoporosis, 58-60, 62-65, 67-69, 131-132, 136

Oxidative Stress, 18, 23, 48, 58-59, 68, 83-91, 93, 95-99, 137, 145-146, 155, 157-158, 160-161, 163, 191, 199-200, 211-215, 217-218, 226-227, 233, 237-241, 255, 266

P

Pathogenesis, 17, 29, 31, 48, 50, 53-54, 56, 58-59, 62, 67-68, 75-76, 87, 89, 96, 144, 158, 191, 199, 211-213, 215, 217-218, 222, 224, 257, 262-264

Pathophysiology, 31, 33, 70, 74, 214, 219, 246, 248, 257

Pentraxin 3, 27-28, 32-35

Periodontitis, 185-189, 191-192, 212

Polymorphism, 48, 56, 83, 139, 142, 144, 183, 268

Polyphenol, 95-96, 99, 200, 213

Polypoidal Choroidal Vasculopathy, 49, 56

Porphyromonas Gingivalis, 185, 191

S

Selenium, 18

Serum Amyloid Protein, 27

Smooth Muscle Cell, 70

Spinal Cord Injury, 114, 119, 126-127

Subretinal Fibrosis, 49, 51-55, 83

T

T Cell, 1, 4-7, 9-10, 47, 57, 101-113, 115, 121, 126, 137-138, 156, 165, 172-176, 178-184, 202-205, 207-210, 220-221, 224, 239, 241, 253

Thymectomy, 101-108, 110-111

Thymic Activity, 101, 111

True Memory, 172, 176

U

Urinary Tract Infection, 114, 117, 121, 126

V

Vascular Disease, 1, 16, 59, 203, 205

Vascular Endothelial Growth, 27, 31, 57

Vascular Tone, 70

www.ingramcontent.com/pod-product-compliance
Lightning Source LLC
Chambersburg PA
CBHW061331190326
41458CB00011B/3967